NEWLY REVISED AND EXPANDED

THE COMPLETE & UP-TO-DATE

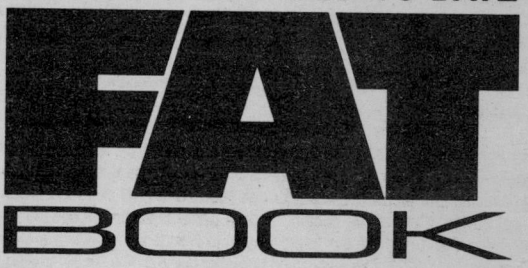

A GUIDE TO THE FAT, CALORIES, AND FAT PERCENTAGES IN YOUR FOOD

KAREN J. BELLERSON

Avery Publishing Group

Garden City Park, New York

SOURCES
Food manufacturers and processors direct, as well as their product labels.
United States Department of Agriculture Handbook No. 8, revised, "Composition of Foods, Raw, Processed, Prepared," sections 8-1 through 8-22; Agriculture Handbook No. 456, "Nutritive Value of American Foods in Common Units"; Home and Garden Bulletin No. 232, "Nutrition and Your Health: Dietary Guidelines for Americans."
Individual fast food chains.

Cover designers: Rudy Shur and William Gonzalez
In-house editors: Amy C. Tecklenburg, Dara Stewart, Karen Hay, and Jennifer L. Santo
Typesetters: Amy C. Tecklenburg and Dara Stewart, with thanks to Evan Schwartz

Avery Publishing Group, Inc.
120 Old Broadway
Garden City Park, NY 11040
1–800–548–5757

Contents

To our darling little Brandon Clark—
A most loving, joyful WELCOME!

Acknowledgments

Many thanks to Rudy Shur, Amy Tecklenburg, Dara Stewart, Karen Hay, and Jennifer Santo at Avery Publishing Group, as well as a special thank-you to Jackie Gallagher, for their hard-working, diligent contributions to the complicated mechanics of this book and helping to create a valuable nutritional resource of such complexity: *The Complete and Up-to-Date Fat Book.*

My thanks go also to those food manufacturers who continue to make nutritional information about their products available, and who have listened to consumers' desires for more and tastier healthy food choices.

And for all of you who continue to take the time to write to me (whether it be to ask questions and/or make comments, or to offer suggestions): Your letters are all invaluable to me. Thank you so very much for allowing me to play a small part in your endeavors to pursue a healthier, nutritionally sound lifestyle!

Preface

"Dare to be wise; begin! He who postpones the hour of living rightly is like the rustic who waits for the river to run dry before he crosses it."

— Horace

Thank you for joining me once again in the pursuit of healthy eating habits, this time for my third revision of *The Complete and Up-To-Date Fat Book.*

Keeping up with all the new "tastier-than-ever" low-fat/no-fat food products flooding the grocery shelves today is, to put it mildly, like the "Never-Ending Story." Just when I think I've come close to gathering all the necessary nutritional data, another batch of new products shows up on the shelves (sometimes replacing products that made their debut just months before!). It certainly keeps me on my toes, and I love it! I have learned about some wonderful products that I might not have been aware of, except for the ongoing research necessary to bring you the most *complete and up-to-date* nutritional information possible.

The one constant in my research remains the countless studies that continue to prove the relationship between a high-fat diet (a diet in which more than 30 percent of daily calories come from fat) and a higher risk of developing life-threatening diseases such as cancer, heart disease, stroke, diabetes, and high blood pressure (hypertension). Professionals throughout the health-care field continue to promote the very real health benefits of a low-fat nutritional lifestyle, while ongoing studies continue to show a direct correlation between a high-fat diet and disease.

Now more than ever, we have nutritional watchdogs such as the Center for Science in the Public Interest (CSPI) *Nutrition Action Health Letter,* the *Tufts University Diet & Nutrition Letter,* the *Harvard Health Letter,* the *Mayo Clinic Health Letter, Consumer Reports on Health,* and *Environmental Nutrition* (to mention just a few) that take our nutritional well-being very seriously. They not only inform us as to what products help to make up a healthy, nutritionally sound lifestyle, they also inform us about products that warrant further inspection before being included in our eating plans. Also, when they come across products that appear to offer little or no nutritional benefit and/or unhealthy side effects, they take action aimed at seeing that either the products are brought up to a healthy par or that the manufacturers are made to warn consumers of harmful side effects—or, if necessary, they do what they can to keep such products off our grocery shelves entirely. Still and all, we must acknowledge and remain aware of the fact that *even the wisest of nutritional choices cannot counteract the effects of unhealthy personal habits,* such as smoking, overindulgence in alcoholic beverages, lack of exercise, and a stress-filled lifestyle.

My goal for *The Complete and Up-to-Date Fat Book* continues to be to keep you as nutritionally up to date as possible concerning the food products available to you, the consumer, whether they are found on your grocery shelves, made at home, or eaten in the fast-food restaurant of your choice.

Wishing you the best of good health,

Karen J. Bellerson

Introduction

"The single most influential dietary change one can make to lower the risk of these diseases [cardiovascular disease, diabetes, and certain forms of cancer] is to reduce intake of foods high in fats and to increase the intake of foods high in com-plex carbohydrates and fiber."

— *The Surgeon General's Report on Nutrition and Health*

"It is calculated that, if intake of dietary fat were reduced from the present 40 percent of total calorie intake to 25 percent, about 9,000 lives would be saved annually."

— National Cancer Institute, *Annual Review of Public Health*

"Eating less fat can reduce the risk of colon, prostate, and breast cancer."

— National Research Council, "Diet and Health"

For decades, studies have shown the influence of diet on the development of disorders such as high blood pressure, diabetes, osteoarthritis, heart disease, and some forms of cancer. Much of what we know today about the diet-disease relationship dates back to World War II, when the incidence of death from heart attacks among the people of Western Europe declined in great numbers while the war was going on. The cause of this dramatic decline was found to be the rationing of foods such as meat, dairy products, and eggs during the war. Once the war was over and these foods were once again available, the incidence of heart disease again rose. In-depth studies were begun in earnest to find out about the negative effects of these foods.

Countless studies continue to prove that there is a very real relationship between our diet and the risk of developing a life-threatening disease. In response to these findings, the United States Department of Agriculture (USDA) replaced the Four Basic Food Groups (milk, meat, vegetables and fruits, and breads and cereals) with the new Food Guide Pyramid (see Figure 1) as a formula for a healthy diet.

Notice that fats, oils, and sweets are the smallest part of the new Food Guide Pyramid. This reflects advice from major health organizations recommending a diet consisting of 55 to 60 percent carbohydrates, 15 percent protein, and *no*

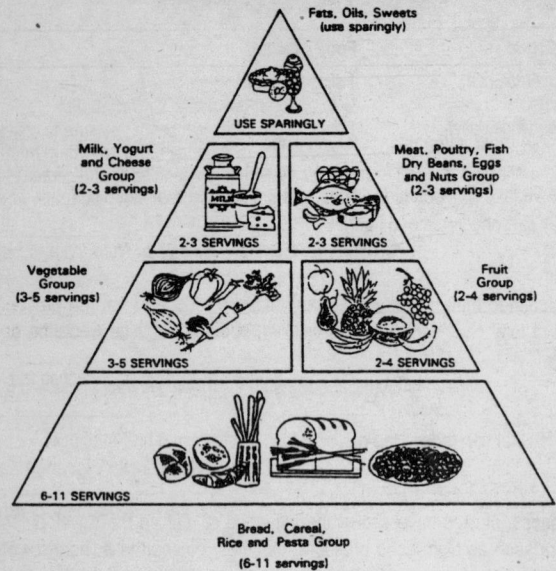

Figure 1. The Food Guide Pyramid

more than 30 percent fat. There are some experts who feel that only 25 percent or less of our calories should come from fat, in order to lower our risk of heart disease and some kinds of cancer.

The Food Guide Pyramid can help you plan a healthy, balanced diet that meets your individual nutritional needs and takes into account your particular food likes and dislikes. When making choices based on the Food Guide Pyramid's recommendations, remember to keep a *balance* by making your choices from all six food categories. In doing this you will find you are automatically eating a *variety* of foods each day. Also, bear in mind *moderation,* in order to keep your consumption of calories, fat (total and saturated), sodium, and sugar in line.

To keep moderation in mind, you need to know what the USDA considers a serving size for each of the categories of food shown. If you eat a portion of a certain food that is larger than the indicated serving size, that adds up to more than one serving for that particular food group and should be counted as such. Table 1 shows USDA serving sizes for the various types of foods in the Food Pyramid.

Table 1. Serving Sizes for Food Categories

Food Group	Food Amount
Bread, cereal, rice, and pasta (6–11 servings daily)	1 slice of bread ½ hamburger roll, bagel, English muffin 1 ounce of ready-to-eat cereal (be sure to check labels, as 1 ounce may equal anywhere from ¼ cup to 2 cups, depending on the cereal) ½ cup of cooked cereal, rice, or pasta 3 or 4 plain crackers (small)
Vegetables (3–5 servings daily)	1 cup of raw leafy vegetables ½ cup of other vegetables, cooked or chopped raw ¾ cup of vegetable juice
Fruit (2–4 servings daily)	1 medium apple, banana, orange, nectarine, or peach ½ cup of chopped raw, cooked, or canned fruit ¾ cup of fruit juice
Milk, yogurt, and cheese (2–3 servings daily)	1 cup of milk or yogurt 1½ ounces of natural cheese 2 ounces of processed cheese
Meat, poultry, fish, and dry beans, (2–3 servings daily)	2–3 ounces of cooked lean meat, poultry, or fish 1½ cups of cooked dry beans 2–3 eggs 4–6 tablespoons of peanut butter

Okay, you're convinced that you need to get the fat out of your diet, but where do you begin? Before we go into some simple guidelines, let's look at a few basic facts about fat.

FAT: A NECESSARY NUTRIENT

The fact is that we need some fat in our diets. Adults need a minimum daily intake of 15 to 25 grams of dietary fat to meet the body's needs. *Children under the age of two years should not have their dietary fat restricted, because it may interfere with their development.*

Our bodies use fat in numerous ways—ways most of us are unaware of. We use fat in manufacturing antibodies to fight disease. Fats act as carriers for the fat-soluble vitamins (A, D, E, and K). Fat is one of the body's three nutrient energy sources, and it also aids in digestion by slowing down the stomach's secretions of hydrochloric acid. This is what produces that satisfying feeling of fullness after a meal. Fat deposits in the body cushion, protect, and hold in place vital organs such as the kidneys, heart, and liver, and also give the body its shape. Fat is the body's insulation against environmental temperature changes. As you can see, fat is a vital nutrient, and should not be totally eliminated from our diets!

All fats are composed of building blocks called *fatty acids.* There are two types of fatty acids: the nonessential fatty acids, which our body is able to manufacture, and the essential fatty acids, which we cannot make and have to get through our diets. Essential fatty acids are necessary for normal growth; for healthy skin, blood, arteries, and nerves; and for keeping the metabolism running smoothly.

CHOLESTEROL AND LIPOPROTEINS (LDL AND HDL)

The main reason to be concerned with the fat in your diet is that fat—both the amount and the type—affects blood cholesterol. Cholesterol is a white, waxy, fatty substance found in all foods that come from animal sources, particularly organ meats such as brains, kidney, and liver. Because plants do not have the ability to manufacture cholesterol, there is no cholesterol found in plants; this includes oils that come from vegetable sources. While cholesterol is not a fatty acid, it is a fatlike substance and is often referred to as a fat.

Cholesterol is essential to our well-being. We need it to help build cell membranes, to produce hormones (estrogen, progesterone, and testosterone), and to manufacture bile acids that are needed to eliminate excess cholesterol from the body. However, if we have more cholesterol than we need in our blood, it clogs up the arteries. For the average person, about 75 percent of the cholesterol found in the body—all the body needs—is manufactured in the liver, even if he or she eats no animal products. The other 25 percent comes from the diet.

Cholesterol is carried through the bloodstream by molecules called lipoproteins. The cholesterol manufactured by the liver is carried to the cells that need it by *low-density lipoproteins (LDLs).* High levels of LDLs in the bloodstream can result in clogged arteries, causing high blood pressure, stroke, or heart disease. This is why LDL is referred to as the "bad cholesterol"—or, as I call it, the "lethal cholesterol." LDL levels can be reduced through a proper diet.

Now we come to the high-density lipoproteins (HDLs), the "good cholesterol" (I refer to it as the "healthy cholesterol"). HDLs pick up excess cholesterol from different body tissues and carry it back to the liver. It is then metabolized by the liver, processed through the intestines, and eliminated from the body. High levels of HDL are associated with a *decreased* risk of coronary heart disease. HDL levels can be raised through regular exercise. *Total cholesterol,* which represents the sum of the total of LDL plus HDL, is also important.

TYPES OF DIETARY FATS IN INDIVIDUAL FOODS

In addition to being classified as essential or nonessential, because of differences in their chemical structure, the fatty acids in the foods we eat fall into three categories. These are polyunsaturated, monounsaturated, and saturated. Most foods contain a combination of all three kinds of dietary fat. However, there is usually a higher content of only one of these types of fats. The percentage of each type of fat contained in any individual food is what makes one food a healthier choice than another food.

Polyunsaturated Fats

Polyunsaturated fats are found in most foods. Omega-3 polyunsaturated fats are found primarily in certain fish, and omega-6 polyunsaturated fats are mainly found in nuts, oils from plants, seeds, and soybeans. These fats are liquid at room temperature. Polyunsaturated fats reduce blood cholesterol, but if eaten in excess may also lower the level of protective "good cholesterol," or HDL. (*See* Cholesterol and Lipoproteins, page 4.) Some studies speculate that there is a link between a high consumption of polyunsaturated fats and breast cancer.

Foods in which polyunsaturated fats are the main type of fat include those listed below. Please note that all of the foods listed here are *not* necessarily high-fat foods. They are simply higher in the polyunsaturated fats than in other types.

- Bagels
- Barbecue sauce
- Bluefish
- Brazil nuts
- Chickpeas (garbanzo beans)
- Cod
- Corn chips
- Cornmeal
- French bread
- Haddock
- Herring
- Italian bread
- Lentils
- Mackerel
- Mussels
- Oysters
- Oatmeal bread
- Pine nuts
- Popcorn (air-popped)
- Potato chips
- Potato salad (made with mayonnaise)
- Pumpernickel
- Pumpkin seeds
- Rainbow trout
- Raisin bread
- Refried beans
- Rye bread
- Salad dressings (most types)
- Salmon
- Sardines
- Scallops
- Sesame seeds
- Soybeans
- Squash
- Squash seeds
- Sunflower seeds
- Sweet potatoes
- Tofu
- Tuna salad (made with mayonnaise)
- Vegetable and nut oils (see the table on page 459)
- Walnuts
- Whitefish

Monounsaturated Fats

Monounsaturated fats are found in most foods, but mainly in vegetable and nut oils such as canola (rapeseed), olive, and peanut. These fats also are liquid at room temperature. Monounsaturated fats reduce total blood cholesterol while not having the side effect of lowering the protective "good cholesterol," HDL.

The following foods have *higher* contents of monounsaturated fats than other types. Those foods marked with an asterisk (*) are also high in saturated fats.

- Almonds
- Animal fats*
  (most types)
- Avocados
- Beef* (leaner cuts)
- Biscuits
- Bread* (most types)
- Brownies
- Cake* (most types)
- Cashews
- Chestnuts
- Chicken
- Cookies*
  (most types)
- Croissants*
- Donuts*
  (most types)

- Eggs*
  Fruitcake
- Gingerbread
- Hazelnuts
- Lard*
- Macadamia nuts
- Margarine
  (stick types)
- Muffins*
- Oatmeal
- Ocean perch
- Pastry (including
  pie crust)
- Peanut butter
- Peanuts
- Pecans

- Pies* (most types)
- Pistachios
- Popcorn (popped in
  vegetable oil)
- Piork*
- Sausage*
  (most types)
- Spaghetti (with
  tomato sauce)
- Taco*
- Veal* (leaner cuts)
- Vegetable and
  nut oils (see the
  table on page 459))
- Vegetable
  shortening

Saturated Fats

Foods containing saturated fats include all meat and dairy products. The tropical oils coconut, palm, and palm kernel, although of plant origin, are also high in saturated fat. Cocoa butter, the oil used in making chocolate, is a highly saturated fat source as well. (This is why I recommend substituting powdered cocoa in recipes that call for chocolate.) Saturated fats are generally solid at room temperature. *Saturated fats—even more than dietary cholesterol—raise total blood cholesterol.*

The following foods are higher in saturated fats than other types. Other foods high in these fats appear the list of high-monounsaturated-fat foods. In those foods marked with asterisks (*), while monounsaturated fats predominate, there are also significant amounts of saturated fats.

- Beef (fattier cuts)
- Beef tallow
- Boston brown bread
  canned)

- Butter
- Cheese
  (most types)
- Cheesecake

- Chili (with beef)
- Chocolate
- Cocoa butter
- Cocoa mixes

- Coconut
- Coconut products
- Cottage cheese (4-percent fat)
- Cream
- Cream soups (most types)
- Custard (baked)
- Duck
- Eggnog
- Fried foods (fried in saturated oils)
- Garlic spread
- Granola
- Gravy (brown, packaged)
- Hot dogs
- Ice cream
- Lamb
- Luncheon meats
- Malts

- Milk (whole, 2-percent, and 1-percent)
- Nondairy creamer
- Nondairy whipped topping
- Pies (cream types)
- Pizza
- Pompano
- Popcorn (most microwave types)
- Pork (fattier cuts)
- Puddings
- Quiche
- Sauces (butter-, egg-, and/or milk-based, such as béarnaise, hollandaise, white, or cheese sauce)

- Seaweed
- Shakes
- Snack cakes (most types, and those with chocolate frosting)
- Sour cream
- Turkey (dark meat or self-basting)
- Veal (fattier cuts)
- Vegetable and nut oils (particularly coconut, palm, and palm kernel; see the table on page 459)

Remember, the essential fatty acids—the ones that must be obtained through the diet—are *un*saturated. This means we can get all the fat we need from unsaturated fats; *there is no biological need for saturated fat!*

Hydrogenated Fats and Trans Fatty Acids

You may have read of, and been confused by, the term "trans fatty acids." Trans fatty acids are simply a type of fat formed when liquid polyunsaturated or monounsaturated oils are subjected to a process called *hydrogenation*. This is a process of adding hydrogen to an oil in order to convert it into a form that is solid or semisolid at room temperature, so that it can be used in processed foods such as baked goods, nondairy creamers, and whipped toppings. The hydrogenation of these unsaturated fats causes them to act like saturated fats in the bloodstream, raising blood cholesterol and LDL. Take note, however, that the amount of trans fatty acids in foods is included in the amount of total fat (but *not* in the amount of saturated fat) on the labels of products such as margarines, shortenings, chips, and baked products. Be aware that both polyunsaturated and monounsaturated fats can be hydrogenated. When reading product labels, watch for the words "hydrogenated" or "partially hydrogenated," which indicate the presence of trans fatty acids.

"Fake Fats"

For many years, we have been reading and hearing about the ongoing research in the area of "fake fats," or fat substitutes. Manufacturers have been eager to develop a no-calorie substitute for fat that would have the characteristics of fat: the texture, "mouth feel," and flavor, as well as the ability to stand up under a wide range of manufacturing processes.

Even the United States Department of Agriculture has scientists working on the development of an acceptable fat replacement. Dr. George Inglett, a research chemist at the department's Agricultural Research Service (ARS) National Center for Agricultural Utilization Research in Peoria, Illinois (and developer of Oatrim-10, an earlier fat substitute), has developed a fat substitute known as Z-Trim. Z-Trim is a purified insoluble fiber made of microscopic plant cell wall fragments (from byproducts such as seed hulls, oats, soybeans, peas, and rice, or bran from corn or wheat) that can be dried to a white powder. When the powder absorbs water, it swells to provide the smooth mouth feel of fat. Since Z-Trim is made of natural dietary fiber, it is not upsetting to the digestive system when consumed in ordinary amounts. ARS plans to license Z-Trim to private companies for commercial development. Fantesk, which uses biopolymers and water to mimic fat in food products, is another fat substitute developed at the National Center for Agricultural Utilization Research. It has been licensed for use in ice cream and processed meat products. Products containing Fantesk are expected to hit market shelves soon.

Simplesse is one of the better known fake fats. Made up of egg whites and milk protein, it has been on the market for several years. Unlike fat, which contains 9 calories per gram, Simplesse contains only 1 to 2 calories per gram. Simplesse breaks down when heated, however, so it can be used only in frozen foods and salad dressings. Because Simplesse consists largely of protein and contains only the fat found in skim milk, the safety of its use, like that of Z-Trim and Fantesk, has not been questioned by the FDA.

Procter & Gamble scientists have been working on their fake fat, Olestra, for twenty-five years or so. They made their first submission to the FDA in 1987, only to have to go back to the drawing board over and over again. Finally, after P&G had spent over $200 million in research costs and produced more than 150,000 pages of supporting data, the FDA gave the green light to Olestra (marketed under the trade name Olean) in January of 1996.

Olestra is a chemically engineered variation of natural fat made from sugar and vegetable oil. It is reported to be virtually fat-free and can withstand being cooked at high temperatures without breaking down. Although Olestra has the taste and consistency of fat, it cannot be digested or absorbed by the body like fat. This "passing through the body undigested" has made this fake fat quite controversial among health-care professionals and others within the public health community.

When the FDA cleared Olestra for the manufacture of salty, savory snack foods only (until long-term effect studies can be done), there were both cheers and boos to be heard across the nation. Enthusiastic cheers came from those who focused on the new and improved low-fat and fat-free products they hoped to see on the grocery shelves, and, perhaps, on the possibility of one day being able to use Olestra in their own home recipes. (Moreover, let's not forget to mention those who stand to gain a great deal of money from the manufacture of such a product!) The boos came from nutritional watchdogs who focused on the possible side effects of consuming foods containing Olestra. Those very real concerns, the basis for the controversy surrounding the FDA approval, are:

• Since Olestra cannot be absorbed by the body, some of the fat-soluble vitamins A, D, E, and K, if eaten at the same time as Olestra, will be dissolved in the Olestra and will also pass through the body. Vitamins eaten at least two hours before or after the Olestra is eaten should not be affected. (P&G plans on adding vitamins A, D, E, and K to Olestra-containing foods to make up for any vitamin loss that may occur.)

• Olestra sharply decreases the levels of some carotenoids in the bloodstream. Carotenoids, a group of more than 500 related compounds found in fruits and vegetables (beta-carotene and lycopene are the best known) are also fat soluble. Large quantities of carotenoids from fruits and vegetables are associated with lower rates of cancer; low levels of carotenoids in the bloodstream are associated with heart disease and stroke.

• Because Olestra is not digested or absorbed, it can cause gastrointestinal side effects such as gas, diarrhea, and, most unpleasant, "anal leakage." The latter may occur as Olestra travels through the body and is eliminated from the body in the form of a greasy liquid.

Because of these concerns, and so that consumers will know if any of the foods they purchase contain Olestra (Olean), the FDA is requiring P&G to make sure that all foods containing Olestra are packaged in containers that carry the following statement:

> This product contains Olestra. Olestra may cause abdominal cramp-
> ng and loose stools. Olestra inhibits the absorption of some vitamins
> and other nutrients. Vitamins A, D, E, and K have been added.

FOOD LABELS: "NUTRITION FACTS"

As you walk down the aisles of your supermarket, make it a practice to look at the wide variety of foods offered. This is a great way to discover the literally hundreds of new food products flooding the market each year from our industrious food manufacturers. Before you buy, read labels and decide if a particular food is going to fit in with your ultimate goal of a healthy eating lifestyle.

Although the standard food label offers a lot of nutritional information (see Figure 2), people often tell me they are confused by it. The "% Daily Values" column in the label especially seems to cause confusion. Some consumers make the mistake of assuming that the "% Daily Value" across from "Total Fat" represents the percentage of calories that come from fat. Don't be misled; it has nothing to do with the percentage of calories from fat. Rather, the daily values are reference numbers that show what percentage of a 2,000 calorie daily diet is met by the corresponding nutrients. Thus, in the label in Figure 2, the "5%" that appears opposite "Total Fat" means that one serving of the product provides 5 percent of daily fat intake. Of course, if you eat more or less than 2,000 calories a day, the "% Daily Value" will not reflect the true percentages of daily diet for you. However, you can still use these numbers to get a general idea of a particular food's nutritional value relative to an average daily diet to help you determine if it is a food you want to include in your eating plans. Remember that the guidelines shown on food labels are for healthy adults and children two years of age or older. A low-fat diet may be harmful to children younger than two years of age.

Also potentially confusing are the many descriptive words that appear on the fronts of food labels, words such as "lite," "reduced-calorie," "low-fat," and "no-sodium." I offer the following definitions in hopes it will lessen that confusion:

• *Cholesterol-free.* A food product containing less than 2 milligrams of cholesterol and 2 grams (or less) of saturated fat per serving. Note that this in no way indicates that the product is fat-free!

• *Extra lean.* A food product containing less than 5 grams of total fat, less than 2 grams of saturated fat, and less than 95 milligrams of cholesterol per serving.

• *Fat-free.* A food product containing less than 0.5 grams of fat per serving.

• *High-fiber.* A food product containing 5 grams or more of fiber per serving.

• *Lean.* A food product containing less than 10 grams of total fat, 4 grams of saturated fat, and 95 milligrams of cholesterol per serving.

• *Less.* A food product, altered or not, that contains 25 percent less of a nutrient or of calories than the referenced food.

• *Light (lite).* A food product containing one-third fewer calories or no more than half the fat of the higher-calorie, higher-fat version; or containing no more than half the sodium of the higher-sodium version.

• *Low saturated fat.* A food product containing 1 gram or less of saturated fat per serving.

• *Low-calorie.* A food product containing 40 or fewer calories per serving.

• *Low-fat.* A food product containing 3 grams of fat or less per serving.

   Note: Because of a special exemption, 2-percent milk will continue to be referred to as "low-fat," even though it does not meet the FDA criteria for a low-fat food.

• *Reduced.* A nutritionally altered product containing 25 percent less of a nutrient or of calories than the regular or referenced product.

   On the following page is a sample and explanation of the most widely used food label (see Figure 2). There are also other styles of the food label that are smaller. These are used when the larger label cannot be made to fit on the packaging. Canned meats and vegetables and refrigerated bakery items are some of the products that often carry the smaller labels. The smaller labels show the same nutritional information as the larger version, but in a slightly different format. If a product's package is too small for any type of readable label (for example, certain types of candies), the manufacturer must list an address or telephone number that consumers may contact to request nutritional information.

   Another style of food label is used for food products that are to have ingredients added to them by the consumer during preparation in order to create a finished product. Boxed pancake mix is an example of such a product. These labels show the nutritional information for one serving of the packaged contents "as packaged" and separate nutritional information for one serving of the finished product with the added ingredients included.

CAUTION: "FAT-FREE" PRODUCTS CAN BE HAZARDOUS TO YOUR WEIGHT!

The grocery shelves are carrying more and more fat-free products, and fat consumption decreased from 40 percent of daily calories in the 1960s to 34 percent of daily calories in 1990. Yet these changes have not had the expected effect on the weight of the population. Why? A clue may lie in the following: The percentage of Americans concerned about their fat intake climbed from 16 percent in 1987 to 65 percent in 1995, according to the Food Marketing Institute, while only 13 percent of us appeared to be concerned about our calorie intake. Is it any wonder, then, that the National Center for Health Statistics reports that 33

Nutrition Facts

Serving Size ½ cup (114g)

Servings Per Container 4

Amount Per Serving

Calories 90   Calories from Fat 30

	% Daily Value*
Total Fat 3g	5%
Saturated Fat 0g	0%
Cholesterol 0mg	0%
Sodium 300mg	13%
Total Carbohydrate 13g	4%
Dietary Fiber 3g	12%
Sugars 3g	
Protein 3g	

Vitamin A 80% • Vitamin C 60% • Calcium 4% • Iron 4%

*Percent Daily Values are based on a 2,000 calorie diet. Your Daily Values may be higher or lower depending on your calorie needs:

Nutrient		2,000 Calories	2,500 Calories
Total Fat	Less than	65g	80g
Sat Fat	Less than	20g	25g
Cholesterol	Less than	300mg	300mg
Sodium	Less than	2,400mg	2,400mg
Total Carbohydrate		300g	375g
Fiber		25g	30g

Calories per gram:

Fat 9 • Carbohydrates 4 • Protein 4

Figure 2. Sample Food Product Label

percent more of us are obese (defined as 30 percent or more over our healthy weight) than just fifteen years before?

Although the biggest culprit behind this statistic appears to be a lack of exercise, it is becoming more and more evident that consumers are seeing fat-free products as being *totally* healthy. Forgotten is the fact that fat-free foods still contain calories—in some cases, as many as (if not more than) their higher-fat counterparts (sugar is sometimes used to compensate for the flavor lost in cutting out the fat). Remember this: Both the amount of fat *and* the number of calories we consume are important. *Don't* buy the myth that "calories don't count!" If you eat more calories than you burn, regardless of the source, you will gain weight. Whether the extra calories come from fat, from carbohydrates, or from protein, you will store them as body fat!

Studies strongly suggest that when we eat low-fat or fat-free foods, we tend to make up for the missing fat calories by eating bigger portions of either the low-fat or fat-free foods, or of other foods. So while fat-free products are of a higher quality than they were a few years ago, and they offer us a viable way to cut the amount of fat we consume, portion control is still very much in order. You might try keeping things in perspective by reminding yourself that while a one-and-a-half-ounce serving of "fat-free" cake has less than 0.5 grams of fat, it still has almost the same number of calories as a tablespoon of butter!

GUIDELINES FOR REDUCING THE FAT IN YOUR DIET

As mentioned earlier, fat is needed for healthy body functions and should not be totally eliminated from the diet. The Surgeon General's Report on Nutrition and Health conveyed, "Adults need a minimum daily intake of 15 to 25 grams of fat to meet these necessities."

However, the American Heart Association; the American Health Foundation; the American Cancer Society; the National Heart, Lung, and Blood Institute; the National Center for Nutrition and Dietetics; the American Diabetes Association; and the Surgeon General all recommend that no more than 30 percent of our daily calories should come from fat, and no more than one third of those fats (or 10 percent of our daily calories) should be saturated fats. Below I will show you how to calculate these percentages.

THE FAT GRAM BUDGET FORMULA

Fortunately, since you have decided to reduce your dietary fat, there is a simple formula that will let you know exactly how many fat grams you should allow yourself on a daily basis. To find out your maximum daily allowance, multiply your daily calorie intake by .3, and divide that total by 9 (there are 9 calories in each gram of fat). For a daily intake of 1,500 calories, your equation would look like this:

$$1500 \times .3 = 450; 450 \div 9 = 50$$

To make calculating your daily fat allowance even easier, I have listed the fat gram budgets for specific daily calorie intakes. Table 2 shows 10-percent, 20-percent, and 30-percent maximum daily fat gram budgets for diets of 1,200 to 3,000 calories per day. Note that the data in Table 2 have been rounded off by dropping all decimal places. It begins at a daily intake of 1,200 calories, as it is not recommended that anyone eat fewer than 1,200 calories (for women) or

Table 2. Maximum Daily Fat Gram Budget

Daily Calorie Intake	Fat Grams Allowed			Daily Calorie Intake	Fat Grams Allowed		
	10%	20%	30%		10%	20%	30%
1,200	13	27	40	2,200	24	49	73
1,300	14	29	43	2,300	26	51	76
1,400	16	31	46	2,400	27	53	80
1,500	17	33	50	2,500	28	56	83
1,600	18	36	53	2,600	29	58	86
1,700	19	38	56	2,700	30	60	90
1,800	20	40	60	2,800	31	62	93
1,900	21	42	63	2,900	32	64	96
2,000	22	44	66	3,000	33	67	100
2,100	23	47	70				

1,500 calories (for men), in order to ensure that her or his daily nutritional needs are met. In using your daily fat gram budget, always remember that just because you have budgeted "X" amount of fat grams for the day, *you don't have to eat that amount of fat.* Just make sure not to go over budget!

Of course, to calculate your daily fat gram budget, you need to know your daily calorie intake. If you don't already know this, just use *The Complete and Up-to-Date Fat Book* to keep a diary for three or four days. Write down everything you eat and drink for these days, add up the totals, then divide by the number of days you kept track.

People often ask me how to find out how many calories they *should* be consuming on a daily basis. Table 3 will give you a general idea of what your daily calorie consumption should be, making it easier for you to figure your fat gram budget. Remember, though, that we all have different metabolisms, so the appropriate amount of daily calories for you may vary slightly either way.

MAKING SMARTER, HEALTHIER CHOICES

The following are some tips to keep in mind as you take stock of your eating habits and begin your quest for better nutrition by reducing your intake of dietary fat:

• Beef and pork have become leaner than ever before because the animals are fed a less fattening diet and are taken to market sooner (before they have had a chance to build up a store of fat). The results are so lean that you can choose from some cuts of beef or pork and have little more fat than a skinless breast of chicken! Stay with the following cuts and *keep your cooked portions to 3 ounces,*

Table 3. Daily Calorie Requirements

Age/Sex/Activity Level	Calorie Requirements
Minimum calories for adequate nutrition	1,000–1,200
Sedentary women	1,600
Moderately active women; children 4–6 years; women 51 and over	1,800
Active women; sedentary men; teen girls; children 7–10 years	2,000–2,200
Very active women; average men 50 and over; boys 11–14 years	2,200–2,600
Active men; teen boys	2,600–2,800
Active to very active men 25–50; athletes in training	3,000–4,000

Source: U.S. Department of Health and Human Services, Food and Drug Administration, FDA Special Report May 1993

prepared without added fat (all cuts should be boneless and trimmed of all visible fat):

Beef (USDA Select)	Pork	Veal
chuck arm pot roast	cured ham (lean)	cutlets
eye of round	loin roast	sirloin
flank steak	sirloin chops	tenderloin
top round	tenderloin	
top sirloin	top loin	

• Familiarize yourself with the number of grams of fat and the percentage of calories from fat of the foods you eat most often so that it becomes "second nature" to compute your fat consumption.

• Once you are familiar enough with where the fat is located in the foods you eat, make your fat gram budget an average covering three to four days instead of focusing on each meal. This allows some flexibility, which is important for healthy lifelong habit changes.

• Don't forget the fat-free or reduced-fat mayonnaise on the market today when putting together a macaroni, potato, tuna, or turkey salad.

• Use a reduced-fat or fat-free margarine or spread instead of butter or regular margarine or spread. These come in spreadable, squeezable, and sprayable forms.

• Use canned evaporated skim milk as a substitute for heavy cream, and low-fat or skim milk in place of whole milk or cream in your recipes.

• There is a great selection of low-fat and fat-free salad dressings on the market today. They come in many flavors and styles. Try them until you find one or more to your taste. Remember that you can save as many as 6 to 10 grams of fat *per tablespoon* by not using regular salad dressings!

• Instead of rich desserts like ice cream, try the wide range of frozen yogurt desserts available in your grocery store's freezer section. Again, because of the wide range of tastes, you may have to try more than one or two to find the ones for you. There are also "lighter" ice creams available in a wide range of such gourmet flavors as caramel nut fudge sundae and mocha almond fudge. The low-fat and fat-free bakery goods now on the market give us almost unlimited choices for our sweet tooth. Remember, though: Moderation!

• Substitute low-fat, reduced-fat, or fat-free cheese for those cheeses higher in fat. The fat saved here is between 6 and 10 grams per ounce!

• Most breads are low in fat (1 gram per slice), but be careful when you reach for a croissant to make that sandwich. Croissants can have as many as 14 grams of fat in them.

• Try dry cereals for a great-tasting snack. Most of them have 0 to 3 grams of fat per serving. Do read the labels on granola-type cereals, most of which are higher in fat.

• Canadian bacon is a tasty lower-fat substitute for bacon. Bacon bits also have less fat, and can be used as a pizza topping, too.

• While ten French fries have 8 grams of fat, a 1.5-ounce package of potato chips has a whopping 15 grams of fat!

• You can thicken sauces without fat by substituting puréed vegetables for cream or whole milk.

• Make your own bread coatings with plain bread crumbs and your choice of spices. Dip food into skim milk, buttermilk, or egg whites before coating and baking in a hot oven.

• Instead of nondairy creamer, try powdered low-fat or skim milk.

• Reduce the amount of oil or melted butter in your recipes by a third to a half, replacing the amount reduced with water or fruit juice. Try to buy only those commercial mixes to which you add the fat or oil, so you can control the amount.

• Instead of pan-frying or deep-frying, try basting your meat, fish, or poultry with wine, lemon juice or other fruit juices, broth, tomato juice, or low-fat or fat-free salad dressing to keep it from drying out.

• Instead of using whole eggs, replace each yolk with two egg whites or a low-fat egg substitute. Omelettes can be made with one whole egg and an additional egg white or two.

• Whenever using oil, make sure it's the least saturated oil available to you, and remember that although it may be low in saturated fat, *all oils have 14 grams of fat for each tablespoon.* (See Oils, pages 459–460.)

• Cocoa powder is an excellent low-fat substitute for baking chocolate, which is high in fat. Three tablespoons of cocoa equal one square of baking chocolate.

• Instead of using cooking oil or shortening, use a nonstick skillet sprayed with a small amount of cooking spray. Or use a paper towel to spread a small amount of oil over the surface of the frying pan.

These simple changes can easily be made. Learn the low-fat substitutes to use in your cooking at home, and stay from too many "bought" high-fat bakery products. Read your labels! Once you have learned to recognize the fat content of the foods available to you by using *The Complete and Up-to-Date Fat Book,* making healthier eating choices will become a way of life!

LET'S GET STARTED!

By following the suggestions in this book just *a little at a time* and educating yourself about the sources of dietary fat, you will be on your way to a healthy, low-fat lifestyle. Using *The Complete and Up-to-Date Fat Book,* check the fat content of the foods you usually eat against your daily fat gram budget and see what you may need to change or replace with a lower-fat food. Then, find appropriate low-fat substitutes for these higher-fat foods to bring you in line with your budget. Sound easy? With the wide range of choices of lower-fat foods on the market today, it's easier than ever!

You will be startled by exactly how much dietary fat you have been eating. You may even find that if a favorite food takes a big enough bite (no pun intended) out of your daily fat gram budget, you will want that favorite food less often and will automatically begin to make more nutritionally-sound food selections!

FOOD FOR THOUGHT

According to the USDA, the following foods are America's top ten fat sources:

1. Margarine.
2. Whole milk.
3. Shortening.
4. Mayonnaise and salad dressing.
5. American cheese.
6. Ground beef.
7. Reduced-fat milk.

8. Eggs.
9. Butter.
10. Vanilla ice cream.

This list does not mean that these foods are the ten foods highest in fat. It means these are the most often consumed high-fat foods. If you eat any of the foods on this list, this is a great place to start in finding lower fat substitutes.

WRITE IT DOWN

In the beginning, as you acquaint yourself with *The Complete and Up-to-Date Fat Book,* you will find that keeping a daily account of your food intake is invaluable. Keep track of everything you eat and drink as you begin to count up the fat grams and calories for each day. This way, you will be able to get a better idea of exactly what you are eating and where you need to make adjustments. Keeping close track of your eating habits, as you begin to form new ones, will also enable you to:

• Recognize your eating patterns.

• Gain control over what you eat.

• Budget your fat grams and calories more realistically.

• Think twice about deviating from a healthy low-fat lifestyle.

• Take pride in seeing your progress in writing.

At the back of this book you will find a Personal Food Diary to help you get started on recording your new eating habits.

GET ACQUAINTED WITH *THE COMPLETE AND UP-TO-DATE FAT BOOK*

Although extreme care has been taking in recording all data in *The Complete and Up-to-Date Fat Book,* you may come across an occasional discrepancy between the information here and the nutritional data on product labels or other sources of nutritional information. There are a number of reasons why this might occur.

First, manufacturers are given a slightly flexible range in which they are able to round off their data and still be in accordance with governmental regulations on product labeling. For example, if a certain product contains 2.3 grams of fat, the manufacturer can list the fat content as 2 grams, dropping the .3. The same is done with data on calories. If a product serving has 134 calories, the manufacturer can list the calorie content as either 130 or 135. Wherever possible, I have kept the nutritional data intact without rounding off either fat or calorie content.

Second, when I gathered data from product labels and compared this with data I received directly from manufacturers, occasionally there was a difference between the two because the product label listed the nutritional data of an old product formula while the manufacturer provided up-to-date data that reflected a recent change in the product formula. In these cases, data obtained directly from the manufacturer were always used. Product serving sizes can also change and cause a change in nutritional data. So be sure, when comparing products, that you are comparing the same serving size—that is, a quarter cup of one product against a quarter cup of another.

Other differences can be caused by differences in the analytical methods and sampling techniques used by the different nutritional sources.

As you can see, data in this book are listed in four columns. "Amount" means the serving size of food served or used in a recipe. Remember that any deviation in serving size will cause a change in the rest of the data given in all of the other columns. The fat content of each food is expressed as the number of fat grams per serving (the measurement used for dietary fat). The calorie column needs no explanation.

In the fourth column, I have listed the percentage of calories from fat under "% Fat Calories" for all foods listed. If you need to figure the percentage of fat in a food not listed, the formula is:

1. Multiply the number of fat grams by 9 to get total fat calories (TFC).
2. Divide TFC by the total calorie content of your chosen food.

EXAMPLE: 1 ounce cheddar cheese contains 9 fat grams and 110 calories
9 (fat grams) x 9 (calories per gram) = 81 (TFC)
81 (TFC) ÷ 110 (total calories) = 0.73, or 73 percent

Since a high-fat food is defined as any food in which 30 percent or more of the calories come from fat, this cheddar cheese would be considered a high-fat food.

Some of the data in the "% Fat Calories" column have been rounded off, as mentioned, and the percentage might be off *slightly,* but not to the point that it matters. For example, all oils and fats get 100 percent of their calories from fat. However, if you look at the listing for a fat such as butter, you will see that if you calculated the percentage of calories from fat (11 fat grams x 9 ÷ 100 calories = 99 percent), this would deviate slightly from the "% Fat Calories" listed (100 percent). Because we know that all oils and fats contain 100 percent fat calories, I did not want to mislead you by using the rounded-off data and listing 99% instead of the absolute 100%.

You will find both generic and brand name products in these tables. The listing of a product by brand name is not necessarily meant as an endorsement. If brand name products are not listed, it is because there was no nutritional data available at the time, and they were omitted for that reason only. Also included are products available in wholesale clubs and through wholesale food distributors. These are identified as "food service products."

HOW TO USE THIS BOOK

The Complete and Up-to-Date Fat Book is an in-depth and comprehensive reference. As you shop for and prepare low-fat foods, this book will be an invaluable source of information.

Serving size, fat grams, total calories, and percentage of calories from fat are provided for every product listed. In most cases, the foods are listed alphabetically for easy reference. Some types of foods, where appropriate, are listed in groups, such as Frozen Entrée/Dinner, Mexican Food, Asian Food, and so on. Following the A-to-Z food list, you will find a separate section on fast foods, organized alphabetically by fast-food franchise.

Since cereals and soups are frequently prepared with milk, quick-reference charts for adding milk can be found in these sections. Also, because it is important to choose the least saturated oil available when using oil in food preparation, I have prepared charts on pages 459–460 that show the percentages of saturated, polyunsaturated, and monounsaturated fats contained in the most commonly used fats and oils.

As far as style, the book is organized with main headings for food capitalized and bold. In some cases, bold (but smaller) subheadings with solid boxes before them have been added for clarity. Descriptions of foods are in upper/lower case, with brand names in parentheses.

If you are unable to find a particular food, look for the listing of a similar food. The nutritional data should be close, if not exactly the same. When comparing foods, make sure you are comparing the same serving size. Also, be sure you are comparing weight measure against weight measure and volume measure against volume measure. The Table of Equivalent Measures (see page 21) should help you, not only in comparing serving sizes, but in making your exchanges easier as well. Finally, note that all servings of cooked vegetables are drained of liquid, unless otherwise noted.

You will find *The Complete and Up-to-Date Fat Book* a valuable companion as you begin to take control of your eating habits. And you will discover that adopting a low-fat lifestyle reaps many rewards—rewards such as more energy, better sleep, lower grocery bills, more control over your weight, and, perhaps most important, vibrant health!

EXPLANATION OF ABBREVIATIONS AND SYMBOLS USED

~	=	approximately	pkg	=	package
<	=	less than	pkt	=	packet
"	=	inch	sec	=	second
–	=	trace amount or less	Tbs	=	tablespoon
dia	=	diameter	tsp	=	teaspoon
lb	=	pound	w/	=	with
oz	=	ounce	w/o	=	without

Regarding dishes noted as "homemade," the data listed assume the use of standard ingredients in preparation; no low-fat substitutes were used in these recipes. The data listed are to be used as a guideline for the dish as you might make it in your home. Data on boxed mix dishes assume that they are prepared according to package directions and, unless noted otherwise, without using low-fat substitute ingredients.

TABLE OF EQUIVALENT MEASURES

VOLUME

1 tablespoon	=	½ fluid ounce	⅔ cup	=	10⅔ tablespoons
		3 teaspoons	¾ cup	=	6 fluid ounces
1 fluid ounce	=	2 tablespoons			12 tablespoons
¼ cup	=	2 fluid ounces	1 pint	=	2 cups
		4 tablespoons			16 fluid ounces
⅓ cup	=	5⅓ tablespoons	1 quart	=	2 pints
1 cup	=	½ pint			4 cups
		8 fluid ounces			32 fluid ounces
		16 tablespoons	1 gallon	=	4 quarts
½ cup	=	4 fluid ounces			8 pints
		8 tablespoons			

WEIGHT

1 ounce	=	28.35 grams	12 ounces	=	¾ pound
100 grams	=	3.5 ounces	1 pound	=	16 ounces
4 ounces	=	¼ pound			454 grams
8 ounces	=	½ pound			

A

Food and Description	Amount	Fat Grams	Total Calories	% Fat Calories
ABALONE				
fried	3 oz	5.8	161	32%
raw	3 oz	1.0	90	10%
ACEROLA/raw	1 medium	–	2	–
	1 cup	–	31	–
ACEROLA JUICE	8 fl oz	0.7	51	12%
ACORN				
dried	1 oz	8.9	145	55%
raw	1 oz	6.8	105	58%
ACORN FLOUR (See FLOUR)				
ADZUKI BEAN				
(Arrowhead Mills) raw	¼ cup	0.5	150	3%
(Eden)	½ cup	–	110	–
generic				
boiled	½ cup	<1.0	147	3%
raw	½ cup	<1.0	325	1%
sweetened/canned	½ cup	<1.0	351	1%
Yokan	¼" slice	–	35	–
AGAR (See SEAWEED)				
ALBACORE (See TUNA)				
ALE (See BEER, ALE, & MALT LIQUOR)				
ALEWIFE/HERRING/raw	4 oz	5.6	144	35%
ALFALFA SPROUTS/raw	1 cup	–	10	–
ALLIGATOR/raw	3 oz	3.0	200	14%
ALLSPICE	1 tsp	–	6	–
ALMOND				
(Azar)				
sliced	1 oz	15.0	170	79%
slivered	1 oz	15.0	170	79%
(Beer Nuts)	1 oz	14.0	180	70%
(Blue Diamond)				
blanched/whole	1 oz	15.0	190	71%
chopped/natural	1 oz	15.0	180	75%
dried/whole	1 oz	15.0	180	75%
roasted/salted	1 oz	17.0	190	81%
slivered	1 oz	15.0	190	71%
Smokehouse	1 oz	17.0	180	85%
(Dole)	1 oz	14.0	170	74%

Food and Description	Amount	Fat Grams	Total Calories	% Fat Calories
generic				
dried				
blanched				
pieces	1 cup	76.0	850	80%
whole	1 oz	15.0	166	81%
unblanched				
pieces	1 cup	49.0	555	79%
slivered/packed	1 cup	70.5	795	80%
whole	1 oz	15.0	167	81%
dry-roasted	1 oz	15.0	167	81%
blanched	1 oz	15.0	167	81%
hickory smoked	1 oz	15.0	166	81%
unblanched	1 oz	15.0	167	81%
oil-roasted				
blanched	1 oz	16.0	174	83%
toasted	1 oz	14.0	167	75%
unblanched	1 oz	16.0	176	82%
(Lance) smoked	¾ oz	10.0	130	69%
(Planters)	1 oz	15.0	170	79%
Gold Measure/slivered	2 oz	31.0	340	82%
honey-roasted	1 oz	14.0	160	79%
ALMOND BUTTER				
(Erewhon)	1 Tbs	8.0	90	80%
generic				
honey & cinnamon	1 Tbs	8.0	96	75%
	½ cup	65.0	755	77%
plain	1 Tbs	9.5	100	86%
	1 cup	74.0	790	84%
(Hain)				
natural/raw	2 Tbs	18.0	190	85%
toasted-blanched	2 Tbs	19.0	220	78%
(Roaster Fresh) unsalted	1 oz	16.0	184	78%
(Spanky's)	1 oz	17.0	190	80%
(Westbrae Natural)				
crunchy	2 Tbs	17.0	190	80%
smooth	2 Tbs	17.0	190	80%
ALMOND FILLING				
(Odense) marizipan	2 Tbs	4.0	500	7%
(Solo)	2 Tbs	2.5	120	19%
ALMOND MEAL/partially defatted	1 oz	5.0	116	39%
ALMOND PASTE	1 Tbs	7.7	127	55%
	1 cup	62.0	1010	55%
ALMOND POWDER				
full-fat	1 oz	15.0	168	80%
	1 cup	34.0	385	80%
partially defatted	1 oz	5.0	112	40%
	1 cup	10.0	255	35%
ALOE VERA JUICE	2 oz	–	5	–

Food and Description	Amount	Fat Grams	Total Calories	% Fat Calories
AMARANTH				
(Arrowhead Mills) Fast Menu vegetarian cuisine	1 cup	–	160	–
generic				
cooked	½ cup	–	14	–
raw	1 cup	–	7	–
AMARANTH FLOUR (See FLOUR)				
AMARANTH SEED	¼ cup	2.0	170	11%
ANASAZI BEAN				
(Arrowhead Mills) dry	¼ cup	0.5	150	3%
(Bean Cuisine) dry	½ cup	1.0	115	8%
ANCHOVY, EUROPEAN				
canned/in oil	5 fish	1.9	42	41%
fresh/raw	3 oz	4.0	62	58%
ANCHOVY PASTE	1 tsp	0.8	14	51%
ANISE	1 tsp	–	7	–
APPLE (See also APPLE, CARAMEL)				
canned				
generic/sliced/sweetened	½ cup	0.5	68	7%
(Luck's) fried				
plain	½ cup	–	130	–
w/cinnamon	½ cup	–	120	–
(Musselman's)				
chips	4 oz	–	50	–
diced	4 oz	–	50	–
rings/green or red	4 oz	–	100	–
sliced				
dessert	4 oz	–	70	–
sweetened				
in syrup	4 oz	–	50	–
in water	4 oz	–	50	–
unpeeled	4 oz	–	90	–
whole				
baked	1 apple	–	110	–
sweetened/peeled-cored	1 apple	–	90	–
(S&W)				
rings	2 pieces	–	25	–
spiced crab	1 piece	–	35	–
(TreeTop) sliced	5 oz	–	40	–
dried				
(Del Monte) sliced	⅓ cup	–	80	–
generic				
cooked				
w/sugar	1 cup	–	232	–
w/o sugar	1 cup	–	144	–
uncooked	10 rings	–	155	–
	1 cup	–	209	–
(Mariani)	¼ cup	–	150	–

Food and Description	Amount	Fat Grams	Total Calories	% Fat Calories
(Nature's Favorite) chips				
cinnamon	1 oz	5.0	120	38%
Golden Delicious	1 oz	5.0	120	38%
original	1 oz	5.0	120	38%
(Sun Maid) chunks	¼ cup	–	110	–
(Weight Watchers) chips	¾ oz	–	70	–
fresh				
cooked/w/o skin	1 cup	0.6	91	6%
microwaved/sliced				
peeled	½ cup	0.5	65	7%
unpeeled	½ cup	0.5	50	9%
raw				
(Dole)	1 medium	1.0	80	11%
w/skin				
sliced	1 cup	–	64	6%
whole	1 medium	0.5	81	6%
w/o skin				
sliced	1 cup	–	62	–
whole	1 medium	–	72	–
APPLE, CARAMEL				
(Classic Kettle)				
almond chocolate	¼ apple	16.0	320	45%
peanut chocolate	¼ apple	12.0	260	42%
pecan chocolate	¼ apple	17.0	320	48%
toffee walnut chocolate	¼ apple	14.0	310	41%
triple chocolate chunk	¼ apple	12.0	300	36%
APPLE BUTTER				
(Dutch Girl)	1 Tbs	–	35	–
(Eden)	1 Tbs	–	25	–
generic	1 Tbs	<1.0	33	3%
	1 cup	2.0	525	3%
(Kozlowski Farms)	1 Tbs	–	30	–
(Mary Ellen)	1 Tbs	–	35	–
(Smucker's)				
cider	1 Tbs	–	45	–
Simply Fruit	1 Tbs	–	45	–
spiced	1 Tbs	–	45	–
APPLE CIDER (See CIDER)				
APPLE DUMPLING (See PASTRY)				
APPLE JUICE/NECTAR				
bottled, boxed, or canned				
(Campbell's) Juice Bowl/apple	6 fl oz	–	110	–
(Dole)	10 fl oz	–	160	–
(Indian Summer)	6 fl oz	–	90	–
(Knudsen)				
apple	8 fl oz	–	110	–
Thirst Quencher				
natural apple	8 fl oz	–	120	–

Food and Description	Amount	Fat Grams	Total Calories	% Fat Calories
nectar	8 fl oz	–	120	–
(Kraft) pure 100%	6 fl oz	–	80	–
(Libby's)				
Juicy Juice	4.23 fl oz	–	60	–
Juicy Pouch	4.23 fl oz	–	60	–
(Martinelli's) sparkling	6 fl oz	–	100	–
(Minute Maid)	8 fl oz	–	112	–
	8.45 fl oz	–	120	–
(Mott's)				
In-a-Minute unfrozen concentrate	2 fl oz	–	120	–
natural	8 fl oz	–	120	–
	9.5 fl oz	–	140	–
	10 fl oz	–	150	–
(Musselman's)				
enriched, w/100% vitamin C	6 fl oz	–	90	–
original	6 fl oz	–	90	–
(Ocean Spray) unsweetened	6 fl oz	–	90	–
(President's Choice) Cox's Orange Pippin	8 fl oz	–	120	–
(Red Cheek)				
natural style	8 fl oz	–	120	–
100% pure	8 fl oz	–	120	–
(S&W)	8 fl oz	–	120	–
(Season's) best	6 fl oz	–	80	–
	8 fl oz	–	120	–
	10 fl oz	–	140	–
	11.5 fl oz	–	160	–
(Seneca)	8 fl oz	–	110	–
country apple	8 fl oz	–	110	–
Granny Smith	8 fl oz	–	110	–
(Sippin' Pak) from concentrate	8.45 fl oz	–	110	–
(Snapple) apple crisp	10 fl oz	–	140	–
(Sunglo)	8.45 fl oz	–	130	–
(TreeTop)				
country style	8.45 fl oz	–	120	–
	10 fl oz	–	140	–
	11.5 fl oz	–	170	–
fiber rich	4 fl oz	–	70	–
	8 fl oz	–	150	–
(TreeSweet)	8 fl oz	–	120	–
(Tropicana)	8 fl oz	–	110	–
(Welch's)				
juice	8 fl oz	–	120	–
	10 fl oz	–	140	–
	11.5 fl oz	–	160	–
Juicemakers	8 fl oz	–	120	–
(White House)	6 fl oz	–	90	–

Food and Description	Amount	Fat Grams	Total Calories	% Fat Calories
frozen				
(Birds Eye)	6 fl oz	–	80	–
(Minute Maid)	8 fl oz	–	110	–
(Seneca)	8 fl oz	–	120	–
country style	8 fl oz	–	120	–
Granny Smith	8 fl oz	–	110	–
(Sunkist)	8 fl oz	–	80	–
(TreeTop)				
country style	8 fl oz	–	120	–
original	8 fl oz	–	120	–
(Welch's) juice cocktail	8 fl oz	–	160	–

APPLE JUICE BLEND/DRINK

(NOTE: Unless stated otherwise, data are for prepared serving amounts.)

Food and Description	Amount	Fat Grams	Total Calories	% Fat Calories
bottled, boxed, or canned				
(Betty Crocker) Squeezit 100/ Acrobat Apple	7 fl oz	–	90	–
(Dole)				
Apple Berry Burst	8 fl oz	–	120	–
apple-cranberry	10 fl oz	–	160	–
(Fruitopia) Apple Raspberry Embrace	8 fl oz	–	75	–
(Hi-C) Jammin' Apple	8.45 fl oz	–	120	–
(Knudsen)				
apple-boysenberry juice	8 fl oz	–	120	–
Thist Quencher/apple-cranberry	8 fl oz	–	130	–
(Libby's) Juicy Juice				
apple-grape	8 fl oz	–	100	–
	8.45 fl oz	–	130	–
(Minute Maid) apple-grape	8 fl oz	–	125	–
(Mott's)				
apple juice drink	9.5 fl oz	–	150	–
	10 fl oz	–	160	–
apple-cranberry juice				
In-a-Minute unfrozen concentrate	2 fl oz	–	170	–
ready to drink	8 fl oz	–	120	–
	9.5 fl oz	–	150	–
	10 fl oz	–	180	–
apple-grape juice	8 fl oz	–	120	–
apple-raspberry juice	6 fl oz	–	85	–
	8.45 fl oz	–	125	–
	9.5 fl oz	–	135	–
	10 fl oz	–	140	–
(Seneca)				
apple juice cocktail	8 fl oz	–	110	–
apple-cranberry juice	8 fl oz	–	120	–
(TreeTop)				
apple-apricot juice	4 fl oz	–	90	–
	8 fl oz	–	160	–

Food and Description	Amount	Fat Grams	Total Calories	% Fat Calories
apple-cranberry juice	10 fl oz	–	190	–
	11.5 fl oz	–	230	–
apple-grape juice	5.5 fl oz	–	90	–
	8.45 fl oz	–	140	–
	11.5 fl oz	–	190	–
apple-orange-banana juice	4 fl oz	–	80	–
	8 fl oz	–	170	–
apple-pear juice	5.5 fl oz	–	80	–
	8 fl oz	–	120	–
	8.45 fl oz	–	120	–
	10 fl oz	–	140	–
	11.5 fl oz	–	170	–
apple-raspberry juice	5.5 fl oz	–	80	–
	8.45 fl oz	–	120	–
	10 fl oz	–	140	–
	11.5 fl oz	–	160	–
(Tropicana) Twister/apple-raspberry-blackberry	8 fl oz	–	130	–
	11.5 fl oz	–	180	–
(Welch's)				
apple-cranberry drink	11.5 fl oz	–	210	–
apple-orange-pineapple drink	11.5 fl oz	–	210	–
Cocktail-In-A-Box				
apple-grape-cherry	8.45 fl oz	–	150	–
apple-grape-raspberry	8.45 fl oz	–	150	–
Juice Cocktail				
apple	8 fl oz	–	140	–
apple-cranberry	8 fl oz	–	150	–
apple-grape-cherry	8 fl oz	–	150	–
apple-orange-pineapple	8 fl oz	–	150	–
frozen				
(Dole) Apple Berry Burst	8 fl oz	–	120	–
(Mott's) Fruit Basket Juice Cocktail				
apple	8 fl oz	–	120	–
apple-raspberry	8 fl oz	–	130	–
(TreeTop)				
apple-cranberry juice	8 fl oz	–	130	–
apple-grape juice	8 fl oz	–	130	–
apple-pear juice	8 fl oz	–	120	–
apple-raspberry juice	8 fl oz	–	110	–
(Welch's) Orchard Juice Blend				
apple-grape-cherry	8 fl oz	–	140	–
apple-grape-raspberry	8 fl oz	–	140	–
APPLESAUCE				
(Del Monte)				
lite	½ cup	–	50	–
sweetened	½ cup	–	90	–
generic/canned				
sweetened	1 cup	–	194	–

Food and Description	Amount	Fat Grams	Total Calories	% Fat Calories
unsweetened	1 cup	–	106	–
(Mott's)				
chunky	5 oz	–	110	–
cinnamon	5 oz	–	120	–
fruit snacks				
cinnamon	4 oz	–	90	–
Dutch apple spice	4 oz	–	70	–
strawberry	4 oz	–	80	–
sweetened	4 oz	–	90	–
(Musselman's)				
applesauce				
chunky	½ cup	–	80	–
deluxe cinnamon	½ cup	–	100	–
natural	½ cup	–	50	–
regular	½ cup	–	80	–
unsweetened	½ cup	–	50	–
Fruit 'N Sauce/apple-cherry	½ cup	–	100	–
(Nutradiet) unsweetened	½ cup	–	55	–
(S&W) Gravenstein				
sweetened	½ cup	–	90	–
unsweetened	½ cup	–	50	–
(Seneca)				
cinnamon	4.5 oz	–	100	–
Golden Delicious	4.5 oz	–	100	–
McIntosh	4.5 oz	–	60	–
100% natural	4.5 oz	–	100	–
regular	4.5 oz	–	100	–
(TreeTop)				
cinnamon	4 oz	–	90	–
	½ cup	–	100	–
original	4 oz	–	90	–
	½ cup	–	100	–
unsweetened	4 oz	–	70	–
	½ cup	–	70	–
(Wilderness)				
raspberry	½ cup	–	82	–
strawberry	½ cup	–	90	–
APRICOT				
candied	1 oz	–	96	–
canned				
(Del Monte) halves/unpeeled				
in heavy syrup	½ cup	–	100	–
in light syrup	½ cup	–	60	–
generic				
peeled				
in juice	1 cup	–	119	–
in water	1 cup	–	51	–

Food and Description	Amount	Fat Grams	Total Calories	% Fat Calories
unpeeled				
in heavy syrup	1 cup	–	214	–
in light syrup	1 cup	–	160	–
in water	1 cup	–	65	–
(Libby's) unpeeled/lite	½ cup	–	60	–
(S&W) whole/peeled/in heavy syrup	½ cup	–	110	–
dried				
(Ann's House of Nuts) Turkish	5 pieces	–	90	–
(Del Monte) sun-dried	⅓ cup	–	80	–
(Dole) Sun Giant Turkish	6 pieces	–	90	–
generic				
cooked	½ cup	<1.0	106	2%
uncooked	½ cup	0.6	155	3%
(Mariani)				
California	¼ cup	–	140	–
Mediterranean	¼ cup	–	140	–
(Sun Maid)	¼ cup	–	140	–
fresh	3 medium	0.5	51	9%
	1 cup	0.6	74	7%
frozen/sweetened	½ cup	–	119	–
APRICOT FILLING (Solo)	2 Tbs	–	80	–
APRICOT JUICE/NECTAR/bottled, boxed, or canned				
(Del Monte)	6 fl oz	–	100	–
generic				
juice/unsweetened	8 fl oz	–	123	–
nectar	8 fl oz	–	140	–
(Kern's)	11.5 fl oz	–	220	–
(Knudsen)	8 fl oz	–	105	–
(Libby's)	6 fl oz	–	110	–
(S&W)	5.5 fl oz	–	100	–
	8 fl oz	–	140	–
	12 fl oz	–	210	–
APRICOT JUICE/NECTAR BLEND/bottled or canned				
(Kern's)				
apricot-mango	11.5 fl oz	–	220	–
apricot-pineapple	11.5 fl oz	–	220	–
(Seneca) apricot nectar cocktail	8 fl oz	–	140	–
ARMADILLO/raw	3 oz	4.0	150	24%
ARROWHEAD/plant				
cooked	medium corm	0.5	9	50%
raw	medium corm	0.5	12	38%
ARTICHOKE (See also JERUSALEM ARTICHOKE)				
canned or jarred				
(Cara Mia) marinated				
crowns	1 oz	–	12	–
hearts	1 oz	2.0	27	67%

Food and Description	Amount	Fat Grams	Total Calories	% Fat Calories
(Progresso) hearts				
marinated	⅓ cup	14.0	160	79%
regular	2 pieces	–	35	–
(Reese)				
bottoms	2 pieces	–	35	–
hearts	3 pieces	–	30	–
(S&W)				
bottoms/in water	3 pieces		25	
hearts				
in water	3 pieces	–	30	–
marinated	2 pieces	2.0	20	90%
fresh				
(Dole)	1 large	–	23	–
generic				
cooked	1 medium	–	53	–
hearts/cooked	½ cup	–	37	–
raw	1 medium	–	65	–
frozen				
(Birds Eye) hearts/deluxe	½ cup	–	30	–
(C&W) hearts	3 oz	–	25	–
generic/cooked	½ cup	–	36	–
ARTICHOKE HEART (See ARTICHOKE)				
ARUGULA				
fresh/chopped	½ cup	<1.0	2	13%
	1 lb	1.5	105	13%

ASIAN FOOD (See also FROZEN ENTRÉE/DINNER; PASTA ENTRÉE/DINNER; RICE DISH; VEGETARIAN FOODS; individual listings)

■ **BEEF DISHES** (See also Chow Mein; Fried Rice; Sweet & Sour in this section)

(Chun King)				
beef pepper Oriental/divider pak entrée/prepared	1 cup	2.5	100	23%
pepper steak				
frozen entrée	13 oz	4.0	300	12%
stir-fry entrée/prepared	6 oz	17.0	250	61%
generic/canned				
beef pepper Oriental	¾ cup	2.0	80	23%
(La Choy)				
beef pepper Oriental				
bi-pack/prepared	1 cup	3.0	100	27%
frozen entrée	8 oz	–	90	–
noodles w/beef/bi-pack/prepared	1 cup	1.0	150	6%
noodles w/vegetables & beef/entrée	1 cup	3.5	155	20%
pepper steak/Dinner Classic	⅓ pkg	–	40	–
(Van de Kamp's) frozen/beef Mandarin	11 oz	10.0	310	29%

■ **CHICKEN DISHES** (See also Chow Mein; Fried Rice; Sweet & Sour in this section)

(Chun King) frozen entrée				
imperial chicken	13 oz	10.0	460	20%

Food and Description	Amount	Fat Grams	Total Calories	% Fat Calories
walnut chicken	13 oz	19.0	460	37%
(La Choy) canned/prepared				
chicken teriyaki	1 cup	3.0	110	25%
noodles w/chicken	1 cup	4.0	160	23%
noodles w/vegetables & chicken	1 cup	3.0	160	17%
spicy chicken Szechwan	1 cup	3.0	100	27%
■ CHOP SUEY				
homemade/USDA Standard Home Recipe				
w/beef & pork	1 cup	17.0	300	51%
w/beef w/o noodles	1 cup	17.0	300	51%
■ CHOW MEIN (See also Vegetables in this section)				
beef				
(Chun King) canned/prepared				
divider pak entrée	1 cup	1.5	110	12%
stir-fry entrée	6 oz	19.0	290	59%
generic/canned	¾ cup	1.0	70	13%
homemade/USDA Standard Home Recipe	1 cup	17.0	300	51%
(La Choy) canned/prepared	1 cup	2.0	105	17%
chicken				
(Chun King)				
canned/prepared				
divider pak entrée	1 cup	4.5	110	37%
stir-fry entrée	6 oz	11.0	220	45%
frozen entrée	13 oz	14.0	370	34%
generic/canned	¾ cup	3.0	80	34%
homemade/USDA Standard Home Recipe	¾ cup	10.0	255	35%
(La Choy)				
canned/prepared	1 cup	4.0	110	33%
entrée	1 cup	3.5	80	39%
frozen entrée	8 oz	5.0	150	30%
pork				
(Chun King) canned/prepared	1 cup	4.5	110	37%
homemade/USDA Standard Home Recipe				
w/noodles	1 cup	24.7	432	51%
w/o noodles	¾ cup	14.0	223	57%
(La Choy) canned/prepared	1 cup	2.0	80	23%
shrimp				
(Chun King) canned/prepared	1 cup	2.5	110	37%
homemade/USDA Standard Home Recipe/w/noodles	¾ cup	3.9	141	25%
(La Choy) canned/prepared	1 cup	1.0	50	18%
vegetable				
(La Choy) frozen entrée	8 oz	2.5	90	25%
■ EGG FOO YOUNG				
(Chun King) canned/prepared	5 oz	8.0	140	51%

Food and Description	Amount	Fat Grams	Total Calories	% Fat Calories
homemade/USDA Standard Home Recipe	~5 oz	10.0	150	60%
■ EGG ROLL				
(Chun King) frozen				
chicken	8 pieces	8.0	260	28%
pork & shrimp	8 pieces	11.0	290	34%
shrimp	8 pieces	8.0	260	28%
homemade/USDA Standard Home Recipe/w/o meat	2.25 oz	5.9	102	52%
(Jeno's) frozen				
chicken	3 oz	9.0	190	43%
shrimp & cheese	3 oz	8.0	190	38%
(La Choy) frozen				
mini				
chicken	4.8 oz	7.0	280	23%
	14 pieces	11.0	430	23%
lobster	4.8 oz	7.0	270	23%
	14 pieces	11.0	410	24%
pork & shrimp	4.8 oz	8.0	280	26%
	14 pieces	12.0	430	25%
shrimp	4.8 oz	6.0	270	20%
	14 pieces	9.0	410	20%
regular				
meat & shrimp	3.75 oz	9.0	240	34%
	4.8 oz	12.0	320	34%
mu shu pork	1 piece	7.0	190	33%
pork	1 piece	6.0	170	32%
pork & shrimp	5 oz	10.0	300	30%
shrimp	1 piece	4.0	150	24%
sweet & sour	1 piece	4.0	180	20%
restaurant style/chicken	3 oz	5.0	170	26%
(Pagoda Cafe) frozen				
chicken	1 piece	5.0	160	28%
pork & shrimp	1 piece	7.0	170	37%
(Schwan's) frozen				
chicken	2 pieces	7.0	220	29%
pork	2 pieces	11.0	240	41%
shrimp	2 pieces	4.5	180	23%
■ EGG ROLL WRAPPER				
(Azumaya Pasta)	2 wrappers	–	130	–
(Nasoya)	2 wrappers	–	120	–
■ FORTUNE COOKIE				
(La Choy)	4 cookies	–	112	–
■ FRIED RICE (See also RICE DISH)				
(Chun King) frozen				
w/chicken	8 oz	6.0	270	20%
w/pork	8 oz	5.0	290	19%

Food and Description	Amount	Fat Grams	Total Calories	% Fat Calories
(Kan Tong) dry				
chicken	2 oz	3.5	190	17%
pork	2 oz	1.0	190	5%
shrimp	2 oz	1.0	190	5%
spicy chicken	2 oz	1.0	190	5%
traditional	2 oz	3.0	190	14%
vegetable	2 oz	0.5	190	2%
(La Choy)	1 cup	1.0	235	4%
(Ling Ling) frozen				
vegetable	1 cup	4.0	140	26%
(Tyson)				
chicken breast tenders/fat-free	1 cup	–	180	–
pork	1 cup	3.0	100	27%
■ **NOODLE** (See also PASTA; PASTA ENTRÉE/DINNER)				
(Chun King) chow mein	½ cup	6.0	140	39%
generic				
Chinese cellophane/long rice/dry	2 oz	–	200	–
chow mein/cooked	1 cup	14.0	240	53%
rice/canned	½ cup	5.0	130	35%
soba/buckwheat				
cooked	4 oz	–	115	–
dry	2 oz	0.5	195	2%
somen/wheat				
cooked	4 oz	–	149	–
dry	2 oz	0.5	205	2%
udon/wheat				
cooked	4 oz	0.5	115	4%
dry	2 oz	0.7	160	4%
(La Choy)				
chow mein	½ cup	6.0	135	40%
crispy wide	½ cup	8.0	150	35%
rice	½ cup	3.0	120	23%
■ **PORK DISH** (See also Chow Mein; Fried Rice; Sweet & Sour in this section)				
(La Choy) frozen entrée				
spicy pork	3 oz	9.0	200	41%
■ **POTSTICKERS**				
(Ling Ling) frozen				
chicken & vegetable dumplings				
dumplings only	5 pieces	7.0	280	23%
w/1 Tbs sauce	1 serving	7.0	300	21%
(Pagoda Cafe) frozen	8 pieces	20.0	400	45%
■ **SAUCES & SEASONINGS** (See also SAUCE; SEASONINGS)				
(Chun King)				
hot teriyaki sauce	1 Tbs	–	17	–
soy sauce	1 Tbs	–	10	–
(Contadina)				
sweet 'n sour sauce	2 Tbs	1.0	40	23%

Food and Description	Amount	Fat Grams	Total Calories	% Fat Calories
generic/soy sauce				
shoyu	1 Tbs	–	9	–
	¼ cup	–	30	–
tamari	1 Tbs	–	11	–
	¼ cup	–	35	–
(House Of Tsang)				
oil				
hot chili sesame	1 tsp	5.0	45	100%
Mongolian Fire Oil	1 tsp	5.0	45	100%
pure sesame	1 tsp	5.0	45	100%
Singapore curry	1 tsp	5.0	45	100%
wok	1 Tbs	14.0	130	100%
sauce				
Bangkok padang	1 Tbs	2.5	45	50%
classic stir-fry	1 Tbs	1.0	25	36%
hoisin sauce	1 tsp	–	15	–
Hong Kong BBQ	1 tsp	–	10	–
Korean teriyaki	1 Tbs	0.5	30	15%
Mandarin marinade	1 Tbs	–	18	–
Saigon sizzle	1 Tbs	1.0	40	23%
soy sauce				
dark	1 Tbs	–	17	–
ginger	1 Tbs	–	10	–
ginger-flavored	1 Tbs	–	20	–
light	1 Tbs	–	5	–
low-sodium	1 Tbs	–	5	–
mushroom	1 Tbs	–	10	–
spicy brown bean	1 tsp	–	15	–
sweet & sour concentrate	1 tsp	–	10	–
sweet & sour stir-fry	1 Tbs	–	35	–
Szechuan spicy stir-fry	1 Tbs	0.5	20	23%
vegetables & sauce				
Cantonese classic	½ cup	1.0	70	13%
Hong Kong sweet & sour	½ cup	1.0	160	6%
Szechaun hot & spicy	½ cup	1.0	70	13%
Tokyo teriyaki	½ cup	–	100	–
(Kikkoman)				
chow mein seasoning				
lite	1 Tbs	–	10	–
regular	1 pkg	–	100	–
soy sauce				
lite	1 Tbs	–	10	–
regular	1 Tbs	–	10	–
teriyaki/baste & glaze	1 Tbs	–	25	–
(La Choy)				
bead molasses	1 Tbs	–	50	–
brown gravy sauce	¼ cup	–	275	–
plum	1 Tbs	–	25	–

Food and Description	Amount	Fat Grams	Total Calories	% Fat Calories
soy sauce/lite	1 Tbs	–	15	–
stir-fry				
Mandarin soy sauce	½ cup	–	70	–
sweet & sour	½ cup	–	140	–
Szechwan	½ cup	–	80	–
teriyaki	½ cup	–	95	–
sweet & sour				
duck sauce	2 Tbs	–	60	–
original	2 Tbs	–	60	–
teriyaki				
lite	1 Tbs	–	18	–
original	1 Tbs	–	16	–
(S&B Sunbird)				
Oriental seasonings/dry				
beef & broccoli	¾ Tbs	–	20	–
Chinese barbecue	½ Tbs	–	10	–
Chinese chicken salad	½ Tbs	–	15	–
chop suey	1 Tbs	–	20	–
chow mein	2 tsp	–	15	–
fried rice	½ Tbs	–	12	–
honey teriyaki	2 tsp	–	15	–
hot & spicy	½ Tbs	–	14	–
kung pao chicken	¾ Tbs	–	20	–
lemon chicken stir-fry	½ Tbs	–	10	–
orange beef	½ Tbs	–	13	–
stir-fry	1 Tbs	–	15	–
sukiyaki	½ tsp	–	15	–
sweet & sour	½ Tbs	–	15	–
tomato beef	¾ Tbs	–	25	–
teriyaki marinade	½ Tbs	–	10	–
■ SEA VEGETABLES				
(Eden)				
hiziki sea vegetable	¼ cup	–	30	–
sushi nori sea vegetable	1 sheet	–	10	–
■ SEAFOOD DISHES (See also Chow Mein; Fried Rice in this section)				
homemade/USDA Standard Home recipe				
teriyaki shrimp	¾ cup	1.0	174	5%
(La Choy) frozen/shrimp entrée	3 oz	5.0	170	26%
	4.8 oz	6.0	270	20%
(Pagoda Cafe) frozen/Cafe Rangoon	8 pieces	22.0	440	45%
■ SEASONINGS (See SAUCES & SEASONINGS in this section)				
■ STIR-FRY				
(Birds Eye) frozen				
broccoli	1 cup	–	30	–
easy recipe				
Oriental	2¼ cups	4.0	210	17%
teriyaki	2 cups	2.5	210	11%
pepper	3 oz	–	25	–

Food and Description	Amount	Fat Grams	Total Calories	% Fat Calories
sugar snap pea	¾ cup	–	35	–
(C&W) frozen/vegetable stir-fry dinner				
w/basmati rice	1 cup	–	220	–
w/Oriental noodles	1 cup	2.5	200	11%
(Green Giant) frozen/Create A Meal!				
broccoli	2⅓ cups	3.5	120	26%
lo mein	2⅓ cups	0.5	160	3%
sweet & sour	1¾ cup	–	130	–
Szechuan	1¾ cup	5.0	150	30%
teriyaki	1¾ cup	–	100	–
vegetable almond	1¾ cup	4.5	150	27%
(Pictsweet) frozen/international combinations				
Chinese	¾ cup	–	30	–
Oriental	¾ cup	–	30	–
Singapore	¾ cup	–	30	–
(Tyson) fat-free chicken breast tenders	1 cup	–	100	–
■ SUKIYAKI				
(Chun King) stir-fry entrée/prepared	6 oz	17.0	260	59%
■ SUSHI				
homemade/USDA Standard Home Recipe/w/vegetables	4.5 oz	–	181	–
■ SWEET & SOUR				
chicken				
generic/canned/prepared	¾ cup	2.0	120	15%
(La Choy) canned/prepared	1 cup	2.0	160	11%
dinner				
(La Choy) Dinner Classic	¼ pkg	–	90	–
noodles w/chicken				
(La Choy) entrée	1 cup	3.0	255	11%
pork				
(Chun King) frozen entrée	13 oz	6.0	450	12%
homemade/USDA Standard Home Recipe	¾ cup	7.7	187	37%
(La Choy) frozen entrée	8 oz	8.0	250	29%
(Van de Kamp's) frozen	11 oz	15.0	430	31%
■ TACO SNACK				
(La Choy) frozen entrée	4.8 oz	12.0	330	33%
■ VEGETABLES/VEGETABLE DISHES (See also Chow Mein; Fried Rice; Sea Vegetables; Stir-Fry in this section)				
(Chun King)				
Chinese pea pods	3 oz	1.5	35	38%
chow mein vegetables/divider pak entrée/prepared	⅔ cup	–	15	–
water chestnuts				
sliced	16 slices	–	10	–
	8 oz	0.5	179	3%

Food and Description	Amount	Fat Grams	Total Calories	% Fat Calories
whole	8.5 oz	0.5	190	2%
(Empress)				
bamboo shoots/sliced	2 oz	–	13	–
water chestnuts				
sliced	2 oz	–	14	–
whole	2 oz	–	14	–
generic				
bamboo shoots	1 cup	<1.0	25	18%
water chestnuts/sliced	½ cup	–	35	–
(La Choy)				
bamboo shoots	2 Tbs	–	3	–
	¼ cup	–	6	–
bean sprouts	1 cup	–	10	–
Chinese mixed	⅔ cup	–	10	–
chop suey vegetables	½ cup	–	15	–
noodles w/vegetables entrée	1 cup	1.0	130	7%
vegetable frozen entrée	3 oz	4.0	170	21%
water chestnuts				
sliced	2 Tbs	–	10	–
	¼ cup	–	18	–
whole	2 medium	–	10	–
▨ WON TON				
generic/fried	½ cup	8.0	110	65%
▨ WON TON ROLL				
(Schwan's) frozen/pizza	5 pieces	16.0	390	37%
▨ WON TON SOUP (*See* SOUP)				
▨ WON TON WRAPPER				
(Azumaya)	1 wrapper	–	23	–
(Nasoya)	1 wrapper	–	23	–
ASPARAGUS				
canned				
(Del Monte) tender green				
cut spears	½ cup	–	20	–
extra-long spears	½ cup	–	20	–
salad tips	½ cup	–	20	–
spears	½ cup	–	20	–
tips	/2 cup	–	20	–
generic	½ cup	0.8	24	29%
(Green Giant)				
cut spears				
50% less sodium	½ cup	–	20	–
regular	½ cup	–	20	–
extra-long spears	4.5 oz	–	20	–
Harvest Fresh				
cuts	⅔ cup	–	25	–
spears	4.5 oz	–	20	–
(LeSueur) extra-large spears	4.5 oz	–	20	–
(Reese) white spears	⅓ can	–	20	–

Food and Description	Amount	Fat Grams	Total Calories	% Fat Calories
(S&W)				
blended	6 pieces	–	15	–
colossal	3 pieces	–	10	–
(Seneca)	½ cup	–	20	–
(Stokely)				
green	½ cup	–	20	–
no salt or sugar added	½ cup	–	20	–
(Thank You) whole spears	½ cup	–	25	–
fresh				
cooked				
cuts w/tips	½ cup	–	22	–
(Dole) spears	5 spears	–	18	–
spears	4 spears	–	15	–
raw				
cuts w/tips	½ cup	–	15	–
spears	4 spears	–	13	–
frozen				
(Birds Eye)				
cuts	3.3 oz	–	25	–
spears	3.3 oz	–	25	–
(C&W) spears	2.6 oz	–	20	–
ASPARAGUS SOUP, CREAM OF (*See* SOUP)				
AVOCADO				
fresh/raw				
California				
mashed	1 cup	36.0	407	80%
whole	1 medium	30.8	324	86%
Florida	1 medium	27.0	340	72%

B

Food and Description	Amount	Fat Grams	Total Calories	% Fat Calories
BABY FOOD (*See also* BABY/INFANT FORMULA)				

(NOTE: The nutritional needs of young children differ from those of older children and adults. A low-fat nutrition program is not recommended for any child under two years of age, as it may interfere with his or her development.)

■ (Beech-Nut)				
Stage 1				
cereal				
barley/dry	¼ cup	–	60	–

Food and Description	Amount	Fat Grams	Total Calories	% Fat Calories
oatmeal/dry	¼ cup	2.0	60	30%
oatmeal & apples	4 oz	–	70	–
rice/dry	¼ cup	–	60	–
fruit				
applesauce/Golden Delicious	2.5 oz	–	50	–
bananas				
Chiquita	2.5 oz	–	70	–
	4 oz	–	110	–
w/pears & apples	4 oz	–	90	–
peaches/yellow cling	2.5 oz	–	60	–
	4 oz	–	70	–
pears/Bartlett	4 oz	–	70	–
juice				
apple	4 fl oz	–	60	–
pear	4 fl oz	–	60	–
white grape	4 fl oz	–	100	–
meat				
beef & broth	2.5 oz	6.0	90	60%
chicken & broth	2.5 oz	3.0	70	39%
lamb & broth	2.5 oz	3.0	60	45%
turkey & broth	2.8 oz	6.0	90	60%
veal & broth	2.5 oz	2.0	70	30%
vegetables				
carrots/sweet	4 oz	–	50	–
green beans	4 oz	–	35	–
peas/tender sweet	4 oz	–	60	–
squash/butternut	4 oz	–	50	–
sweet potatoes	4 oz	–	80	–
Stage 2				
cereal				
mixed/dry	¼ cup	1.0	60	15%
mixed cereal & apples	4 oz	–	70	–
oatmeal & apples	4 oz	–	70	–
rice cereal & apples	4 oz	–	70	–
rice cereal & bananas	4 oz	–	70	–
desserts				
apple, peach, & strawberry	4 oz	–	100	–
apple, pear, & banana	4 oz	–	90	–
banana yogurt	4 oz	2.0	120	15%
banana-pineapple	4 oz	–	100	–
cottage cheese w/pears	4 oz	1.0	120	8%
Dutch apple	4 oz	–	100	–
flan de banana	4 oz	–	110	–
flan de vanilla	4 oz	3.0	120	23%
fruit	4 oz	–	80	–
mixed fruit w/yogurt	4 oz	–	100	–
vanilla custard pudding	4 oz	3.0	120	23%

Food and Description	Amount	Fat Grams	Total Calories	% Fat Calories
dinners				
beef & egg noodle	4 oz	6.0	100	54%
beef supreme	4 oz	9.0	130	62%
chicken & rice	4 oz	3.0	80	34%
chicken noodle	4 oz	4.0	70	51%
chicken soup	4 oz	4.0	90	40%
macaroni & beef w/vegetables	4 oz	6.0	110	49%
turkey dinner supreme	4 oz	4.0	90	40%
turkey rice	4 oz	3.0	70	39%
vegetable beef	4 oz	5.0	100	45%
vegetable chicken	4 oz	3.0	80	34%
vegetable ham	4 oz	3.0	80	34%
fruit				
apples & bananas	4 oz	–	60	–
apples & blueberries	4 oz	–	70	–
apples & cherries	4 oz	–	80	–
apples & pears	4 oz	–	80	–
apples & plums	4 oz	–	70	–
apples, pears, & bananas	4 oz	–	90	–
apricots w/pears & apples	4 oz	–	90	–
peaches & bananas	4 oz	–	70	–
pears & raspberries	4 oz	–	80	–
juice				
apple-banana	4 fl oz	–	70	–
apple-cherry	4 fl oz	–	70	–
apple-cranberry	4 fl oz	–	60	–
apple-grape	4 fl oz	–	60	–
mixed	4 fl oz	–	70	–
vegetables				
corn & sweet potatoes	4 oz	1.0	80	11%
garden vegetables	4 oz	–	50	–
Stage 3				
cereal/oatmeal & pears w/cinnamon	6 oz	–	90	–
desserts				
cottage cheese w/pears	6 oz	2.0	180	10%
fruit	6 oz	–	120	–
mixed fruit w/yogurt	6 oz	–	170	–
vanilla custard pudding	6 oz	6.0	190	28%
dinners				
beef & egg noodle	6 oz	6.0	130	42%
chicken noodle	6 oz	4.0	110	33%
macaroni & beef	6 oz	6.0	130	42%
spaghetti & beef	6 oz	6.0	130	42%
turkey rice	6 oz	3.0	100	27%
vegetable beef	6 oz	6.0	130	42%
vegetable chicken	6 oz	4.0	110	33%
fruit				
apples & bananas	6 oz	–	90	–

Food and Description	Amount	Fat Grams	Total Calories	% Fat Calories
apples & cherries	6 oz	–	110	–
applesauce	6 oz	–	100	–
apricots	6 oz	–	130	–
bananas/Chiquita	6 oz	–	160	–
peaches	6 oz	–	100	–
pears/Bartlett	6 oz	–	110	–
juice/orange	4 fl oz	–	60	–
vegetables				
carrots	6 oz	–	70	–
green beans	6 oz	–	50	–
sweet potatoes	6 oz	–	110	–
Table Time/microwave				
chicken & stars	6 oz	7.0	150	42%
macaroni & cheese	6 oz	12.0	200	54%
spaghetti rings in meat sauce	6 oz	6.0	160	34%
turkey stew w/rice	6 oz	7.0	150	42%
vegetable stew w/beef	6 oz	3.0	110	25%
■ (Earth's Best)				
cereal				
brown rice	0.5 oz	–	60	–
mixed grain	0.5 oz	–	60	–
dinners				
meat				
chicken & stars	6 oz	2.0	100	18%
sweet potato & chicken	4 oz	4.0	80	45%
vegetable beef	4 oz	4.0	80	45%
vegetable beef pilaf	6 oz	2.0	100	18%
vegetable turkey	4 oz	2.0	60	30%
vegetarian				
macaroni & cheese	4 oz	5.0	100	45%
pasta dinner	4 oz	3.0	70	39%
potato & green bean	4 oz	3.0	80	34%
rice & lentil	4 oz	1.0	60	15%
spaghetti w/cheese	6 oz	4.0	120	30%
spring vegetables & pasta	6 oz	2.0	90	20%
summer vegetables	4 oz	2.0	70	26%
vegetable souffle	6 oz	3.0	105	26%
fruit				
apples	4 oz	–	50	–
apples & apricots	4 oz	–	60	–
apples & bananas	4 oz	–	50	–
apples & blueberries	4 oz	–	50	–
apples & plums	4 oz	–	50	–
bananas	4 oz	–	70	–
orchard fruit/chunky	6 oz	–	80	–
pears	4 oz	–	50	–
pears & raspberries	4 oz	–	50	–

Food and Description	Amount	Fat Grams	Total Calories	% Fat Calories
fruit & grains				
apple-cinnamon oatmeal	6 oz	1.0	100	9%
peach-apricot muesli	6 oz	1.0	100	9%
peaches, oatmeal, & bananas	4 oz	1.0	60	15%
plums, bananas, & rice	4 oz	–	70	–
prunes & oatmeal	4 oz	–	90	–
juice				
apple	4 fl oz	–	70	–
apple-banana	4 fl oz	–	70	–
apple-grape	4 fl oz	–	70	–
pear	4 fl oz	–	70	–
vegetables				
carrots	4 oz	–	25	–
corn & butternut squash	4 oz	1.0	60	15%
potatoes & vegetables/country	6 oz	2.0	90	20%
green beans & rice	4 oz	–	45	–
mixed				
garden	4 oz	–	45	–
golden harvest	6 oz	1.0	80	11%
peas & brown rice	4 oz	1.0	70	13%
spinach & potatoes	4 oz	–	50	–
squash/winter	4 oz	–	35	–
sweet potato pudding	6 oz	2.0	130	14%
sweet potatoes	4 oz	–	50	–
yogurt breakfasts				
apple yogurt	4 oz	2.0	90	20%
blueberry yogurt	4 oz	2.0	90	20%
■ (Gerber)				
baked goods				
Biter Biscuits	1 biscuit	0.5	45	10%
zwieback toast	1 toast	1.0	30	30%
1st Foods				
cereal				
barley	4 Tbs	0.5	60	8%
oatmeal	4 Tbs	0.5	60	8%
rice	4 Tbs	0.5	60	8%
fruit				
applesauce	2.5 oz	–	40	–
bananas	2.5 oz	–	70	–
peaches	2.5 oz	–	30	–
pears	2.5 oz	–	40	–
prunes	2.5 oz	–	70	–
juice				
apple	4 fl oz	–	60	–
pear	4 fl oz	–	60	–
white grape	4 fl oz	–	80	–
vegetables				
carrots	2.5 oz	–	25	–

Food and Description	Amount	Fat Grams	Total Calories	% Fat Calories
green beans	2.5 oz	–	25	–
peas	2.5 oz	–	35	–
squash	2.5 oz	–	25	–
sweet potatoes	2.5 oz	–	50	–
2nd Foods				
cereal				
high protein/dry	4 Tbs	1.0	60	15%
mixed				
plain/dry	4 Tbs	1.0	50	18%
w/applesauce & bananas	4 oz	1.0	90	10%
w/bananas/dry	4 Tbs	1.0	60	15%
oatmeal				
w/applesauce & bananas	4 oz	1.0	90	10%
w/bananas/dry	4 Tbs	1.0	60	15%
rice				
w/applesauce & bananas	4 oz	–	90	–
w/bananas/dry	4 Tbs	1.0	60	15%
desserts				
banana yogurt	4 oz	0.5	80	6%
banana-apple	4 oz	–	80	–
cherry-vanilla pudding	4 oz	–	80	–
Dutch apple	4 oz	1.5	90	15%
fruit	4 oz	–	90	–
Hawaiian delight	4 oz	–	100	–
mixed fruit yogurt	4 oz	–	90	–
peach cobbler	4 oz	–	90	–
vanilla custard pudding	4 oz	1.0	100	9%
dinners				
regular				
beef egg noodle	4 oz	3.0	70	39%
chicken noodle	4 oz	1.0	60	15%
macaroni & cheese	4 oz	2.5	70	32%
macaroni tomato beef	4 oz	1.0	70	13%
turkey rice	4 oz	1.0	60	15%
vegetable bacon	4 oz	4.0	90	40%
vegetable beef	4 oz	2.5	70	32%
vegetable chicken	4 oz	1.5	70	19%
vegetable ham	4 oz	2.0	70	26%
vegetable turkey	4 oz	1.0	50	18%
simple recipe				
apples & chicken	4 oz	1.5	70	19%
apples & ham	4 oz	1.0	80	11%
apples & turkey	4 oz	1.5	80	17%
broccoli & chicken	4 oz	1.5	50	27%
carrots & beef	4 oz	3.0	70	39%
green beans & turkey	4 oz	1.5	60	23%
fruit				
apple-blueberry	4 oz	–	60	–

Food and Description	Amount	Fat Grams	Total Calories	% Fat Calories
applesauce	4 oz	–	60	–
applesauce-apricot	4 oz	–	60	–
apricots w/tapioca	4 oz	–	80	–
banana-pineapple w/tapioca	4 oz	–	60	–
bananas w/tapioca	4 oz	–	90	–
peaches	4 oz	–	70	–
pear-pineapple	4 oz	–	60	–
pears	4 oz	–	60	–
plums w/tapioca	4 oz	–	80	–
prunes w/tapioca	4 oz	–	90	–
juice				
apple-banana	4 fl oz	–	60	–
apple-cherry	4 fl oz	–	60	–
apple-cranberry	4 fl oz	–	60	–
apple-grape	4 fl oz	–	60	–
apple-peach	4 fl oz	–	60	–
apple-plum	4 fl oz	–	60	–
apple-prune	4 fl oz	–	70	–
mixed fruit	4 fl oz	–	60	–
orange	4 fl oz	–	60	–
juice w/lowfat yogurt				
apple	4 oz	1.0	90	10%
banana	4 oz	1.5	110	12%
mixed fruit	4 oz	1.5	90	15%
meat				
beef	2.5 oz	3.0	70	39%
chicken	2.5 oz	6.0	90	60%
ham	2.5 oz	4.0	80	45%
lamb	2.5 oz	3.5	70	45%
turkey	2.5 oz	4.5	80	51%
veal	2.5 oz	3.5	70	45%
vegetables				
beets	4 oz	–	45	–
carrots	4 oz	–	35	–
corn/creamed	4 oz	0.5	70	19%
green beans	4 oz	–	35	–
mixed				
garden	4 oz	0.5	45	10%
regular	4 oz	–	50	–
peas	4 oz	0.5	50	9%
spinach/creamed	4 oz	1.0	50	18%
squash	4 oz	–	35	–
sweet potatoes	4 oz	–	70	–
3rd Foods				
cereal				
mixed				
w/apples & bananas	6 oz	1.0	140	6%

Food and Description	Amount	Fat Grams	Total Calories	% Fat Calories
w/apricots & yogurt	6 oz	1.0	140	6%
w/peaches & yogurt	6 oz	1.0	140	6%
oatmeal				
w/apples & cinnamon	6 oz	1.0	140	6%
w/apples & yogurt	6 oz	1.0	130	7%
rice w/mixed fruit	6 oz	0.5	130	3%
desserts				
blueberry buckle	6 oz	–	130	–
cherry cobbler	6 oz	–	140	–
Dutch apple	6 oz	2.0	130	14%
fruit	6 oz	–	120	–
Hawaiian delight	6 oz	–	150	–
peach cobbler	6 oz	–	130	–
raspberry cobbler	6 oz	–	140	–
vanilla custard pudding	6 oz	1.5	150	9%
dinners				
beef egg noodle	6 oz	3.5	110	29%
chicken noodle	6 oz	1.5	90	15%
lasagna w/meat sauce	6 oz	3.0	100	27%
spaghetti in tomato sauce w/beef/Italian	6 oz	2.0	130	19%
turkey & rice	6 oz	1.5	90	15%
vegetable bacon	6 oz	6.0	130	42%
vegetable ham	6 oz	3.0	100	27%
vegetable pasta	6 oz	2.0	100	18%
vegetables/mixed				
& beef	6 oz	3.5	110	29%
& turkey	6 oz	2.5	90	25%
vegetables & chicken/homestyle	6 oz	1.5	80	17%
fruit				
apple-banana	6 oz	–	130	–
apple-blueberry	6 oz	–	80	–
applesauce	6 oz	–	80	–
apricots w/tapioca	6 oz	–	120	–
bananas				
w/pineapple & tapioca	6 oz	–	90	–
w/tapioca	6 oz	–	130	–
bananas & strawberries w/tapioca	6 oz	–	130	–
fruit salad	6 oz	–	160	–
peaches	6 oz	–	110	–
pears	6 oz	–	90	–
plums w/tapioca	6 oz	–	130	–
juice				
apple-carrot	4 fl oz	–	50	–
apple-sweet potato	4 fl oz	–	60	–
orange-carrot	4 fl oz	–	50	–
pineapple-carrot	4 fl oz	–	60	–

Food and Description	Amount	Fat Grams	Total Calories	% Fat Calories
meat				
beef	2.5 oz	3.0	70	39%
chicken	2.5 oz	6.0	100	54%
turkey	2.5 oz	5.0	90	50%
vegetables				
broccoli-carrots-cheese	6 oz	2.0	80	23%
carrots	6 oz	–	80	–
green beans w/rice	6 oz	–	70	–
mixed vegetables	6 oz	–	70	–
peas w/rice	6 oz	0.5	90	5%
squash	6 oz	0.5	80	6%
sweet potatoes	6 oz	0.5	100	5%
Graduates				
baked goods				
arrowroot cookies	1 cookie	1.0	25	36%
banana cookies	1 cookie	1.0	35	26%
cinnamon-graham animal crackers	2 crackers	1.0	35	26%
pretzels	1 pretzel	–	50	–
cereal				
apple-cinnamon finger snacks	¾ cup	1.0	80	11%
apple-cinnamon oatmeal/dry	8 Tbs	2.0	110	16%
banana-apple finger snacks	¾ cup	1.0	80	11%
peaches & vanilla oatmeal/dry	8 Tbs	2.0	110	16%
finger foods				
Finger Sticks				
chicken	2.5 oz	6.0	100	54%
meat	2.5 oz	7.0	110	57%
turkey	2.5 oz	5.0	90	50%
Fruit Dices				
apples	4.5 oz	–	60	–
peaches	4.5 oz	–	70	–
pears	4.5 oz	–	70	–
Vegetable Dices				
carrots	2.5 oz	–	15	–
green beans	2.5 oz	–	20	–
peas	2.5 oz	0.5	40	11%
potatoes	2.5 oz	–	40	–
juice				
apple w/calcium	6 fl oz	–	90	–
apple-banana w/calcium	6 fl oz	–	100	–
apple-cherry w/calcium	6 fl oz	–	90	–
apple-grape w/calcium	6 fl oz	–	90	–
fruit punch w/calcium	6 fl oz	–	100	–
main dishes				
chicken stew w/noodles	6 oz	3.0	120	23%
macaroni & beef	6 oz	3.5	140	23%
pasta shells & cheese	6 oz	4.5	140	29%

Food and Description	Amount	Fat Grams	Total Calories	% Fat Calories
spaghetti w/mini meatballs & sauce	6 oz	4.0	150	24%
tomato sauce w/cheese ravioli	6 oz	3.5	170	19%
turkey stew w/rice	6 oz	2.0	100	18%
vegetable stew w/beef	6 oz	2.0	120	15%
Tropical Foods				
fruit				
banana-vanilla	4 oz	1.0	100	9%
guava	4 oz	–	80	–
mango	4 oz	–	80	–
mango-banana w/tapioca & passion fruit juice	4 oz	–	80	–
papaya	4 oz	–	70	–
peach-mango	4 oz	–	80	–
juice				
guava w/mixed fruit	4 fl oz	–	70	–
mango w/mixed fruit	4 fl oz	–	70	–
mixed tropical	4 fl oz	–	70	–
orange-banana pineapple	4 fl oz	–	80	–
papaya w/mixed fruit	4 fl oz	–	70	–
■ **(Growing Healthy) frozen**				
1st Bites				
cereal				
mixed w/bananas	4 oz	1.0	80	11%
rice w/bananas & apples	4 oz	–	70	–
fruit				
applesauce	4 oz	1.0	80	11%
apricots	4 oz	1.0	90	10%
peaches	4 oz	–	80	–
2nd Bites				
chicken	4 oz	7.0	160	39%
vegetables/garden	4 oz	–	45	–
vegetables & chicken	4 oz	1.0	70	13%
vegetables & turkey	4 oz	2.0	90	20%
strained foods				
applesauce	4 oz	1.0	80	11%
apricots	4 oz	1.0	110	8%
chicken	4 oz	6.0	160	34%
turkey	4 oz	7.0	130	48%
3rd Bites				
pasta, chicken, & vegetables	6 oz	1.0	130	7%
vegetables & chicken	6 oz	2.0	110	16%
■ **(Health Valley)**				
brown rice cereal/100% organic	1 Tbs	1.0	60	15%
sprouted baby cereal/100% organic	1 Tbs	1.0	60	15%
■ **(Healthy Times)**				
biscuits for teethers				
maple	2 biscuits	3.0	97	28%

Food and Description	Amount	Fat Grams	Total Calories	% Fat Calories
vanilla	2 biscuits	3.0	92	29%
cereal				
brown rice/dry	4 Tbs	–	60	–
oatmeal w/bananas/dry	4 Tbs	–	60	–
child's 1st cookie/arrowroot toddlers' cookies				
maple	1 cookie	3.0	109	25%
vanilla	1 cookie	3.0	106	25%
■ (Heinz)				
beginner foods				
fruit				
applesauce	3.5 oz	–	70	–
bananas w/tapioca	3.5 oz	–	105	–
peaches	3.5 oz	–	80	–
pears	3.5 oz	–	75	–
vegetables				
carrots	3.5 oz	–	30	–
green beans	3.5 oz	–	30	–
peas	3.5 oz	0.5	55	8%
squash	3.5 oz	–	35	–
sweet potatoes	3.5 oz	–	70	–
cereal				
barley/instant	3.5 oz	3.7	370	9%
mixed/instant	3.5 oz	4.9	373	12%
rice/instant	3.5 oz	4.0	375	10%
junior foods				
desserts				
Dutch apple	3.5 oz	0.5	70	6%
fruit	3.5 oz	–	65	–
peach cobbler	3.5 oz	–	75	–
tutti-frutti	3.5 oz	–	70	–
vanilla custard	3.5 oz	1.0	75	12%
dinners				
beef vegetable stew	3.5 oz	2.0	75	24%
chicken noodle	3.5 oz	2.0	55	33%
chicken 'n rice w/garden vegetables	3.5 oz	1.5	60	23%
chicken vegetable stew	3.5 oz	2.0	60	30%
macaroni dinner w/tomatoes & beef	3.5 oz	1.0	50	18%
macaroni & beef	3.5 oz	1.0	60	15%
macaroni & cheese	3.5 oz	2.0	80	23%
pasta & vegetables in cheese sauce	3.5 oz	1.5	70	19%
spaghetti/tomato beef	3.5 oz	1.5	55	25%
spaghetti w/meat sauce	3.5 oz	1.0	60	15%
turkey w/rice & garden vegetables	3.5 oz	0.5	55	8%
vegetable bacon	3.5 oz	2.0	60	30%
vegetable beef	3.5 oz	2.0	50	36%
vegetable chicken	3.5 oz	2.0	60	30%
vegetable ham	3.5 oz	1.0	50	18%

Food and Description	Amount	Fat Grams	Total Calories	% Fat Calories
vegetable turkey	3.5 oz	2.0	50	36%
fruit				
apples & blueberries	3.5 oz	–	50	–
apples & cranberries w/tapioca	3.5 oz	–	70	–
applesauce	3.5 oz	–	50	–
apricot w/tapioca	3.5 oz	–	65	–
bananas & pineapple w/tapioca	3.5 oz	–	65	–
bananas w/tapioca	3.5 oz	–	70	–
peaches	3.5 oz	–	70	–
pears	3.5 oz	–	60	–
plums	3.5 oz	–	70	–
meat				
beef w/broth	3.5 oz	7.0	125	50%
chicken w/broth	3.5 oz	9.5	145	59%
vegetables				
broccoli & carrots w/cheese	3.5 oz	1.0	50	18%
carrots	3.5 oz	–	25	–
corn/creamed	3.5 oz	0.5	65	7%
green beans/creamed	3.5 oz	–	40	–
peas	3.5 oz	–	60	–
squash	3.5 oz	–	35	–
sweet potato	3.5 oz	–	70	–
strained foods				
cereal				
mixed w/apples & bananas	3.5 oz	–	70	–
oatmeal w/apples & bananas	3.5 oz	0.6	76	7%
rice w/apples & bananas	3.5 oz	–	70	–
desserts				
banana & apple	3.5 oz	–	70	–
banana pudding	3.5 oz	0.5	75	6%
banana yogurt	3.5 oz	0.5	80	–
custard pudding	3.5 oz	1.0	75	12%
Dutch apple	3.5 oz	1.0	90	10%
fruit	3.5 oz	–	65	–
Hawaiian delight	3.5 oz	–	70	–
mixed fruit w/yogurt	3.5 oz	0.5	75	6%
peach cobbler	3.5 oz	–	75	–
peach yogurt	3.5 oz	0.5	80	6%
pear yogurt	3.5 oz	0.5	80	6%
tutti-frutti	3.5 oz	–	70	–
vanilla custard	3.5 oz	1.0	75	12%
dinners				
beef & egg noodle	3.5 oz	2.0	50	36%
chicken noodle	3.5 oz	2.0	55	33%
macaroni & cheese	3.5 oz	3.0	85	34%
turkey rice	3.5 oz	1.0	50	18%
turkey w/vegetables	3.5 oz	1.0	50	18%
vegetable bacon	3.5 oz	2.0	50	36%

Food and Description	Amount	Fat Grams	Total Calories	% Fat Calories
vegetable beef	3.5 oz	3.0	50	54%
vegetable beef dumpling	3.5 oz	1.5	50	27%
vegetable ham	3.5 oz	0.5	35	13%
vegetable turkey	3.5 oz	2.0	50	36%
fruit				
apples & apricots	3.5 oz	–	55	–
apples & cranberries	3.5 oz	–	70	–
apples & pears	3.5 oz	–	55	–
applesauce	3.5 oz	–	50	–
apricots w/tapioca	3.5 oz	–	65	–
bananas & pineapple w/tapioca	3.5 oz	–	65	–
bananas w/tapioca	3.5 oz	–	75	–
peaches	3.5 oz	–	70	–
pears	3.5 oz	–	60	–
pears & pineapple	3.5 oz	–	60	–
plums w/tapioca	3.5 oz	–	70	–
prunes w/tapioca	3.5 oz	–	90	–
juice				
apple	3.5 fl oz	–	50	–
	4.2 fl oz	–	70	–
apple-banana	3.5 fl oz	–	50	–
apple-cherry	3.5 fl oz	–	45	–
apple-cranberry	3.5 fl oz	–	50	–
apple-grape	3.5 fl oz	–	45	–
apple-peach	3.5 fl oz	–	45	–
apple-pineapple	3.5 fl oz	–	45	–
apple-prune	3.5 fl oz	–	50	–
mixed fruit	3.5 fl oz	–	50	–
orange	3.5 fl oz	–	50	–
orange-apple	3.5 fl oz	–	50	–
pear	3.5 fl oz	–	50	–
	4.2 fl oz	–	70	–
white grape	3.5 fl oz	–	60	–
meat				
beef w/broth	3.5 oz	7.0	125	50%
chicken & apples	3.5 oz	1.0	60	15%
chicken w/broth	3.5 oz	9.5	145	59%
ham & apples	3.5 oz	1.0	60	15%
turkey & apples	3.5 oz	0.5	60	8%
turkey w/broth	3.5 oz	8.0	140	40%
soup/chicken	3.5 oz	2.0	50	36%
vegetables				
beets	3.5 oz	–	40	–
broccoli & chicken	3.5 oz	1.0	40	23%
carrots	3.5 oz	–	25	–
carrots & beef	3.5 oz	3.0	60	45%
corn/creamed	3.5 oz	0.5	65	7%
green beans	3.5 oz	–	25	–

Food and Description	Amount	Fat Grams	Total Calories	% Fat Calories
green beans & turkey	3.5 oz	0.5	40	11%
mixed	3.5 oz	0.5	45	10%
peas	3.5 oz	0.5	60	8%
squash	3.5 oz	–	35	–
sweet potatoes	3.5 oz	–	70	–

BABY/INFANT FORMULA

(NOTE: A low-fat nutrition program is not recommended for any child under two years of age, as the nutritional needs of young children differ from those of older children and adults.)

Food and Description	Amount	Fat Grams	Total Calories	% Fat Calories
(Alimentum) hypoallergenic/ liquid ready to feed	5 fl oz	5.5	100	50%
(Bonamil)				
liquid	5 fl oz	5.4	100	49%
liquid ready to feed	5 fl oz	5.4	100	49%
powder/prepared	5 fl oz	5.4	100	49%
(Carnation)				
Alsoy				
liquid	5 fl oz	5.5	100	50%
powder/prepared	5 fl oz	5.5	100	50%
Good Start				
liquid	5 fl oz	5.1	100	46%
liquid ready to feed	5 fl oz	5.1	100	46%
powder/prepared	5 fl oz	5.1	100	46%
Follow-Up				
liquid	5 fl oz	4.1	100	37%
liquid ready to feed	5 fl oz	4.1	100	37%
powder/prepared	5 fl oz	4.1	100	37%
soy/prepared	5 fl oz	5.5	100	50%
(Enfamil)				
liquid ready to feed				
w/iron	5 fl oz	5.3	100	48%
w/low iron	5 fl oz	5.3	100	48%
Next Step/toddler				
regular	5 fl oz	5.0	100	45%
soy	5 fl oz	4.4	100	40%
powder/prepared				
w/iron	5 fl oz	5.3	100	48%
w/low iron	5 fl oz	5.3	100	48%
(Gerber) powder/prepared				
regular	5 fl oz	5.3	100	48%
soy	5 fl oz	5.3	100	48%
(Isomil)				
liquid	5 fl oz	5.5	100	50%
liquid ready to feed	5 fl oz	5.5	100	50%
powder/prepared	5 fl oz	5.5	100	50%
(Lactofree)				
liquid	5 fl oz	5.5	100	50%
powder/prepared	5 fl oz	5.5	100	50%

Food and Description	Amount	Fat Grams	Total Calories	% Fat Calories
(Nursoy) liquid concentrate	5 fl oz	5.3	100	48%
(ProSobee)				
liquid	5 fl oz	5.3	100	48%
liquid ready to feed	5 fl oz	5.3	100	48%
powder/prepared	5 fl oz	5.3	100	48%
(Similac)				
liquid ready to feed				
w/iron	5 fl oz	5.4	100	49%
w/low iron	5 fl oz	5.4	100	49%
powder/prepared				
w/iron	5 fl oz	5.4	100	49%
w/low iron	5 fl oz	5.4	100	49%
Toddler's Best Beverage				
berry	8 fl oz	8.0	160	45%
chocolate	8 fl oz	8.0	160	45%
vanilla	8 fl oz	8.0	160	45%
(SMA)				
liquid				
w/iron	5 fl oz	5.3	100	48%
w/low iron	5 fl oz	5.3	100	48%
powder/prepared/w/iron	5 fl oz	5.3	100	48%
BACON (*See also* BACON, CANADIAN STYLE; BACON BITS, CHIPS, & PIECES; BACON SUBSTITUTE; LUNCHEON MEAT)				
(Butterball) turkey bacon	2 slices	2.5	70	32%
generic				
pork breakfast strips/medium-sliced				
cooked	3 slices	12.0	160	68%
raw	3 slices	24.0	265	82%
regular				
all types/cooked/yield from 1 lb raw	4.5 oz	59.5	735	73%
medium-sliced				
cooked	3 slices	9.0	110	74%
raw	3 slices	37.0	380	88%
thick-sliced/raw	1 slice	20.5	210	88%
(Hillshire Farm) country smoked	1 slice	12.0	120	90%
(Hormel) cooked				
Black Label				
center cut	3 slices	4.5	60	68%
low-salt	2 slices	4.5	60	68%
regular	2 slices	4.5	60	68%
microwave	2 slices	5.0	70	64%
Old Smokehouse				
Range	2 slices	9.0	100	90%
Red Label	2 slices	7.0	80	79%
(Kahn's) American Beauty/cooked	2 slices	9.0	100	81%
(Louis Rich) turkey bacon	1 slice	2.5	30	75%
(Mr. Turkey) turkey bacon	1 slice	2.0	25	72%

Food and Description	Amount	Fat Grams	Total Calories	% Fat Calories
(Oscar Mayer) cooked				
⅛" thick cut	1 slice	5.0	60	75%
center cut	3 slices	7.0	90	70%
lower sodium	2 slices	4.0	60	60%
original	2 slices	5.0	60	75%
(Schwan's) thick-sliced	1 slice	6.0	70	77%
BACON, CANADIAN STYLE				
generic/1-oz slices				
cold	2 slices	4.0	89	40%
heated	2 slices	3.9	86	41%
(Hormel) Black Label/1-oz slices/cooked	2 slices	3.0	70	39%
(Jones) Canadian style/uncooked	3 slices	3.0	70	39%
(Oscar Mayer), cooked	2 slices	1.5	50	27%
BACON BITS, CHIPS, & PIECES				
imitation				
(Betty Crocker) BacOs				
bits	1 Tbs	1.0	30	30%
chips	1 Tbs	1.0	30	30%
(Durkee)				
bits	1 Tbs	1.0	25	36%
chips	1 Tbs	1.0	25	36%
(McCormick/Schilling)				
Bac'n Bits	1 Tbs	<1.0	25	18%
Bac'n Chips	1 Tbs	<1.0	25	18%
(Molly McButter) sprinkles	½ tsp	–	4	–
(Produce Partners) crumbles	1 Tbs	1.5	30	45%
(Tone's) bits	1 Tbs	1.0	30	30%
real				
(Hormel)				
bits	1 Tbs	1.5	30	30%
pieces	1 Tbs	1.5	25	54%
(Oscar Mayer) bits	1 Tbs	1.5	25	54%
BACON SUBSTITUTE (*See also* BACON BITS, CHIPS, & PIECES; VEGETARIAN FOODS)				
(Oscar Mayer) Lean 'N Tasty beef breakfast strips	1 slice	4.0	45	80%
(Sizzlean) cooked	2 strips	5.0	70	64%
(Swift Premium) Sizzling breakfast, lunch, & dinner strips				
beef & turkey	1 slice	6.0	70	77%
pork & turkey	1 slice	6.0	70	77%
BAGEL				
(Dunkin' Donuts)				
cinnamon-raisin	1 bagel	1.0	340	3%
onion	1 bagel	1.0	320	3%
plain	1 bagel	1.0	330	3%
(International-Bialys)				
garlic	1.5 oz	<1.0	110	4%

Food and Description	Amount	Fat Grams	Total Calories	% Fat Calories
onion	1.5 oz	<1.0	110	4%
plain	1.5 oz	<1.0	110	4%
(Lender's)				
frozen				
cinnamon-raisin				
Big 'N Crusty	1 bagel	2.0	230	8%
original	1 bagel	1.0	150	6%
egg				
Big 'N Crusty	1 bagel	2.0	230	8%
New York Style	1 bagel	2.0	220	8%
original	1 bagel	1.0	150	6%
garlic	1 bagel	1.0	150	6%
oat bran	1 bagel	1.0	150	6%
onion				
Big 'N Crusty	1 bagel	2.0	230	8%
New York Style	1 bagel	2.0	220	8%
original	1 bagel	1.0	150	6%
plain				
Big 'N Crusty	1 bagel	2.0	230	8%
New York Style	1 bagel	2.0	220	8%
poppy	1 bagel	1.0	150	6%
pumpernickel	1 bagel	1.0	150	6%
raisin/New York Style	1 bagel	2.0	220	8%
raisin & honey	1 bagel	1.0	150	6%
rye	1 bagel	1.0	150	6%
sesame	1 bagel	1.0	150	6%
soft				
egg	1 bagel	3.0	200	14%
plain	1 bagel	3.0	200	14%
raisin	1 bagel	3.0	200	14%
(Pepperidge Farm) food service/				
Bountiful Bagels				
cinnamon-raisin	1 bagel	1.5	300	5%
onion	1 bagel	1.5	290	5%
plain	1 bagel	1.5	300	5%
poppy	1 bagel	1.5	300	5%
sesame	1 bagel	1.0	300	3%
The Works	1 bagel	1.5	300	5%
(Roman Meal) original	1 bagel	1.0	220	4%
(Rubschlager) sandwich	1 bagel	2.0	90	20%
(Sara Lee)				
food service				
bagelette	1 bagel	–	80	–
cinnamon & raisin	2.3 oz	0.5	180	3%
	3 oz	1.0	240	4%
egg	3 oz	2.0	240	8%
onion	2.3 oz	0.5	180	3%
	3 oz	1.0	230	4%

Food and Description	Amount	Fat Grams	Total Calories	% Fat Calories
plain	2.3 oz	0.5	180	3%
	3 oz	1.0	230	4%
wheat 'n honey	2.3 oz	1.0	180	5%
fresh				
blueberry				
mini	1 bagel	–	80	–
regular	1 bagel	1.0	280	3%
cinnamon-raisin				
mini	1 bagel	–	80	–
regular	1 bagel	1.0	290	3%
egg	1 bagel	2.0	280	6%
onion	1 bagel	1.0	280	3%
plain				
mini	1 bagel	–	80	–
regular	1 bagel	1.0	280	3%
rye	1 bagel	1.0	280	3%
frozen				
blueberry	1 bagel	1.5	210	6%
cinnamon-raisin	1 bagel	1.0	220	4%
egg	1 bagel	1.5	220	6%
oat bran	1 bagel	1.0	210	4%
onion	1 bagel	–	210	–
plain	1 bagel	0.5	210	2%
poppy seed	1 bagel	1.0	210	4%
sesame seed	1 bagel	1.5	210	6%
(Thomas')				
egg	1 bagel	1.0	160	6%
multigrain	1 bagel	1.0	150	6%
onion	1 bagel	1.0	150	6%
plain	1 bagel	1.0	150	6%
(Western) Big Bagels				
blueberry	4.3 oz	1.0	330	3%
cinnamon-raisin	4.3 oz	1.0	315	3%
plain	4.3 oz	1.0	330	3%
BAGEL CHIPS				
(Burns & Ricker) Bagel Crisps				
cinnamon-raisin	5 chips	4.0	130	28%
fat-free original	5 chips	–	100	–
garlic	5 chips	4.0	130	28%
onion	5 chips	4.0	130	28%
plain	5 chips	4.0	130	28%
sea salt	5 chips	4.0	130	28%
sesame	5 chips	6.0	130	36%
(New York Style)				
cinnamon-raisin	3 chips	4.0	130	28%
garlic				
bite-size	28 chips	4.0	140	26%
regular	3 chips	4.0	130	28%

Food and Description	Amount	Fat Grams	Total Calories	% Fat Calories
original	3 chips	6.0	140	39%
sea salt	3 chips	4.0	140	29%
(Sara Lee)				
cinnamon-raisin	6 chips	5.0	130	35%
garlic	6 chips	5.0	130	35%
plain	6 chips	5.0	130	35%
sour cream & onion	6 chips	5.0	130	35%
BAKE & FRY MIX (*See also* SEASONINGS; TEMPURA BATTER)				
(Arrowhead) biscuit mix	2 oz	1.0	100	9%
(Bisquick)				
original	2 oz	8.0	240	30%
reduced fat	½ cup	4.0	210	17%
(Calhoun Bend Mill) mix only				
chicken & shrimp fry	4 Tbs	–	35	–
fish fry				
mild	4 Tbs	–	35	–
spicy	4 Tbs	–	30	–
(Fearn)				
brown rice	½ cup	2.0	215	8%
rice	½ cup	1.0	260	4%
whole wheat	½ cup	2.0	210	9%
(Golden Dipt)				
all-purpose batter mix	¼ cup	–	120	–
beer batter	¼ cup	–	120	–
breading/frying mix	¼ cup	0.5	120	4%
Cajun style fish fry	1⅓ Tbs	–	40	–
chicken				
frying mix/extra crispy	1½ Tbs	–	60	–
herbs & spices	2 Tbs	–	60	–
hot 'n spicy	2 Tbs	–	60	–
original homestyle	2 Tbs	–	50	–
corn dog batter	¼ cup	–	120	–
cracker meal	¼ cup	0.5	140	3%
fish & chips batter	¼ cup	–	120	–
fish fry	1⅓ Tbs	–	40	–
funnel cake	¼ cup	1.0	110	8%
hushpuppy				
deluxe	¼ cup	–	150	–
jalapeño	1¼ oz	–	120	–
w/onion	¼ cup	–	150	–
onion ring mix	¼ cup	–	120	–
seafood fry	1⅔ Tbs	–	60	–
tempura batter	¼ cup	–	120	–
(Hain) whole wheat	⅓ cup	1.0	140	6%
(Jiffy)	1 oz	3.0	115	24%
(Krusteaz)				
bake & fry baking crepe mix				
mix only	2 Tbs	1.0	80	11%

Food and Description	Amount	Fat Grams	Total Calories	% Fat Calories
prepared	2 crepes	3.0	100	27%
bake & fry mix	⅓ cup	6.0	180	30%
(Martha White) Recip-Ease	½ cup	8.0	240	30%
(Pioneer) biscuit & baking mix/low-fat	¼ cup	0.5	150	3%
(Produce Partners)				
vegetable batter mix	¼ cup	0.5	120	4%
Zebbie's onion ring batter mix	¼ cup	0.5	120	4%
BAKING BITS, CHIPS, CHUNKS, & PIECES				
(Baker's) baking chocolate				
bars				
German sweet	2 squares	3.5	60	52%
semisweet	1 square	9.0	130	62%
unsweetened	1 square	14.0	140	90%
white	1 square	14.0	140	90%
chips				
milk chocolate, 55 chips per ounce	½ oz	4.0	70	51%
semisweet, 55 chips per ounce	½ oz	3.5	60	52%
(Champion) Chocolate Naps	1 oz	14.0	140	90%
(Flavorite) candy coating				
chocolate	1 cube	16.0	300	48%
vanilla	1 cube	16.0	300	48%
(Ghirardelli) baking chocolate				
bars				
bittersweet	3 sections	15.0	210	64%
classic white	3 sections	15.0	240	56%
semisweet	3 sections	14.0	210	60%
sweet dark	3 sections	14.0	210	60%
unsweetened	3 sections	23.0	210	99%
chips				
classic white	2 Tbs	4.0	80	45%
Flickettes	2 Tbs	4.0	70	51%
milk chocolate	2 Tbs	3.5	70	45%
semisweet	2 Tbs	4.0	70	51%
(Hershey)				
bits for baking				
chocolate & Reese's peanut butter	1 Tbs	3.0	70	39%
Skor English toffee	1 Tbs	4.0	60	60%
chips				
butterscotch	1 Tbs	4.0	80	45%
chocolate				
semisweet				
mini	1 Tbs	4.0	80	45%
regular	1 Tbs	4.0	80	45%
sweet	1 Tbs	4.5	80	51%
Reese's peanut butter	1 Tbs	4.0	80	45%
raspberry	1 Tbs	4.0	80	45%
vanilla	1 Tbs	4.0	80	45%
chunks/semisweet chocolate	6 pieces	4.0	80	45%

Food and Description	Amount	Fat Grams	Total Calories	% Fat Calories
(M&M★Mars) M&M Baking Bits				
milk chocolate	0.5 oz	3.0	70	39%
semisweet chocolate	0.5 oz	3.5	70	45%
(Nestle)				
baking bars/chocolate				
Choco Bake	½ oz	8.0	80	56%
premier white	½ oz	5.0	80	56%
semisweet	½ oz	4.0	70	51%
unsweetened	½ oz	7.0	80	79%
baking morsels				
butterscotch	1 Tbs	4.0	80	45%
chocolate				
milk	1 Tbs	4.0	70	51%
mint	1 Tbs	4.0	70	51%
semisweet				
mini	1 Tbs	4.0	70	51%
regular	1 Tbs	4.0	70	51%
rainbow	1 Tbs	3.0	70	39%
BAKING CHOCOLATE (See BAKING BITS, CHIPS, CHUNKS, & PIECES)				
BAKING POWDER				
(Calumet)	1 tsp	–	4	–
(Davis)	1 Tbs	–	15	–
generic	1 tsp	–	5	–
BAKING SODA	1 tsp	–	5	–
BALSAM PEAR/raw	1 cup	–	15	–
leaf tips				
cooked	½ cup	–	10	–
raw	½ cup	–	7	–
pods				
cooked	½ cup	–	12	–
raw	½ cup	–	8	–
BAMBOO SHOOT (See also ASIAN FOOD)				
canned	1 cup	<1.0	25	18%
fresh				
cooked	1 cup	–	15	–
raw	½ cup	–	21	–
BANANA				
dried	¼ cup	0.5	90	5%
freeze-dried/chips	½ cup	8.0	250	29%
fresh				
red				
whole	1 medium	<1.0	120	2%
sliced	½ cup	<1.0	70	3%
yellow				
mashed	1 cup	1.0	210	4%
whole	1 medium	0.5	105	4%
(Chiquita)	1 medium	–	110	–
(Dole)	1 medium	1.0	120	8%

Food and Description	Amount	Fat Grams	Total Calories	% Fat Calories
powdered	1 Tbs	–	20	–
BANANA, COOKING OR BAKING (*See* PLANTAIN)				
BANANA NECTAR/NECTAR BLEND				
(Kern's)				
banana	11.5 fl oz	–	190	–
banana-pineapple	11.5 fl oz	–	220	–
BARBECUE LOAF (*See* LUNCHEON MEAT)				
BARBECUE SAUCE (*See also* SAUCE; SEASONINGS)				
(Annie's)	2 Tbs	0.5	45	10%
(Bill Johnson's)				
hickory	2 Tbs	–	40	–
hot & spicy	2 Tbs	–	40	–
mesquite	2 Tbs	–	40	–
original	2 Tbs	–	40	–
(Bull's Eye)				
original	2 Tbs	–	60	–
steakhouse style	2 Tbs	–	50	–
(Chris' & Pitt's)	1 Tbs	–	15	–
(Estee)	1 Tbs	–	18	–
(Featherweight)	1 Tbs	–	14	–
(French's) Cattleman's				
mild	1 Tbs	–	25	–
smoky	1 Tbs	–	25	–
(Healthy Choice)				
hickory	2 Tbs	–	25	–
original	2 Tbs	–	25	–
(Heinz)				
Barbecue Select				
hickory	2 Tbs	–	35	–
original	2 Tbs	–	40	–
Thick & Rich				
Cajun	2 Tbs	–	35	–
chunky	2 Tbs	–	30	–
Hawaiian	2 Tbs	–	40	–
hickory smoke	2 Tbs	–	35	–
mesquite	2 Tbs	–	30	–
mushroom	2 Tbs	–	30	–
old-fashioned	2 Tbs	–	35	–
onion	2 Tbs	–	30	–
original	2 Tbs	–	35	–
Texas Hot	2 Tbs	–	30	–
(Hunt's)				
Dijon/mild	2 Tbs	–	40	–
hickory				
bold	2 Tbs	–	45	–
regular	2 Tbs	–	40	–
hickory & brown sugar	2 Tbs	–	75	–

Food and Description	Amount	Fat Grams	Total Calories	% Fat Calories
honey				
hickory	2 Tbs	–	40	–
mustard	2 Tbs	–	50	–
hot & spicy	2 Tbs	–	50	–
light	2 Tbs	–	25	–
mesquite	2 Tbs	–	40	–
mild	2 Tbs	–	40	–
original				
bold	2 Tbs	–	45	–
regular	2 Tbs	–	40	–
teriyaki	2 Tbs	–	50	–
(K.C. Masterpiece)				
bold	2 Tbs	–	60	–
hickory	2 Tbs	–	60	–
honey Dijon	2 Tbs	1.0	50	18%
honey teriyaki	2 Tbs	1.0	60	15%
mesquite	2 Tbs	–	60	–
original				
no salt	2 Tbs	–	60	–
regular	2 Tbs	–	60	–
spicy	2 Tbs	–	60	–
(Kingsford) Masterpiece				
mesquite	1 Tbs	–	30	–
original	1 Tbs	–	30	–
(Kraft)				
regular				
Char-Grill	2 Tbs	1.0	60	15%
garlic	2 Tbs	–	40	–
hickory smoke				
hot	2 Tbs	–	40	–
regular	2 Tbs	–	40	–
w/onion bits	2 Tbs	–	50	–
honey	2 Tbs	–	50	–
hot	2 Tbs	–	40	–
Italian seasonings	2 Tbs	0.5	45	10%
Kansas City style	2 Tbs	–	45	–
mesquite smoke	2 Tbs	–	40	–
onion bits	2 Tbs	–	50	–
original				
extra rich	2 Tbs	–	50	–
regular	2 Tbs	–	40	–
salsa style	2 Tbs	–	40	–
teriyaki	2 Tbs	1.0	60	15%
Thick 'N Spicy				
hickory smoke	2 Tbs	–	50	–
honey	2 Tbs	–	60	–
Kansas City style	2 Tbs	–	60	–
mesquite smoke	2 Tbs	–	50	–

Food and Description	Amount	Fat Grams	Total Calories	% Fat Calories
original	2 Tbs	–	50	–
(Lawry's) California Grill/orange	¼ cup	1.0	35	26%
(Lea & Perrins)				
bold & spicy	2 Tbs	–	50	–
original	2 Tbs	–	50	–
tomato, garlic, & herbs	2 Tbs	–	40	–
(Maull's)				
beer-flavor (nonalcoholic)	1 Tbs	<1.0	20	23%
	3.5 oz	3.5	140	23%
genuine	1 Tbs	<1.0	20	23%
Kansas City style	1 Tbs	<1.0	30	15%
lite	1 Tbs	<1.0	12	38%
onion	1 Tbs	<1.0	20	23%
smoky	1 Tbs	<1.0	20	23%
	3.5 oz	3.5	140	23%
sweet/mild	1 Tbs	<1.0	30	15%
	3.5 oz	3.5	210	15%
sweet/smoky	1 Tbs	<1.0	30	15%
	3.5 oz	3.5	210	15%
w/onion bits	1 Tbs	<1.0	20	23%
	3.5 oz	3.5	140	23%
(Newman's Own) Bandito Diavalo/spicy	2 Tbs	2.0	70	26%
(Ott's)				
original	1 Tbs	–	14	–
smoky	1 Tbs	–	14	–
(Open Pit)				
hickory smoke	1 Tbs	–	25	–
hickory thick 'n tangy	1 Tbs	–	25	–
hot 'n tangy	1 Tbs	–	25	–
mesquite 'n tangy	1 Tbs	–	25	–
original				
regular	1 Tbs	–	25	–
w/onions	1 Tbs	–	25	–
sweet 'n tangy	1 Tbs	–	25	–
(Texas Best)				
Bill's Recipe	2 Tbs	–	20	–
Cajun	2 Tbs	3.0	45	60%
Hawaiian	2 Tbs	–	60	–
honey mustard	2 Tbs	1.0	50	18%
mesquite	2 Tbs	–	45	–
original recipe	2 Tbs	2.5	40	56%
sweet & sour	2 Tbs	0.5	60	8%
BARLEY (See also BABY FOOD; CEREAL)				
(Arrowhead Mills)				
flakes/rolled	¼ cup	1.0	110	8%
hulless	¼ cup	1.0	140	6%
pearled	¼ cup	0.5	170	3%

Food and Description	Amount	Fat Grams	Total Calories	% Fat Calories
generic				
pearled				
cooked	4 oz	0.5	139	2%
	1 cup	0.7	193	3%
dry	1 oz	<1.0	100	4%
	1 cup	2.0	704	3%
raw	1 oz	0.7	100	6%
	1 cup	4.0	651	6%
(Manischewitz) egg/plain	¼ cup	3.0	220	12%
(Quaker/Scotch)				
pearled/quick	⅓ cup	1.0	170	5%
regular/medium	¼ cup	1.0	170	5%
BARLEY MALT				
(Eden)	1 Tbs	–	60	–
BARRACUDA				
baked or broiled	3 oz	5.0	135	33%
breaded & fried	3 oz	7.5	169	40%
BASIL				
dried				
generic				
crumbled	1 tsp	–	3	–
	1 Tbs	–	10	–
ground	1 tsp	–	5	–
(McCormick/Schilling)	¼ tsp	–	1	–
fresh	2 Tbs	–	1	–
BASS				
black				
cooked-dry heat	3 oz	14.5	215	61%
raw	3 oz	1.0	80	11%
freshwater/raw	3 oz	3.0	97	28%
mixed species/raw	3 oz	3.0	97	28%
striped/cooked-dry heat	3 oz	2.0	82	22%
BAY LEAF/crumbled	1 tsp	–	5	–
BEAN (See individual bean listings)				
BEAN DISH (See also BEANS, BAKED & VARIETY; FROZEN ENTRÉE/DINNER; MEXICAN FOOD; individual bean listings)				
can, jar, or microwave container				
generic				
four-bean salad	½ cup	–	100	–
three-bean salad	½ cup	7.0	153	41%
(Green Giant) three bean salad	½ cup	–	70	–
(Hanover) four-bean salad	½ cup	–	80	–
(Hormel) beef & wieners	7.5 oz	13.0	290	40%
(Kid's Kitchen) beans & wieners microwave cup	1 cup	13.0	310	38%
(Libby's) Diner beans w/franks	1 container	16.0	330	44%
(Luck's)				
beans w/sliced hot dogs	1 cup	16.0	390	37%

Food and Description	Amount	Fat Grams	Total Calories	% Fat Calories
mixed bean salad seasoned w/pork	7.25 oz	5.0	200	23%
(Read) four-bean salad	½ cup	–	110	–
(S&W) bean salad				
deli style	½ cup	–	80	–
dill garden	½ cup	–	50	–
marinated	½ cup	–	70	–
marinated garden	½ cup	–	50	–
(Seneca) three-bean salad	½ cup	–	60	–
homemade/USDA Standard Home Recipe				
three-bean salad	1 cup	15.0	300	45%
BEAN SOUP (*See* SOUP)				
BEAN SPROUTS (*See also* individual bean listings)				
canned				
(LaChoy) drained	⅔ cup	–	8	–
fresh				
kidney				
boiled	4 oz	<1.0	37	12%
raw	1 cup	<1.0	53	8%
mung				
boiled	½ cup	–	13	–
canned				
(Arrowhead Mills)	½ cup	–	25	–
raw	4 oz	–	40	–
stir-fried	½ cup	–	31	–
navy				
boiled	1 cup	<1.0	88	5%
raw	4 oz	<1.0	70	6%
pinto				
boiled	4 oz	–	25	–
raw	4 oz	1.0	70	13%
soy				
boiled	½ cup	2.0	38	47%
raw	10 sprouts	0.6	12	45%
stir-fried	4 oz	8.0	143	50%
BEANS, BAKED & VARIETY (*See also* BEAN DISH; MEXICAN FOOD)				
(B&M) baked beans				
barbecue	½ cup	2.0	170	10%
brick oven	½ cup	2.0	180	10%
extra hearty	½ cup	2.0	190	9%
red kidney	½ cup	2.0	170	10%
w/honey	½ cup	1.5	170	8%
yellow eye	½ cup	2.0	170	10%
(Bush's Best)				
baked beans				
homestyle	½ cup	2.0	150	12%
w/onions	½ cup	2.0	150	12%
pork & beans				
deluxe	½ cup	2.0	160	11%

Food and Description	Amount	Fat Grams	Total Calories	% Fat Calories
Fanci Pak	½ cup	2.0	160	11%
vegetarian	½ cup	2.0	140	13%
(Campbell's)				
baked beans				
barbecue	½ cup	3.0	130	21%
brown sugar & bacon	½ cup	5.0	150	30%
home style	½ cup	3.0	130	21%
New England	½ cup	5.0	150	30%
old fashioned/in molasses & brown sugar sauce	½ cup	5.0	150	30%
vegetarian	½ cup	2.0	110	16%
pork & beans	½ cup	3.0	120	23%
(Friend's) baked				
original	½ cup	1.0	170	5%
red kidney	½ cup	1.0	160	6%
generic/baked				
w/beef	½ cup	4.6	160	26%
w/brown sugar	½ cup	2.5	145	16%
w/crumbled bacon	½ cup	4.0	160	23%
w/franks	½ cup	8.0	180	40%
w/molasses & brown sugar	½ cup	1.5	135	10%
w/pork	½ cup	2.0	135	13%
w/pork & sweet sauce	½ cup	2.0	140	13%
(Green Giant)				
baked				
in sauce	½ cup	1.5	160	8%
w/onions	½ cup	1.5	150	9%
barbecue	½ cup	0.5	140	3%
honey bacon flavored	½ cup	0.5	160	3%
Italian	½ cup	1.0	130	7%
pork & beans w/tomato sauce	½ cup	1.0	120	8%
(Hanover)				
baked beans				
barbecue	½ cup	2.0	140	13%
brown sugar & bacon	½ cup	3.0	170	16%
vegetarian	½ cup	–	130	–
pork & beans	½ cup	1.5	120	11%
(Health Valley) baked/honey				
no salt	½ cup	–	110	–
regular	½ cup	–	110	–
(Heartland) baked/Iron Kettle	½ cup	1.0	150	6%
(Heinz) vegetarian in tomato sauce	½ cup	0.5	130	3%
homemade/USDA Standard Home Recipe				
baked/made w/white beans, molasses, brown sugar, salt pork, & spices	½ cup	6.5	190	31%
barbecue	½ cup	<1.0	120	4%
(Hunt's)				
Big John's Beans & Fixins	½ cup	3.5	130	24%

Food and Description	Amount	Fat Grams	Total Calories	% Fat Calories
pork & beans	½ cup	1.0	130	7%
(Joan of Arc)				
baked				
in sauce	½ cup	1.5	160	8%
w/onions	½ cup	1.5	150	9%
barbecue	½ cup	0.5	140	3%
honey bacon flavored	½ cup	0.5	160	3%
Italian	½ cup	1.0	130	7%
pork & beans w/tomato sauce	½ cup	1.0	120	8%
(Libby's)				
pork & molasses	½ cup	2.0	140	13%
pork & tomato sauce	½ cup	2.0	140	13%
vegetarian	½ cup	1.0	130	7%
(Luck's) pork & beans in tomato sauce	½ cup	1.0	150	6%
(S&W)				
baked				
brick oven	½ cup	0.5	160	3%
honey mustard	½ cup	–	130	–
maple sugar	½ cup	0.5	150	3%
sweet bacon	½ cup	1.5	140	10%
barbecue/Texas Style	½ cup	1.5	140	10%
Pinquitos	½ cup	0.5	80	6%
(Stagg) baked	½ cup	2.5	145	16%
(Van Camp's)				
baked				
deluxe	1 cup	4.0	320	11%
regular	1 cup	2.0	260	7%
Beanee Weenee	1 cup	7.0	326	19%
brown sugar	1 cup	5.0	290	16%
pork & beans	1 cup	2.0	216	8%
vegetarian style	1 cup	1.0	205	4%
BEAR				
simmered	4 oz	15.0	295	46%
simmered/diced	1 cup	19.0	365	47%
BEAVER				
roasted	4 oz	6.0	190	28%
roasted/diced	1 cup	7.5	230	29%
BEECHNUT/dried	1 oz	14.0	164	77%

BEEF

(NOTE: All serving sizes are for cooked portions, unless otherwise stated. "Lean" means beef trimmed of separable fat before cooking. "Lean & fat" means untrimmed and cooked or eaten as purchased. In most cases, 4 ounces of raw beef yields approximately 3 ounces cooked. Prime cuts have the most fat; choice cuts less; and select cuts the least.)

■ **BEEF CUTS/FRESH**

brisket/all grades/braised
flat half
lean
0" fat

0" fat	3 oz	5.0	160	28%

Food and Description	Amount	Fat Grams	Total Calories	% Fat Calories
¼" fat	3 oz	8.0	190	38%
lean & fat				
¼" fat	3 oz	24.0	310	70%
½" fat	3 oz	25.0	315	71%
whole				
lean				
0" fat	3 oz	9.0	185	44%
¼" fat	3 oz	11.0	210	47%
lean & fat				
¼" fat	3 oz	27.0	330	74%
½" fat	3 oz	28.0	330	76%
chuck				
arm pot roast/braised				
lean				
0" fat				
choice	3 oz	7.5	187	36%
select	3 oz	5.0	170	26%
¼" fat				
choice	3 oz	8.0	190	38%
select	3 oz	6.0	175	31%
lean & fat				
¼" fat				
choice	3 oz	16.0	250	58%
select	3 oz	12.0	220	49%
½" fat				
choice	3 oz	23.0	305	68%
select	3 oz	20.0	280	64%
blade roast/braised				
lean				
0" fat				
choice	3 oz	12.0	225	48%
select	3 oz	10.0	205	44%
¼" fat				
choice	3 oz	12.0	225	48%
select	3 oz	10.0	205	44%
lean & fat				
¼" fat				
choice	3 oz	24.0	310	70%
select	3 oz	20.0	280	64%
½" fat				
choice	3 oz	26.0	330	71%
select	3 oz	24.0	310	70%
roast or steak/braised				
lean				
choice	3 oz	15.6	218	64%
select	3 oz	8.7	187	42%
lean & fat				
choice	3 oz	31.0	364	77%

Food and Description	Amount	Fat Grams	Total Calories	% Fat Calories
select	3 oz	25.8	321	72%
stew meat				
boneless/braised or stewed				
lean	3 oz	8.0	183	39%
lean & fat	3 oz	20.0	279	65%
corned beef				
boneless/roasted	3 oz	25.8	316	74%
flank/braised				
lean/0" fat/choice	3 oz	8.5	175	44%
lean & fat/0" fat/choice	3 oz	10.5	195	48%
ground				
extra-lean				
baked				
medium	3 oz	14.0	215	59%
well-done	3 oz	13.5	235	52%
broiled				
medium	3 oz	14.0	215	59%
well-done	3 oz	13.0	225	52%
pan-fried				
medium	3 oz	14.0	220	57%
well-done	3 oz	14.0	225	56%
lean				
baked				
medium	3 oz	15.5	230	61%
well-done	3 oz	15.5	250	56%
broiled				
medium	3 oz	15.5	230	61%
well-done	3 oz	15.0	240	56%
pan-fried				
medium	3 oz	16.0	235	61%
well-done	3 oz	15.0	235	57%
regular				
baked				
medium	3 oz	18.0	245	66%
well-done	3 oz	18.0	270	60%
broiled				
medium	3 oz	17.5	245	64%
well-done	3 oz	16.5	250	59%
pan-fried				
medium	3 oz	19.0	260	66%
well-done	3 oz	16.0	245	59%
loin/top/broiled				
lean				
¼" fat				
choice	3 oz	8.5	185	41%
select	3 oz	6.5	165	35%
½" fat				
choice	3 oz	8.0	175	41%

Food and Description	Amount	Fat Grams	Total Calories	% Fat Calories
select	3 oz	6.5	165	35%
lean & fat				
¼" fat				
choice	3 oz	18.0	255	64%
select	3 oz	14.5	225	58%
½" fat				
choice	3 oz	16.5	245	61%
select	3 oz	14.0	220	57%
London broil/100% lean				
choice/braised	3 oz	6.0	167	32%
porterhouse/braised				
lean/¼" fat/choice	3 oz	9.0	185	44%
lean & fat/¼" fat/choice	3 oz	19.0	260	66%
rib				
large end/roasted				
lean/0" fat				
choice	3 oz	13.0	215	54%
select	3 oz	10.0	190	47%
lean & fat				
¼" fat				
choice	3 oz	27.0	326	76%
select	3 oz	23.0	290	71%
½" fat				
choice	3 oz	26.0	315	74%
select	3 oz	25.0	305	74%
small end/broiled				
lean				
0" fat				
choice	3 oz	10.0	190	47%
select	3 oz	7.5	170	40%
¼" fat				
choice	3 oz	11.0	200	50%
select	3 oz	8.0	180	40%
lean & fat				
¼" fat				
choice	3 oz	24.0	300	72%
select	3 oz	20.5	275	67%
whole/roasted				
lean				
¼" fat				
choice	3 oz	12.0	210	54%
select	3 oz	9.0	180	45%
½" fat				
choice	3 oz	12.0	200	54%
select	3 oz	10.0	190	47%
lean & fat				
¼" fat				
choice	3 oz	26.0	320	73%

Food and Description	Amount	Fat Grams	Total Calories	% Fat Calories
select	3 oz	22.5	290	70%
½" fat				
choice	3 oz	27.5	330	75%
select	3 oz	25.0	310	73%
rib eye/broiled				
lean/0" fat/choice	3 oz	10.0	190	47%
lean & fat/0" fat/choice	3 oz	19.0	260	66%
ribs/short/braised				
lean/choice	3 oz	15.0	250	54%
lean & fat/choice	3 oz	36.0	400	81%
round				
bottom/roasted				
lean				
0" fat				
choice	3 oz	6.5	165	35%
select	3 oz	4.5	145	28%
¼" fat				
choice	3 oz	7.0	170	37%
select	3 oz	5.0	155	29%
lean & fat				
0" fat				
choice	3 oz	8.0	175	41%
select	3 oz	5.0	150	30%
¼" fat				
choice	3 oz	14.0	220	57%
select	3 oz	11.0	200	50%
eye of/roasted				
lean				
¼" fat				
choice	3 oz	5.0	150	30%
select	3 oz	3.5	140	23%
½" fat				
choice	3 oz	6.0	160	34%
select	3 oz	5.0	150	30%
lean & fat				
¼" fat				
choice	3 oz	12.0	205	53%
select	3 oz	9.5	185	46%
½" fat				
choice	3 oz	12.0	210	51%
select	3 oz	11.5	200	52%
full cut/broiled				
lean				
¼" fat				
choice	3 oz	6.5	165	35%
select	3 oz	4.5	145	28%
lean & fat/¼" fat/choice	3 oz	11.5	205	50%

Food and Description	Amount	Fat Grams	Total Calories	% Fat Calories
tip/roasted				
lean				
0" fat				
choice	3 oz	5.5	155	32%
select	3 oz	4.5	145	28%
¼" fat				
choice	3 oz	6.0	160	34%
select	3 oz	5.5	155	32%
lean & fat				
¼" fat				
choice	3 oz	12.5	210	54%
select	3 oz	10.5	195	48%
½" fat				
choice	3 oz	13.0	220	53%
select	3 oz	12.0	205	53%
top/broiled				
lean				
¼" fat				
choice	3 oz	5.0	160	28%
select	3 oz	3.5	145	22%
½" fat				
choice	3 oz	5.5	165	30%
select	3 oz	4.5	155	26%
lean & fat				
¼" fat				
choice	3 oz	9.0	190	47%
select	3 oz	7.0	175	36%
½" fat				
choice	3 oz	8.0	180	40%
select	3 oz	7.0	180	35%
rump roast/roasted				
lean				
choice	3 oz	7.9	177	40%
select	3 oz	6.0	162	33%
lean & fat				
choice	3 oz	23.0	295	70%
select	3 oz	19.9	269	67%
shank crosscuts/simmered				
lean/choice	3 oz	5.5	175	28%
lean & fat/¼" fat/choice	3 oz	12.5	225	50%
sirloin				
top/broiled				
lean				
¼" fat				
choice	3 oz	7.0	175	36%
select	3 oz	5.5	160	31%
½" fat				
choice	3 oz	8.0	180	40%

Food and Description	Amount	Fat Grams	Total Calories	% Fat Calories
select	3 oz	6.5	170	34%
lean & fat				
¼" fat				
choice	3 oz	14.0	230	55%
select	3 oz	12.0	219	51%
½" fat				
choice	3 oz	16.0	240	60%
select	3 oz	15.0	235	57%
wedge-bone/broiled				
lean				
choice	3 oz	6.0	178	30%
prime	3 oz	10.0	201	45%
select	3 oz	7.0	170	37%
lean & fat				
choice	3 oz	16.0	240	56%
prime	3 oz	19.0	271	63%
select	3 oz	15.0	232	58%
steak/broiled				
club/choice				
lean & fat	3 oz	34.5	386	30%
porterhouse/choice				
lean	3 oz	9.0	185	44%
lean & fat	3 oz	18.0	254	64%
T-bone/choice				
lean	3 oz	9.0	185	44%
lean & fat/¼" fat	3 oz	18.0	255	64%
tenderloin/roasted				
lean				
¼" fat				
choice	3 oz	14.5	265	49%
select	3 oz	9.0	180	43%
½" fat				
choice	3 oz	10.0	190	47%
select	3 oz	8.5	180	43%
lean & fat				
¼" fat				
choice	3 oz	22.5	290	70%
select	3 oz	21.0	275	69%
½" fat				
choice	3 oz	19.5	265	66%
select	3 oz	17.5	245	64%
■ BEEF CUTS, LEAN/BRAND NAME				
(Bill Bailey's) fresh marinated bottom sirloin tip roast w/BBQ flavor	4 oz	14.0	220	57%
(Dakota Lean) raw				
chuck roast	3 oz	2.0	80	23%
eye of round	3 oz	2.0	80	23%
flank	3 oz	1.0	80	11%

Food and Description	Amount	Fat Grams	Total Calories	% Fat Calories
ground	3 oz	2.0	90	20%
rib eye	3 oz	2.0	90	20%
round/outside	3 oz	1.0	80	11%
round/top	3 oz	1.0	80	11%
sirloin tip	3 oz	3.0	90	30%
strip loin	3 oz	2.0	90	20%
tenderloin	3 oz	1.0	70	13%
(Kirkland) fresh/frozen				
ground beef				
chubs	4 oz	10.0	180	50%
patties/78% lean	1 patty	25.0	310	72%
ground sirloin patties	1 patty	23.0	330	63%
(Lean & Free) raw				
burger	4 oz	9.5	175	49%
cube steak	4 oz	1.0	110	8%
rib eye	4 oz	2.5	120	19%
round steak	4 oz	1.0	110	8%
sirloin steak	4 oz	1.5	110	12%
sirloin tip	4 oz	1.0	110	8%
strip steak/loin	4 oz	2.0	115	16%
T-bone	4 oz	2.5	125	18%
tenderloin steak/fillet	4 oz	2.5	120	19%
top round	4 oz	4.5	135	30%
(TriFoods) Steak-Umm sandwich steaks	1 steak	17.0	190	81%
▦ **BEEF CUTS, ORGAN/OTHER**				
brain				
fried	3 oz	13.5	167	73%
simmered	3 oz	10.6	136	70%
heart/braised	3 oz	4.8	148	29%
kidney/simmered	3 oz	2.9	122	21%
liver				
braised	3 oz	4.0	137	26%
fried	3 oz	6.8	184	33%
lung/braised	3 oz	3.0	102	27%
pancreas/braised	3 oz	14.7	232	57%
spleen/braised	3 oz	4.0	123	29%
sweetbread/braised	3 oz	19.7	272	65%
thymus/braised	3 oz	21.0	273	69%
tongue				
braised/medium fat	3 oz	22.0	208	95%
simmered	3 oz	17.6	241	66%
tripe				
(Armour Star) canned	3 oz	1.5	90	15%
raw	4 oz	4.0	111	32%
BEEF, DRIED/SMOKED (*See also* LUNCHEON MEAT)				
dried or chipped	2.5 oz	4.0	145	25%
smoked/chopped	1 oz	1.0	38	24%
BEEF BROTH (*See* SOUP)				

Food and Description	Amount	Fat Grams	Total Calories	% Fat Calories

BEEF DISH/ENTRÉE (*See also* ASIAN FOOD; FROZEN ENTRÉE/DINNER; HAMBURGER; MEXICAN FOOD; PASTA ENTRÉE/DINNER; RICE DISH; individual listings)

Food and Description	Amount	Fat Grams	Total Calories	% Fat Calories
canned				
(Armour Star)				
beef stew	1 cup	12.0	220	49%
corned beef hash	1 cup	30.0	440	61%
roast beef hash	1 cup	25.0	400	56%
roast beef in gravy	½ cup	4.0	150	24%
(Chef Boyardee)				
Beefaroni				
beef	1 cup	5.0	230	20%
w/beef	1 cup	7.0	260	24%
mini ravioli	1 cup	5.0	230	20%
Sir Chomps-A-Lot	1 cup	4.0	210	17%
(Dinty Moore)				
American Classics				
beef stew	1 bowl	13.0	260	45%
pot roast	1 bowl	3.0	210	13%
roast beef w/mashed potatoes	1 bowl	5.0	240	19%
Salisbury steak	1 bowl	14.0	310	41%
other				
beef stew	1 cup	14.0	230	55%
meatball stew	1 cup	16.0	270	53%
(Heinz)				
beef stew	7.5 oz	9.0	210	34%
goulash	7.5 oz	11.0	240	41%
(Hormel)				
beef goulash	7.5 oz	11.0	230	43%
cubed beef	½ cup	3.0	130	21%
roast beef w/gravy	2 oz	2.0	60	30%
(Libby's)				
corned beef	2 oz	7.0	120	53%
corned beef hash	1 cup	36.0	490	66%
roast beef hash	1 cup	33.0	460	65%
roast beef w/gravy	⅔ cup	3.0	140	19%
(Mary Kitchen)				
corned beef hash	7.5 oz	22.0	350	57%
	1 cup	24.0	390	55%
Fiesta hash	1 cup	23.0	410	50%
roast beef hash	7.5 oz	21.0	348	54%
	1 cup	24.0	390	55%
frozen				
(Armanino) cocktail meatballs	7 pieces	17.0	220	70%
(Morton) beef pot pie	7 oz	17.0	310	49%
(Schwan's)				
beef patty				
4-oz patty	1 patty	23.0	280	74%

Food and Description	Amount	Fat Grams	Total Calories	% Fat Calories
3.75-oz patty	1 patty	11.0	180	55%
beef patty melt	1 patty	27.0	340	71%
beef tips & gravy	1 cup	6.0	220	25%
Big Sam beef steak	6 oz	7.0	210	30%
breaded beef steak fingers	5 pieces	5.0	160	28%
breaded cubed beef steak	4 oz	20.0	290	62%
chopped BBQ beef	½ cup	8.0	220	33%
chopped beef steaks	5.3 oz	31.0	390	72%
creamed chipped beef	1 cup	17.0	310	49%
dinner steak	7 oz	32.0	440	65%
Phili style beef sandwich steak	3 slices	5.0	140	32%
pizza patty	1 patty	26.0	300	78%
sirloin ball tip steak	6 oz	12.0	250	43%
sirloin fillet of beef steak	4 oz	6.0	150	36%
(Swanson) beef pot pie	1 pie	19.0	380	45%
homemade/USDA Standard Home Recipe				
beef bourguignon	¾ cup	8.0	194	37%
beef pot pie/9" dia	⅓ pie	30.0	515	52%
beef stew	1 cup	11.0	220	45%
beef stroganoff w/noodles	1 cup	20.0	342	53%
beef Wellington	4 oz	18.0	325	50%
corned beef hash	1 cup	21.5	344	56%
creamed dried beef	¾ cup	18.0	275	59%
stuffed green pepper				
w/beef & bread crumbs	1 medium	10.5	325	29%
w/beef, bread crumbs, & rice	½ pepper	13.0	219	53%
microwave container				
(Chef Boyardee) microwave bowl				
beef ravioli/main meal	1 bowl	5.0	270	17%
beef stew	1 bowl	11.0	220	45%
Beefaroni				
w/beef	1 bowl	3.0	190	14%
w/meat sauce	1 bowl	3.0	180	15%
chili w/beans	1 bowl	14.0	300	42%
meat tortellini				
main meal	1 bowl	4.0	300	12%
regular	1 bowl	2.5	220	10%
rice w/beef & vegetables	1 bowl	7.0	250	25%
Sir Chomps-A-Lot	1 bowl	2.0	180	10%
(Dinty Moore) microwave cup				
beef stew	1 cup	10.0	190	47%
burger stew/hearty	1 cup	13.0	240	49%
corned beef hash	1 cup	22.0	350	57%
meatball stew	1 cup	15.0	250	54%
(Hormel) micro cup meal				
beef stew	1 cup	9.0	180	45%
(Libby's) Diner				
beef ravioli	1 container	9.0	230	35%

Food and Description	Amount	Fat Grams	Total Calories	% Fat Calories
beef stew	1 container	20.0	290	62%
(Luck's) microwave bowl/beef stew	7.5 oz bowl	1.0	130	7%
(Lunch Bucket) beef stew/hearty mix	1 container	9.0	170	48%
(Betty Crocker) Hamburger Helper				
beef noodle				
mix only	⅔ cup	1.5	120	11%
prepared	1 cup	10.0	260	35%
beef Romanoff				
mix only	⅔ cup	1.5	150	9%
prepared	1 cup	11.0	290	34%
beef stew/homestyle				
mix only	½ cup	0.5	110	4%
prepared	1 cup	10.0	250	36%
beef taco				
mix only	½ cup	2.0	160	11%
prepared	1 cup	11.0	300	33%
beef teriyaki				
mix only	⅓ cup	1.0	170	5%
prepared	1 cup	10.0	320	28%
cheddar 'n bacon				
mix only	⅔ cup	5.0	170	26%
prepared	1 cup	16.0	350	41%
cheeseburger macaroni				
mix only	⅓ cup	4.0	170	21%
prepared	1 cup	13.0	320	39%
cheesy shells				
mix only	½ cup	6.0	180	30%
prepared	1 cup	16.0	340	42%
chili macaroni				
mix only	⅓ cup	1.0	140	6%
prepared	1 cup	10.0	290	31%
fettuccine Alfredo				
mix only	½ cup	4.0	150	24%
prepared	1 cup	14.0	310	41%
hamburger stew				
mix only	⅔ cup	0.5	100	5%
prepared	1 cup	10.0	250	36%
Italian				
cheesy				
mix only	½ cup	3.0	150	18%
prepared	1 cup	14.0	330	38%
rigatoni/homestyle				
mix only	⅓ cup	1.0	150	6%
prepared	1 cup	10.0	290	31%
zesty				
mix only	⅓ cup	1.0	160	6%
prepared	1 cup	11.0	320	31%

Food and Description	Amount	Fat Grams	Total Calories	% Fat Calories
lasagna				
mix only	⅔ cup	0.5	140	3%
prepared	1 cup	10.0	280	32%
meat loaf				
mix only	1.5 Tbs	0.5	50	9%
prepared	⅙ loaf	15.0	280	48%
mushroom & wild rice				
mix only	¼ cup	2.5	170	13%
prepared	1 cup	13.0	350	33%
nacho cheese				
mix only	½ cup	3.0	160	17%
prepared	1 cup	14.0	340	37%
pizza pasta w/cheese topping				
mix only	½ cup	2.0	150	12%
prepared	1 cup	11.0	290	34%
Pizzabake				
mix only	⅓ cup	1.5	140	10%
prepared	⅙ pizza	10.0	270	33%
rice Oriental				
mix only	¼ cup	0.5	160	3%
prepared	1 cup	10.0	310	29%
Salisbury/homestyle				
mix only	⅔ cup	1.0	140	6%
prepared	1 cup	10.0	280	32%
spaghetti				
mix only	½ cup	1.0	150	6%
prepared	1 cup	11.0	300	33%
stroganoff				
mix only	⅔ cup	3.0	170	16%
prepared	1 cup	14.0	350	36%
Swedish meatballs/homestyle				
mix only	⅔ cup	7.0	170	37%
prepared	1 cup	16.0	320	45%
three cheese				
mix only	½ cup	6.0	180	30%
prepared	1 cup	16.0	350	41%
(Borden) Hamburger Mate				
beef noodle				
mix only	1.5 oz	1.5	150	9%
prepared	1 cup	110.0	300	33%
burger 'n cheese				
mix only	1.5 oz	2.5	160	14%
prepared	1 cup	12.0	320	34%
chili-tomato				
mix only	1.5 oz	1.0	160	6%
prepared	1 cup	11.0	320	31%
twists & tomato sauce				
mix only	1.5 oz	0.5	160	3%

Food and Description	Amount	Fat Grams	Total Calories	% Fat Calories
prepared	1 cup	11.0	320	31%

BEEF JERKY, STICKS, & STRIPS (*See also* SAUSAGE STICK)

Food and Description	Amount	Fat Grams	Total Calories	% Fat Calories
(Bridgford)				
jerky				
hot 'n spicy	1.25 oz	2.0	100	18%
original	1.25 oz	2.0	110	16%
teriyaki	1.25 oz	1.0	90	10%
sticks				
bacon & beef	1 oz	12.0	140	77%
beef	1 oz	12.0	140	77%
beef & cheese	1.5 oz	14.0	170	74%
(Eagle)				
beef stick	1 oz	9.0	110	8%
kippered beefsteak strip				
hot	0.8 oz	0.5	50	9%
regular	0.8 oz	0.5	50	9%
(Frito Lay) Rustlers Roundup				
beef jerky				
5 per pkg	1 pkg	1.5	20	67%
6.3 per pkg	1 pkg	2.0	30	60%
Spicy Stick				
9 per pkg	1 pkg	4.0	50	72%
13 per pkg	1 pkg	6.0	70	77%
(Hickory Farms) original	1 oz	3.0	100	27%
(Lance)				
beef & cheese	1.5 oz	11.0	150	66%
beef jerky				
jumbo	9/16 oz	4.0	70	51%
regular	0.25 oz	2.0	30	60%
beef snack				
jumbo	1 oz	13.0	150	78%
regular	0.63 oz	8.0	100	72%
supersize	0.46 oz	6.0	70	77%
	0.5 oz	7.0	80	79%
(Pacific Gold) natural				
hot & spicy	1 oz	1.0	90	10%
original	1 oz	1.0	80	11%
teriyaki	1 oz	1.0	80	11%
(Pemmican)				
Arrowhead	0.7 oz	3.0	70	39%
jalapeño	1.3 oz	3.0	110	25%
natural	1 oz	2.0	80	23%
	1.3 oz	3.0	110	25%
peppered	1.3 oz	3.0	110	25%
Steaker's				
pouch	1.1 oz	1.0	80	11%
strips	1 strip	1.0	40	23%
tabasco	1.3 oz	3.0	110	25%

Food and Description	Amount	Fat Grams	Total Calories	% Fat Calories
Tender Brave	1 oz	2.0	80	23%
Tender Chief	1 oz	2.0	80	23%
Tender Tomahawk	0.25 oz	1.0	20	45%
Tender Trail	1 oz	1.0	80	11%
Tender Tribe	1 oz	1.0	80	11%
teriyaki	1 oz	2.0	80	23%
	1.3 oz	2.0	100	18%
(Slim Jim)				
Big Jerk	0.25 oz	1.0	25	36%
Giant Jerk	0.63 oz	2.0	60	30%
original	0.14 oz	1.0	20	45%
Super Jerk				
regular	0.31 oz	1.0	30	30%
tabasco	0.31 oz	1.0	30	30%
(Tombstone)				
beef jerky	1 stick	–	35	–
beef sticks	1 stick	10.0	110	82%
Snappy Sticks	1 stick	10.0	110	82%
BEEF SPREAD (*See* LUNCHEON MEAT)				
BEEF SAUSAGE (*See* LUNCHEON MEAT; SAUSAGE)				
BEEF SEASONING (*See* SEASONINGS)				
BEEF SOUP (*See* SOUP)				
BEEF TALLOW (*See also* SUET, BEEF)	1 Tbs	12.8	115	100%
	1 cup	205.0	1849	100%
BEER, ALE, & MALT LIQUOR				
(Amber Key) light				
repeal	12 fl oz	–	106	–
3.2	12 fl oz	–	106	–
(Amstel) Light	12 fl oz	–	95	
(Anheuser-Busch)				
light	12 fl oz	–	75	–
natural light	12 fl oz	–	110	–
regular	12 fl oz	–	153	–
(Arctic Ice)				
light				
repeal	12 fl oz	–	121	–
3.2	12 fl oz	–	111	–
original				
repeal	12 fl oz	–	148	–
3.2	12 fl oz	–	111	–
(Augsburger)				
bock	12 fl oz	–	169	–
dark	12 fl oz	–	169	–
golden	12 fl oz	–	169	–
red	12 fl oz	–	159	–
(Beck's)				
dark	12 fl oz	–	156	–
light	12 fl oz	–	132	–

Food and Description	Amount	Fat Grams	Total Calories	% Fat Calories
regular	12 fl oz	–	143	–
(Black Horse)	12 fl oz	–	158	–
(Blatz LA) Old Style	12 fl oz	–	73	–
(Budweiser)				
dry	12 fl oz	–	130	–
ice	12 fl oz	–	148	–
ice light	12 fl oz	–	96	–
light	12 fl oz	–	110	–
regular	12 fl oz	–	148	–
(Busch)				
light	12 fl oz	–	110	–
nonalcoholic	12 fl oz	–	60	–
regular	12 fl oz	–	143	–
(Carling's) Black Label	12 fl oz	–	136	–
(Carlsburg)				
light	12 fl oz	–	110	–
regular	12 fl oz	–	149	–
(Champale) extra dry	12 fl oz	–	169	–
(Cheers) nonalcoholic	12 fl oz	–	55	–
(Classic)	12 fl oz	–	144	–
(Colt 45)	12 fl oz	–	156	–
(Coors)				
dry	12 fl oz	–	94	–
Extra Gold	12 fl oz	–	118	–
light	12 fl oz	–	105	–
regular	12 fl oz	–	135	–
(Coqui) malt liquor	12 fl oz	–	208	–
(Corona) light	12 fl oz	–	105	–
(Cutter)	12 fl oz	–	76	–
(Elephant) malt liquor	12 fl oz	–	208	–
(Elk Mountain)				
amber ale	12 fl oz	–	201	–
red	12 fl oz	–	159	–
(Foster's) lager	12 fl oz	–	120	–
(Gablinger's)	12 fl oz	–	96	–
generic				
ale	12 fl oz	–	155	–
light	12 fl oz	–	100	–
near beer	12 fl oz	–	32	–
regular	12 fl oz	–	146	–
stout	12 fl oz	–	120	–
(Genesee)				
bock	12 fl oz	–	156	–
Genny Ice	12 fl oz	–	156	–
Genny N/A/nonalcoholic	12 fl oz	–	70	–
Genny Red	12 fl oz	–	148	–
light	12 fl oz	–	96	–
regular	12 fl oz	–	148	–

Food and Description	Amount	Fat Grams	Total Calories	% Fat Calories
12 Horse Ale	12 fl oz	–	152	–
(Goebel)	12 fl oz	–	131	–
(Guinness) extra stout	12 fl oz	–	192	–
(Hamm's)				
light	12 fl oz	–	96	–
regular	12 fl oz	–	136	–
(Heidelberg) light	12 fl oz	–	115	–
(Heileman's)				
Black Label	12 fl oz	–	156	–
Old Style				
light	12 fl oz	–	110	–
regular	12 fl oz	–	147	–
Special Export				
dark	12 fl oz	–	155	–
light	12 fl oz	–	115	–
regular	12 fl oz	–	151	–
(Heineken)				
regular	12 fl oz	–	152	–
special dark	12 fl oz	–	192	–
(Herman Joseph's)	12 fl oz	–	157	–
(Hofbrau) dark reserve	12 fl oz	–	204	–
(JW Dundee's) honey brown lager	12 fl oz	–	150	–
(Keystone)				
dry	12 fl oz	–	125	–
ice	12 fl oz	–	131	–
light	12 fl oz	–	106	–
original	12 fl oz	–	118	–
(KGA)				
ice	12 fl oz	–	154	–
regular	12 fl oz	–	138	–
(KGAL)	12 fl oz	–	110	–
(Killian's)				
brown				
repeal	12 fl oz	–	187	–
3.2	12 fl oz	–	131	–
regular	12 fl oz	–	124	–
(King Cobra)	12 fl oz	–	176	–
(Kingsbury) nonalcoholic malt	12 fl oz	–	60	–
(Knickerbocker)	12 fl oz	–	140	–
(Kronenbourg)	12 fl oz	–	170	–
(LA)	12 fl oz	–	112	–
(Lite)				
genuine draft	12 fl oz	–	98	–
ultra	12 fl oz	–	77	–
(Löwenbrau)				
dark special	12 fl oz	–	158	–
regular	12 fl oz	–	157	–
special	12 fl oz	–	158	–

Food and Description	Amount	Fat Grams	Total Calories	% Fat Calories
(Michelob)				
classic dark	12 fl oz	–	164	–
dry	12 fl oz	–	133	–
golden draft	12 fl oz	–	151	–
golden draft light	12 fl oz	–	110	–
light	12 fl oz	–	134	–
regular	12 fl oz	–	160	–
(Mickeys) malt liquor	12 fl oz	–	156	–
(Miller)				
genuine draft	12 fl oz	–	147	–
High Life	12 fl oz	–	147	–
Lite	12 fl oz	–	96	–
Magnum	12 fl oz	–	162	–
Sharp's/nonalcoholic	12 fl oz	–	58	–
(Milwaukee's Best) light	12 fl oz	–	98	–
(Minnesota's Best)	12 fl oz	–	138	–
(Molson) light	12 fl oz	–	109	–
(Moussy) nonalcoholic	11.1 fl oz	–	50	–
(MSB&T)	12 fl oz	–	150	–
(Msia)	12 fl oz	–	145	–
(MS Blonde) lager	12 fl oz	–	150	–
(Nordik Wolf) light	12 fl oz	–	110	–
(O'Doul's)	12 fl oz	–	70	–
(Old Milwaukee)				
ice	12 fl oz	–	154	–
light	12 fl oz	–	110	–
nonalcoholic	12 fl oz	–	72	–
red	12 fl oz	–	136	–
regular	12 fl oz	–	145	–
(Olympia) gold light	12 fl oz	–	70	–
(Ortlieb's)	12 fl oz	–	140	–
(Pabst)				
Blue Ribbon	12 fl oz	–	135	–
low-calorie	12 fl oz	–	110	–
nonalcoholic	12 fl oz	–	55	–
Old English malt liquor	12 fl oz	–	151	–
(Piels)				
light	12 fl oz	–	127	–
regular	12 fl oz	–	133	–
(Pilsner) natural	12 fl oz	–	145	–
(Primo)	12 fl oz	–	138	–
(Prior) double dark	12 fl oz	–	171	–
(Rainier)	12 fl oz	–	142	–
(Red Bull) malt liquor	12 fl oz	–	192	–
(Red Light)	12 fl oz	–	106	–
(Red River Valley) lager	12 fl oz	–	163	–
(Red White & Blue) light	12 fl oz	–	115	–
(Red Wolf)	12 fl oz	–	157	–

Food and Description	Amount	Fat Grams	Total Calories	% Fat Calories
(Rheingold)				
light	12 fl oz	–	96	–
regular	12 fl oz	–	148	–
(St. Pauli Girl)				
dark	12 fl oz	–	156	–
light	12 fl oz	–	144	–
(Schaefer)				
light	12 fl oz	–	112	–
regular	12 fl oz	–	138	–
(Schlitz)				
ice	12 fl oz	–	145	–
ice light	12 fl oz	–	121	–
light	12 fl oz	–	120	–
malt liquor	12 fl oz	–	177	–
regular	12 fl oz	–	145	–
(Schmidt)				
light	12 fl oz	–	96	–
regular	12 fl oz	–	142	–
select nonalcoholic malt	12 fl oz	–	80	–
(Silver Thunder)	12 fl oz	–	165	–
(Steinlager)	12 fl oz	–	138	–
(Stroh's)				
American lager	12 fl oz	–	145	–
light	12 fl oz	–	115	–
Signature	12 fl oz	–	158	–
(Tiger Head) ale	12 fl oz	–	166	–
(XXXX)	12 fl oz	–	133	–
(Ziegen) bock	12 fl oz	–	152	–
(Zima) gold	12 fl oz	–	132	–
BEERWURST (*See* SAUSAGE)				
BEET				
canned or jarred				
(Del Monte)				
pickled/sliced/crinkle style	½ cup	–	80	–
regular				
sliced	½ cup	–	35	–
whole	½ cup	–	35	–
(Freshlike)				
pickled/small	½ cup	–	40	–
regular				
sliced	½ cup	–	40	–
small	½ cup	–	40	–
whole	½ cup	–	40	–
generic				
Harvard/sliced	½ cup	–	89	–
pickled	½ cup	–	75	–
(Green Giant)				
Harvard	⅓ cup	–	60	–

Food and Description	Amount	Fat Grams	Total Calories	% Fat Calories
regular				
sliced				
no salt added	½ cup	–	35	–
regular	½ cup	–	35	–
whole	½ cup	–	35	–
(LeSueur) baby/whole	½ cup	–	35	–
(Libby's)				
pickled				
sliced	½ cup	–	80	–
whole	½ cup	–	35	–
regular/sliced	½ cup	–	35	–
(S&W)				
pickled				
party sliced	1 oz	–	15	–
sliced	½ cup	–	30	–
whole	1 oz	–	15	–
regular				
julienne	½ cup	–	30	–
whole/small	½ cup	–	30	–
(Seneca)				
Harvard	½ cup	–	90	–
pickled	1 oz	–	20	–
(Stokely)				
pickled				
canned	½ cup	–	100	–
jar	½ cup	–	90	–
regular				
cut	½ cup	–	40	–
diced	½ cup	–	40	–
sliced	½ cup	–	40	–
whole	½ cup	–	40	–
fresh				
cooked				
sliced	½ cup	–	26	–
whole	2 medium	–	30	–
raw				
sliced	½ cup	–	38	–
whole	2 medium	–	70	–
BEET GREENS/fresh				
cooked	½ cup	–	20	–
raw	½ cup	–	4	–
BEET JUICE	6 oz	–	75	–
BERLINER SAUSAGE (*See* SAUSAGE)				
BERRIES, MIXED				
(C&W) berry medley/frozen-sweetened/ w/red raspberries, whole strawberries, Marion blackberries, blueberries	1 cup	–	60	–

Food and Description	Amount	Fat Grams	Total Calories	% Fat Calories
BERRY DRINK/BLEND (*See also* BERRY JUICE/JUICE BLEND; FRUIT PUNCH; SOFT DRINK; SOFT DRINK MIX; individual drink listings)				
bottled, boxed, or canned				
(Betty Crocker)				
Squeezit	7 fl oz	–	110	–
Squeezit 100	7 fl oz	–	100	–
(Hawaiian Punch)				
Very Berry	6 fl oz	–	90	–
(Hi-C)				
Boppin' Berry				
can	7.7 fl oz	–	110	–
drink box	8.45 fl oz	–	130	–
pet	8 fl oz	–	120	–
wild berry				
pet	8 fl oz	–	120	–
frozen or chilled				
(Chiquita)				
Berry Apple Orchard	8 fl oz	–	120	–
Light/cranberry-raspberry-strawberry	8 fl oz	–	35	–
BERRY JUICE/JUICE BLEND (*See also* BERRY DRINK/BLEND; individual juice listings)				
bottled, boxed, or canned				
(Capri Sun)				
red berry	6.75 fl oz	–	100	–
Yo Yogi Berry	6.75 fl oz	–	100	–
(Heinke's) nectar	8 fl oz	–	120	–
(Knudsen) Oregon berry	8 fl oz	–	100	–
(Libby's) Juicy Juice	8 fl oz	–	130	–
frozen				
(Hi-C) Five Alive/berry citrus	8 fl oz	–	120	–
BIRCH BEER (*See* SOFT DRINK)				
BISCOTTI (*See* COOKIE)				
BISCUIT (*See also* BAKE & FRY MIX: BREAKFAST SANDWICH)				
frozen				
(Bridgeford) heat & serve	1 biscuit	6.0	180	30%
homemade/USDA Standard Home Recipe				
buttermilk/1½" high/2½" dia	1 biscuit	9.0	212	38%
plain/1½" high/2½" dia	1 biscuit	9.0	212	38%
mix				
(Arrowhead Mills) biscuit mix				
mix only	¼ cup	1.0	120	8%
(Betty Crocker) Gold Medal biscuit mix				
mix only	⅓ cup	7.0	180	35%
prepared	2 biscuits	7.0	180	35%
generic				
buttermilk	1 biscuit	7.0	190	38%
plain	1 biscuit	7.0	190	38%
(Jiffy) buttermilk				
mix only	⅓ cup	4.0	160	23%

Food and Description	Amount	Fat Grams	Total Calories	% Fat Calories
prepared	1 biscuit	4.5	170	24%
(Krusteaz)				
baking mix				
mix only	⅓ cup	6.0	180	30%
prepared	2 biscuits	6.0	180	30%
cinnamon-raisin				
mix only	⅜ cup	11.0	290	34%
prepared w/glaze	3" biscuit	11.0	290	34%
(Martha White) Bix Mix	⅓ cup	5.0	160	28%
packaged ready to serve				
(Arnold) old-fashioned	2 biscuits	5.0	130	35%
(Awrey's)				
country	1 biscuit	5.0	160	28%
round	1 biscuit	3.0	80	34%
sliced	1 biscuit	5.0	160	28%
square	1 biscuit	3.0	80	34%
unsliced	1 biscuit	5.0	160	28%
(Oroweat)				
Australian toaster	1 biscuit	4.5	180	23%
cinnamon-raisin	1 biscuit	5.0	200	23%
refrigerated				
(Pillsbury)				
1869				
baking powder	1 biscuit	5.0	100	45%
buttermilk	1 biscuit	5.0	100	45%
Ballard Extra Lights Oven Ready				
buttermilk	3 biscuits	2.0	150	12%
plain	3 biscuits	2.0	150	12%
Big Country				
butter tastin'	1 biscuit	4.0	100	36%
buttermilk	1 biscuit	4.0	100	36%
Southern style	1 biscuit	4.0	100	36%
Grands!				
butter	1 biscuit	10.0	200	45%
buttermilk	1 biscuit	10.0	200	45%
cinnamon-raisin	1 biscuit	8.0	200	36%
flaky	1 biscuit	9.0	190	43%
homestyle	1 biscuit	9.0	190	43%
Southern style	1 biscuit	10.0	200	45%
Hungry Jack				
butter tastin' flaky	2 biscuits	7.0	170	37%
buttermilk/flaky	2 biscuits	7.0	170	37%
flaky	2 biscuits	7.0	170	37%
fluffy	2 biscuits	8.0	180	40%
honey tastin' flaky	2 biscuits	7.0	180	35%
Southern style flaky	2 biscuits	7.0	170	37%
Pillsbury				
butter	3 biscuits	2.5	150	15%

Food and Description	Amount	Fat Grams	Total Calories	% Fat Calories
buttermilk	3 biscuits	2.5	150	15%
country	3 biscuits	2.5	150	15%
tender layer buttermilk	3 biscuits	4.5	160	25%
BLACK BEAN				
(Eden)	½ cup	–	100	–
(Fantastic Foods) instant				
mix only	⅓ cup	1.5	160	8%
prepared	½ cup	1.5	160	8%
generic				
boiled	½ cup	<1.0	113	4%
raw	½ cup	1.5	330	4%
(Goya) frijoles negros	½ cup	0.5	90	5%
(Green Giant)	½ cup	–	100	–
(Joan of Arc)	½ cup	–	100	–
(Progresso)	½ cup	1.0	130	7%
(S&W)				
50% less salt	½ cup	–	70	–
regular	½ cup	–	70	–
(Sun Vista)	½ cup	1.0	70	13%
BLACK BEAN SOUP (See SOUP)				
BLACK CHERRY DRINK/bottled	8 fl oz	–	130	–
BLACK CHERRY JUICE/bottled, boxed, or canned				
(Knudsen) Thirst Quencher	8 fl oz	–	180	–
(Smucker's)	8 fl oz	–	130	–
BLACK TURTLE BEAN				
(Hain)	4 oz	–	170	–
BLACK TURTLE BEAN SOUP (See SOUP)				
BLACKBERRY (See also BERRIES, MIXED)				
canned				
in heavy syrup	½ cup	<1.0	94	5%
in juice	½ cup	<1.0	41	11%
in water	1 cup	1.5	60	23%
fresh	½ cup	<1.0	40	7%
	1 lb	2.0	240	7%
frozen/no sugar	½ cup	<1.0	97	5%
BLACKBERRY JUICE				
generic/canned	8 fl oz	2.0	92	20%
(Smucker's)	8 fl oz	1.5	91	15%
BLACK-EYED PEA				
canned				
(Bush's Best)				
regular	½ cup	–	70	–
seasoned w/bacon	½ cup	1.0	190	5%
(Glory) Southern style	½ cup	0.5	60	8%
(Green Giant)	½ cup	1.0	90	10%
(Luck's) seasoned w/pork	½ cup	3.0	130	21%
(Trappey's) w/bacon	½ cup	1.5	110	12%

Food and Description	Amount	Fat Grams	Total Calories	% Fat Calories
dried				
mature				
boiled	½ cup	0.6	100	5%
raw	½ cup	1.0	131	7%
young pods w/seeds				
boiled	1 cup	–	32	–
raw	1 cup	–	42	–
frozen				
(Freshlike)	3.3 oz	1.0	130	7%
generic/cooked	½ cup	1.0	114	8%
	10 oz	2.0	400	5%
(Pictsweet)	½ cup	1.0	110	8%
(Veg-All)	3.3 oz	1.0	130	7%
BLINTZ (See FROZEN ENTRÉE/DINNER)				
BLONDIE (See BROWNIE/BLONDIE)				
BLOOD SAUSAGE (See SAUSAGE)				
BLUEBERRY (See also BERRIES, MIXED)				
canned				
generic				
in heavy syrup	1 cup	<1.0	225	2%
in water	2 cup	<1.0	94	5%
(S&W) wild Maine/in heavy syrup	⅓ cup	–	70	–
fresh	2 cups	<1.0	82	6%
frozen				
(C&W)	¾ cup	–	70	–
generic				
no sugar added	1 cup	<1.0	88	5%
	3.5 oz	<1.0	50	9%
sweetened	1 cup	<1.0	190	2%
BLUEBERRY JUICE				
(Knudsen) Thirst Quencher/Maine coast	8 fl oz	–	90	–
BLUEFISH/raw	3 oz	3.6	105	31%
BOLOGNA (See LUNCHEON MEAT)				
BORAGE/fresh				
cooked	½ cup	1.0	25	36%
raw	½ cup	<1.0	9	50%
BORSCHT (See SOUP)				
BOYSENBERRY				
canned				
in heavy syrup	1 cup	–	226	–
in water	1 cup	–	90	–
fresh	½ lb	–	125	–
frozen				
no sugar added	1 cup	–	66	–
sweetened	1 cup	–	144	–
BOYSENBERRY JUICE/NECTAR				
(Knudsen) nectar	8 fl oz	–	110	–
(Smucker's) juice	8 fl oz	–	120	–

Food and Description	Amount	Fat Grams	Total Calories	% Fat Calories
BRAN (*See also* CEREAL)				
corn/dry	½ cup	0.5	85	5%
oat				
generic				
cooked	¼ cup	1.0	45	20%
dry	½ cup	3.0	115	23%
(Golden Harvest)	1 oz	2.0	90	20%
(Hodgson Mill)	¼ cup	3.0	120	23%
(Mother's) prepared	½ cup	3.0	150	18%
(Quaker) prepared	½ cup	3.0	150	18%
rice				
generic/dry	½ cup	8.5	130	59%
(Golden Harvest)	½ cup	8.0	120	60%
(Uncle Ben's)	½ cup	9.0	100	81%
wheat				
(Arrowhead Mills)	⅓ cup	1.0	30	30%
generic/dry	½ cup	1.5	65	21%
(Hodgson Mill)	¼ cup	1.0	30	30%
(Kretchmer) toasted	¼ cup	1.0	30	30%
BRANDY (*See* LIQUEUR)				
BRATWURST (*See* SAUSAGE)				
BRAZIL NUT				
dried	1 oz	19.0	186	91%
shelled	1 oz	19.0	190	90%
	1 cup	93.0	920	91%
(Diamond)	1 oz	19.0	190	90%
BREAD (*See also* BAGEL; BISCUIT; BREADSTICK; CROISSANT; MUFFIN; ROLL)				
■ **BROWN & SERVE**				
(Arnold) Francisco sourdough	1 oz	0.5	70	6%
(Colombo)				
sourdough				
French/round	½" slice	0.5	120	4%
French sourdough	1½" slice	–	130	–
garlic/plain	3" slice	9.0	190	43%
Luigi's loaves	1" slice	1.0	130	7%
(Earth Grains) pizza rounds	1 round	4.0	210	17%
(Pepperidge Farm) European Bake Shoppe				
Italian	⅛ loaf	2.0	130	14%
(Wonder) du jour				
Austrian	1 slice	1.0	70	13%
French	1 slice	1.0	70	13%
■ **CANNED**				
(B&M)				
plain	½" slice	0.5	130	3%
raisin	½" slice	0.5	130	3%
(Friends)				
plain	½" slice	0.5	130	3%
raisin	½" slice	0.5	130	3%

Food and Description	Amount	Fat Grams	Total Calories	% Fat Calories
generic				
Boston/3¼" x ½" slice	1 slice	1.0	95	10%
(S&W) New England recipe	½" slice	1.0	90	10%
■ **FROZEN**				
(Bridgeford) dough/baked				
French	2 slices	1.0	150	6%
honey wheat	1 slice	1.0	75	12%
white	1 slice	1.0	75	12%
(Cole's) mini loaf/garlic butter-flavored	1 slice	3.0	90	39%
(Mama Bella) homestyle garlic				
original/1" slice	2 slices	8.0	150	48%
Romano cheese/1" slice	2 slices	9.0	160	51%
(Marie Callender's)				
cornbread	1 piece	3.0	150	18%
honey butter added	1 Tbs	5.0	50	90%
(Pepperidge Farm)				
garlic	⅙ loaf	10.0	160	56%
garlic & olive oil loaves/reduced fat	2½" slice	7.0	170	37%
garlic Parmesan	⅙ loaf	7.0	160	39%
Monterey Jack/jalapeño cheese	⅙ loaf	10.0	200	45%
mozzarella garlic	⅙ loaf	10.0	200	45%
sourdough garlic	⅙ loaf	9.0	180	45%
two cheddar cheese	⅙ loaf	11.0	210	47%
(Rhodes) dough/baked				
honey wheat	1 slice	2.0	130	14%
Italian	1 slice	2.0	130	14%
raisin	1 slice	2.0	140	13%
sweet	1 slice	3.0	150	18%
white	1 slice	2.0	140	13%
(Rich's) dough/baked				
white	1 slice	2.0	150	12%
(Schwan's)				
dough/baked				
wheat				
honey	2 oz	1.5	130	10%
stone ground	2 oz	1.5	130	10%
white	2 oz	1.5	130	10%
ready to heat				
garlic 5 cheese	3.38 oz	20.0	340	53%
hushpuppies	3 pieces	6.0	180	30%
■ **HOMEMADE**				
USDA Standard Home Recipe (Note: If milk was an ingredient, whole milk was used in preparation)				
banana	1 slice	6.0	195	28%
corn pone/9" dia	⅛ pone	3.0	122	22%
cornbread/3" square	1 piece	5.0	170	26%
date nut	1 slice	3.0	100	27%
Irish soda	1 slice	3.0	175	15%

Food and Description	Amount	Fat Grams	Total Calories	% Fat Calories
pumpkin	1 slice	7.0	200	32%
raisin	1 slice	2.0	135	13%
spoonbread w/whole ground cornmeal	2 oz	7.0	117	54%
white	1 slice	2.0	110	16%
whole wheat	1 slice	2.0	125	14%
■ **MIX**				
(Arrowhead Mills) mix only				
cornbread	¼ cup	1.0	120	8%
kamut	⅓ cup	1.0	140	6%
multigrain	⅓ cup	1.0	160	6%
rye	⅓ cup	0.5	160	3%
spelt	⅓ cup	1.0	150	6%
white	⅓ cup	0.5	150	3%
whole wheat	⅓ cup	1.0	150	3%
(Aunt Patsy) mix only				
cornbread	¼ cup	–	130	–
sourdough beer	¼ cup	–	130	–
(Ballard)				
cornbread				
mix only	1/18 pkg	1.5	110	12%
prepared	1 piece	2.5	130	17%
(Calhoun Bend Mill)				
cornbread/country style/prepared	1 piece	<1.0	146	3%
Mexican/mix only	¼ cup	0.5	120	4%
hushpuppy/mix only	2 Tbs	–	150	–
(Daily Bread Co.) Quick Loaf/fat-free/mix only				
cinnamon-raisin	3 Tbs	–	120	–
garlic & herb	3 Tbs	–	120	–
honey oatmeal	3 Tbs	–	120	–
onion dill	3 Tbs	–	120	–
nine-grain	3 Tbs	–	120	–
wheat/cracked/hearty	3 Tbs	–	120	–
(Dromedary) mix only				
cheddar cheese	1/9 pkg	2.5	140	16%
cornbread	1/10 pkg	2.5	140	16%
date nut	1/12 pkg	7.0	180	35%
gingerbread	⅙ pkg	4.0	260	14%
Italian herb	1/9 pkg	2.5	140	16%
sourdough	1/9 pkg	2.0	140	13%
wheat/stone-ground	1/9 pkg	2.0	140	13%
white/country	1/9 pkg	1.0	140	6%
(Krusteaz)				
cinnamon-raisin/prepared	1 slice	2.5	180	13%
cornbread/fat-free				
mix only	¼ cup	–	120	–
prepared	2 pieces	–	120	–
cornbread/original				
mix only	¼ cup	2.5	110	20%

Food and Description	Amount	Fat Grams	Total Calories	% Fat Calories
prepared/2" x 2" piece	1 piece	3.0	120	23%
cornbread & muffin/fat-free honey				
mix only	¼ cup	–	120	–
prepared/2" x 3" piece	1 piece	–	120	–
dill rye	1 slice	2.0	150	12%
gingerbread				
mix only	⅓ cup	3.0	190	14%
prepared	⅛ cake	3.5	200	16%
honey wheat berry	1 slice	2.0	150	12%
Italian herb	1 slice	2.0	150	12%
sourdough	1 slice	2.0	150	12%
wheat/cracked	1 slice	2.0	150	12%
white/country	1 slice	2.0	150	12%
(Marie Callender's) cornbread/mix only	¼ cup	4.0	150	24%
(Martha White) cornbread				
buttermilk/prepared	⅕ pan	3.0	140	19%
Cotton Pickin				
mix only	¼ pkg	3.0	140	19%
prepared	⅕ loaf	3.0	140	19%
Mexican/prepared	⅙ pan	3.0	120	23%
(Pillsbury)				
bread machine mix/prepared				
wheat/cracked	1/12 loaf	2.0	130	14%
white/crusty	1/12 loaf	2.0	130	14%
gingerbread mix/prepared	⅛ pkg	5.0	220	20%
quickbread mix				
apple-cinnamon				
mix only	1/12 pkg	1.5	140	10%
prepared	1 slice	6.0	180	30%
banana				
mix only	1/12 pkg	1.5	130	10%
prepared	1 slice	6.0	170	32%
blueberry				
mix only	1/12 pkg	1.5	140	10%
prepared	1 slice	6.0	180	30%
carrot				
mix only	1/12 pkg	1.0	110	8%
prepared	1 slice	5.0	140	32%
cranberry				
mix only	1/12 pkg	1.5	140	10%
prepared	1 slice	4.0	160	23%
date				
mix only	1/12 pkg	1.5	150	9%
prepared	1 slice	4.0	180	20%
nut				
mix only	1/12 pkg	3.5	150	21%
prepared	1 slice	6.0	170	32%

Food and Description	Amount	Fat Grams	Total Calories	% Fat Calories
pumpkin				
mix only	½₂ pkg	1.5	130	10%
prepared	1 slice	6.0	170	32%
(Zia Foods) cornbread/blue cornmeal	1 piece	6.0	110	49%
■ PACKAGED/READY TO SERVE				
(Arnold)				
August Brothers				
onion rye				
plain	1 slice	1.0	80	11%
w/seeds	1 slice	1.0	90	10%
pumpernickel				
16-oz loaf	1 slice	1.0	80	11%
24-oz loaf	1 slice	1.0	90	10%
rye				
thin w/o seeds	2 slices	1.0	90	10%
w/seeds				
16-oz loaf	1 slice	1.0	80	11%
24-oz loaf	1 slice	1.0	90	10%
w/o seeds				
16-oz loaf	1 slice	1.0	80	11%
24-oz loaf	1 slice	1.0	90	10%
rye n' pump	1 slice	1.0	90	10%
sliced stick	2 slices	1.0	110	8%
sourdough	1 slice	1.0	110	8%
Texas toast	1 slice	3.0	150	18%
Arnold				
bakery light				
country bran	2 slices	1.0	80	11%
golden wheat	2 slices	0.5	80	6%
Italian	2 slices	1.0	80	11%
oatmeal	2 slices	1.0	80	11%
soft rye	2 slices	1.0	80	11%
sourdough	2 slices	0.5	80	6%
white/premium	2 slices	0.5	80	6%
bakery soft				
rye				
seeded	1 slice	1.0	80	11%
unseeded	1 slice	1.0	80	11%
Bran'nola				
country oat	1 slice	2.5	90	25%
honey wheat berry	1 slice	1.5	90	15%
nutty grains	1 slice	2.5	90	25%
original	1 slice	2.0	90	20%
7-grain white	1 slice	2.0	90	20%
12-grain	1 slice	2.0	90	20%
wheat				
dark	1 slice	2.0	90	20%
hearty	1 slice	3.0	90	30%

Food and Description	Amount	Fat Grams	Total Calories	% Fat Calories
Brick Oven				
wheat				
8-oz loaf	2 slices	2.5	110	20%
1-lb loaf	2 slices	3	110	25%
2-lb loaf	1 slice	2	80	23%
white				
8-oz loaf	2 slices	2.5	120	19%
1-lb loaf	2 slices	2.5	130	17%
2-lb loaf	1 slice	1.5	80	17%
Country				
buttermilk	1 slice	2.0	100	18%
potato	1 slice	2.0	100	18%
soft rye	1 slice	1.0	70	13%
soft white	1 slice	1.5	80	17%
wheat	1 slice	1.5	90	15%
white	1 slice	1.5	100	14%
other				
cranberry	1 slice	1.0	70	13%
honey wheat berry	1 slice	1.0	70	13%
100% stone-ground whole wheat				
1-lb-4-oz loaf	1 slice	1.0	60	15%
2-lb loaf	1 slice	1.5	100	14%
pumpernickel	1 slice	1.0	80	11%
raisin & cinnamon	1 slice	1.0	70	13%
rye				
deli	1 slice	0.5	80	6%
dill	1 slice	1.0	80	11%
Francisco				
French bread	1 oz	1.0	70	13%
French stick	1 oz	1.0	70	13%
Italian sliced bread	2 slices	1.0	110	8%
Italian sliced stick	1 slice	0.5	70	6%
Italian stick	1 oz	1.0	70	13%
sourdough/24-oz loaf	1 slice	1.0	90	10%
Levy's				
melba thin sliced rye	1 slice	1.0	90	10%
pumpernickel	1 slice	0.5	80	6%
Real Jewish Rye				
w/seeds	1 slice	1.0	70	13%
w/o seeds	1 slice	0.5	70	6%
Middle East pita pocket bread				
garlic	1 pita	2.0	160	11%
onion	1 pita	2.0	150	12%
white				
4" dia	1 pita	–	70	–
4 per pkg	1 pita	1.0	210	4%
6 per pkg	1 pita	0.5	140	3%
wheat/4" dia	1 pita	–	70	–

Food and Description	Amount	Fat Grams	Total Calories	% Fat Calories
whole wheat				
4 per pkg	1 pita	1.5	200	7%
6 per pkg	1 pita	1.0	140	6%
Real Jewish/rye				
Dijon	1 slice	1.0	80	11%
melba thin	2 slices	1.0	90	10%
regular				
w/seeds	1 slice	1.0	70	13%
w/o seeds				
1-lb loaf	1 slice	1.0	70	13%
2-lb loaf	1 slice	0.5	70	6%
Savoni's Italian bread	1 slice	0.5	60	8%
Sunmaid raisin bread	1 slice	1.0	70	13%
Sunny Valley				
wheat/enriched	1 slice	1.5	100	14%
white/enriched	1 slice	1.5	100	14%
August Brothers (*See* (Arnold) in this section)				
(Aunt Hattie's)				
buttermilk	1 slice	–	70	–
potato/homestyle	1 slice	1.5	80	17%
wheat				
homestyle	1 slice	2.0	80	23%
soft	1 slice	1.0	70	13%
stone-ground whole	1 slice	1.0	100	9%
white/homestyle	1 slice	2.0	80	23%
Bran'nola (*See* (Arnold); (Brownberry) in this section)				
(Brownberry)				
bakery light				
country bran	2 slices	1.0	80	11%
golden wheat	2 slices	0.5	80	6%
Italian	2 slices	1.0	80	11%
oatmeal	2 slices	1.0	80	11%
soft rye	2 slices	1.0	80	6%
white/premium	2 slices	0.5	80	6%
Bran'nola				
country oat	1 slice	2.5	90	25%
nutty grains	1 slice	2.5	90	25%
original				
24-oz loaf	1 slice	2.0	90	20%
3-lb loaf	1 slice	2.0	90	20%
7-grain white	1 slice	2.0	90	20%
wheat				
dark	1 slice	2.0	90	20%
hearty	1 slice	3.0	90	30%
Francisco International				
French/twin	1 slice	1.0	80	11%
Italian/thick-sliced	2 slices	1.0	110	8%
sliced stick	1 slice	–	100	–

Food and Description	Amount	Fat Grams	Total Calories	% Fat Calories
sourdough	1 slice	1.0	90	10%
Hearth				
grain	1 slice	1.5	90	15%
rye	1 slice	1.5	90	15%
wheat	1 slice	1.0	90	10%
Natural				
cinnamon	1 slice	2.0	80	23%
dill	1 slice	1.0	70	13%
health nut	1 slice	1.5	70	19%
oatmeal	1 slice	1.0	70	13%
pumpernickel rye	1 slice	0.5	70	6%
rye				
caraway	1 slice	1.0	70	13%
unseeded				
regular	1 slice	1.0	70	13%
thin-sliced	2 slices	1.0	100	9%
12-grain	2 slices	2.5	110	20%
wheat				
24-oz loaf	1 slice	1.0	80	11%
3-lb loaf	1 slice	1.0	80	11%
white	2 slices	1.5	120	11%
whole bran	1 slice	1.0	60	15%
other				
orange-raisin	1 slice	1.0	70	13%
raisin-cinnamon	1 slice	1.0	70	13%
raisin-walnut	1 slice	2.5	80	28%
soft oatmeal	1 slice	1.5	70	19%
wheat				
apple honey	1 slice	1.0	60	15%
country	1 slice	1.5	90	15%
soft				
16-oz loaf	2 slices	2.0	110	16%
24-oz loaf	1 slice	–	80	–
3-lb loaf	1 slice	2.0	80	23%
white				
country	1 slice	1.5	90	15%
soft				
16-oz loaf	2 slices	2.0	110	16%
24-oz loaf	1 slice	1.5	80	17%
(Country Hearth)				
European butter sesame	1 slice	1.0	70	13%
granola	1 slice	1.0	75	12%
honey nugget	1 slice	1.0	70	13%
Indian	1 slice	1.0	100	9%
old-fashioned buttermilk	1 slice	1.0	70	13%
old-fashioned sandwich	1 slice	1.0	75	12%
old-fashioned wheat	1 slice	1.0	70	13%
7 whole grain	1 slice	1.0	80	11%

Food and Description	Amount	Fat Grams	Total Calories	% Fat Calories
stone-ground whole wheat	1 slice	1.0	70	13%
wheat berry	1 slice	1.0	70	13%
(Earth Grains)				
barley bran	1 slice	1.0	70	13%
Canadian oat	1 slice	1.0	70	13%
French	1 slice	1.0	70	13%
gold'n bran	1 slice	1.0	70	13%
honey 'n bran	1 slice	1.0	70	13%
honey multigrain	1 slice	1.0	70	13%
honey oat & nut	1 slice	2.0	80	23%
honey oatberry	1 slice	1.0	70	13%
oat & nut	1 slice	2.0	80	23%
oat bran	1 slice	2.0	80	23%
raisin-cinnamon swirl	1 slice	2.0	80	23%
rye				
dark	1 slice	1.0	70	13%
deli	1 slice	1.0	70	13%
extra sour	1 slice	1.0	80	11%
Jewish	1 slice	1.5	80	17%
Russian style	1 slice	1.0	80	11%
sourdough	1 slice	1.0	70	13%
wheat berry	1 slice	1.5	100	14%
yogurt bran	1 slice	1.0	70	13%
(Father Sam's) pocket bread				
cinnamon-raisin	1 pita	–	150	–
Magic Pockets	1 pita	–	170	–
wheat				
medium	½ pita	–	110	–
mini	1 pita	–	100	–
white				
large	¼ pita	–	140	–
medium	½ pita	–	110	–
mini	1 pita	–	110	–
Francisco (See (Arnold); (Brownberry) in this section)				
generic				
black	1 slice	–	64	–
bran	1 slice	2.9	110	24%
buttermilk/homestyle	1 slice	1.0	75	12%
cheese	1 slice	1.0	72	13%
cinnamon-raisin	1 slice	1.0	80	11%
cracked wheat	1 slice	1.0	75	12%
egg	1 slice	2.0	115	16%
French/5" x 2½" x 1"	1 slice	1.0	80	11%
garlic	2 slices	3.8	100	34%
gluten	1 slice	1.0	70	13%
high-calcium				
dark	1 slice	<1.0	60	8%
light	1 slice	<1.0	65	7%

Food and Description	Amount	Fat Grams	Total Calories	% Fat Calories
hushpuppies	1 piece	7.0	145	43%
Indian (Navajo) fry				
5" dia	1 piece	8.0	295	24%
10.5" dia	1 piece	14.0	525	24%
Italian/4½" x 3¼" x ¾"	1 slice	1.0	85	11%
low-sodium	1 slice	0.8	70	10%
mixed-grain	1 slice	1.0	70	13%
oat bran				
reduced calorie	1 slice	<1.0	55	8%
regular	1 slice	1.0	70	13%
oatmeal				
reduced calorie	1 slice	<1.0	60	8%
regular	1 slice	1.0	70	13%
pita				
sesame/6½" dia	1 pita	1.0	140	6%
white				
6½" dia	1 pita	0.5	165	3%
8½" dia	1 pita	1.0	232	4%
whole wheat				
6½" dia	1 pita	1.0	170	6%
8½" dia	1 pita	2.0	200	9%
potato	1 slice	0.8	70	10%
pumpernickel	1 slice	1.0	80	11%
raisin	1 slice	1.0	80	11%
rice bran	1 slice	1.0	70	13%
rye				
reduced calorie	1 slice	<1.0	55	8%
regular	1 slice	1.0	80	11%
seven-grain	1 slice	1.0	65	14%
sourdough	1 slice	0.8	72	10%
triticale	1 slice	0.5	60	8%
Vienna/4¾" x 4" x ½"	1 slice	1.0	70	13%
wheat berry	1 slice	1.0	75	12%
wheat bran	1 slice	1.0	90	10%
wheat germ	1 slice	1.0	75	13%
white				
reduced calorie	1 slice	<1.0	60	8%
regular	1 slice	1.0	65	14%
whole wheat	1 slice	1.0	70	13%
(Grant's Farm)				
buttermilk	1 slice	1.0	80	11%
honey cracked	1 slice	1.0	70	13%
oat bran	1 slice	1.0	70	13%
oatmeal & toasted almonds	1 slice	2.0	80	11%
pumpernickel rye	1 slice	1.0	70	13%
stone-ground wheat & 7 grain	1 slice	1.0	70	13%
wheat berry	1 slice	1.0	70	13%

Food and Description	Amount	Fat Grams	Total Calories	% Fat Calories
(Hearth Farms)				
buttermilk wheat	1 slice	0.5	60	8%
buttermilk white	1 slice	0.5	70	6%
deli rye	1 slice	1.0	100	9%
honey 'n nut oat bran	1 slice	1.0	100	9%
honey wheat berry	1 slice	1.0	90	10%
multigrain	1 slice	1.5	100	14%
whole wheat	1 slice	1.0	90	10%
(Kangaroo) pocket bread				
breakfast				
cinnamon-raisin	1 loaf	–	65	–
wheat-oat bran	1 loaf	–	60	–
sandwich	1 loaf	–	75	–
(King's Hawaiian) center slice	½" slice	4.0	180	20%
Levy's (See (Arnold) in this section)				
Master's Best (See (Orowheat) in this section)				
Middle East (See (Arnold) in this section)				
(Monk's Bread)				
cinnamon	1 slice	2.0	70	26%
golden rice bran	1 slice	1.0	70	13%
Hi-Fibre	1 slice	1.0	50	18%
raisin	1 slice	2.0	70	26%
sunflower & bran	1 slice	1.0	70	13%
(Mrs. Wright's)				
French/enriched	1 slice	1.0	70	13%
grain/unsalted	1 slice	1.0	70	13%
honey bran	1 slice	1.0	90	10%
honey wheat berry	1 slice	1.0	70	13%
Jewish rye w/seeds	1 slice	1.0	60	15%
lite	1 slice	–	40	–
multimeal/sandwich	1 slice	1.0	70	13%
old fashioned Italian	1 slice	1.0	100	9%
Old World style black	1 slice	1.0	60	15%
raisin	1 slice	1.0	70	13%
sandwich				
supersoft	1 slice	1.0	60	15%
wheat	1 slice	1.0	80	11%
wheat				
crushed				
regular	1 slice	1.0	80	11%
sandwich	1 slice	1.0	70	13%
homestyle butter top	1 slice	1.0	70	13%
roundtop	1 slice	1.0	80	11%
white				
homestyle butter top	1 slice	1.0	80	11%
supersoft	1 slice	1.0	80	11%
unsalted	1 slice	1.0	80	11%

Food and Description	Amount	Fat Grams	Total Calories	% Fat Calories
(Natural Hearth)				
buttermilk	1 slice	1.0	70	13%
7-grain	1 slice	1.5	100	14%
stone-ground whole wheat	1 slice	1.0	60	15%
wheat berry	1 slice	1.0	70	13%
(Oatmeal Goodness)				
oatmeal				
cinnamon	1 slice	2.0	90	20%
light	1 slice	0.5	40	11%
wheat	1 slice	2.0	90	20%
oatmeal & sunflower seeds	1 slice	2.0	90	20%
oatmeal bran	1 slice	2.0	90	20%
(Oroweat)				
Master's Best				
deli rye	2 slices	1.5	130	10%
northern oat	1 slice	3.0	100	27%
3-seed	1 slice	3.5	90	35%
winter wheat	1 slice	3.0	90	30%
Orowheat				
country oat/light	1 slice	–	40	–
oatnut	1 slice	2.0	100	18%
100% whole wheat/light	1 slice	–	40	–
rye				
dark	1 slice	1.0	70	13%
extra sour	1 slice	1.0	70	13%
hearty/light	1 slice	–	40	–
Jewish	1 slice	1.0	70	13%
Russian	1 slice	1.0	70	13%
9-grain/light	1 slice	–	40	–
sourdough/light	1 slice	–	40	–
(Pepperidge Farm)				
Bakery Breads				
apple walnut	1 slice	2.0	80	23%
cinnamon	1 slice	2.5	80	28%
cracked wheat/thin-sliced	1 slice	1.0	70	13%
golden swirl	1 slice	2.5	90	25%
honey bran	1 slice	1.0	90	10%
honey wheat berry/hearty	1 slice	1.5	100	14%
oat/hearty crunchy	1 slice	2.0	100	18%
oatmeal				
light	3 slices	1.0	140	6%
regular	1 slice	1.0	80	11%
thin	1 slice	1	60	15%
pumpernickel				
classic dark	1 slice	1.0	80	11%
party slices	8 slices	1.5	110	12%
raisin w/cinnamon	1 slice	1.5	80	17%
russet potato/hearty	1 slice	1.5	90	15%

Food and Description	Amount	Fat Grams	Total Calories	% Fat Calories
rye				
Jewish				
seeded	1 slice	1.0	80	11%
seedless family	1 slice	1.0	80	11%
onion	1 slice	1.0	80	11%
party rye slices	8 slices	1.5	110	12%
thin-sliced Dijon	2 slices	1.5	100	14%
7-grain				
hearty slice	1 slice	1.5	100	14%
light	3 slices	1.0	140	6%
sourdough/light	3 slices	1.0	130	7%
Vienna				
light	3 slices	1.0	130	7%
thick-sliced	1 slice	1.0	70	13%
wheat				
light	3 slices	1.0	130	7%
natural	1 slice	1.5	90	15%
regular				
family 2-lb loaf	1 slice	1.0	70	13%
1.5-lb loaf	1 slice	1.5	90	15%
sesame/hearty	1 slice	1.5	100	14%
very thin sliced	3 slices	2.0	110	16%
white				
country/hearty	1 slice	1.0	90	10%
hearty	1 slice	1.0	90	10%
large family thin	1 slice	1.5	80	17%
sandwich	2 slices	2.0	130	14%
thin	1 slice	1.5	80	17%
toasting	1 slice	3.0	90	30%
very thin	3 slices	1.5	110	12%
whole wheat thin	1 slice	1.0	60	15%
European Bake Shoppe breads				
French style	⅛ loaf	1.5	130	10%
French/enriched	⅛ of 2 loaves	1.5	130	10%
sourdough/twin	⅛ of 2 loaves	1.5	130	10%
food service breads				
multigrain/restaurant	1 slice	1.5	100	14%
pita				
wheat	1 pocket	1.0	160	6%
white	1 pocket	1.0	150	6%
pumpernickel	1 slice	1.0	80	11%
round top wheat/restaurant	1 slice	1.5	100	14%
round top white/restaurant	1 slice	1.0	90	10%
rye				
Dijon	1 slice	1.0	80	11%
seedless	1 slice	1.0	80	11%
Texas toast	1 slice	2.0	110	16%
white/restaurant	1 slice	1.5	100	14%

Food and Description	Amount	Fat Grams	Total Calories	% Fat Calories
natural whole grain breads				
crunchy grain	1 slice	1.5	90	15%
9 grain	1 slice	1.0	90	10%
100% whole wheat	1 slice	1.0	90	10%
soft breads				
oatmeal	1 slice	0.5	60	8%
100% whole wheat	1 slice	0.5	60	8%
toasting bread	1 slice	0.5	110	4%
(Rainbo)				
family recipe split top				
grain	1 slice	1.0	70	13%
oat	1 slice	1.0	70	13%
wheat				
honey buttered	1 slice	1.0	70	13%
regular	1 slice	1.0	70	13%
stone-ground	1 slice	1.0	70	13%
white	1 slice	1.0	80	11%
regular				
milk/old-fashioned	1 slice	1.0	70	13%
sourdough/light	1 slice	0.5	40	11%
thin	1 slice	1.0	70	13%
wheat/light	1 slice	<1.0	40	11%
white				
iron kids	1 slice	1.0	60	15%
light	1 slice	<1.0	40	11%
(Roman Meal)				
light				
oat bran	2 slices	1.0	80	11%
100% whole wheat	2 slices	1.0	80	11%
7-grain	2 slices	1.0	80	11%
wheat				
hearty	2 slices	1.0	80	11%
regular	2 slices	1.0	80	11%
wheat berry	2 slices	1.0	80	11%
white	2 slices	1.0	80	11%
original				
round top	1 slice	1.0	70	13%
sandwich	2 slices	1.5	110	12%
w/oat bran	1 slice	1.0	70	13%
premium				
honey nut oat bran	1 slice	2.0	75	24%
honey oat bran	1 slice	1.0	70	13%
100% whole wheat	1 slice	1.0	65	14%
100% whole-grain	1 slice	1.0	90	10%
raisin	1 slice	1.0	70	13%
7-grain	1 slice	1.0	70	13%
wheat/natural	1 slice	1.0	90	10%

Food and Description	Amount	Fat Grams	Total Calories	% Fat Calories
(Rubschlager)				
cocktail breads				
honey whole grain	3 slices	1.0	80	11%
pumpernickel	3 slices	1.0	80	11%
rye	3 slices	1.5	80	17%
regular				
Komissbrot/German-style	1 slice	1.0	70	13%
pumpernickel				
Danish	1 slice	1.0	70	13%
Westphalian	1 slice	0.5	70	6%
rye				
Jewish deli	1 slice	1.0	70	13%
marble	2 slices	1.5	110	12%
sandwich	1 slice	2.0	90	20%
Swedish limpa	1 slice	1.0	60	15%
sandwich				
malt	1 slice	2.0	90	20%
rye	1 slice	2.0	90	20%
wheat	1 slice	2.0	90	20%
whole-grain/European-style	1 slice	2.0	80	23%
(Sahara) (*See* (Thomas') in this section)				
(Sara Lee) pita bread				
plain	1 pita	1.0	160	6%
whole wheat	1 pita	1.0	160	6%
(Sunbeam)				
family	2 slices	2.0	120	15%
king				
round top	2 slices	2.0	120	15%
sandwich	2 slices	2.0	120	15%
w/buttermilk	2 slices	2.0	120	15%
one-pound	1 slice	1.0	70	13%
(The Great Dakotas Baking Co.)				
blueberry walnut	1 slice	3.5	100	32%
pesto	1 slice	1.0	80	11%
raisin walnut-wheat	1 slice	3.5	100	32%
(Thomas')				
date nut loaf	1 slice	2.0	80	23%
Sahara pita bread				
oat	1 pita	1.0	130	7%
onion	1 pita	0.5	140	3%
original				
large, 4 per pkg	1 pita	1.0	220	4%
mini, 8 per pkg	1 pita	–	70	–
regular, 6 or 12 per pkg	1 pita	1.0	150	6%
sourdough	1 pita	0.5	150	3%
whole wheat				
mini, 8 per pkg	1 pita	0.5	60	9%
regular, 6 per pkg	1 pita	1.0	130	7%

Food and Description	Amount	Fat Grams	Total Calories	% Fat Calories
(Wolferman's) toasting breads				
cinnamon & raisin	1 slice	1.0	120	8%
heartland harvest	1 slice	1.0	110	8%
honey nut	1 slice	1.5	120	11%
oatmeal cinnamon	1 slice	2.0	120	15%
original	1 slice	–	110	–
sourdough	1 slice	–	110	–
(Wonder)				
DiCarlo				
French/Parisian	1 slice	1.0	70	13%
sourdough	1 slice	1.0	70	13%
Good Hearth				
buttermilk	1 slice	1.0	70	13%
French sourdough	1 slice	2.0	100	18%
honey wheat	1 slice	1.0	90	10%
honey whole grain	1 slice	1.0	100	9%
Home Pride				
butter top	1 slice	1.0	70	13%
regular	1 slice	1.0	70	13%
soft	1 slice	1.0	70	13%
100% whole wheat				
regular	1 slice	1.0	70	13%
soft	1 slice	1.0	70	13%
7-grain	1 slice	1.0	70	13%
stone-ground	1 slice	1.0	70	13%
wheat				
light	1 slice	–	40	–
regular	1 slice	1.0	70	13%
Wonder				
cinnamon-raisin	1 slice	1.0	80	11%
French				
light	2 slices	–	80	–
regular	1 slice	1.0	70	13%
Hollywood				
dark	1 slice	1.0	70	13%
light	1 slice	1.0	70	13%
Italian				
family	1 slice	1.0	70	13%
light	2 slices	1.0	80	11%
light/fat-free	1 slice	–	40	–
multigrain/beefsteak	1 slice	1.0	70	13%
Oatmeal Goodness	1 slice	2.0	90	20%
rye				
beefsteak				
hearty	1 slice	1.0	70	13%
light/fat-free	1 slice	–	40	–
mild	1 slice	1.0	70	13%
onion	1 slice	1.0	70	13%

Food and Description	Amount	Fat Grams	Total Calories	% Fat Calories
regular	1 slice	1.0	70	13%
soft				
wheat berry	1 slice	1.0	70	13%
Braun's Old Allegheny	1 slice	1.0	70	13%
regular	1 slice	1	70	13%
sourdough				
light	2 slices	–	80	–
light/fat-free	1 slice	–	40	–
wheat				
beefsteak				
hearty	1 slice	1.0	70	13%
soft	1 slice	1.0	70	13%
country grain	1 slice	1.0	70	13%
cracked	1 slice	1.0	70	13%
family	1 slice	1.0	70	13%
fresh & natural	1 slice	1.0	70	13%
golden/country style	1 slice	0.5	70	6%
high-fiber	1 slice	–	40	–
light/fat-free	1 slice	–	40	–
white				
beefsteak robust	1 slice	1.0	70	13%
calcium-enriched				
light	2 slices	1.0	80	11%
regular	1 slice	1.0	70	13%
high-fiber	1 slice	–	40	–
light	2 slices	–	80	–
light/fat-free	1 slice	–	40	–
regular	1 slice	–	70	13%
large loaf	1 slice	1.0	80	11%
small loaf	2 slices	1.5	110	12%
thin sandwich				
regular	1 slice	1.0	60	15%
w/buttermilk	1 slice	1.0	70	13%
■ REFRIGERATED				
(Pillsbury)				
cornbread twists	1 twist	6.0	130	42%
French loaf	⅛ loaf	1.0	150	6%
pipin' hot loaf	⅙ loaf	0.5	110	4%
BREAD COATING (See BAKE & FRY MIX; SEASONINGS)				
BREAD CRUMBS (See also BAKE & FRY MIX; SEASONINGS)				
(Contadina)	⅓ cup	1.5	100	14%
(Devonsheer)				
Italian	¼ cup	2.0	100	18%
plain	¼ cup	1.5	100	14%
(Friday's) seasoned	1 oz	–	56	–
generic				
plain	1 oz	1.0	110	8%
	1 cup	5.0	425	12%

Food and Description	Amount	Fat Grams	Total Calories	% Fat Calories
seasoned	1 oz	1.0	105	9%
	1 cup	3.0	440	6%
(Kellogg's) corn flake crumbs	2 Tbs	–	40	–
(Old London)				
plain	¼ cup	1.5	100	14%
seasoned	¼ cup	2.0	100	18%
(Progresso)				
lemon-herb	¼ cup	1.0	100	9%
plain	¼ cup	1.5	100	14%
seasoned	¼ cup	2.0	100	18%
tomato-basil	¼ cup	1.5	120	11%
BREAD CUBES (See CROUTONS; STUFFING/DRESSING)				
BREAD PUDDING (See PUDDING & MOUSSE)				
BREAD STUFFING (See also STUFFING/DRESSING)				
dry	1 cup	31.0	500	56%
moist	1 cup	26.0	420	56%
BREADFRUIT/raw	¼ small	–	99	–
	1 cup	0.5	227	2%
BREADSTICK				
(Angonoa)				
mini				
cheese	1 oz	2.0	110	16%
pizza	1 oz	2.0	120	15%
sesame	1 oz	4.0	120	30%
whole wheat	1 oz	4.0	120	30%
regular				
cheese	1 oz	2.0	110	16%
garlic	1 oz	2.0	120	15%
Italian	1 oz	2.0	120	15%
onion	1 oz	3.0	120	23%
sesame royal	1 oz	4.0	120	30%
(Continental Baking)				
Bread du Jour sourdough	1 piece	1.0	130	7%
(Fattorie & Pandea)				
traditional	3 pieces	1.0	60	15%
whole wheat	3 pieces	1.0	60	15%
generic/brown & serve				
garlic	1 piece	<1.0	70	6%
Italian soft	1 piece	1.0	80	11%
(Lance)				
cheese	4 pieces	1.0	50	18%
garlic	4 pieces	1.0	50	18%
plain	4 pieces	1.0	50	18%
sesame	4 pieces	2.0	60	30%
(Oroweat)				
cheese	1 oz	2.0	110	16%
garlic	1 oz	2.0	113	16%
plain	1 oz	2.0	110	16%

Food and Description	Amount	Fat Grams	Total Calories	% Fat Calories
sesame	1 oz	2.0	120	15%
(Pepperidge Farm)				
brown & serve	1 piece	1.5	150	9%
cheddar cheese/thin	7 pieces	2.5	70	32%
onion/thin	7 pieces	2.0	70	26%
sesame/thin	7 pieces	1.5	60	23%
(Pillsbury) soft/refrigerated	1 piece	2.5	110	20%
(Stella D'Oro)				
garlic				
deli/fat-free	5 pieces	–	60	–
Grissini/fat-free	3 pieces	–	60	–
regular	1 piece	1.0	35	26%
traditional/fat-free	2 pieces	–	70	–
onion	1 piece	1.0	40	23%
original				
deli/fat-free	5 pieces	–	60	–
Grissini/fat-free	3 pieces	–	60	–
traditional/fat-free	2 pieces	–	70	–
pizza	1 piece	1.0	43	21%
sesame				
low-fat	2 pieces	1.0	70	13%
sodium-free	1 piece	3.0	50	54%
wheat	1 piece	1.0	40	21%
(Toufayan) soft				
cinnamon-raisin	1 piece	2.0	110	16%
onion	1 piece	2.0	110	16%
plain	1 piece	2.0	110	16%

BREAKFAST BAR (*See* GRANOLA/GRANOLA-TYPE BAR)
BREAKFAST DRINK (*See also* NUTRITIONAL SUPPLEMENT)
(NOTE: Unless otherwise noted, mixes are prepared according to package directions)

Food and Description	Amount	Fat Grams	Total Calories	% Fat Calories
(Alba) Dairy Shake				
chocolate	8 fl oz	–	70	–
double fudge	8 fl oz	–	70	–
vanilla	8 fl oz	–	70	–
(Carnation) Instant Breakfast				
liquid ready to drink				
cafe mocha	10 fl oz	2.5	220	10%
milk chocolate/creamy	10 fl oz	2.5	220	10%
French vanilla	10 fl oz	3.0	200	14%
strawberry creme	10 fl oz	3.0	220	12%
powdered mix				
cafe mocha				
mix only	1 envelope	0.5	130	3%
prepared w/8 oz skim milk	9 fl oz	1.0	220	4%
chocolate malt/classic				
no sugar added				
mix only	1 envelope	1.5	70	19%
prepared w/8 oz skim milk	9 fl oz	3.0	160	17%

Food and Description	Amount	Fat Grams	Total Calories	% Fat Calories
regular				
mix only	1 envelope	1.5	130	10%
prepared w/8 oz skim milk	9 fl oz	3.0	220	12%
French vanilla				
no sugar added				
mix only	1 envelope	–	70	–
prepared w/8 oz skim milk	9 fl oz	1.0	150	6%
regular				
mix only	1 envelope	–	130	–
prepared w/8 oz skim milk	9 fl oz	1.0	220	4%
milk chocolate/creamy				
no sugar added				
mix only	1 envelope	1.0	70	13%
prepared w/8 oz skim milk	9 fl oz	2.0	160	11%
regular				
mix only	1 envelope	1.0	130	7%
prepared w/8 oz skim milk	9 fl oz	2.0	220	8%
strawberry creme				
no sugar added				
mix only	1 envelope	–	70	–
prepared w/8 oz skim milk	9 fl oz	1.0	150	6%
regular				
mix only	1 envelope	–	130	–
prepared w/8 oz skim milk	9 fl oz	1.0	220	4%
(Lucerne) Instant Breakfast				
chocolate	1 serving	1.0	130	7%
coffee	1 serving	–	130	–
vanilla	1 serving	–	130	–
(Pillsbury) Instant Breakfast				
chocolate-chocolate malt				
mix only	1 pkg	1.0	140	6%
prepared w/8 oz skim milk	1 serving	1.5	220	6%
strawberry				
mix only	1 pkg	1.0	140	6%
prepared w/8 oz skim milk	1 serving	1.5	220	6%
vanilla				
mix only	1 pkg	1.0	140	6%
prepared w/8 oz skim milk	1 serving	1.5	220	6%
BREAKFAST SANDWICH (*See also* individual FAST FOOD listings)				
(Amy's) breakfast burrito ranchero	6 oz	5.0	230	20%
(Bob Evans) Snackwich				
ham & cheese bagel	2 bagels	6.0	240	23%
sausage biscuit	2 biscuits	28.0	300	84%
sausage burrito	2 burritos	19.0	340	50%
(Don Miguel) frozen				
bacon & egg	1 sandwich	27.0	520	47%
sausage	1 sandwich	27.0	510	48%
smoked ham	1 sandwich	17.0	420	36%

Food and Description	Amount	Fat Grams	Total Calories	% Fat Calories
(Hormel)				
biscuits				
sausage	1 biscuit	22.0	350	57%
sausage & cheese	1 biscuit	26.0	410	57%
sausage & egg	1 biscuit	24.0	390	55%
steak	1 biscuit	14.0	320	39%
muffins				
Canadian bacon, egg, & cheese	1 muffin	9.0	260	31%
sausage, egg, & cheese	1 muffin	23.0	390	53%
(Jimmy Dean)				
bagels				
ham & Swiss	1 bagel	5.0	230	20%
ham, egg, & cheese	1 bagel	10.0	270	33%
sausage & cheese	1 bagel	19.0	330	52%
sandwiches				
chicken	2 sandwiches	13.0	280	42%
sausage/pork	2 sandwiches	21.0	330	57%
sausage/turkey & pork/lite	2 sandwiches	10.0	220	41%
steak/beef	2 sandwiches	10.0	280	32%
(Krusteaz) Breakfast In A Biscuit				
ham & cheese	1 biscuit	8.0	260	28%
sausage	1 biscuit	13.0	290	40%
veggie	1 biscuit	7.0	240	26%
(Owens) Border Breakfasts				
sandwiches				
ham 'n cheese	1 sandwich	6.0	150	36%
sausage	1 sandwich	14.0	210	60%
smoked sausage	1 sandwich	12.0	200	54%
tacos				
ham	2 tacos	6.0	90	60%
sausage	2 tacos	12.0	190	57%
(Schwan's) frozen				
Bright Starts				
bacon singles	1 sandwich	25.0	440	51%
breakfast burrito	1 burrito	17.0	280	55%
Western singles	1 sandwich	24.0	420	51%
other				
cinnamon-raisin	1 biscuit	15.0	300	45%
ham steak 'n egg muffin	1 muffin	10.0	250	36%
sausage & biscuit	1 twin pack	23.0	340	61%
sausage & gravy biscuit	1 biscuit	15.0	350	39%
(Swanson) Great Starts				
biscuits				
egg, bacon, & cheese	1 biscuit	19.0	360	48%
egg, sausage, & cheese	1 biscuit	30.0	490	55%
burritos				
bacon	1 burrito	11.0	250	40%
ham & cheese	1 burrito	6.0	210	26%

Food and Description	Amount	Fat Grams	Total Calories	% Fat Calories
hot w/spicy	1 burrito	7.0	220	29%
original	1 burrito	8.0	200	36%
pizza w/cheese & pepperoni	1 burrito	9.0	240	34%
sausage	1 burrito	12.0	240	45%
muffin/egg & Canadian bacon	1 muffin	15.0	290	47%
(Weight Watchers)				
bagel sandwich/ham & cheese	1 sandwich	5.0	200	23%
English muffin sandwich	1 sandwich	7.0	230	27%
omelet sandwich				
classic	1 sandwich	5.0	220	20%
garden vegetable	1 sandwich	6.0	220	25%
sausage biscuit	1 sandwich	11.0	230	43%
BREATH MINT (See CANDY)				
BREWER'S YEAST (See YEAST)				
BROAD BEAN				
canned	½ cup	<1.0	91	5%
fresh				
boiled	½ cup	<1.0	93	5%
raw				
immature	8 oz	1.0	238	4%
mature	8 oz	3.8	766	5%
BROCCOLI (See also BROCCOLI DISH)				
fresh				
cooked				
chopped	½ cup	–	23	–
florets				
(Dole)	3 oz	0.5	25	18%
spears				
(Dole)	1 medium	1.0	40	23%
raw/chopped	½ cup	–	12	–
frozen				
(Birds Eye)				
chopped	3.3 oz	–	25	–
cuts	3.3 oz	–	25	–
florets	3.3 oz	–	25	–
spears				
baby deluxe	3.3 oz	–	30	–
regular	3.3 oz	–	25	–
(C&W)				
florets	5 florets	–	25	–
microwave Brocclettes	1 cup	–	30	–
generic				
chopped	10 oz	<1.0	75	10%
spears	10 oz	1.0	85	11%
(Green Giant)				
chopped/select poly bag	¾ cup	–	25	–
cuts				
plain poly bag	1 cup	–	25	–

Food and Description	Amount	Fat Grams	Total Calories	% Fat Calories
regular	⅔ cup	–	25	–
florets	1⅓ cups	–	25	–
spears				
regular	3.5 oz	–	25	–
select poly bag	3 oz	–	25	–
(Pictsweet) spears	3.3 oz	–	25	–
(Seneca)	1 cup	–	25	–
(Stokely) cuts	3 oz	–	25	–

BROCCOLI DISH (*See also* FROZEN ENTRÉE/DINNER; VEGETABLES, MIXED; VEGETARIAN FOODS)

frozen				
(Birds Eye)				
broccoli stir-fry	1 cup	–	30	–
butter sauce combinations/spears	3.3 oz	2.0	45	40%
generic/spears w/butter sauce	½ cup	–	58	–
(Green Giant)				
broccoli in cheese-flavored sauce	⅔ cup	2.5	70	32%
spears in butter sauce	4 oz	1.5	50	27%
(Pepperidge Farm) vegetables in pastry				
broccoli w/cheese	1 pastry	14.0	240	53%
(Stokely) Singles				
broccoli in cheese sauce	4 oz	4.0	80	45%

BROCCOLI SOUP (*See* SOUP)
BROTWURST (*See* SAUSAGE)
BROWNIE/BLONDIE (*See also* CAKE; CAKE, SNACK; COOKIE)

frozen				
(Weight Watchers)				
à la mode	6.42 oz	4.0	190	19%
cheesecake	3.5 oz	6.0	200	27%
chocolate frosted	1.25 oz	3.0	100	27%
peanut butter fudge	1.23 oz	2.5	110	20%
homemade/USDA Standard Home Recipe				
butterscotch/1¾" x 1¾" x ⅞"	1 brownie	5.0	115	39%
plain	~1 oz	7.0	115	55%
w/nuts	~1 oz	8.0	105	69%
mix				
(Arrowhead Mills) prepared				
fat-free	1 brownie	–	120	–
regular	1 brownie	<1.0	110	4%
wheat-free	1 brownie	2.0	120	15%
(Betty Crocker)				
brownies				
caramel				
mix only	⅛ pkg	2.0	130	14%
prepared	1 brownie	9.0	190	43%
chocolate chip				
mix only	⅛ pkg	3.5	140	23%
prepared	1 brownie	10.0	200	45%

Food and Description	Amount	Fat Grams	Total Calories	% Fat Calories
cookies & cream				
mix only	1/18 pkg	3.0	140	19%
prepared	1 brownie	10.0	200	45%
dark chocolate fudge				
mix only	1/18 pkg	2.0	130	14%
prepared	1 brownie	8.0	190	38%
frosted				
mix only	1/18 pkg	3.5	170	19%
prepared	1 brownie	10.0	230	43%
fudge/prepared				
low-fat	1 brownie	2.5	130	17%
regular				
family size	1 brownie	9.0	200	41%
regular size	1 brownie	8.0	190	38%
German chocolate				
mix only	1/18 pkg	3.0	160	17%
prepared	1 brownie	9.0	220	37%
hot fudge				
mix only	1/18 pkg	4.0	140	26%
prepared	1 brownie	9.0	190	43%
original				
mix only	1/18 pkg	2.0	140	13%
prepared	1 brownie	9.0	200	41%
peanut butter candies w/Reese's Pieces				
mix only	1/18 pkg	3.5	150	21%
prepared	1 brownie	10.0	210	43%
walnut				
mix only	1/18 pkg	4.0	140	26%
prepared	1 brownie	11.0	200	50%
white chocolate swirl				
mix only	1/18 pkg	3.5	150	21%
prepared	1 brownie	10.0	210	43%
microwave brownie sundaes/mix only				
caramel	1/4 pkg	13.0	400	29%
cookies & cream	1/4 pkg	15.0	380	36%
hot fudge	1/4 pkg	15.0	390	35%
(Duncan Hines)				
chewy recipe fudge				
19.8-oz box				
mix only	1/18 pkg	3.0	130	21%
prepared	1 brownie	7.0	160	39%
12.9-oz box				
mix only	1/12 pkg	3.0	130	21%
prepared	1 brownie	7.0	160	39%
dark chocolate flavor fudge				
regular				
mix only	1/18 pkg	3.0	120	23%

Food and Description	Amount	Fat Grams	Total Calories	% Fat Calories
prepared	1 brownie	8.0	170	42%
w/milk chocolate chunks				
mix only	1/20 pkg	4.0	140	26%
prepared	1 brownie	7.0	160	39%
double fudge				
mix only	1/20 pkg	3.0	140	20%
prepared	1 brownie	7.0	170	37%
milk chocolate chunk				
mix only	1/20 pkg	4.0	140	26%
prepared	1 brownie	7.0	170	37%
peanut butter				
mix only	1/20 pkg	3.5	130	24%
prepared	1 brownie	8.0	160	45%
turtle				
mix only	1/18 pkg	4.0	140	26%
prepared	1 brownie	6.0	160	34%
walnut				
mix only	1/20 pkg	4.5	140	29%
prepared	1 brownie	8.0	170	42%
(Estee)	1/8 pkg	4.0	100	36%
(Obie's)				
deluxe fudge/2¼" square	1 brownie	–	120	–
(Pillsbury)				
deluxe mixes				
chocolate				
mix only	1/20 pkg	3.0	140	19%
prepared	1 brownie	7.0	180	35%
cream cheese swirl				
mix only	1/20 pkg	5.0	140	32%
prepared	1 brownie	9.0	180	45%
fudge				
15-oz box				
mix only	1/16 pkg	2.5	110	20%
prepared	1 brownie	6.0	150	36%
21.5-oz box				
mix only	1/20 pkg	2.5	130	17%
prepared	1 brownie	8.0	180	35%
hot fudge				
mix only	1/24 pkg	3.5	130	24%
prepared	1 brownie	7.0	160	39%
Lovin' Lites fudge				
mix only	1/16 pkg	3.0	150	18%
prepared	1 brownie	3.5	160	20%
walnut				
mix only	1/18 pkg	5.0	140	32%
prepared	1 brownie	9.0	180	45%
SnackWell's/fudge	1 brownie	2.5	150	15%

Food and Description	Amount	Fat Grams	Total Calories	% Fat Calories
ready to serve				
(Dolly Madison)				
low-fat	1.48 oz	3.0	150	18%
regular				
individual	2.96 oz	11.0	340	29%
multi-pack	1.6 oz	6.0	180	30%
(Drake's) fudge nut/reduced fat	1 brownie	2.5	170	13%
(Dunkin' Donuts)				
blondie w/chocolate chips	1 blondie	13.0	300	39%
fudge brownie	1 brownie	13.0	290	40%
peanut butter blondie	1 blondie	18.0	330	49%
(Eagle) fudge w/chocolate chips	1 brownie	11.0	260	38%
(Entenmann's) fudge/fat-free	1/10 strip	–	110	–
(Famous Amos) chocolate/fat-free	1 brownie	–	130	–
(Frookie) fudge/fat-free	1 brownie	–	110	–
generic				
chocolate w/frosting	~3/4 oz	4.0	100	36%
plain	1 oz	5.0	115	39%
	2 oz	9.0	230	35%
w/nuts	1 oz	10.0	250	36%
(Greenfield) fat-free				
apple spice blondie	1 blondie	–	120	–
chocolate chip blondie	1 blondie	–	120	–
homestyle	1 brownie	–	120	–
(Health Valley) w/fudge filling/fat-free	1 brownie	–	110	–
(Hostess) Brownie Bites				
light, low-fat	1 brownie	2.5	140	16%
plain	5 brownies	14.0	260	48%
w/walnuts	5 brownies	15.0	270	50%
(Lance) Fudge Nut	2 3/4 oz	13.0	340	34%
(Little Debbie)				
fudge	1.2 oz	13.0	270	43%
	2.5 oz	15.0	310	44%
	3.59 oz	21.0	450	42%
light, low-fat	1.9 oz	3.0	190	14%
(Pepperidge Farm)				
blondie	1 blondie	–	120	–
chocolate	1 brownie	–	120	–
chocolate chip	1 brownie	–	120	–
(Sara Lee) fresh fudge nut	1 brownie	14.0	160	79%
(Tastykake) fudge walnut	1 brownie	17.0	370	41%
refrigerated				
(Pillsbury) fudge	1 brownie	6.0	160	34%
BRUSSELS SPROUTS				
fresh				
cooked	1/2 cup	–	30	–
raw	1/2 cup	–	20	–
(Dole)	1/2 cup	–	19	–

Food and Description	Amount	Fat Grams	Total Calories	% Fat Calories
frozen				
(Birds Eye)				
baby	3.3 oz	–	35	–
regular	3.3 oz	–	35	–
(C&W) petite	10 sprouts	–	30	–
generic	½ cup	–	33	–
(Green Giant)	½ cup	–	25	–
(Freshlike)	3.3 oz	–	35	–
(Pictsweet)				
regular	3.3 oz	–	35	–
express microwave	2.5 oz	–	30	–
(Stokely)	3 oz	–	35	–
BRUSSELS SPROUTS DISH				
(Green Giant) baby, in butter sauce	⅔ cup	1.5	60	23%
(Stokely) singles, in butter sauce	4 oz	1.0	50	18%
BUCKWHEAT GROATS/KASHA				
(Arrowhead Mills) brown	¼ cup	1.0	140	6%
(Wolff's) roasted kernels/cooked	½ cup	1.0	170	5%
BUFFALO/BISON				
cooked				
(Denver Buffalo Co.)				
buffalo burgers	4 oz	5.2	130	36%
ground	4 oz	17.0	250	61%
dried	4 oz	2.0	149	12%
raw	4 oz	1.6	112	13%
roasted	3 oz	2.0	148	12%
BULGUR/HARD RED WINTER WHEAT				
cooked				
(Arrowhead Mills)	¼ cup	1.0	160	6%
generic	1 cup	<1.0	152	3%
dry/canned				
seasoned	1 cup	4.5	246	17%
unseasoned	1 serving	0.9	227	4%
uncooked	1 cup	3.0	600	5%
BUN (See PASTRY; ROLL)				
BURBOT/raw	3 oz	0.7	76	8%
BURDOCK ROOT				
cooked	1 cup	<1.0	110	4%
raw	1 cup	<1.0	85	5%
BURGER (See BEEF; BUFFALO; HAMBURGER; TURKEY; VEGETARIAN FOODS)				
BURGER MIX (See BEEF DISH/ENTRÉE; VEGETARIAN FOODS)				
BURRITO (See BREAKFAST SANDWICH; MEXICAN FOOD; VEGETARIAN FOODS)				
BUTTER (See also BUTTER BLEND, BUTTER-FLAVORED SEASONING; MARGARINE, MARGARINE SPREAD, & SPRAY)				
(Breakstone)				
stick/salted or unsalted	1 Tbs	11.0	100	100%
whipped/salted or unsalted	1 Tbs	7.0	70	100%

Food and Description	Amount	Fat Grams	Total Calories	% Fat Calories
(Darigold)				
stick/salted or unsalted	1 tsp	4.0	35	100%
whipped/salted or unsalted	1 tsp	3.0	25	100%
generic				
stick/salted or unsalted	1 pat	4.0	36	100%
	1 Tbs	11.0	100	100%
	½ cup	92.0	810	100%
whipped/salted or unsalted	1 pat	3.0	27	100%
	1 Tbs	9.0	81	100%
	½ cup	61.0	542	100%
(Hotel Bar)	1 tsp	4.0	35	100%
(Keller's)	1 tsp	4.0	35	100%
(Land O'Lakes)				
light				
stick/salted or unsalted	1 Tbs	5.5	50	100%
whipped	1 Tbs	4.0	35	100%
stick/salted or unsalted	1 Tbs	11.0	100	100%
whipped/salted or unsalted	1 Tbs	7.0	60	100%
BUTTER BEAN (See also LIMA BEAN)				
canned				
(Bush Bros)				
baby	½ cup	–	120	–
green	½ cup	–	110	–
large	½ cup	–	100	–
speckled	½ cup	–	110	–
(Green Giant)	½ cup	–	90	–
(Joan of Arc)	½ cup	–	90	–
(Luck's) speckled/seasoned w/pork	½ cup	3.0	140	19%
(S&W) tender cooked/dry	½ cup	–	70	–
(Trappey's) large white	½ cup	1.0	80	11%
(Van Camp's)	1 cup	1.0	160	6%
BUTTER BLEND (See also HONEY BUTTER)				
(Blue Bonnet)				
stick w/tub	1 Tbs	11.0	90	100%
	4 oz	44.0	360	100%
(Buttery Blend) liquid	1 Tbs	14.0	120	100%
(Kraft) Touch of Butter				
bowl	1 Tbs	6.0	50	100%
squeeze bottle	1 Tbs	9.0	80	100%
stick/50% fat	1 Tbs	10.0	90	100%
(Land O'Lakes) Country Morning Blend				
stick				
light	1 Tbs	6.0	50	100%
regular/salted or unsalted	1 Tbs	11.0	100	100%
tub				
light	1 Tbs	6.0	50	100%
regular	1 Tbs	11.0	100	100%

Food and Description	Amount	Fat Grams	Total Calories	% Fat Calories
BUTTERBUR				
cooked	½ cup	<1.0	8	56%
raw	1 cup	<1.0	13	35%
BUTTERFISH/raw	3 oz	6.8	124	49%
BUTTER-FLAVORED SEASONING (*See also* SEASONINGS)				
(Best O' Butter)				
cheddar cheese flavor	½ tsp	<1.0	6	60%
garlic buttery	½ tsp	<1.0	4	90%
original	½ tsp	<1.0	4	90%
sour cream flavor	½ tsp	<1.0	4	90%
(Butter Buds)				
butter-flavored mix	1 Tbs	–	6	–
butter-flavored salt	any amount	–	–	–
(Molly McButter) sprinkles				
butter	1 tsp	–	5	–
cheese	1 tsp	–	5	–
garlic & herb	1 tsp	–	5	–
BUTTERNUT/dried	1 oz	16.0	174	83%

C

Food and Description	Amount	Fat Grams	Total Calories	% Fat Calories
CABBAGE (*See also* SWAMP CABBAGE)				
canned or jarred				
(Aunt Nellie's)				
pickled	1 cup	<1.0	260	2%
red/sweet & sour	2 Tbs	–	15	–
(S&W) red/sweet & sour	2 Tbs	–	15	–
fresh				
Chinese/bok choy/napa				
cooked	½ cup	–	10	–
raw/shredded	½ cup	–	5	–
(Dole)	½ cup	–	5-6	–
Danish				
shredded	½ cup	–	20	–
whole/2-lb head	1 head	2.0	225	8%
red/raw/shredded	½ cup	–	10	–
(Dole)	3 oz	–	25	–
Savoy/raw	1 cup	–	12	–
spoon/raw	1 cup	–	37	–

Food and Description	Amount	Fat Grams	Total Calories	% Fat Calories
white				
cooked	½ cup	–	16	–
raw/shredded	½ cup	–	12	–
CABBAGE DISH (*See also* ASIAN FOOD; FROZEN ENTRÉE/DINNER)				
homemade/USDA Standard Home Recipe				
coleslaw/made w/regular mayonnaise	⅔ cup	10.0	150	60%
stuffed cabbage	~5 oz	18.0	310	52%
CACTUS				
(Embassa)	⅔ cup	–	5	–
(La Costena)				
Napolitos tender cactus	1 cup	–	20	–
CAKE (*See also* BROWNIE; CAKE, SNACK; DONUT; MUFFIN; PASTRY; POPCORN BARS & CAKES; RICE CAKES)				
■ **FROZEN OR REFRIGERATED**				
(ChefPierre) food service products				
cheesecake/10" dia				
French cream	1/10 cake	28.0	410	61%
dessert cups				
Boston cream pie	1 cup	11.0	310	32%
strawberry shortcake	1 cup	9.0	210	39%
layer cake/9" dia				
apple spice	1/21 cake	17.0	310	49%
carrot	1/18 cake	20.0	340	53%
chocolate cream	1/18 cake	11.0	260	38%
chocolate gold	1/18 cake	12.0	300	36%
coconut	1/18 cake	14.0	310	41%
double chocolate	1/20 cake	14.0	320	39%
German chocolate	1/20 cake	15.0	310	44%
lemon cream	1/16 cake	12.0	290	37%
walnut cream	1/16 cake	12.0	290	37%
(Pepperidge Farm)				
layer cake				
chocolate fudge	⅙ cake	16.0	300	48%
chocolate fudge stripe	⅙ cake	14.0	290	43%
coconut	⅙ cake	14.0	300	42%
devil's food	⅙ cake	14.0	290	43%
German chocolate	⅙ cake	16.0	300	48%
golden	⅙ cake	14.0	290	43%
strawberry stripe	⅙ cake	13.0	310	38%
vanilla	⅙ cake	13.0	290	40%
pound cake/all butter	⅕ cake	13.0	290	40%
special recipe cake				
Boston creme pie	⅛ cake	9.0	260	31%
chocolate mousse	⅛ cake	10.0	250	36%
deluxe carrot	⅛ cake	16.0	310	46%
lemon mousse	⅛ cake	12.0	250	43%
pineapple cream	1/9 cake	10.0	240	39%
strawberry cream	1/9 cake	9.0	230	35%

Food and Description	Amount	Fat Grams	Total Calories	% Fat Calories
(Sara Lee)				
food service				
brunch cake/apple	1/21 cake	15.0	290	47%
Cake Sensations				
Best Banana Chocolate Chip	1/4 cake	27.0	590	41%
Chocolate Razz	1/4 cake	28.0	590	43%
Tropical Tidal Wave	1/4 cake	24.0	540	40%
World's Greatest Carrot	1/4 cake	37.0	700	48%
cheesecake				
French cream				
round	1/10 cake	22.0	360	55%
tray pack	1/6 cake	24.0	390	55%
old-fashioned				
butter pecan	1/6 cake	31.0	440	63%
chocolate marble	1/6 cake	30.0	430	63%
creamy	1/6 cake	31.0	420	66%
double chocolate	1/6 cake	27.0	420	58%
homestyle	1/4 cake	16.0	280	51%
New York style				
plain	1/6 cake	28.0	410	61%
crumb cake				
blueberry	1 cake	5.0	180	25%
French	1 cake	4.5	180	23%
Desserts Elite				
cheesecake				
caramel pecan	1/4 cake	37.0	520	64%
fudge truffle	1/4 cake	32.0	460	63%
mocha swirl	1/6 cake	35.0	500	63%
white chocolate tuxedo	1/4 cake	28.0	420	60%
chocolate torte	1/20 torte	24.0	370	58%
flourless chocolate indulgence	1/4 cake	34.0	520	59%
flourless lemon torte	1/4 torte	31.0	510	55%
Irish cream mousse cake	1/12 cake	23.0	430	48%
homestyle cake				
apple cranberry	1/5 cake	14.0	320	39%
banana chocolate chip	1/5 cake	12.0	320	34%
blueberry yogurt	1/5 cake	11.0	300	33%
lemon poppy seed	1/4 cake	10.0	300	30%
iced sheet cake				
banana	1/24 cake	10.0	290	31%
carrot	1/32 cake	15.0	290	47%
chocolate	1/22 cake	13.0	310	38%
coconut	1/22 cake	14.0	320	39%
German chocolate	1/20 cake	14.0	300	42%
orange	1/22 cake	13.0	310	38%
individually wrapped cake				
banana	1 cake	10.0	240	38%
brownie	1 piece	11.0	230	43%

Food and Description	Amount	Fat Grams	Total Calories	% Fat Calories
carrot	1 cake	15.0	260	52%
chocolate	1 cake	9.0	200	9%
pound	1 cake	9.0	190	9%
layer cake				
old-fashioned				
carrot				
precut	1/14 cake	27.0	490	50%
uncut	1/21 cake	18.0	330	49%
chocolate				
precut	1/14 cake	18.0	370	44%
uncut	1/16 cake	16.0	320	45%
German chocolate				
precut	1/14 cake	23.0	430	48%
uncut	1/20 cake	17.0	300	51%
whipped cream				
Black Forest	1/14 cake	10.0	210	43%
carrot cream	1/12 cake	15.0	260	52%
celebration/6" dia	1/6 cake	15.0	280	48%
chocolate delight	1/10 cake	15.0	280	54%
coconut breeze	1/12 cake	14.0	250	50%
lemon chiffon	1/12 cake	12.0	240	45%
peach 'n cream	1/14 cake	9.0	200	41%
raspberry dream	1/12 cake	11.0	260	38%
strawberry cloud	1/14 cake	9.0	210	39%
walnut cream	1/10 cake	15.0	280	48%
pound cake				
original/large	1/8 cake	13.0	300	39%
reduced fat/large	1/8 cake	3.5	220	14%
retail				
carrot cake	1/8 cake	17.0	320	48%
cheesecake				
cherry cream	1/4 cake	12.0	350	31%
chocolate swirl	1/4 cake	14.0	330	38%
French	1/6 cake	21.0	350	54%
original	1/4 cake	18.0	350	46%
strawberry	1/4 cake	12.0	330	33%
strawberry French	1/6 cake	14.0	320	39%
coffee cake				
butter streusel	1/6 cake	12.0	220	49%
crumb coffee	1/8 cake	9.0	220	37%
pecan	1/6 cake	12.0	220	49%
layer cake				
double chocolate	1/8 cake	13.0	260	45%
flaky coconut	1/8 cake	14.0	280	45%
fudge golden	1/8 cake	13.0	270	43%
German chocolate	1/8 cake	15.0	280	48%
pound cake				
regular	1/4 cake	16.0	320	45%

Food and Description	Amount	Fat Grams	Total Calories	% Fat Calories
strawberry swirl	¼ cake	11.0	290	34%
(Weight Watchers)				
caramel fudge à la mode	6.07 oz	3.0	180	15%
cheesecake				
brownie	3.5 oz	6.0	200	27%
toasted almond amaretto	3 oz	5.0	170	26%
triple chocolate	3.15 oz	5.0	200	23%
▣ HOMEMADE				
USDA Standard Home Recipe				
angel food	1/12 cake	–	140	–
Boston creme pie	1/8 cake	12.0	290	37%
caramel/8" dia				
w/caramel icing	1/12 cake	12.0	315	34%
w/o icing	1/12 cake	10.0	218	42%
carrot w/cream cheese frosting/ 10" dia	1/10 cake	21.0	385	49%
cheesecake/9" dia	1/12 cake	18.0	280	58%
chocolate/9" dia				
w/chocolate icing	1/12 cake	16.0	385	40%
w/o icing	1/12 cake	13.0	272	43%
chocolate torte/8½" dia	1/16 cake	22.0	317	63%
coffeecake				
cheese w/crumb topping	1/6 cake	12.0	260	42%
cinnamon w/crumb topping	1/9 cake	15.0	260	52%
fruit	1/8 cake	5.0	160	28%
cottage pudding				
w/chocolate sauce	3 oz	8.7	315	25%
w/o sauce	3 oz	8.0	251	29%
devil's food w/chocolate icing/9" dia	1/16 cake	8.0	235	31%
fruitcake/dark/7½" dia	1/32 cake	7.0	165	38%
gingerbread/8" square	1/9 cake	4.0	175	21%
pineapple upside down	1/9 cake	14.0	365	35%
pound cake/8½" x 3½" x 3¼"	1/17 cake	5.0	120	38%
prune whip/baked				
cold	1 cup	–	203	–
hot	1 cup	–	140	–
sheet cake/9" square				
w/no-cook white frosting	1/9 cake	14.0	445	28%
w/o frosting	1/9 cake	12.0	314	334%
spice w/brown sugar frosting/9" dia	1/10 cake	16.0	411	35%
sponge/tube/9¾" dia	1/12 cake	3.8	196.0	17%
white/9" dia				
w/coconut frosting	1/16 cake	10.0	289	31%
w/white frosting	1/16 cake	9.0	260	28%
yellow/9" dia				
w/caramel frosting	1/16 cake	9.5	293	29%
w/chocolate frosting	1/16 cake	11.0	245	40%

Food and Description	Amount	Fat Grams	Total Calories	% Fat Calories
■ **MIX**				
(Betty Crocker)				
Classic Dessert				
Boston creme pie/prepared	1/10 pie	4.5	200	20%
chocolate pudding cake				
mix only	1/8 pkg	3.0	160	17%
prepared	1/8 cake	3.5	170	19%
date bar/prepared	1 bar	7.0	160	39%
gingerbread fun kit/prepared	2 pieces	4.5	150	27%
golden pound cake				
mix only	1/8 pkg	11.0	270	37%
prepared	1/8 cake	13.0	290	40%
lemon chiffon cake				
mix only	1/16 pkg	2.5	140	16%
prepared	1/16 cake	3.0	140	19%
lemon pudding cake				
mix only	1/8 pkg	3.0	160	17%
prepared	1/8 cake	4.0	180	20%
pineapple upside down cake				
mix only	1/6 pkg	10.0	350	26%
prepared	1/6 cake	15.0	400	34%
Super Moist				
angel food/prepared				
chocolate swirl	1/12 cake	–	150	–
confetti	1/12 cake	–	150	–
lemon custard	1/12 pkg	–	140	–
one-step white	1/12 pkg	–	140	–
traditional	1/12 pkg	–	130	–
butter chocolate				
mix only	1/12 pkg	4.5	190	21%
prepared	1/12 cake	13.0	270	43%
butter pecan				
mix only	1/12 pkg	3.5	180	18%
prepared	1/12 cake	11.0	250	40%
butter yellow				
mix only	1/12 pkg	2.0	170	11%
prepared	1/12 cake	11.0	260	38%
carrot cake				
mix only	1/10 pkg	4.0	210	17%
prepared	1/10 cake	13.0	300	39%
cherry chip				
mix only	1/10 pkg	4.5	210	19%
prepared	1/10 cake	12.0	280	39%
chocolate chip				
mix only	1/12 pkg	4.0	180	20%
prepared	1/12 cake	14.0	280	45%
chocolate fudge				
mix only	1/12 pkg	4.0	180	20%

Food and Description	Amount	Fat Grams	Total Calories	% Fat Calories
prepared	1/12 cake	11.0	250	40%
devil's food				
light				
mix only	1/10 pkg	3.0	210	13%
prepared	1/10 cake	4.5	230	18%
regular				
mix only	1/12 pkg	4.5	180	23%
prepared	1/12 cake	12.0	250	43%
double chocolate swirl				
mix only	1/12 pkg	4.5	180	23%
prepared	1/12 cake	12.0	250	43%
French vanilla				
mix only	1/12 pkg	3.0	180	15%
prepared	1/12 cake	10.0	250	36%
fudge marble				
mix only	1/12 pkg	3.5	180	18%
prepared	1/12 cake	11.0	250	40%
German chocolate				
mix only	1/12 pkg	4.0	180	20%
prepared	1/12 cake	11.0	250	40%
golden vanilla				
mix only	1/12 pkg	4.0	180	20%
prepared	1/12 cake	14.0	280	45%
lemon				
mix only	1/12 pkg	3.5	180	18%
prepared	1/12 cake	11.0	250	40%
milk chocolate				
mix only	1/12 pkg	4.5	180	23%
prepared	1/12 cake	12.0	250	43%
party swirl				
mix only	1/12 pkg	3.5	180	18%
prepared	1/12 cake	11.0	250	40%
peanut chocolate swirl				
mix only	1/12 pkg	4.0	180	20%
prepared	1/12 cake	10.0	240	38%
rainbow chip				
mix only	1/12 pkg	4.0	180	20%
prepared	1/12 cake	11.0	250	40%
sour cream white				
mix only	1/10 pkg	5.0	210	21%
prepared	1/10 cake	12.0	280	39%
spice				
mix only	1/12 pkg	4.0	180	20%
prepared	1/12 cake	11.0	250	40%
strawberry swirl				
mix only	1/10 pkg	3.0	200	14%
prepared	1/10 cake	12.0	290	37%

Food and Description	Amount	Fat Grams	Total Calories	% Fat Calories
white				
light				
mix only	1/10 pkg	3.5	210	15%
prepared	1/10 cake	3.5	210	15%
regular				
mix only	1/12 pkg	4.0	180	20%
prepared	1/12 cake	10.0	240	38%
white chocolate swirl				
mix only	1/12 pkg	3.5	180	18%
prepared	1/12 cake	11.0	250	40%
yellow				
light				
mix only	1/10 pkg	3.0	210	13%
prepared	1/10 cake	4.5	230	18%
regular				
mix only	1/12 pkg	2.5	170	13%
prepared	1/12 cake	10.0	250	36%
Supreme Dessert Bar				
caramel oatmeal				
mix only	1/20 pkg	6.0	160	34%
prepared	1 bar	8.0	180	40%
chocolate chunk				
mix only	1/20 pkg	5.0	150	30%
prepared	1 bar	9.0	180	45%
chocolate peanut butter				
mix only	1/20 pkg	5.0	150	30%
prepared	1 bar	7.0	170	37%
easy layer				
mix only	1/20 pkg	5.0	150	30%
prepared	1 bar	8.0	170	42%
raspberry				
mix only	1/20 pkg	4.0	150	24%
prepared	1 bar	6.0	170	32%
strawberry swirl cheesecake				
mix only	1/24 pkg	6.0	130	42%
prepared	1 bar	10.0	180	50%
Sunkist lemon				
mix only	1/24 pkg	3.5	130	24%
prepared	1 bar	4.0	140	26%
Sweet Rewards/fat-free/prepared				
apple cinnamon	1/8 cake	–	170	–
Chiquita banana	1/8 cake	–	170	–
chocolate	1/8 cake	–	160	–
lemon	1/8 cake	–	170	–
(Dromedary) pound cake				
mix only	1/8 pkg	10.0	260	35%
prepared	1/12 cake	11.0	250	40%

Food and Description	Amount	Fat Grams	Total Calories	% Fat Calories
(Duncan Hines)				
angel food				
mix only	½12 pkg	–	140	–
prepared	½12 cake	–	140	–
banana supreme				
mix only	½12 pkg	4.0	180	20%
prepared	½12 cake	11.0	250	40%
butter recipe fudge				
mix only	½10 pkg	6.0	220	25%
prepared	½10 cake	17.0	320	48%
butter recipe golden				
mix only	½10 pkg	5.0	230	20%
prepared	½10 cake	16.0	320	45%
caramel				
mix only	½12 pkg	4.0	180	20%
prepared	½12 cake	11.0	250	40%
devil's food				
mix only	½12 pkg	4.0	180	20%
prepared	½12 cake	15.0	290	47%
Dutch dark fudge				
mix only	½12 pkg	4.0	180	20%
prepared	½12 cake	15.0	290	47%
French vanilla				
mix only	½12 pkg	4.0	180	20%
prepared	½12 cake	11.0	250	40%
fudge marble				
mix only	½12 pkg	4.0	180	20%
prepared	½12 cake	11.0	250	40%
lemon supreme				
mix only	½12 pkg	4.0	180	20%
prepared	½12 cake	11.0	250	40%
orange supreme				
mix only	½12 pkg	4.0	180	20%
prepared	½12 cake	11.0	250	40%
pineapple supreme				
mix only	½12 pkg	4.0	180	20%
prepared	½12 cake	11.0	250	40%
raspberry				
mix only	½12 pkg	4.0	180	20%
prepared	½12 cake	11.0	250	40%
spice				
mix only	½12 pkg	4.0	180	20%
prepared	½12 cake	11.0	250	40%
strawberry supreme				
mix only	½12 pkg	4.0	180	20%
prepared	½12 cake	11.0	250	40%
Swiss chocolate				
mix only	½12 pkg	4.0	180	20%

Food and Description	Amount	Fat Grams	Total Calories	% Fat Calories
prepared	1/12 cake	15.0	290	47%
white				
mix only	1/12 pkg	4.0	180	20%
prepared	1/12 cake	10.0	240	38%
yellow				
mix only	1/12 pkg	4.0	180	20%
prepared	1/12 cake	10.0	240	38%
(Estee) prepared				
chocolate	1/5 cake	4.0	190	19%
lemon	1/5 cake	4.0	200	18%
pound cake	1/5 cake	4.0	200	18%
white	1/5 cake	4.0	200	18%
(Jell-O) no-bake dessert/cheesecake				
blueberry				
mix only	1/8 pkg	4.0	220	16%
prepared	1/8 cake	12.0	320	34%
cherry				
mix only	1/8 pkg	4.0	230	59%
prepared	1/8 cake	12.0	330	33%
homestyle				
mix only	1/6 pkg	4.0	220	16%
prepared	1/6 cake	15.0	360	38%
real				
mix only	1/6 pkg	5.0	220	20%
prepared	1/6 cake	16.0	350	41%
strawberry				
mix only	1/8 pkg	4.0	240	15%
prepared	1/8 cake	12.0	340	32%
(Pillsbury)				
bundt cake				
chocolate caramel nut				
mix only	1/16 pkg	7.0	180	35%
prepared	1/16 cake	18.0	190	56%
double hot fudge				
mix only	1/16 pkg	5.0	180	25%
prepared	1/16 cake	16.0	280	51%
strawberry cream cheese				
mix only	1/16 pkg	5.0	190	24%
prepared	1/16 cake	17.0	300	51%
deluxe bar				
apple streusel				
mix only	1/24 pkg	4.5	130	31%
prepared	1 bar	6.0	150	36%
lemon cheesecake				
mix only	1/24 pkg	9.0	170	48%
prepared	1 bar	10.0	180	50%
Moist Supreme				
angel food/prepared	1/12 cake	–	140	–

Food and Description	Amount	Fat Grams	Total Calories	% Fat Calories
banana				
mix only	½ pkg	4.0	180	20%
prepared	½ cake	11.0	260	38%
butter recipe				
mix only	½ pkg	3.0	170	16%
prepared	½ cake	12.0	260	42%
butter recipe chocolate				
mix only	½ pkg	4.0	180	20%
prepared	½ cake	13.0	270	43%
carrot				
mix only	½ pkg	4.0	180	20%
prepared	½ cake	12.0	260	42%
chocolate				
mix only	½ pkg	4.0	180	20%
prepared	½ cake	11.0	250	40%
chocolate chip				
mix only	½ pkg	5.0	190	24%
prepared	½ cake	10.0	240	38%
dark chocolate				
mix only	½ pkg	4.0	180	20%
prepared	½ cake	11.0	250	40%
devil's food				
Lovin' Lites				
mix only	⅒ pkg	4.5	210	19%
prepared	⅒ cake	5.0	230	20%
regular				
mix only	½ pkg	4.0	180	20%
prepared	½ cake	14.0	270	47%
French vanilla				
mix only	½ pkg	5.0	220	20%
prepared	½ cake	13.0	300	39%
fudge swirl				
mix only	½ pkg	4.5	200	20%
prepared	½ cake	10.0	250	36%
Funfetti				
mix only	½ pkg	4.5	190	21%
prepared	½ cake	9.0	240	34%
German chocolate				
mix only	½ pkg	4.0	180	20%
prepared	½ cake	11.0	250	40%
lemon				
mix only	⅒ pkg	4.0	210	17%
prepared	⅒ cake	13.0	300	39%
strawberry				
mix only	½ pkg	4.0	180	20%
prepared	½ cake	11.0	260	38%
sunshine vanilla				
mix only	½ pkg	5.0	190	24%

Food and Description	Amount	Fat Grams	Total Calories	% Fat Calories
prepared	1/12 cake	12.0	260	42%
white				
Lovin' Lites				
mix only	1/10 pkg	4.0	210	17%
prepared	1/10 cake	5.0	230	20%
regular				
mix only	1/12 pkg	5.0	220	20%
prepared	1/12 cake	11.0	280	35%
white 'n fudge swirl				
mix only	1/12 pkg	4.5	200	20%
prepared	1/12 cake	10.0	250	36%
yellow				
Lovin' Lites				
mix only	1/10 pkg	4.0	220	16%
prepared	1/10 cake	5.0	230	20%
regular				
mix only	1/12 pkg	4.0	180	20%
prepared	1/12 cake	10.0	240	38%
Pillsbury Plus				
angel food/prepared	1/10 cake	–	150	–
banana				
mix only	1/12 pkg	4.0	180	20%
prepared	1/12 cake	11.0	260	38%
butter recipe				
mix only	1/12 pkg	3.0	170	16%
prepared	1/12 cake	12.0	260	42%
butter recipe chocolate				
mix only	1/12 pkg	4.0	180	20%
prepared	1/12 cake	13.0	270	43%
carrot				
mix only	1/12 pkg	4.5	190	21%
prepared	1/12 cake	12.0	260	42%
chocolate				
mix only	1/12 pkg	4.5	180	23%
prepared	1/12 cake	12.0	260	42%
chocolate chip				
mix only	1/12 pkg	5.0	190	24%
prepared	1/12 cake	10.0	240	38%
dark chocolate				
mix only	1/12 pkg	4.5	180	23%
prepared	1/12 cake	12.0	250	4%
devil's food				
Lovin' Lites				
mix only	1/10 pkg	4.5	210	19%
prepared	1/10 cake	5.0	230	20%
regular				
mix only	1/12 pkg	4.0	180	23%
prepared	1/12 cake	14.0	270	47%

Food and Description	Amount	Fat Grams	Total Calories	% Fat Calories
French vanilla				
mix only	1/12 pkg	6.0	230	23%
prepared	1/12 cake	15.0	320	42%
fudge swirl				
mix only	1/12 pkg	5.0	200	23%
prepared	1/12 cake	12.0	270	40%
Funfetti				
mix only	1/12 pkg	4.5	190	21%
prepared	1/12 cake	9.0	240	34%
German chocolate				
mix only	1/12 pkg	4.0	180	20%
prepared	1/12 cake	11.0	250	40%
lemon				
mix only	1/10 pkg	4.0	210	17%
prepared	1/10 cake	13.0	310	38%
strawberry				
mix only	1/12 pkg	4.0	180	20%
prepared	1/12 cake	11.0	260	38%
sunshine vanilla				
mix only	1/12 pkg	5.0	190	24%
prepared	1/12 cake	12.0	260	42%
white				
Lovin' Lites				
mix only	1/10 pkg	4.0	210	17%
prepared	1/10 cake	5.0	230	20%
regular				
mix only	1/10 pkg	5.0	220	20%
prepared	1/10 cake	11.0	280	35%
white 'n fudge				
mix only	1/12 pkg	4.5	200	20%
prepared	1/12 cake	10.0	250	36%
yellow				
Lovin' Lites				
mix only	1/10 pkg	4.0	220	16%
prepared	1/10 cake	5.0	230	20%
regular				
mix only	1/12 pkg	4.0	180	20%
prepared	1/12 cake	11.0	250	40%
Streusel Swirl/cinnamon				
mix only	1/16 pkg	5.0	210	21%
prepared	1/16 cake	11.0	260	38%
(Robin Hood) pouch				
devil's food				
mix only	1/5 pkg	5.0	190	50%
prepared	1/5 cake	17.0	310	49%
yellow				
mix only	1/5 pkg	4.0	190	19%
prepared	1/5 cake	13.0	280	42%

Food and Description	Amount	Fat Grams	Total Calories	% Fat Calories
(Royal) No-Bake				
cheesecake				
original				
mix only	⅙ pkg	5.0	230	20%
prepared	⅙ cake	15.5	380	37%
whipped/lite				
mix only	⅛ pkg	4.0	120	30%
prepared	⅛ cake	5.0	190	24%
Mississippi mud				
mix only	⅙ pkg	6.0	250	22%
prepared	⅙ cake	14.5	370	35%
(Vermont Country Maple) prepared				
chocolate	1 slice	2.0	290	6%
gingerbread	1 slice	1.0	270	3%
■ READY TO SERVE				
(Awrey's)				
Best Wishes/6" dia	¼ cake	9.0	150	54%
Black Forest torte	¹⁄₁₄ cake	21.0	350	54%
carrot cake				
supreme/iced	1 slice	12.0	210	51%
3-layer/cream cheese icing	¹⁄₁₂ cake	23.0	390	53%
chocolate/2-layer w/white icing	¹⁄₁₂ cake	15.0	270	50%
coconut & yellow cake/3-layer	¹⁄₁₂ cake	21.0	350	54%
coconut butter cream cake	1 slice	9.0	160	51%
double chocolate cake				
iced	1 slice	6.0	130	42%
3-layer	¹⁄₁₂ cake	14.0	310	41%
2-layer	¹⁄₁₂ cake	11.0	250	40%
double chocolate torte	¹⁄₁₄ cake	15.0	340	40%
German chocolate cake				
iced	2" square	9.0	260	31%
3-layer	¹⁄₁₂ cake	18.0	350	46%
golden pound cake	¹⁄₁₄ loaf	5.0	130	35%
lemon & yellow cake/2-layer	¹⁄₁₂ cake	17.0	290	53%
lemon cake/3-layer	¹⁄₁₂ cake	19.0	320	53%
milk chocolate & yellow cake/2-layer	¹⁄₁₂ cake	17.0	290	53%
Neapolitan torte	¹⁄₁₄ cake	22.0	380	52%
orange cake				
frosty w/icing	1 slice	8.0	150	
3-layer	¹⁄₁₂ cake	17.0	320	48%
pistachio torte	¹⁄₁₂ cake	22.0	370	54%
sponge cake	2" square	3.0	80	34%
strawberry supreme torte	¹⁄₁₄ cake	12.0	270	40%
walnut torte	¹⁄₁₄ cake	19.0	320	53%
(Entenmann's)				
fat-free				
apple spice cake	⅛ cake	–	130	–
banana loaf	⅛ cake	–	150	–

Food and Description	Amount	Fat Grams	Total Calories	% Fat Calories
blueberry crunch coffeecake	⅛ cake	–	140	–
carrot cake	⅛ cake	–	170	–
chocolate crunch	⅛ cake	–	130	–
chocolate loaf	⅛ loaf	–	130	–
cinnamon apple coffeecake	⅛ cake	–	130	–
creme filled chocolate	1 slice	–	160	–
fudge iced chocolate cake	⅙ cake	–	210	–
fudge iced gold cake	⅙ cake	–	220	–
golden chocolatey chip loaf	⅛ loaf	–	130	–
golden French crumb cake	⅛ cake	–	140	–
golden loaf	⅛ loaf	–	120	–
Louisiana crunch	⅙ cake	–	220	–
marble loaf	⅛ loaf	–	130	–
mocha iced chocolate	⅙ cake	–	200	–
raisin loaf	⅛ loaf	–	140	–
original				
all butter French crumb	⅛ cake	10.0	210	43%
all butter loaf	⅙ loaf	10.0	220	41%
banana crunch	⅛ cake	9.0	220	37%
carrot cake	⅛ cake	16.0	290	50%
cheese coffeecake	⅑ cake	8.0	190	39%
cheese filled crumb coffeecake	⅛ cake	10.0	210	43%
chocolate fudge	⅙ cake	14.0	310	41%
crumb coffeecake	1/10 cake	12.0	250	43%
Louisiana crunch	⅙ cake	13.0	310	38%
marble loaf	⅛ loaf	10.0	200	45%
marshmallow iced devil's food cake	⅙ cake	18.0	350	46%
raisin loaf	⅛ loaf	9.0	220	37%
sour cream chip & nut loaf	⅛ loaf	14.0	240	24%
thick fudge golden cake	⅙ cake	16.0	330	44%
(Formagg) Le Creme				
amaretto almond	2 oz	6.0	115	47%
pineapple	2 oz	6.0	115	47%
plain	2 oz	6.0	115	47%
strawberry	2 oz	6.0	115	47%
(Sara Lee) retail/fresh				
angel food/fat-free	⅕ cake	–	210	–
chocolate fudge/reduced fat	⅙ cake	3.0	250	11%
chocolate loaf/reduced fat	¼ cake	6.0	260	21%
golden loaf/reduced fat	¼ cake	6.0	250	22%
pound cake	¼ cake	12.0	290	37%

CAKE, SNACK

■ HOMEMADE

USDA Standard Home Recipe (Note: Homemade cakes were made with vegetable shortening. Homemade frostings were made with margarine.)

cupcake				
chocolate				
w/chocolate frosting	1 cupcake	8.0	175	41%

Food and Description	Amount	Fat Grams	Total Calories	% Fat Calories
w/o frosting	1 cupcake	5.0	103	44%
white				
w/chocolate frosting	1 cupcake	8.0	186	39%
w/white frosting	1 cupcake	6.0	165	33%
w/o frosting	1 cupcake	5.0	114	35%
yellow				
w/chocolate frosting	1 cupcake	8.0	195	37%
w/o frosting	1 cupcake	5.0	125	36%
■ READY TO SERVE				
(Dolly Madison)				
angel food ring	2 oz	1.5	160	8%
apple crumb cake				
2 per pkg	2 piece	10.0	330	27%
6 per pkg	1 piece	5.0	170	26%
bar cakes				
angel food				
mini	1 piece	1.5	180	8%
regular	2 oz	1.5	160	8%
devil's food	2.8 oz	14.0	330	38%
spice	2.8 oz	17.0	350	44%
white	2.8 oz	14.0	320	39%
buttercrumb cake				
2 per pkg	2 pieces	11.0	340	29%
3 per pkg	1 piece	6.0	180	30%
6 per pkg	1 piece	6.0	170	32%
cake delights				
2 per pkg	2 pieces	12.0	280	39%
6 per pkg	1 piece	6.0	140	39%
carrot cake/individual	1 piece	8.0	360	20%
cinnamon swirl coffee	1 piece	6.0	170	32%
coconut layer cake	3 oz	9.0	300	27%
coffeecake	2 pieces	11.0	270	37%
creme boat				
2 per pkg	2 pieces	9.0	300	27%
3 per pkg	1 piece	13.0	430	27%
4 per pkg	2 pieces	10.0	320	28%
creme cakes				
3 per pkg	3 pieces	12.0	340	32%
4 per pkg	4 pieces	15.0	420	32%
7 per pkg	3 pieces	12.0	320	34%
10 per pkg	3 pieces	12.0	330	33%
crumb cake/low-fat				
2 per pkg	2 pieces	3.0	280	9%
6 per pkg	1 piece	1.5	140	10%
cupcakes				
chocolate				
2 per pkg	2 pieces	10.0	390	23%
3 per pkg	1 piece	5.0	190	24%

Food and Description	Amount	Fat Grams	Total Calories	% Fat Calories
6 per pkg	1 piece	5.0	190	24%
8 per pkg	1 piece	5.0	190	24%
spice				
2 per pkg	2 pieces	20.0	470	38%
3 per pkg	1 piece	10.0	230	39%
6 per pkg	1 piece	10.0	230	39%
dessert roll				
lemon	1 piece	2.5	260	8%
plain	1 piece	2.0	230	8%
Flips				
banana flip	1 piece	15.0	410	33%
devil's food flip	1 piece	14.0	380	33%
sweet potato flip	1 piece	15.0	310	44%
German chocolate cake				
6 per pkg	1 piece	9.0	220	37%
2 per pkg	2 pieces	19.0	450	38%
Goggles	2 pieces	10.0	420	21%
Koo Koo's	2 pieces	17.0	400	38%
pound cake				
mini	1 piece	13.0	370	32%
½ ring	3 oz	13.0	360	33%
whole ring	2.5 oz	11.0	310	32%
shortcake	1 piece	2.0	110	16%
squares				
raspberry				
2 per pkg	2 pieces	15.0	370	36%
3 per pkg	3 pieces	22.0	560	35%
6 per pkg	1 piece	7.0	190	33%
snack				
2 per pkg	2 pieces	19.0	400	43%
3 per pkg	3 pieces	29.0	610	43%
6 per pkg	1 piece	10.0	210	43%
Zingers				
chocolate				
4 per pkg	4 pieces	14.0	470	27%
7 per pkg	2 pieces	8.0	280	26%
12 per pkg	2 pieces	8.0	260	26%
raspberry				
3 per pkg	3 pieces	17.0	440	35%
4 per pkg	2 pieces	11.0	300	33%
7 per pkg	2 pieces	11.0	290	34%
12 per pkg	2 pieces	11.0	300	33%
yellow				
3 per pkg	3 pieces	12.0	400	27%
4 per pkg	4 pieces	15.0	530	25%
(Drake)				
Boston creme	1 piece	8.0	170	42%

Food and Description	Amount	Fat Grams	Total Calories	% Fat Calories
coffee cakes				
low-fat	1 piece	1.5	100	14%
original	1 piece	6.0	130	42%
Devil Dogs	1 piece	7.0	170	37%
Funny Bones	2 pieces	12.0	300	36%
Ring Dings	2 pieces	14.0	320	39%
Sunny Doodles				
40% less fat	2 pieces	4.5	180	23%
original	2 pieces	8.0	220	33%
Yankee Doodles	2 pieces	9.0	220	37%
Yodels	2 pieces	16.0	280	51%
generic				
devil's food cupcake w/creme filling	1 cake	4.0	105	34%
(Hostess)				
angel food ring	⅙ cake	3.0	150	18%
apple spice lights	1 cake	1.0	130	7%
Brownie Bites				
plain	5 pieces	14.0	260	48%
walnut	5 pieces	15.0	270	50%
Chocodiles	1 cake	11.0	240	41%
chocolate lights	2 cakes	3.0	270	10%
Chocolicious	2 cakes	14.0	370	34%
crumb coffeecake				
cinnamon/light	3 cakes	1.5	260	5%
original	3 cakes	14.0	360	35%
cupcakes				
chocolate	2 cupcakes	12.0	360	30%
orange	2 cupcakes	10.0	320	28%
dessert cups	1 cake	2.0	90	20%
Ding Dongs	2 cakes	17.0	320	48%
fruit loaf	1 piece	10.0	350	26%
Ho Ho's	3 cakes	18.0	370	43%
holiday fruitcake	⅛ cake	14.0	490	26%
holiday cakes	2 cakes	6.0	320	17%
King Dons	2 cakes	17.0	320	48%
Lil' Angels	1 cake	2.0	90	20%
pound cake	⅕ cake	16.0	350	41%
Snoballs	2 cakes	11.0	350	28%
Suzy Q's				
banana	1 cake	10.0	240	38%
original	1 cake	9.0	220	33%
Tiger Tails	1 cake	6.0	160	34%
Twinkies				
banana	2 cakes	13.0	300	39%
devil's food	2 cakes	12.0	300	36%
lights	2 cakes	3.0	260	10%
original	2 cakes	10.0	310	29%

Food and Description	Amount	Fat Grams	Total Calories	% Fat Calories
(Lance) fig				
fat-free	½ piece	–	100	–
original	½ piece	2.0	110	16%
(Little Debbie)				
angel cake/low-fat	1 pkg	1.0	120	8%
apple coffee streusel cake	1 pkg	7.0	230	27%
banana twins	1 pkg	10.0	250	36%
Be My Valentine cake				
chocolate				
boxed	1 pkg	13.0	270	43%
individual pkg	1 pkg	17.0	340	45%
vanilla/boxed	1 pkg	14.0	280	45%
cherry cordial	1 pkg	8.0	170	42%
Choc-O-Jel	1 pkg	7.0	150	42%
chocolate chip cake	1 pkg	14.0	270	47%
chocolate chip cupcake	1 pkg	15.0	290	47%
chocolate twins	1 pkg	9.0	250	33%
Christmas cake	1 pkg	13.0	260	45%
Christmas tree cake	1 pkg	10.0	190	47%
coconut creme cake	1 pkg	10.0	210	43%
coconut rounds	1 pkg	7.0	140	45%
coffeecake	1 pkg	7.0	230	27%
devil creme cake				
boxed	1 pkg	8.0	190	38%
individual pkg	1 pkg	16.0	370	39%
devil squares	1 pkg	13.0	270	43%
Easter basket cakes				
chocolate	1 pkg	14.0	290	43%
vanilla	1 pkg	15.0	310	44%
fancy cakes	1 pkg	15.0	300	45%
Figaroos/low-fat	1 pkg	2.5	150	15%
frosted fudge cake				
boxed	1 pkg	10.0	180	50%
individual pkg	1 pkg	14.0	270	47%
fudge rounds	1 pkg	6.0	140	39%
golden creme cake				
boxed	1 pkg	7.0	170	37%
individual pkg	1 pkg	12.0	280	39%
holiday cake roll				
cherry creme	1 pkg	13.0	270	43%
chocolate	1 pkg	14.0	300	42%
vanilla	1 pkg	16.0	310	46%
marshmallow supreme	1 pkg	5.0	130	35%
Nutty Bar	1 pkg	17.0	290	53%
oatmeal creme pie	1 pkg	8.0	170	42%
oatmeal lights/low-fat	1 pkg	2.5	130	17%
peanut butter & jelly sandwich	1 pkg	5.0	130	35%
peanut butter bar	1 pkg	15.0	270	50%

Food and Description	Amount	Fat Grams	Total Calories	% Fat Calories
peanut cluster	1 pkg	11.0	190	52%
raisin creme pie	1 pkg	5.0	140	32%
snack cake				
chocolate	1 pkg	17.0	360	43%
vanilla	1 pkg	18.0	370	44%
spice cake				
boxed	1 pkg	15.0	300	45%
individual pkg	1 pkg	13.0	270	43%
Star Crunch	1 pkg	6.0	140	39%
strawberry shortcake roll				
boxed	1 pkg	8.0	240	30%
individual pkg	1 pkg	11.0	290	34%
Swiss cake roll				
boxed	1 pkg	12.0	260	42%
2.7-oz pkg	1 pkg	15.0	320	42%
3.2-oz pkg	1 pkg	18.0	380	43%
Tiger Cake	1 pkg	15.0	310	44%
Zebra Cake				
boxed	1 pkg	16.0	330	44%
individual pkg	1 pkg	18.0	370	44%
(TastyKake)				
Creamies				
banana	1 cake	7.0	170	37%
chocolate	1 cake	7.0	180	35%
sprinkled	1 cake	6.0	150	36%
	2 cakes	11.0	310	32%
vanilla	1 cake	8.0	190	38%
witchy good treats	1 cake	6.0	150	36%
	2 cakes	11.0	310	32%
cupcakes				
mini/creme-filled				
butter cream	2 cakes	4.0	110	33%
	4 cakes	7.0	230	27%
chocolate iced	2 cakes	4.0	110	33%
	4 cakes	7.0	220	29%
chocolate iced vanilla	2 cakes	4.0	110	33%
	4 cakes	8.0	220	33%
koffee kake	2 cakes	4.0	110	33%
	4 cakes	9.0	210	39%
regular				
butter cream iced	2 cakes	8.0	250	29%
chocolate				
iced	2 cakes	8.0	250	29%
plain	2 cakes	6.0	220	25%
	3 cakes	9.0	330	25%
Koffee Kake	2 cakes	9.0	240	34%
Kreme Kup	2 cakes	6.0	190	28%

Food and Description	Amount	Fat Grams	Total Calories	% Fat Calories
Tasty Too/creme-filled				
chocolate	2 cakes	3.0	200	14%
vanilla	2 cakes	4.0	210	17%
juniors				
chocolate	1 cake	13.0	360	33%
coconut	1 cake	8.0	320	23%
Koffee Kake	1 cake	9.0	270	30%
pound Kake	1 cake	13.0	320	37%
Krimpets				
butterscotch iced	2 cakes	5.0	210	21%
	3 cakes	8.0	320	23%
jelly filled	2 cakes	3.0	190	14%
	3 cakes	4.0	280	13%
Kreme Krimpies	2 cakes	8.0	230	31%
	3 cakes	12.0	340	32%
strawberry iced	2 cakes	5.0	210	21%
	3 cakes	8.0	320	23%
Tasty Too				
jelly-filled	2 cakes	1.5	180	8%
lemon-filled	2 cakes	2.0	180	10%
Kandy Kakes				
chocolate	3 cakes	13.0	270	43%
	4 cakes	17.0	360	43%
coconut	3 cakes	13.0	260	45%
	4 cakes	17.0	350	44%
frosty	3 cakes	11.0	260	38%
	4 cakes	15.0	350	39%
peanut butter	3 cakes	14.0	280	45%
	4 cakes	19.0	370	46%

CAKE FROSTING/ICING (See also CAKE/COOKIE DECORATION)

Food and Description	Amount	Fat Grams	Total Calories	% Fat Calories
(Betty Crocker)				
mix				
creamy frosting				
coconut pecan				
mix only	3 Tbs	4.0	120	30%
prepared	2 Tbs	8.0	160	45%
chocolate fudge				
mix only	3 Tbs	1.5	110	12%
prepared	2 Tbs	4.5	140	29%
vanilla				
mix only	3 Tbs	1.5	110	12%
prepared	2 Tbs	4.0	130	28%
fluffy frosting/white				
mix only	3 Tbs	–	100	–
prepared	2 Tbs	–	100	–
ready to spread				
creamy deluxe				
butter cream	2 Tbs	6.0	160	34%

Food and Description	Amount	Fat Grams	Total Calories	% Fat Calories
butter pecan	2 Tbs	6.0	150	36%
caramel chocolate chip	2 Tbs	6.0	140	39%
cherry	2 Tbs	5.0	140	32%
chocolate chip cookie dough	2 Tbs	6.0	160	34%
chocolate chocolate chip	2 Tbs	7.0	150	42%
chocolate Swiss almond	2 Tbs	6.0	150	36%
chocolate w/dinosaurs/party	2 Tbs	5.0	150	30%
dark chocolate				
light	2 Tbs	1.0	120	8%
regular	2 Tbs	6.0	150	30%
milk chocolate				
light	2 Tbs	1.0	120	8%
regular	2 Tbs	6.0	150	36%
strawberry cream cheese	2 Tbs	6.0	150	36%
vanilla				
light	2 Tbs	0.5	120	4%
regular	2 Tbs	5.0	140	32%
w/bears/party	2 Tbs	5.0	140	32%
white chocolate	2 Tbs	5.0	140	32%
whipped deluxe				
cream cheese	2 Tbs	5.0	110	41%
lemon	2 Tbs	5.0	110	41%
strawberry	2 Tbs	5.0	110	41%
vanilla cream	2 Tbs	5.0	110	41%
(Duncan Hines) ready to spread				
berry blue	2 Tbs	5.0	140	32%
butter cream	2 Tbs	5.0	140	32%
caramel	2 Tbs	5.0	140	32%
cream cheese	2 Tbs	5.0	140	32%
chocolate	2 Tbs	5.0	130	35%
chocolate butter cream	2 Tbs	5.0	130	35%
dark chocolate	2 Tbs	5.0	130	35%
grape bubble gum	2 Tbs	5.0	140	32%
kiwi strawberry	2 Tbs	5.0	140	32%
lemon	2 Tbs	5.0	140	32%
mango tangerine	2 Tbs	5.0	140	32%
milk chocolate	2 Tbs	5.0	130	35%
peaches & cream	2 Tbs	5.0	140	32%
raspberries & cream	2 Tbs	5.0	140	32%
strawberries & cream	2 Tbs	5.0	140	32%
vanilla	2 Tbs	5.0	140	32%
wild cherry vanilla	2 Tbs	5.0	140	32%
(Estee) mix/all flavors/mix only	⅕ pkg	–	80	–
homemade/USDA Standard Home Recipe				
boiled	¼ cup	–	74	–
caramel	¼ cup	6.0	306	18%
chocolate	¼ cup	9.5	259	33%
coconut	¼ cup	5.0	300	15%

Food and Description	Amount	Fat Grams	Total Calories	% Fat Calories
white	¼ cup	5.0	300	15%
(Jiffy) mix/prepared				
fudge	¼ cup	4.0	150	24%
white	¼ cup	4.0	150	24%
(Pillsbury) ready to spread				
Creamy Supreme				
caramel pecan	2 Tbs	8.0	150	48%
chocolate	2 Tbs	6.0	140	39%
chocolate fudge				
original	2 Tbs	6.0	140	39%
reduced fat	2 Tbs	3.5	140	23%
coconut pecan	2 Tbs	10.0	160	56%
cream cheese	2 Tbs	6.0	150	36%
creamy candy	2 Tbs	7.0	150	42%
dark chocolate	2 Tbs	6.0	130	42%
French vanilla	2 Tbs	6.0	150	36%
Funfetti				
pink vanilla	2 Tbs	6.0	150	36%
vanilla	2 Tbs	6.0	150	36%
lemon creme	2 Tbs	6.0	150	36%
milk chocolate				
Lovin' Lites	2 Tbs	3.0	130	21%
regular	2 Tbs	6.0	140	39%
milk chocolate swirl w/fudge glaze	2 Tbs	6.0	140	39%
Oreo	2 Tbs	6.0	150	36%
strawberry creme	2 Tbs	6.0	150	36%
vanilla/Lovin' Lites	2 Tbs	3.0	140	19%
vanilla swirl w/fudge glaze	2 Tbs	6.0	150	36%
Frosting Supreme				
caramel pecan	2 Tbs	8.0	150	48%
chocolate	2 Tbs	6.0	140	39%
chocolate fudge				
original	2 Tbs	5.0	140	32%
reduced fat	2 Tbs	3.5	140	23%
coconut almond	2 Tbs	9.0	160	51%
coconut pecan	2 Tbs	10.0	160	56%
creamy candy	2 Tbs	7.0	150	42%
cream cheese	2 Tbs	6.0	150	36%
dark chocolate	2 Tbs	6.0	130	42%
French vanilla	2 Tbs	6.0	160	34%
Funfetti				
chocolate	2 Tbs	6.0	140	39%
pink	2 Tbs	6.0	150	36%
vanilla	2 Tbs	6.0	160	34%
lemon creme	2 Tbs	6.0	150	36%
milk chocolate				
Lovin' Lites	2 Tbs	3.0	130	21%
regular	2 Tbs	6.0	140	39%

Food and Description	Amount	Fat Grams	Total Calories	% Fat Calories
milk chocolate swirl w/fudge glaze	2 Tbs	6.0	140	39%
Oreo	2 Tbs	6.0	150	36%
strawberry creme	2 Tbs	6.0	150	36%
vanilla				
Lovin' Lites	2 Tbs	3.0	140	19%
regular	2 Tbs	6.0	150	36%
vanilla swirl w/fudge glaze	2 Tbs	6.0	150	36%
(Robin Hood) mix				
chocolate				
mix only	2 Tbs	1.5	110	12%
prepared	2 Tbs	5.0	140	32%
(Vermont Country Maple) mix/prepared				
delectable cocoa	1 Tbs	–	50	–
maple butter cream	1 Tbs	–	40	–
CAKE/COOKIE DECORATION (See also CAKE FROSTING/ICING)				
(Dec-A-Cake)				
all sugar crystals	1 tsp	–	15	–
bats/pumpkins	1 tsp	–	20	–
candy cards	4 gm	–	15	–
choco mint trims	1 tsp	0.5	15	30%
choco trims	1 tsp	0.5	15	30%
confetti	1 tsp	–	15	–
dec-a-cone	1 tsp	0.5	15	30%
decorating icing				
chocolate	1 tsp	0.5	20	23%
all other colors	1 tsp	0.5	25	18%
fruit cocktail	9 pieces	–	15	–
fun sprinkles	1 tsp	0.5	15	30%
harvest mix	1 tsp	0.5	15	30%
holiday sprinkles	1 tsp	0.5	15	30%
nonpareils	1 tsp	–	15	–
party imperials	9 pieces	–	15	–
pastel trims	1 tsp	0.5	15	30%
rainbow mix	1 tsp	0.5	15	30%
red/green trim	1 tsp	0.5	15	30%
red/white trim	1 tsp	0.5	15	30%
red/white/pink hearts	1 tsp	–	20	–
variety pack	1 tsp	0.5	15	30%
(McCormick/Schilling)				
decorating gel/all colors	1 tsp	–	25	–
decorating icing/all colors	1 tsp	1.0	35	26%
decors				
chocolate-flavored	1 tsp	1.0	20	45%
cinnamon	1 tsp	–	25	–
fruit flavored	1 tsp	–	25	–
nonpareil	1 tsp	–	15	–
snowflake	1 tsp	–	15	–

Food and Description	Amount	Fat Grams	Total Calories	% Fat Calories
sugar crystals/all colors	1 tsp	–	–	–
CALAMARI (*See* SQUID)				
CALIFORNIA RED BEAN/boiled	½ cup	–	109	–
CANADIAN BACON (*See* BACON, CANADIAN STYLE)				
CANDY				
■ ABRA CA BUBBLE (*See* (Brach's) in this section)				
■ (Allen Wertz)				
Coffee Time				
assorted	1 piece	1.0	30	30%
decaffeinated	1 piece	1.0	20	45%
■ ALMOND JOY (*See* (Hershey) in this section)				
■ ALMOND ROCA (*See* (Brown & Haley) in this section)				
■ ALPINE WHITE (*See* Nestle) in this section)				
■ (Andes)				
cherry jubilee thins	8 pieces	13.0	210	56%
creme de menthe wafers	8 pieces	13.0	210	56%
nut & honey thins	8 pieces	13.0	210	56%
orange mint thins	8 pieces	13.0	200	59%
parfait mints	8 pieces	13.0	210	56%
toasted coconut	8 pieces	13.0	210	56%
toffee crunch thins	8 pieces	12.0	210	51%
■ (Andre Prost)				
Honees Bars				
Eu-Mint	1 piece	–	20	–
Milk-N-Honees	1 piece	–	20	–
original	1 piece	–	20	–
Swedish peppermint creams	14 pieces	3.0	70	16%
Zotz				
Lotz-A-Zotz	1 piece	–	40	–
Mega Zotz	1 piece	–	15	–
pops	1 pop	–	40	–
strings	1 piece	–	15	–
■ A-OK (*See* (Nature's Warehouse) in this section)				
■ BABY RUTH (*See* (Nestle) in this section)				
■ BAR NONE (*See* (Hershey) in this section)				
■ (Beich)				
Laffy Taffy chews				
apple	1 oz	1.0	110	8%
banana	1 oz	1.0	110	8%
grape	1 oz	1.0	110	8%
passion punch	1 oz	1.0	110	8%
strawberry	1 oz	1.0	110	8%
sweet & sour cherry	1 oz	1.0	110	8%
watermelon	1 oz	1.0	110	8%
■ BIT-O-HONEY (*See* (Concorde) in this section)				
■ BLACK COW (*See* (Clark) in this section)				
■ BOUNTY (*See* (M&M★Mars) in this section)				

Food and Description	Amount	Fat Grams	Total Calories	% Fat Calories
■ (Brach's)				
Abra Ca Bubble	1 piece	–	40	–
bells/solid chocolate/foiled	1 oz	8.0	150	48%
bridge mix	14 pieces	8.0	190	38%
butterscotch disks	3 pieces	–	70	–
candy corn				
chickens	6 pieces	–	160	–
corn	26 pieces	–	150	–
rabbits	6 pieces	–	160	–
Chelsea Chips/chocolate-covered	1 oz	6.0	140	39%
cherries				
chocolate creme	1 oz	2.0	110	16%
chocolate-covered	1 oz	2.0	110	16%
dark chocolate covered	2 pieces	3.0	140	19%
milk chocolate covered	2 pieces	3.0	140	19%
chocolate-covered raisins	34 pieces	7.0	170	37%
Christmas ornaments	1 oz	8.0	150	48%
cinnamon candy				
disks	3 pieces	–	70	–
imperials	52 pieces	–	60	–
coffee candy	3 pieces	2.0	70	26%
Cookie Delites	40 pieces	10.0	210	43%
Crazy Pumpkin Heads	1 oz	1.0	100	9%
Double Dippers	15 pieces	14.0	220	57%
Easter eggs				
buttercream/chocolate-covered	1 oz	3.0	120	23%
cherry cream/chocolate-covered	1 oz	2.0	110	16%
coconut cream/chocolate-covered	1 oz	3.0	110	25%
fruit & nut cream/chocolate-covered	1 oz	2.0	110	16%
malted milk				
chocolate	5 pieces	5.0	180	25%
fiesta	5 pieces	5.0	180	25%
maple cream/chocolate-covered	1 oz	2.0	110	16%
marshmallow	1 oz	3.0	120	23%
pastel fiesta	1 oz	3.0	120	23%
PBM	1 oz	10.0	160	56%
solid chocolate	1 oz	8.0	150	48%
solid milk chocolate	8 pieces	11.0	200	50%
Fruit Bunch	3 pieces	–	150	–
Gumdinger gum balls	1 oz	2.0	110	16%
Gummi Bears				
regular	18 pieces	–	130	–
wild 'n fruity	15 pieces	–	130	–
Gummi Worms	5 pieces	–	120	–
heart box candies	1 oz	2.0	110	16%
hearts				
PBM	1 oz	9.0	150	54%

Food and Description	Amount	Fat Grams	Total Calories	% Fat Calories
Valentine	1 oz	2.0	110	16%
Hulachews/dark chocolate covered	1 oz	8.0	140	51%
jelly beans	14 pieces	–	140	–
jelly bird eggs	14 pieces	–	150	–
Jots				
chocolate	1 oz	5.0	130	35%
Christmas	1 oz	5.0	130	35%
mint	1 oz	2.0	120	15%
peanut	1 oz	6.0	140	39%
Jube Jels	1 oz	–	100	–
kisses				
peanut butter	4 pieces	6.0	170	32%
peppermint	4 pieces	2.0	150	12%
Valentine nougat	1 oz	2.0	110	16%
lemon drops	3 pieces	–	60	–
licorice				
red laces	1 oz	–	100	–
red twists	5 pieces	–	150	–
twists	1 oz	1.0	100	9%
Lollydrops	3 pieces	–	70	–
malt balls				
malted milk	15 pieces	9.0	190	43%
milk chocolate covered	1 oz	5.0	130	35%
maple nut goodies	7 pieces	9.0	190	43%
Milk Maid caramels				
chocolate	4 pieces	4.0	150	24%
regular	4 pieces	4.0	150	24%
mint-filled straws	1 oz	1.0	110	8%
mints				
chocolate-covered mints	1 oz	2.0	110	16%
creme de menthe	1 oz	9.0	150	54%
cremes/chocolate-covered	1 oz	2.0	110	16%
dessert	37 pieces	–	160	–
holiday	1 oz	1.0	110	8%
Kentucky	17 pieces	0.5	150	3%
patties/chocolate-covered	1 oz	2.0	110	16%
pearls				
Christmas	1 oz	1.0	110	8%
regular	1 oz	2.0	120	15%
starlight				
regular	3 pieces	–	60	–
spearmint	3 pieces	–	60	–
thin/chocolate-covered	1 oz	2.0	110	16%
Neapolitan coconuts	3 pieces	5.0	160	28%
nonpareils/dark chocolate				
Christmas	1 oz	6.0	140	39%
regular	1 oz	6.0	140	39%

Food and Description	Amount	Fat Grams	Total Calories	% Fat Calories
nougat				
Christmas	1 oz	2.0	110	16%
jelly	4 pieces	2.0	170	11%
nut goodies	1 oz	4.0	130	28%
orange slices	2 pieces	–	130	–
orange sticks/chocolate-covered	1 oz	2.0	110	16%
Orangettes	2 pieces	–	130	–
parfait				
mint	1 oz	9.0	150	54%
peanut	1 oz	10.0	160	56%
party mix	29 pieces	9.0	190	43%
PBM squares	1 oz	9.0	150	54%
peanut clusters				
milk chocolate covered	1 oz	9.0	150	54%
peanut-caramel	3 pieces	14.0	240	53%
regular	3 pieces	15.0	230	59%
peanuts				
chocolate-covered	1 oz	10.0	160	56%
circus	11 pieces	–	260	–
filled	1 oz	1.0	110	8%
French burnt	28 pieces	9.0	190	43%
milk chocolate covered	1 oz	9.0	150	54%
panned	1 oz	7.0	140	45%
petite	1 oz	9.0	150	54%
Putters/milk chocolate covered	1 oz	9.0	150	54%
rabbits				
chocolate-covered	4 pieces	7.0	200	32%
marshmallow	1 oz	3.0	120	23%
robin's eggs/solid milk chocolate	6 pieces	8.0	200	36%
Rocks	7 pieces	–	150	–
Royals	5 pieces	4.0	150	24%
salt water taffy	4 pieces	2.0	140	13%
Santas				
assortment	1 oz	2.0	110	16%
foiled/tray of 8	1 oz	7.0	140	45%
marshmallow	1 oz	3.0	120	23%
PBM	1 oz	10.0	160	56%
Snappy Tarts	6 pieces	–	150	–
Sour Sea Creatures	16 pieces	–	140	–
spearmint leaves	5 pieces	–	140	–
spice drops	12 pieces	–	130	–
Spicettes	12 pieces	–	130	–
Star Brites				
fruit candies	3 pieces	–	45	–
peppermint	3 pieces	–	60	–
stars				
Christmas	10 pieces	11.0	200	50%
chocolate	10 pieces	11.0	200	50%

Food and Description	Amount	Fat Grams	Total Calories	% Fat Calories
milk chocolate	1 oz	8.0	150	48%
Targets	4 pieces	4.0	160	23%
Ting-A-Ling	1 oz	8.0	150	48%
toffee				
butter	3 pieces	2.0	80	23%
Special Treasures International				
amaretto	3 pieces	2.0	80	23%
French vanilla	3 pieces	2.0	80	23%
Suisse mocha	3 pieces	2.0	80	23%
Twisters	5 pieces	1.0	160	6%
vanilla cream/chocolate-covered	1 oz	2.0	110	16%
wild 'n fruity	5 pieces	–	120	–
■ (Breath Savers)				
breath mints/sugar-free				
cinnamon	1 piece	–	10	–
iced mint	1 piece	–	10	–
peppermint	1 piece	–	10	–
spearmint	1 piece	–	10	–
vanilla mint	1 piece	–	10	–
wintergreen	1 piece	–	10	–
■ (Brown & Haley)				
Almond Roca	3 pieces	15.0	210	64%
■ BUNCHA CRUNCH (See (Nestle) in this section)				
■ BUTTERFINGER (See (Nestle) in this section)				
■ (Cadbury)				
Caramello/5-oz bar	5 blocks	9.0	190	43%
chocolate creme egg	1 egg	6.0	180	30%
dairy milk chocolate bar/5 oz	9 blocks	12.0	220	49%
fruit & nut bar/5 oz	9 blocks	11.0	210	47%
roasted almond bar/5 oz	9 blocks	13.0	220	53%
■ (Cambridge)				
Charleston Chew/all flavors	1.875 oz	7.0	230	27%
Junior Mints	1.6 oz	4.0	190	19%
Pom Poms	1.58 oz	6.0	200	27%
Sugar Babies	1.7 oz	2.0	190	9%
Sugar Daddy	1.7 oz	3.0	200	14%
■ CARAMELLO (See (Cadbury) in this section)				
■ (Cellas)				
chocolate-covered cherries				
dark chocolate	2 pieces	4.0	110	33%
milk chocolate	2 pieces	4.0	110	33%
■ (Certs)				
breath mints/sugar-free				
assorted	1 piece	–	5	–
extra flavor peppermint	1 piece	–	5	–
peppermint	1 piece	–	5	–
spearmint	1 piece	–	5	–
wintergreen	1 piece	–	5	–

Food and Description	Amount	Fat Grams	Total Calories	% Fat Calories
■ CHARLESTON CHEW (*See* (Cambridge) in this section)				
■ (Charms)				
blow pop	1 pop	–	80	–
flat pop	1 pop	–	70	–
■ CHUCKLES (*See* (Leaf) in this section)				
■ CHUNKY (*See* (Nestle) in this section)				
■ (Chupa Chups)				
ice-cream-flavored lollipops				
choco vanilla	1 piece	–	50	–
strawberry vanilla	1 piece	–	50	–
vanilla	1 piece	–	50	–
■ (Clark)				
Black Cow/sucker	1 oz	3.0	127	21%
Clark bar	1.76 oz	10.0	240	38%
Slo Poke	1 sucker	2.0	124	15%
■ COFFEE TIME (*See* (Allen Wertz) in this section)				
■ (Concorde)				
Bit-O-Honey				
bar	1 bar	4.0	200	18%
pieces				
jar	1 piece	0.6	32	17%
	5 pieces	3.0	160	17%
twist-wrap	1 piece	0.5	28	16%
	6 pieces	3.0	170	16%
Laffy Taffy	1 piece	0.5	38	12%
	4 pieces	2.0	150	12%
Shock Tarts	1 piece	–	8	–
	8 pieces	0.5	60	8%
Taffy Tarts	1 piece	–	2	–
	27 pieces	0.5	60	8%
■ CRUNCH BAR (*See* (Nestle) in this section)				
■ (Demet's)				
turtles	1 piece	4.5	80	51%
■ DOVE (*See* (M&M★Mars) in this section)				
■ DREAM BAR (*See* (Litesse) in this section)				
■ DUM DUM (*See* (Spangler) in this section)				
■ (Estee)				
butterscotch	2 pieces	–	50	–
candy-coated peanuts	¼ cup	9.0	200	41%
caramel/chocolate & vanilla	5 pieces	5.0	150	30%
chocolate bar				
dark chocolate	7 squares	14.0	200	63%
milk chocolate				
crisp rice	1 bar	26.0	370	63%
plain	7 squares	17.0	230	67%
w/almonds	7 squares	17.0	230	67%
w/fruit & nuts	7 squares	16.0	220	65%
mint	7 squares	14.0	200	63%

Food and Description	Amount	Fat Grams	Total Calories	% Fat Calories
chocolate-covered raisins	¼ cup	6.0	180	60%
fruit & nut mix	¼ cup	12.0	210	51%
gumdrops				
assorted	23 pieces	–	140	–
licorice	23 pieces	–	140	–
gummy bears/assorted	16 pieces	–	140	–
hard candy				
fruit/assorted	5 pieces	–	60	–
mint/assorted	5 pieces	–	60	–
toffee	5 pieces	–	60	–
tropical/assorted	5 pieces	–	60	–
lollipops/assorted fruit	2 lollipops	–	60	–
peanut brittle	1½ oz	9.0	210	39%
peppermint swirl	3 pieces	–	60	–
■ (Farley)				
bridge mix/chocolate	18 pieces	8.0	180	40%
butter toffee	3 pieces	1.0	70	13%
butterscotch discs	3 pieces	–	70	–
candy corn	24 pieces	–	150	–
candy roll	1 roll	–	25	–
chocolate-covered raisins	37 pieces	8.0	180	40%
cinnamon discs	3 pieces	–	70	–
Clearly Fruit hard candies	3 pieces	–	70	–
fruit slices	3 pieces	–	150	–
fruit snacks				
cherry	15 pieces	–	90	–
strawberry	13 pieces	–	90	–
giant jellies	3 pieces	–	120	–
gummy bears	17 pieces	–	130	–
gummy dinos	7 pieces	–	120	–
jelly beans				
itsy bitsy	32 pieces	–	140	–
regular	17 pieces	–	150	–
Kid Pops	1 pop	–	45	–
Kiddie Mix	0.67 oz	–	70	–
orange slices	3 pieces	–	150	–
party mix	3 pieces	–	60	–
peanut clusters/chocolate	3 pieces	16.0	230	63%
peanuts				
chocolate-dipped	17 pieces	13.0	220	53%
circus	5 pieces	–	160	–
French burnt	25 pieces	5.0	180	25%
spice drops	10 pieces	–	140	–
starlight mints	3 pieces	–	60	–
■ (Featherweight)				
Sweet Pretenders				
chewy caramels	5 pieces	5.0	130	30%

Food and Description	Amount	Fat Grams	Total Calories	% Fat Calories
hard candy				
berry patch	5 pieces	–	60	–
butterscotch	2 pieces	–	50	–
orchard blend	5 pieces	–	60	–
peppermint swirls	3 pieces	–	60	–
tropical blend	5 pieces	–	60	–
milk chocolate				
w/almonds	7 squares	17.0	230	67%
w/crisp rice	1 bar	26.0	370	63%
■ 5TH AVENUE (*See* (Hershey) in this section)				
■ GENERIC				
almonds/chocolate-covered	1 oz	12.0	161	67%
butternut	2 oz	13.0	270	43%
butterscotch	1 oz	1.0	113	8%
candy corn	¼ cup	1.0	180	5%
cherries/chocolate-covered	1 piece	3.0	90	30%
chocolate bar				
dark sweet chocolate	1 oz	10.0	150	60%
milk chocolate				
plain	1 oz	9.0	145	50%
w/almonds	1 oz	10.0	150	60%
w/peanuts	1 oz	11.0	155	64%
chocolate discs/sugar-coated	1 oz	5.6	132	38%
chocolate mint patty	1 piece	1.0	50	18%
fudge				
caramel & peanuts	1 oz	5.0	123	37%
chocolate	1 oz	4.5	122	33%
chocolate w/nuts	1 oz	5.9	128	42%
vanilla	1 oz	3.0	113	24%
vanilla w/nuts	1 oz	5.0	120	38%
gumdrops/all flavors	1 oz	–	100	–
hard candy	1 oz	–	110	–
jaw breaker	1 piece	–	20	–
jelly beans/all flavors	1 oz	–	100	–
	1 cup	1.0	807	1%
licorice/black	1 oz	<1.0	100	5%
malt balls/milk chocolate covered	2 pieces	4.0	50	72%
nonpareils/mint	1 oz	9.0	150	54%
peanuts/yogurt-covered	1 pz	9.0	125	65%
penuchii	1 oz	4.0	120	30%
pralines	1 oz	3.0	90	30%
stars/milk chocolate	1 oz	8.0	160	45%
taffy	1 oz	1.0	100	9%
vanilla cream	1 oz	4.8	123	35%
■ (Ghirardelli)				
chocolate bars				
Baby Premier/1.25 oz				
cookies & cream	1 bar	11.0	190	52%

Food and Description	Amount	Fat Grams	Total Calories	% Fat Calories
dark chocolate				
plain	1 bar	12.0	180	60%
w/raspberries	1 bar	12.0	180	60%
milk chocolate				
plain	1 bar	11.0	190	52%
w/almonds	1 bar	12.0	190	57%
w/crisp	1 bar	10.0	180	50%
w/macadamia	1 bar	13.0	190	62%
milk chocolate	1 bar	12.0	180	60%
Premier/2.5 oz				
double chocolate mocha	1 bar	19.0	350	49%
cookies & cream	1 bar	21.0	370	51%
dark chocolate				
plain	4 sections	14.0	210	60%
w/almonds	4 sections	16.0	220	65%
milk chocolate				
plain	4 sections	14.0	220	57%
w/almonds	4 sections	15.0	230	59%
w/crisp	1 bar	20.0	360	50%
w/macadamias	1 bar	26.0	380	62%
w/pecans	4 sections	16.0	230	63%
w/raspberries	4 sections	14.0	210	60%
w/toffee	4 sections	13.0	220	53%
mint chocolate	4 sections	14.0	220	57%
white confection w/raspberries	4 sections	14.0	230	55%
white mocha w/biscotti	2.5 oz bar	22.0	380	52%
Legend Boxes				
almond clusters	3 clusters	16.0	210	69%
milk chocolate wafers	11 pieces	12.0	210	51%
mint chocolate wafers	11 pieces	14.0	220	57%
nonpareils	10 pieces	9.0	190	43%
peanut clusters	3 pieces	15.0	210	64%
■ (Godiva)				
almond butter dome	3 pieces	17.0	240	64%
bouchee au chocolat	1 piece	11.0	210	47%
bouchee ivory raspberry	1 piece	9.0	160	51%
gold ballotin	3 pieces	10.0	210	43%
truffles				
amaretto di Saronno	2 pieces	12.0	210	51%
deluxe liqueur	2 pieces	13.0	210	43%
■ GOOBERS (See (Nestle) in this section)				
■ GOOD & PLENTY (See (Leaf) in this section)				
■ GUMMI BEARS (See (Brach's) in this section)				
■ GUMMY BEARS (See (Hershey) in this section)				
■ (GuyLian)				
chocolate bars/no sugar added				
dark chocolate	8 squares	9.0	112	72%

Food and Description	Amount	Fat Grams	Total Calories	% Fat Calories
milk chocolate				
plain	8 squares	9.0	125	65%
w/hazelnuts	8 squares	10.0	132	68%
■ HATTIE BROOKS (See (Kirkland Confections) in this section)				
■ (Heath)				
Heath Bar				
regular	1.4 oz	13.0	210	56%
snack bar	5 pieces	15.0	240	56%
Sensations	⅕ bag	12.0	210	51%
■ (Hershey)				
Almond Joy	0.69 oz	5.0	90	50%
Bar None	0.67 oz	6.0	100	54%
Cookies 'n' Creme bar/0.6 oz	2 bars	10.0	180	50%
Cookies 'n' Mint				
bar/0.6 oz	1 bar	4.5	90	45%
nuggets/0.35 oz	1 piece	2.5	45	50%
5th Avenue	0.58 oz	3.5	80	39%
Golden Collection solitaires/almonds	1 piece	1.0	15	60%
Gummy Bears/amazin' fruit	1 pouch	–	60	–
Hugs				
plain	1 piece	1.5	25	54%
w/almonds	1 piece	1.5	25	54%
Kisses				
plain	1 piece	1.5	25	54%
w/almonds	1 piece	1.5	20	63%
Kit-Kat	0.56 oz	4.5	80	51%
Krackel	0.3 oz	2.5	45	50%
	0.6 oz	5.0	90	50%
milk chocolate bar				
plain	0.3 oz	2.5	45	50%
	0.6 oz	5.0	90	50%
w/almond nuggets	0.35 oz	3.5	60	53%
w/almonds	0.6 oz	6.0	90	60%
milk chocolate nuggets	1 piece	3.0	50	54%
Mr. Goodbar	0.3 oz	2.5	45	50%
	0.6 oz	5.0	90	50%
Mounds	0.69 oz	5.0	90	50%
Reese's Nutrageous	0.6 oz	5.0	90	50%
	1.6 oz	14.0	240	53%
Reese's peanut butter cup/miniatures	0.275 oz	2.5	40	56%
Reese's Pieces	10 pieces	2.0	40	45%
	0.7 oz	4.0	100	36%
Rolo chocolate caramels	1 piece	1.5	30	45%
	3 pieces	4.0	80	45%
Special Dark	0.3 oz	2.5	45	49%
Symphony				
milk chocolate				
plain	0.6 oz	6.0	100	54%

Food and Description	Amount	Fat Grams	Total Calories	% Fat Calories
w/almonds & toffee chips	0.6 oz	6.0	100	54%
Whatchamacallit	0.58 oz	4.5	80	51%
■ HOMEMADE				
USDA Standard Home Recipe				
divinity/plain	1 oz	–	98	–
truffles	0.5 oz	4.0	59	61%
■ HOT TAMALES (*See* (Leaf) in this section)				
■ JOLLY RANCHERS (*See* (Leaf) in this section)				
■ JUNIOR MINTS (*See* (Cambridge) in this section)				
■ (Kirkland Confections)				
gourmet jelly beans	2 Tbs	–	150	–
Hattie Brooks chocolate peanut clusters	3 pieces	19.0	267	64%
Hattie Brooks chocolate raisins	20 pieces	9.0	180	45%
■ KIT-KAT (*See* (Hershey) in this section)				
■ KRACKEL (*See* (Hershey) in this section)				
■ (Kraft)				
caramels				
chocolate fudgies	5 pieces	5.0	180	25%
original	5 pieces	3.0	170	16%
mints				
butter	7 pieces	–	60	–
party	7 pieces	–	60	–
peanut brittle	5 pieces	5.0	170	26%
■ KUDOS (*See* (M&M★Mars) in this section)				
■ LAFFY TAFFY (*See* (Beich); (Concorde) in this section)				
■ (Lance)				
chews/11 pieces per pkg				
cinnamon	1 pkg	0.5	120	4%
fruit	1 pkg	0.5	120	4%
mint	1 pkg	0.5	120	4%
strawberry	1 pkg	0.5	120	4%
chocolaty peanut bar	1 bar	15.0	270	50%
gum ball pops	1 piece	–	45	–
K-Nuts	4 pieces	15.0	240	56%
peanut bar	1 bar	15.0	270	50%
Pop-A-Lance	1 piece	–	45	–
popcorn 'n' caramel bar	1 bar	–	90	–
starlight mints	3 pieces	–	60	–
suckers/assorted	3 pieces	–	50	–
whistle pop	1 piece	–	70	–
■ (Leaf)				
Chuckles/jellied candies				
fruit flavors	1 oz	–	100	–
jellied eggs	1 oz	–	110	–
Jujubees	1 oz	–	110	–
Juju Softees	1 oz	–	100	–
licorice	1 oz	–	100	–
Good & Plenty	1 oz	<1.0	106	4%

Food and Description	Amount	Fat Grams	Total Calories	% Fat Calories
Hot Tamales	2.12 oz	–	220	–
Jolly Ranchers	3 pieces	–	60	–
Mike & Ike	2.12 oz	–	220	–
Milk Duds	13 pieces	6.0	170	32%
	1.85 oz	8.0	230	31%
Pay Day	1.83 oz	12.0	240	45%
Whoppers	17 pieces	7.0	180	35%
■ LIFE SAVERS (*See* (Planters) in this section)				
■ (Litesse)				
Dream bar	1 oz	3.0	90	30%
■ (M&M ★ Mars)				
Bounty				
dark chocolate	1 oz	8.0	140	51%
milk chocolate	1 oz	8.0	140	51%
Dove				
dark chocolate				
miniatures	7 pieces	14.0	220	55%
single	1.3 oz	12.0	200	54%
6-oz bar	¼ bar	14.0	230	55%
milk chocolate				
miniatures	7 pieces	13.0	230	51%
single	1.3 oz	12.0	200	54%
6-oz bar	¼ bar	13.0	230	51%
Promises				
dark chocolate	6 pieces	14.0	220	57%
milk chocolate	6 pieces	13.0	230	51%
truffles	4 pieces	14.0	210	60%
Kudos				
chocolate chip	1 bar	5.0	120	38%
chocolate chunk	1 bar	3.0	90	30%
low-fat				
blueberry	1 bar	1.5	90	15%
strawberry	1 bar	1.5	80	17%
M&M's milk chocolate mini's	1 bar	2.5	90	25%
milk & cookies	1 bar	5.0	130	35%
nutty fudge	1 bar	5.0	130	35%
peanut butter	1 bar	5.0	130	35%
M&M's				
almond	1.3 oz	11.0	200	50%
baking & decorating pack	0.5 oz	3.0	70	38%
mint	1.68 oz	10.0	230	39%
peanut	1.7 oz	13.0	250	47%
peanut butter	1.6 oz	13.0	240	49%
plain	1.6 oz	10.0	230	39%
Mars Bar/fun size	2 bars	10.0	190	47%
Milky Way				
dark chocolate				
fun size	1 bar	3.0	90	30%

Food and Description	Amount	Fat Grams	Total Calories	% Fat Calories
miniature	5 pieces	7.0	180	35%
single	1.76 oz	8.0	220	33%
lite bar				
full-size/1.57 oz	1 bar	5.0	170	26%
miniatures	1 piece	1.0	30	30%
milk chocolate				
fun size	2 bars	7.0	180	35%
king size	⅓ bar	6.0	160	34%
miniature	5 pieces	7.0	190	33%
single	2.15 oz	11.0	280	35%
reduced fat	1 bar	7.0	140	45%
Skittles				
original				
fun size	3 bags	2.0	180	10%
king size	½ bag	1.5	150	9%
single	2.1 oz	2.5	250	10%
tropical				
fun size	2 bags	1.5	160	8%
single	2.1 oz	2.5	250	10%
wild berry				
fun size	2 bags	1.5	160	8%
single	2.1 oz	2.5	250	10%
Snickers				
munch bar	1.4 oz	15.0	230	59%
original				
fun size	2 bars	9.0	190	43%
king size	⅓ bar	8.0	170	40%
miniature	4 pieces	8.0	170	40%
single	2 oz	14.0	280	45%
peanut butter bar	2 oz	20.0	310	58%
Starburst				
fruit chews				
California	8 pieces	3.0	160	37%
	1 stick	4.5	240	17%
original	8 pieces	3.0	160	37%
	1 stick	5.0	240	19%
strawberry	8 pieces	3.0	160	37%
	1 stick	5.0	240	19%
tropical	8 pieces	3.0	160	37%
	1 stick	5.0	240	19%
jelly beans	5 pieces	–	150	–
trial size	1 bag	–	130	–
3 Musketeers	1.1 oz	4.0	140	26%
	2.12 oz	8.0	260	28%

■ MIKE & IKE (*See* (Leaf) in this section)
■ MILK DUDS (*See* (Leaf) in this section)

| ■ (Milkshake) | 1.8 oz | 7.0 | 220 | 29% |

■ MILKY WAY (*See* (M&M★Mars) in this section)

Food and Description	Amount	Fat Grams	Total Calories	% Fat Calories
■ **MR. GOODBAR** (*See* (Hershey) in this section)				
■ **MOUNDS** (*See* (Hershey) in this section)				
■ **(Nabisco)**				
Peppermint Patty	1 oz	1.0	110	8%
Thin Mint	1 piece	1.0	42	21%
■ **(Natural Touch)**				
Caroby Bars				
almond	4 sections	10.0	150	60%
milk	4 sections	9.0	150	54%
milk-free	4 sections	11.0	160	62%
mint	4 sections	9.0	150	54%
■ **(Nature's Warehouse)**				
A-OK	1 oz	6.0	130	42%
My O My	1 oz	1.5	105	13%
No-How	1 oz	10.0	140	64%
Nut Wit	1 oz	6.0	135	40%
■ **(Nestle)**				
Alpine White chocolate almond bar	1.3 oz	13.0	200	59%
	2.2 oz	23.0	350	59%
Baby Ruth				
fun size	2 bars	9.0	200	40%
regular	2.1 oz	12.0	280	39%
Buncha Crunch	1.4 oz	10.0	200	45%
Butterfinger				
BB's	1.7 oz	10.0	230	39%
fun size	2 bars	8.0	200	36%
regular	2.1 oz	11.0	280	35%
Chunky	1.4 oz	11.0	200	50%
Crunch				
bar				
fun size	4 bars	10.0	200	45%
regular	1.55 oz	12.0	230	47%
spring series	1 disk	9.0	170	48%
Goobers	1.38 oz	13.0	210	56%
milk chocolate bar	1.45 oz	13.0	220	53%
Nest Eggs/crunch	5 pieces	10.0	190	47%
Nips				
chocolate mint	2 pieces	1.5	60	23%
peanut butter parfait	2 pieces	2.0	60	30%
Oh Henry!	1.8 oz	9.0	230	35%
Raisinets	1.58 oz	8.0	200	36%
Sno Caps	2.3 oz	13.0	320	37%
Thousand Grand	1.5 oz	8.0	200	36%
turtles	2 pieces	9.0	160	51%
■ **(Newman's Own)**				
Organics bars				
crisp rice				
espresso sweet dark chocolate	½ bar	15.0	240	56%

Food and Description	Amount	Fat Grams	Total Calories	% Fat Calories
milk chocolate	½ bar	17.0	250	61%
milk chocolate	½ bar	16.0	240	60%
■ NO-HOW (*See* (Nature's Warehouse) in this section)				
■ NUT WIT (*See* (Nature's Warehouse) in this section)				
■ NUTRAGEOUS (*See* (Hershey) in this section)				
■ (Ocean Spray)				
Fruit Waves/cranberry	4 pieces	–	50	–
■ OH HENRY! (*See* (Nestle) in this section)				
■ (Panda)				
licorice	3.5 oz	<1.0	340	1%
raspberry-flavored chew	3.5 oz	<1.0	340	1%
■ PAY DAY (*See* (Leaf) in this section)				
■ (PB Max)				
fun size	2 pieces	12.0	180	60%
regular	2 pieces	15.0	240	56%
■ (Pearson's)				
butter rum	2 pieces	1.5	60	23%
caramel nip	2 pieces	1.5	60	23%
chocolate mint	2 pieces	1.5	60	23%
chocolate parfait	2 pieces	1.5	60	23%
coffee nip	2 pieces	1.5	60	23%
licorice nip	2 pieces	1.5	60	23%
mint patties	5 pieces	2.5	150	15%
peanut butter parfait	2 pieces	1.5	60	23%
■ (Pez)	roll	–	30	–
■ (Planters)				
Life Savers				
candy cane, big tablet	4 pieces	–	60	–
cards 'n candy	4 pieces	–	40	–
Gummy Savers				
five flavor	11 pieces	–	130	–
mixed berry	11 pieces	–	130	–
tangy fruit	11 pieces	–	130	–
variety bag	2 bags	–	120	–
wacky frootz	11 pieces	–	130	–
Holes				
five flavor	20 pieces	–	20	–
island fruits	20 pieces	–	20	–
sour 'n sweet	16 pieces	–	20	–
sunshine fruits	20 pieces	–	20	–
super tart	20 pieces	–	20	–
wild fruits super	20 pieces	–	20	–
Life Savers/regular roll				
butter rum	2 pieces	–	20	–
candy cane	4 pieces	–	40	–
cryst-o-mint	2 pieces	–	20	–
egg-sortment	1 roll	–	40	–
five flavor	2 pieces	–	20	–

Food and Description	Amount	Fat Grams	Total Calories	% Fat Calories
fruits on fire	2 pieces	–	20	–
pep-o-mint	3 pieces	–	20	–
spear-o-mint	3 pieces	–	20	–
sunshine fruits	2 pieces	–	20	–
tangy fruit swirls	4 pieces	–	40	–
tangy fruits	2 pieces	–	20	–
tropical fruits	2 pieces	–	20	–
watermelon	2 pieces	–	20	–
wint-o-green	3 pieces	–	20	–
lollipops/assorted	1 pop	–	40	–
Sack'it				
butter rum	4 pieces	–	60	–
Christmas tin	4 pieces	–	60	–
five flavor	4 pieces	–	60	–
holiday tin	4 pieces	–	60	–
pep-o-mint	4 pieces	–	60	–
tangy fruits	4 pieces	–	60	–
wild cherry	4 pieces	–	60	–
wint-o-green	4 pieces	–	60	–
peanut bar	1.6 oz	14.0	230	54%
peanut brittle	½ cup	7.0	180	35%
peanut butter chocolates	4 pieces	15.0	230	59%
sweet 'n crunchy	1 oz	7.0	140	45%
■ POM POMS (*See* (Cambridge) in this section)				
■ RAISINETS (*See* (Nestle) in this section)				
■ REESE'S (*See* (Hershey) in this section)				
■ RIESEN (*See* (Storck) in this section)				
■ ROLO (*See* (Hershey) in this section)				
■ (Russell Stover)				
almond delights	2 pieces	12.0	210	51%
Ambassadors miniature chocolates	6 pieces	9.0	190	43%
candy jar chocolates	4 pieces	9.0	190	43%
caramels	3 pieces	7.0	170	37%
assorted	3 pieces	8.0	190	38%
English	6 pieces	6.0	180	30%
Santas	1 Santa	11.0	230	43%
squares/soft & creamy	3 pieces	10.0	190	47%
cherry cordials	3 pieces	7.0	170	37%
chocolate assortments				
dark chocolate	3 pieces	8.0	190	38%
gift box				
gold bow	2 pieces	10.0	200	45%
regular	3 pieces	8.0	180	40%
milk chocolate	3 pieces	8.0	190	38%
chocolate-covered nuts	3 pieces	16.0	230	63%
coconut clusters	3 pieces	14.0	230	55%
fudge/German chocolate	1 piece	10.0	190	47%

Food and Description	Amount	Fat Grams	Total Calories	% Fat Calories
mints				
French chocolate				
boxed	4 pieces	14.0	220	57%
individual	1 bar	15.0	240	56%
Mint Dream	1 bar	8.0	160	45%
patties/dark chocolate covered	6 pieces	6.0	180	30%
pecan delights				
boxed	2 pieces	14.0	220	57%
individual	1 bar	20.0	310	58%
pecan roll	1.5 oz	20.0	300	60%
truffles	3 pieces	11.0	200	50%
whips/assorted	2 pieces	7.0	210	30%
■ (Sherwood)				
Cows				
butter n' cream	3 pieces	1.5	71	19%
butter n' toffees				
chocolate-filled	6 pieces	11.0	240	41%
plain	6 pieces	7.0	180	35%
■ SHOCK TARTS (See (Concorde) in this section)				
■ SKITTLES (See (M&M ★ Mars) in this section)				
■ SLO POKE (See (Clark) in this section)				
■ SNICKERS (See (M&M ★ Mars) in this section)				
■ SNO CAPS (See (Nestle) in this section)				
■ (Sorbee)				
sour lemon	1 piece	–	12	–
wintergreen	1 piece	–	12	–
■ (Spangler)				
candy cane	1 piece	–	60	–
chocolate-coated creme center	1 piece	2.0	80	23%
caramel w/nuts	1 piece	6.0	100	54%
cherry w/nuts	1 piece	5.0	110	41%
fudge w/nuts	1 piece	6.0	140	39%
fudge w/pecans	1 piece	7.0	140	45%
maple w/nuts	1 piece	5.0	110	41%
vanilla w/nuts	1 piece	5.0	110	41%
circus peanuts	4 pieces	–	110	–
lollipops				
Dum Dums/all flavors	1 lollipop	–	25	–
Saf-T-Pops	1 lollipop	–	45	–
w/bubble gum center/all flavors	1 lollipop	–	60	–
mint/dark chocolate covered	1 piece	2.0	80	23%
■ STARBURST (See (M&M ★ Mars) in this section)				
■ (Storck)				
Chocolate Riesen	5 pieces	7.0	180	35%
Riesen chocolate chew	1 bar	7.0	180	35%
Werther's original	3 pieces	1.0	60	15%
■ SUGAR BABIES (See (Cambridge) in this section)				
■ SUGAR DADDY (See (Cambridge) in this section)				

Food and Description	Amount	Fat Grams	Total Calories	% Fat Calories
■ (Sweet 'N Low)				
hard candies				
butterscotch	4 pieces	–	30	–
cinnamon	4 pieces	–	30	–
coffee	4 pieces	–	30	–
fancy fruit	4 pieces	–	30	–
fruit	4 pieces	–	30	–
peppermint	4 pieces	–	30	–
watermelon	4 pieces	–	30	–
■ SWEET PRETENDERS (See (Featherweight) in this section)				
■ SYMPHONY (See (Hershey) in this section)				
■ TAFFY TARTS (See (Concorde) in this section)				
■ THOUSAND GRAND (See (Nestle) in this section)				
■ 3 MUSKETEERS (See (M&M★Mars) in this section)				
■ (Tiger's Milk)				
bars				
carob-coated	1.25 oz	6.0	160	34%
cocoa & yogurt fudge	1.25 oz	3.0	120	23%
crunchie	2 oz	3.0	200	14%
light	1.25 oz	3.0	120	23%
peanut butter/light	1.25 oz	3.0	120	23%
peanut butter & honey	1.25 oz	5.0	150	30%
peanut butter crunch	1.25 oz	8.0	170	42%
■ (Tootsie Roll)				
Tootsie Pop				
caramel apple	1 pop	0.5	70	6%
regular	1 pop	–	60	–
Tootsie Roll				
midgees	6 pieces	3.0	160	17%
regular	1 oz	2.0	110	16%
■ TWIX (See (M&M★Mars) in this section)				
■ TWIZZLERS (See (Y&S) in this section)				
■ (Ultra Slim-Fast)				
peanut caramel crunch	1 oz	4.0	120	30%
■ (Velamints)				
breath mints/sugar-free				
cinnamon	1 piece	–	5	–
cocoamint	1 piece	–	5	–
peppermint	1 piece	–	5	–
spearmint	1 piece	–	5	–
■ WERTHER'S (See (Storck) in this section)				
■ WHATCHAMACALLIT (See (Hershey) in this section)				
■ WHOPPERS (See (Leaf) in this section)				
■ (Woody's)				
fudge				
chocolate w/nuts	1 piece	4.0	120	30%
maple walnut	1 piece	4.0	120	30%
mint w/walnuts	1 piece	4.0	120	30%

Food and Description	Amount	Fat Grams	Total Calories	% Fat Calories
vanilla w/walnuts	1 piece	4.0	120	30%
■ (Y&S)				
Twizzlers				
cherry	1 piece	–	30	–
chocolate	1 piece	–	30	–
licorice	1 piece	–	30	–
pull 'n peel cherry twists	1 piece	1.0	110	–
strawberry	1 pieces	–	35	–
■ (York)				
Peppermint Patty/bite-size	1 piece	1.5	60	23%
■ (Zachary)				
creme drops/old-fashioned milk chocolate	3 pieces	3.0	170	16%
■ (Zagnut)	1.8 oz	9.0	230	35%
■ (Zero)	1.4 oz	6.0	170	32%
■ ZOTZ (See (Andre Prost) in this section)				
CANDY APPLE (See APPLE, CARAMEL)				
CANNELLINI BEAN (See KIDNEY BEAN)				
CANTALOUPE/MUSKMELON				
fresh				
cubed	1 cup	<1.0	57	8%
whole/~ 9.5 oz	½ melon	0.7	94	7%
CAPERS				
(Progresso) drained	1 tsp	–	5	–
CAPON				
giblets/simmered	5 oz	7.8	238	30%
meat & skin/roasted	3.5 oz	11.7	229	46%
	~1.5 lb	74.0	1457	46%
meat only/roasted	3.5 oz	8.8	178	44%
CARAMBOLA (See STAR FRUIT)				
CARAWAY SEEDS	1 tsp	–	8	–
CARDAMOM SEEDS				
ground	1 Tbs	0.5	20	23%
whole	1 tsp	–	6	–
CARDOON				
cooked	3 oz	–	19	–
raw/shredded	1 cup	–	35	–
CARIBOU/boneless				
raw	3 oz	5.0	160	28%
roasted	4 oz	5.0	190	24%
roasted/diced	1 cup	6.0	235	23%
CARISSA/NATAL PLUM				
raw	1 medium	–	12	–
CAROB CHIPS				
regular	1 oz	7.0	140	45%
mint	1 oz	7.0	140	45%
CAROB POWDER				
(Chatfield's)	¼ cup	–	96	–
(El Molino)	¼ cup	–	110	–

Food and Description	Amount	Fat Grams	Total Calories	% Fat Calories
CARP (See also CARP ROE)				
breaded & fried	3 oz	12.0	226	48%
cooked-dry heat	3 oz	6.0	138	39%
raw	3 oz	4.8	108	40%
smoked	1 oz	1.8	50	32%
CARP ROE/raw	3 oz	1.7	111	14%
CARROT (See also VEGETABLES, MIXED)				
canned				
(Del Monte) sliced	½ cup	–	35	–
(Freshlike) sliced/crinkle cut	½ cup	–	30	–
generic/sliced/cooked	½ cup	–	35	–
(Green Giant) sliced	½ cup	–	25	–
(LeSueur) whole baby	½ cup	–	35	–
(Libby's)				
diced	½ cup	–	20	–
sliced	½ cup	–	20	–
(S&W)				
julienne	½ cup	0.5	25	18%
sliced	½ cup	0.5	25	18%
whole tiny	½ cup	0.5	25	18%
(Seneca) all styles	½ cup	–	30	–
(Stokely)				
diced/no salt or sugar added	½ cup	–	35	–
sliced	½ cup	–	35	–
(Thank You) fingerling	½ cup	–	30	–
(Veg-All) crinkle cut	½ cup	–	30	–
fresh				
cooked	1 small	–	21	–
raw				
shredded	½ cup	–	24	–
(Dole)	3 oz	1.0	50	18%
whole	1 medium	–	31	–
(Dole)	1 medium	1.0	40	23%
frozen				
(Birds Eye)				
sliced	½ cup	–	35	–
whole baby	½ cup	–	40	–
(C&W)				
Parisienne	⅔ cup	–	40	–
petite tips	⅔ cup	–	35	–
generic	½ cup	–	26	–
(Green Giant) baby cut				
Harvest Fresh	⅔ cup	–	20	–
regular	¾ cup	–	30	–
(Seneca)	¾ cup	–	30	–
(Stokely)				
diced	½ cup	–	35	–
sliced	½ cup	–	35	–

Food and Description	Amount	Fat Grams	Total Calories	% Fat Calories
whole baby	⅔ cup	–	35	–
CARROT JUICE/canned				
generic	6 fl oz	–	75	–
(Hain)	6 fl oz	–	80	–
(Hollywood)	12 fl oz	–	120	–
CASABA MELON/fresh				
cubed	1 cup	–	45	–
whole/8" melon	2" slice	–	45	–
CASHEW				
(Beer Nuts)	1 oz	13.0	170	69%
(Eagle)				
honey-roasted	1 oz	14.0	180	70%
lightly salted	1 oz	14.0	190	66%
(Fisher)				
honey-roasted	1 oz	13.0	150	78%
oil-roasted	1 oz	15.0	170	79%
(Frito Lay)	1½ oz	22.0	270	73%
generic				
dry-roasted/salted or unsalted	1 oz	13.0	163	72%
	1 cup	64.0	790	73%
oil-roasted/salted or unsalted	1 oz	14.0	163	77%
	1 cup	63.0	750	76%
(Guy's) Whole Salted	1 oz	14.0	170	74%
(Lance)	1⅛ oz	16.0	200	72%
(Planters)				
honey-roasted				
Munch 'N Go	2 oz	24.0	310	70%
regular	1 oz	12.0	150	72%
	2 oz	24.0	310	70%
oil-roasted				
fancy	1 oz	14.0	170	74%
	2 oz	29.0	340	77%
halves	1 oz	14.0	170	74%
lightly salted	1 oz	13.0	160	73%
Munch 'N Go	2 oz	28.0	330	76%
nut bag	1 oz	14.0	160	79%
regular	1.48 oz	21.0	250	76%
CASHEW BUTTER				
generic/plain	1 Tbs	8.0	94	77%
	1 oz	14.0	167	75%
(Hain)				
raw	2 Tbs	15.0	190	71%
toasted	2 Tbs	17.0	210	73%
unsalted	2 Tbs	19.0	210	81%
(Roaster Fresh) unsalted	1 oz	14.0	165	76%
(Westbrae) natural				
raw	2 Tbs	17.0	190	81%
roasted	2 Tbs	17.0	190	81%

Food and Description	Amount	Fat Grams	Total Calories	% Fat Calories
CASSAVA				
raw/trimmed	3.5 oz	<1.0	120	3%
	1 lb	2.0	525	3%
CATFISH (*See also* SEAFOOD ENTRÉE/DINNER)				
channel/fresh/meat only				
baked or broiled	3 oz	7.0	149	42%
breaded & fried	3 oz	11.0	194	51%
raw	3 oz	3.6	99	33%
CATSUP/KETCHUP				
(Del Monte) tomato	1 Tbs	–	15	–
generic	1 Tbs	<1.0	15	3%
	1 cup	1.0	290	3%
(Hain) natural				
no salt added	1 Tbs	–	16	–
regular	1 Tbs	–	16	–
(Healthy Choice)	1 Tbs	–	15	–
(Heinz)				
hot	1 Tbs	–	15	–
lite	1 Tbs	–	10	–
regular	1 Tbs	–	15	–
w/onions	1 Tbs	–	20	–
(Hunt's)				
no salt added	1 Tbs	–	16	–
regular	1 Tbs	–	16	–
(Smucker's)	1 Tbs	–	25	–
(Stokely)	1 Tbs	–	20	–
(Weight Watchers)	1 Tbs	–	15	–
(Westbrae) fruit-sweetened				
no salt	1 Tbs	–	10	–
regular	1 Tbs	–	10	–
CAULIFLOWER				
fresh				
cooked	½ cup	–	17	–
raw				
chopped	½ cup	–	12	–
(Dole)	3 oz	0.5	20	23%
whole/medium head	⅙ head	–	18	–
frozen				
(Birds Eye)	½ cup	–	25	–
(Green Giant) florets	1 cup	–	25	–
(Seneca)	1 cup	–	20	–
jarred				
(Mrs. Klein's) hot	1 oz	–	–	–
(Vlasic)				
hot & spicy	1 oz	–	4	–
sweet	1 oz	–	35	–
CAULIFLOWER DISH (*See also* FROZEN ENTRÉE/DINNER; VEGETABLES, MIXED)				
(Birds Eye) frozen w/cheese sauce	½ pkg	5.0	90	50%

Food and Description	Amount	Fat Grams	Total Calories	% Fat Calories
(Green Giant) frozen in cheese-flavored sauce	½ cup	2.5	60	38%
CAULIFLOWER SOUP (*See* SOUP)				
CAVIAR				
general/black or red				
granular	1 Tbs	3.0	40	68%
	1 oz	5.0	71	63%
pressed	1 Tbs	2.8	54	47%
	1 oz	4.7	90	47%
(Romanoff)				
black lumpfish	1 Tbs	1.0	15	60%
black whitefish	1 Tbs	1.5	25	54%
red lumpfish	1 Tbs	1.0	15	60%
CELERIAC/CELERY ROOT/WILD CELERY				
raw	½ cup	–	31	–
	4-5 medium	–	40	–
CELERY				
fresh/medium stalks				
cooked	½ cup	–	11	–
raw	1 stalk	–	6	–
	½ cup	–	9	–
(Dole)	2 stalks	–	20	–
frozen				
(Freshlike)	3.5 oz	–	14	–
(Seneca)	¾ cup	–	10	–
CELERY ROOT (*See* CELERIAC)				
CELERY SEED/whole	1 tsp	0.5	8	56%
	1 Tbs	1.5	25	54%

CELERY SOUP (*See* SOUP)
CEREAL (*See also* BABY FOOD; BARLEY; BULGUR; CORN GRITS)

QUICK REFERENCE: MILK	Amount	Fat Grams	Total Calories	% Fat Calories
Skim/fat-free	¼ cup	–	23	–
	½ cup	–	45	–
1% fat/light	¼ cup	0.5	26	17%
	½ cup	1.0	55	16%
2% fat/reduced fat	¼ cup	1.0	31	29%
	½ cup	2.5	61	37%
Whole	¼ cup	2.0	38	47%
	½ cup	4.0	75	48%

■ **COLD/READY TO EAT**
(Alpen) Swiss style

low-fat	⅔ cup	3.0	200	14%

Food and Description	Amount	Fat Grams	Total Calories	% Fat Calories
original	⅓ cup	2.0	110	16%
	⅔ cup	4.0	220	16%
Alpha-Bits (*See* (Post) in this section)				
(Arrowhead Mills)				
amaranth flakes	1 cup	2.0	130	14%
Apple Corns	1 cup	1.5	150	9%
bran flakes	1 cup	1.0	100	9%
corn flakes	1 cup	–	130	–
Crispy Puffs	1 cup	1.0	80	11%
Maple Corns	1 cup	3.0	190	14%
multigrain flakes	1 cup	1.5	140	10%
Nature O's	1 cup	2.0	130	14%
oat bran flakes	1 cup	2.0	110	16%
puffed corn	1 cup	–	80	–
puffed kamut	1 cup	–	50	–
puffed millet	1 cup	0.5	90	5%
puffed rice	1 cup	–	90	–
puffed wheat	1 cup	0.5	90	5%
spelt flakes	1 cup	1.0	100	9%
wheat bran	¼ cup	0.5	30	15%
wheat germ/raw	3 Tbs	0.5	50	9%
(Back To Nature) granola				
apple blueberry	½ cup	3.0	170	16%
apple strawberry	½ cup	3.0	190	14%
natural	½ cup	3.0	170	16%
raisin	½ cup	2.5	170	13%
(Barbara's)				
Breakfast O's w/oat bran	1¼ cup	2.0	110	16%
blue corn flakes	1 cup	–	110	–
High 5	¾ cup	0.5	100	5%
Brown Rice Crisps	1 cup	<1.0	110	4%
Shredded Spoonfuls/multigrain	¾ cup	1.5	120	11%
shredded wheat biscuits	2 biscuits	1.0	140	6%
Startoons frosted cocoa crunch	1 cup	0.5	110	4%
Basic 4 (*See* (General Mills) in this section)				
Bran'nola (*See* (Post) in this section)				
(Breadshop)				
Cinnamon Grins	¾ cup	0.5	110	4%
granola				
blueberries 'n cream	½ cup	7.5	220	31%
crunchy oat bran	½ cup	8.5	210	36%
raspberries 'n cream	½ cup	7.5	220	31%
strawberries 'n cream	½ cup	7.5	220	31%
super natural w/almonds	½ cup	9.0	220	37%
Kamut 'n Honey	1 cup	0.5	110	4%
Puffs 'n Honey	¾ cup	3.0	120	23%
Cap'n Crunch (*See* (Quaker) in this section)				
Cheerios (*See* (General Mills) in this section)				

Food and Description	Amount	Fat Grams	Total Calories	% Fat Calories
Chex (*See* (Ralston) in this section)				
Common Sense (*See* (Kellogg's) in this section)				
Crispix (*See* (Kellogg's) in this section)				
(El Molino)				
puffed corn	¾ cup	–	50	–
puffed millet	¾ cup	–	50	–
puffed rice	¾ cup	–	50	–
puffed wheat	¾ cup	–	50	–
(Erewhon)				
amaranth/Aztec Corn	1 cup	–	110	–
Apple Stroodles	¾ cup	0.5	110	4%
Banana O's	¾ cup	–	110	–
corn flakes	1¼ cup	2.5	210	11%
crisp brown rice				
low-sodium	1 oz	1.0	110	8%
regular	1 oz	1.0	110	8%
Fruit 'n Wheat	¾ cup	1.0	100	9%
Galaxy Grahams	¾ cup	0.5	100	5%
kamut flakes	1 oz	–	90	–
Poppels	1 cup	1.0	120	8%
raisin bran	1 cup	1.0	170	5%
Right Start				
original	1 cup	–	90	–
w/raisins	1 cup	–	90	–
Super O's	1 oz	–	110	–
wheat flakes	1 oz	1.0	110	8%
(Estee)				
corn flakes	1 oz	–	90	–
raisin bran	1 oz	0.5	90	5%
(Familia) Swiss style muesli				
chocolate	½ cup	10.0	250	36%
no sugar	½ cup	3.0	200	9%
original	½ cup	3.0	210	13%
(Featherweight) corn flakes	1 cup	–	110	–
Froot Loops (*See* (Kellogg's) in this section)				
Fruit & Fibre (*See* (Post) in this section)				
(General Mills)				
Basic 4	1 cup	3.0	210	13%
Body Buddies/natural fruit	1 cup	1.0	120	8%
Booberry	1 cup	1.5	120	4%
Cheerios				
apple cinnamon	¾ cup	2.5	120	19%
frosted	1 cup	1.0	120	8%
honey nut	1 cup	1.5	120	11%
multigrain	1 cup	1.0	110	8%
original	1 cup	2.0	110	16%
Cinnamon Toast Crunch	¾ cup	3.5	130	24%

Food and Description	Amount	Fat Grams	Total Calories	% Fat Calories
Clusters	1 cup	4.0	220	16%
w/almonds/walnuts/pecans	½ cup	2.0	110	16%
Cocoa Puffs	1 cup	1.0	120	8%
corn flakes/country	1 cup	0.5	120	4%
Count Chocula	1 cup	1.0	120	8%
Crispy Wheats & Raisins	1 cup	1.0	190	5%
Fiber One	½ cup	1.0	60	15%
Frankenberry	1 cup	0.5	120	4%
Golden Grahams	¾ cup	1.0	120	8%
Hidden Treasures	¾ cup	2.0	130	14%
Kaboom	1¼ cups	1.5	120	11%
Kix				
berry berry	¾ cup	1.0	120	8%
original	1⅓ cups	1.0	120	8%
Lucky Charms	1 cup	1.0	120	8%
Nature Valley				
low-fat fruit granola	⅔ cup	2.5	210	11%
100% natural cereal				
cinnamon & raisin	¾ cup	8.0	240	30%
fruit & nut	⅔ cup	11.0	250	40%
toasted oat & honey	¾ cup	10.0	250	36%
Oatmeal Crisp				
almond	1 cup	6.0	230	23%
apple cinnamon	1 cup	2.5	210	11%
raisin	1 cup	3.0	210	13%
Reese's Peanut Butter Puffs	¾ cup	3.0	130	21%
Ripple Crisp				
honey bran	1¼ cups	1.0	190	5%
honey corn	¾ cup	0.5	110	4%
S'mores Grahams	¾ cup	1.5	120	11%
Sprinkle Spangles	1 cup	1.0	120	8%
Sun Crunchers	1 cup	3.0	210	13%
Total				
corn flakes	1⅓ cup	0.5	110	4%
raisin bran	1 cup	1.0	180	5%
whole wheat	¾ cup	1.0	180	5%
Triples	1 cup	1.0	120	8%
Trix	1 cup	1.5	120	11%
Wheaties				
Dunk-A-Balls	¾ cup	1.0	110	8%
honey frosted	¾ cup	–	110	–
honey gold	¾ cup	1.5	110	4%
original	1 cup	1.0	110	8%
Raisin Nut Bran	1 cup	4.5	210	19%
(Golden Temple)				
almond raisin/low-fat	1 oz	1.5	110	12%
apple cinnamon/low-fat	1 cup	1.5	110	12%

Food and Description	Amount	Fat Grams	Total Calories	% Fat Calories
granola				
cashew almond	1 oz	3.5	130	24%
cinnamon apple raisin	1 oz	3.5	125	25%
coconut almond	1 oz	7.0	145	43%
fruit 'n nut	1 oz	4.5	130	31%
golden	1 oz	6.0	140	39%
Hawaiian	1 oz	4.0	125	29%
high protein	1 oz	3.5	125	25%
honey almond	1 oz	3.5	130	24%
honey blueberry apple	1 oz	3.5	130	24%
lite 'n crunchy	1 oz	4.5	130	31%
low-fat/sweet home farm	1 oz	2.0	110	16%
maple almond	1 oz	3.5	130	24%
natural blueberry				
coconut-free	1 oz	4.5	130	31%
regular	1 oz	5.0	130	35%
natural delite	1 oz	3.5	130	24%
oat bran				
berries	1 oz	3.5	120	25%
raisins & almonds	1 oz	3.5	120	25%
orange almond	1 oz	4.0	135	27%
raisin apricot date	1 oz	3.5	130	24%
hazelnut boysenberry				
muesli				
lite	1 oz	1.0	100	9%
oat bran				
dates & almonds	1 oz	1.5	110	12%
raisins & hazelnuts	1 oz	1.5	100	14%
sweet home farm crunchy/low-fat	1 oz	2.0	105	17%
Swiss style	1 oz	1.5	105	13%
35% fruit	1 oz	1.0	100	9%
natural foods/low-fat				
apple cinnamon	1 oz	1.0	110	8%
raisin almond	1 oz	1.0	110	8%
strawberry/raspberry	1 oz	1.0	110	8%
oat bran flakes				
almond	1 oz	3.5	120	26%
apple	1 oz	3.5	110	29%
muesli				
dates & almonds	1 oz	1.5	110	12%
raisins & hazelnuts	1 oz	1.5	100	14%
100% natural				
almond	1 oz	4.0	125	29%
apple cinnamon	1 oz	4.0	120	30%
oat bran	1 oz	2.5	70	32%
raisin & almond	1 oz	4.0	120	30%
organic oats	1 oz	5.5	135	37%
6 Grain Crisp/fruit & flaxseed	1 oz	3.5	120	26%

Food and Description	Amount	Fat Grams	Total Calories	% Fat Calories
Sweet Home Farm				
almond	1 oz	4.0	125	29%
raisin	1 oz	1.5	105	13%
Grape-Nuts (*See* (Post) in this section)				
(Health Valley)				
Granola O's/fat-free				
apple cinnamon	¾ cup	–	120	–
almond	¾ cup	–	120	–
honey crunch	¾ cup	–	120	–
Honey Clusters & Flakes				
almond	¾ cup	–	130	–
apple cinnamon	¾ cup	–	130	–
honey crunch	¾ cup	–	130	–
honey sweetened puffed	1 cup	–	80	–
(Healthy Choice)				
multigrain flakes				
original	1 cup	–	100	–
raisins, crunchy oat clusters, & almonds	1¼ cups	2.0	200	9%
multigrain squares	1¼ cups	1.0	190	5%
Heartland (*See* (Pillsbury) in this section)				
homemade/USDA Standard Home Recipe				
granola	¼ cup	7.7	138	50%
(Kashi) puffed cereal				
medley	½ cup	1.0	100	9%
breakfast pilaf	½ cup	3.0	170	11%
regular	1 cup	1.5	70	6%
(Kellogg's)				
All Bran				
original	½ cup	1.0	80	11%
w/extra fiber	½ cup	1.0	50	18%
Apple Jacks	1 cup	–	110	–
Apple Raisin Crisp	1 cup	–	180	–
Bran Buds	⅓ cup	1.0	70	13%
Cinnamon Mini Buns	¾ cup	0.5	120	4%
Cocoa Krispies	¾ cup	0.5	120	4%
Common Sense Oat Bran				
regular	¾ cup	1.0	110	12%
w/raisins	¾ cup	2.5	200	11%
Complete Bran Flakes	¾ cup	0.5	100	5%
corn flakes	1 cup	–	110	–
Corn Pops	1 cup	–	110	–
Cracklin Oat Bran	¾ cup	8.0	230	31%
Crispix	1 cup	–	110	–
Double Dip Crunch	¾ cup	–	110	–
Froot Loops	1 cup	1.0	120	8%
Frosted Bran	¾ cup	–	100	–
Frosted Flakes	¾ cup	–	120	–

Food and Description	Amount	Fat Grams	Total Calories	% Fat Calories
Frosted Krispies	¾ cup	–	110	–
Frosted Mini Wheats				
bite-size	1 cup	1.0	190	5%
regular	1 cup	1.0	190	5%
Fruitful Bran	1¼ cups	1.0	170	5%
Fruity Marshmallow Krispies	¾ cup	–	110	–
granola/low-fat				
w/raisins	⅔ cup	3.0	210	13%
w/o raisins	½ cup	3.0	210	13%
Just Right				
fruit & nut	1 cup	2.0	200	9%
w/crunchy nuggets	1 cup	1.5	210	6%
Kenmei Rice Bran	¾ cup	1.0	110	8%
Mueslix				
crispy blend	⅔ cup	3.0	200	14%
golden crunch w/apples & almonds	¾ cup	5.0	210	21%
Nut & Honey Crunch	⅔ cup	2.0	120	15%
Nut & Honey Crunch O's	⅔ cup	2.5	120	19%
Nutri-Grain				
almond & raisin	1¼ cups	3.0	200	14%
golden wheat	¾ cup	0.5	100	5%
golden wheat & raisin	1¼ cups	1.0	180	5%
nuggets	½ cup	1.0	180	5%
Pop Tart Crunch/frosted strawberry	½ cup	1.0	120	8%
Product 19	1 cup	–	110	–
Raisin Bran	1 cup	1.0	170	5%
Rice Krispies				
apple cinnamon	¾ cup	–	110	–
original	1¼ cup	–	110	–
Rice Krispies Treats	¾ cup	1.5	120	11%
Smacks	¾ cup	0.5	110	4%
Special K	1 cup	–	110	–
Squares				
apple cinnamon	¾ cup	1.0	180	5%
blueberry	¾ cup	1.0	180	5%
raisin	¾ cup	1.0	180	5%
strawberry	¾ cup	1.0	180	5%
(Kolln) Fruit 'N Oat Bran Crunch	1 cup	1.0	110	8%
(Kretschmer)				
toasted wheat bran	¼ cup	1.0	30	30%
wheat germ				
honey crunch	5 tsp	1.0	50	18%
plain	2 Tbs	1.0	50	18%
(Krusteaz)				
corn flakes	1 cup	–	130	–
Crisp Rice	1 cup	–	130	–
Frosted Flakes	¾ cup	–	110	–
Fruit Whirls	¾ cup	1.0	120	8%

Food and Description	Amount	Fat Grams	Total Calories	% Fat Calories
raisin bran	¾ cup	1.5	210	6%
Toasted Oats				
apple cinnamon	¾ cup	2.0	130	14%
honey nut	¾ cup	2.0	120	15%
original	1 cup	2.0	120	15%
Life (*See* (Quaker) in this section)				
(Lifestream)				
berry granola	½ cup	2.5	200	11%
multigrain honey puffs	¾ cup	3.0	130	21%
(Lundberg Family)				
Brown Rice Crunchies	1 cup	1.0	170	5%
rice				
cinnamon raisin	⅓ cup	1.5	190	7%
sweet almond	⅓ cup	3.5	200	16%
(Mayacamas) Just Enough granola/ raisin & cinnamon	1 cup	1.0	130	7%
Mueslix (*See* (Kellogg's) in this section)				
(Nabisco)				
Fruit Wheats				
blueberry	¾ cup	0.5	170	3%
raspberry	¾ cup	0.5	160	3%
strawberry	¾ cup	0.5	170	3%
100% Bran	⅓ cup	0.5	80	6%
shredded wheat				
frosted				
bite-size	1 cup	1.0	190	5%
Wheat Bites	1 cup	1.0	190	5%
original	2 biscuits	0.5	160	3%
spoon-size	1 cup	0.5	170	3%
shredded wheat 'n bran	1¼ cups	1.0	200	5%
Team Flakes	1¼ cups	–	220	–
Nature Valley (*See* (General Mills) in this section)				
(Nature's Path)				
corn flakes	¾ cup	–	115	–
Heritage				
flakes	¾ cup	–	115	–
O's	¾ cup	–	115	–
muesli				
blueberry almond	½ cup	4.0	200	18%
heritage	½ cup	3.0	215	13%
multigrain				
& raisins	⅔ cup	<1.0	110	4%
oatbran flakes	⅔ cup	<1.0	110	4%
rice/millet	¾ cup	1.0	120	8%
(Nectar Sweet)				
granola				
blueberry 'n cream	⅓ cup	4.0	110	33%
raspberry 'n cream	⅓ cup	4.0	110	33%

Food and Description	Amount	Fat Grams	Total Calories	% Fat Calories
strawberry 'n cream	⅓ cup	4.0	110	33%
Crunch Oat Bran	⅓ cup	5.0	110	41%
(New Morning) Oatios				
apple cinnamon	1 cup	2.0	110	16%
plain	1 cup	1.0	110	8%
Nutri-Grain (*See* (Kellogg's) in this section)				
(Pacific Grain)				
Nutty Corn	¾ cup	10.0	220	41%
Nutty Wheat	¾ cup	5.0	220	20%
Pebbles (*See* (Post) in this section)				
(Pillsbury) Heartland				
plain	½ cup	11.0	290	28%
w/raisins				
low-fat	½ cup	3.0	210	13%
regular	½ cup	10.0	290	28%
(Post)				
Alpha-Bits				
original	1 cup	1.0	130	7%
w/marshmallows	1 cup	1.0	120	7%
Banana Nut Crunch	1 cup	6.0	250	22%
Blueberry Mornin	1¼ cups	3.5	230	14%
bran flakes	⅔ cup	0.5	90	5%
Bran'nola				
original	½ cup	3.0	200	14%
raisin	½ cup	3.0	200	14%
Cocoa Pebbles	¾ cup	1.0	120	8%
corn flakes/Post Toasties	1 cup	–	100	–
Crispy Critters	1⅓ cup	–	120	–
Fruit & Fibre				
dates/raisins/walnuts	1 cup	3.0	210	13%
peaches/raisins/almonds	1 cup	3.0	210	13%
pineapple/banana/coconut	⅔ cup	3.0	120	23%
Fruity Pebbles	¾ cup	1.0	110	8%
Golden Crisp	¾ cup	–	110	–
Golden Raisin Crisp	1 cup	3.5	250	13%
Grape-Nuts				
flakes	¾ cup	1.0	100	9%
original	½ cup	1.0	200	5%
Great Grains				
crunchy pecan	⅔ cup	6.0	220	25%
raisin, date, & pecan	⅔ cup	5.0	210	21%
hearty granola	⅔ cup	9.0	280	29%
Honey Bunches of Oats				
regular	¾ cup	1.5	120	11%
w/almonds	¾ cup	3.0	130	21%
Honeycomb	1⅓ cups	–	110	–
raisin bran	1 cup	1.0	190	5%
Product 19 (*See* (Kellogg's) in this section)				

Food and Description	Amount	Fat Grams	Total Calories	% Fat Calories
(Quaker)				
bran/unprocessed	⅓ cup	–	30	–
Crunchy Bran	¾ cup	1.0	90	10%
Cap'n Crunch				
Christmas Crunch	¾ cup	1.5	100	14%
Crunchberries	¾ cup	1.5	100	14%
Deep Sea Crunch	1 cup	2.0	130	14%
peanut butter	¾ cup	2.5	110	20%
regular	¾ cup	1.5	110	12%
Honey Graham Oh's	¾ cup	2.0	110	16%
King Vitaman	1½ cups	1.0	120	8%
Life				
cinnamon	1 cup	2.0	190	9%
plain	¾ cup	1.5	120	11%
Marshmallow Stars	¾ cup	1.5	120	11%
oat bran flakes	1¼ cups	3.0	210	13%
Oat Squares				
cinnamon	1 cup	2.5	230	10%
original	1 cup	3.0	220	12%
100% Natural				
low-fat w/raisins	½ cup	3.0	190	14%
regular				
oats & honey	½ cup	8.0	220	33%
oats, honey, & raisins	½ cup	8.0	220	33%
Popeye				
cocoa blasts	1 cup	1.5	130	10%
fruit curls	1 cup	1.0	120	8%
Jeepers	1⅓ cups	1.0	110	8%
Jeepers crispy corn puffs	1⅓ cups	0.5	110	4%
Oat 'Mmms				
plain	1 cup	2.0	120	15%
toasted	1 cup	1.5	110	12%
puffed rice	1¼ cups	–	50	–
puffed wheat	1¼ cups	–	50	–
Quisp	1 cup	1.5	110	12%
shredded wheat	3 biscuits	1.5	220	6%
Sugar Frosted Flakes	¾ cup	–	110	–
Sweet Puffs	1 cup	0.5	130	3%
Toasted Oatmeal				
honey nut	1 cup	4.5	200	20%
original	¾ cup	1.0	120	8%
(Quinoa) quinoa flakes	⅓ cup	1.0	105	9%
(Ralston)				
Cookie Crisp/chocolate chip	1 cup	1.5	120	11%
Corn Bran	⅔ cup	0.9	109	7%
Corn Chex	1¼ cups	–	110	–
Double Chex	1¼ cups	–	120	–

Food and Description	Amount	Fat Grams	Total Calories	% Fat Calories
fruit muesli				
blueberry pecan	1 cup	2.5	200	11%
cranberry walnut	¾ cup	3.0	200	14%
peach pecan	¾ cup	3.0	200	14%
raspberry almond	¾ cup	3.0	200	14%
strawberry pecan	1 cup	2.5	210	11%
Honey Almond Delight	1 cup	3.0	210	13%
Multi-Bran Chex	1¼ cups	1.0	220	4%
raisin bran	¾ cup	–	120	–
Rice Chex	1 cup	–	120	–
Sun Flakes	¾ cup	1.0	110	8%
Wheat Chex/100% whole wheat	¾ cup	1.0	190	5%
Rice Krispies (*See* (Kellogg's) in this section)				
(Skinner's) raisin bran	½ cup	1.0	100	9%
Special K (*See* (Kellogg's) in this section)				
(Stone Buhr)				
4 Grain Cereal Mates	2 oz	2.0	210	9%
hot apple granola	⅓ cup	1.0	130	7%
(Sun Country) granola				
w/almonds	½ cup	9.0	270	30%
w/raisins & dates	¼ cup	8.0	260	28%
(Sunbelt)				
five whole grains muesli	1.9 oz	2.0	210	9%
granola				
banana nut	1.9 oz	9.0	250	32%
berry basic	1.9 oz	6.0	220	25%
fruit & nut	1.9 oz	7.0	230	27%
low-fat	1.9 oz	3.0	200	14%
(Sunshine) shredded wheat				
bite-size	1 cup	1.5	180	8%
regular	1 biscuit	1.5	170	8%
(S.W. Graham)				
cinnamon	½ cup	–	100	–
plain	½ cup	–	100	–
Team Flakes (*See* (Nabisco) in this section)				
Total (*See* (General Mills) in this section)				
(U.S. Mills) Uncle Sam	1 cup	1.0	110	8%
(Weetabix) whole wheat	2 biscuits	<1.0	100	5%
Wheaties (*See* (General Mills) in this section)				

■ HOT/COOKED

(NOTE: All cereals are either dry or prepared with water per directions on packaging. If milk is used, calorie and fat content increase accordingly. Data on milk are shown in the Quick Reference on page 164. For additional information on milk, see MILK.)

(Arrowhead Mills)				
Bear Mush/dry	¼ cup	1.0	160	6%
Bits of Barley	⅓ cup	1.0	140	6%
bulgur	¼ cup	0.5	150	3%
couscous/dry	¼ cup	–	170	–

Food and Description	Amount	Fat Grams	Total Calories	% Fat Calories
cracked wheat/dry	¼ cup	0.5	140	3%
4 grain plus flax/dry	¼ cup	2.0	150	12%
oat bran/dry	⅓ cup	2.5	150	16%
oatmeal				
instant				
cinnamon raisin almond	1 pkg	3.0	130	21%
maple apple	1 pkg	2.0	130	14%
regular	1 pkg	2.0	110	16%
regular/steel-cut/dry	¼ cup	3.0	170	16%
Rice & Shine/dry	¼ cup	3.0	170	16%
rolled wheat flakes	¼ cup	0.5	110	4%
seven-grain cereal/dry				
regular	⅓ cup	1.5	140	10%
wheat-free	¼ cup	1.5	120	11%
(Cream of the West)				
Montana's 100% roasted wheat	¼ cup	<1.0	110	4%
(Erewhon)				
Barley Plus	1 serving	1.0	110	8%
cream of brown rice/prepared	1 cup	1.0	170	5%
oat bran w/toasted wheat germ	1 oz	2.0	115	16%
oatmeal/instant dry				
apple cinnamon	1 pkg	2.0	130	14%
apple raisin	1 pkg	2.0	140	13%
dates & walnuts	1 pkg	2.5	130	17%
maple spice	1 pkg	2.0	130	14%
raisins dates & nuts	1 pkg	2.5	130	17%
w/added oat bran	1 pkg	3.0	125	22%
(Fantastic Foods) cereal cup/dry				
banana nut barley	1.6 oz	2.5	180	13%
oatmeal				
apple cinnamon	1.9 oz	3.0	210	13%
cranberry orange	1.9 oz	3.0	210	13%
wheat n' berries	⅑ oz	1.0	210	4%
(General Mills) Wheat Hearts/dry	¼ cup	1.0	130	7%
generic				
farina				
cooked	½ cup	–	57	–
	1 cup	–	116	–
dry	1 oz	<1.0	105	1%
	1 cup	1.0	649	1%
oatmeal/regular				
cooked	4 oz	1.0	70	13%
	1 cup	2.0	145	12%
dry	1 oz	1.8	109	15%
	1 cup	5.0	311	14%
(Golden Harvest)				
maple/brown sugar hot fiber cereal	⅓ cup	2.0	100	18%

Food and Description	Amount	Fat Grams	Total Calories	% Fat Calories
(Highspire)				
Maltex	⅓ cup	0.5	170	3%
Wheatena	⅓ cup	1.0	150	6%
(H-O) oatmeal				
instant/dry				
apple cinnamon	1 pkg	2.0	130	14%
maple & brown sugar	1 pkg	2.0	160	11%
oats 'n fiber				
apple & bran	1 pkg	2.0	130	14%
plain	1 pkg	2.0	110	16%
raisin & bran	1 pkg	2.0	150	12%
plain	1 pkg	2.0	110	16%
raisins & spice	1 pkg	2.0	150	12%
sweet 'n mellow	1 pkg	2.0	150	12%
regular				
gourmet	⅓ cup	2.0	100	18%
quick	½ cup	2.0	130	14%
(Holden Foods) farina	3 Tbs	–	100	–
(Krusteaz)				
Ala/dry	¼ cup	0.5	50	9%
farina	3 Tbs	–	100	–
(Lundberg Family)				
hot 'n creamy rice cereal/prepared				
plain	1 serving	1.0	110	8%
w/almonds & nuts	1 serving	1.0	110	8%
(Malt-O-Meal)				
maple brown sugar	1 serving	–	100	–
plain or chocolate	1 serving	–	120	–
plus 40% oat bran	1 serving	2.0	130	14%
(Maypo)				
instant maple	½ cup	2.0	190	9%
Vermont style	⅓ cup	2.0	150	12%
(Mother's)				
multigrain/dry	½ cup	1.5	130	10%
oat bran/dry	½ cup	3.0	150	18%
oatmeal/instant/dry	½ cup	3.0	150	18%
whole wheat hot natural cereal	1 serving	1.0	130	7%
(Nabisco)				
cream of rice/instant/dry	¼ cup	–	170	–
cream of wheat				
instant/dry	¼ cup	1.5	150	3%
mix & eat/prepared				
apple cinnamon	1 serving	–	130	–
brown sugar/cinnamon	1 serving	–	130	–
cinnamon toast	1 serving	–	130	–
maple/brown sugar	1 serving	–	130	–
original	1 serving	–	100	–
quick	3 Tbs	–	120	–

Food and Description	Amount	Fat Grams	Total Calories	% Fat Calories
regular	3 Tbs	–	120	–
(Pathmark) farina/enriched	3 Tbs	–	100	–
(Pritikin) hearty hot cereal				
apple raisin spice	1 pkg	2.5	170	13%
multigrain	1 pkg	1.5	160	8%
(Quaker)				
oat bran/dry	½ cup	3.0	150	18%
oatmeal				
instant				
apple & cinnamon	1 pkg	1.5	130	8%
blueberries & cream	1 pkg	2.5	130	45%
cinnamon & spice	1 pkg	2.0	170	11%
honey nut	1 pkg	3.0	130	21%
maple & brown sugar	1 pkg	2.0	160	12%
peaches & cream	1 pkg	2.0	130	14%
regular	1 pkg	2.5	130	18%
raisin & spice	1 pkg	2.0	160	12%
raisins, dates, & walnuts	1 pkg	2.5	130	26%
strawberries & cream	1 pkg	2.0	130	14%
regular				
old-fashioned	½ cup	3.0	150	18%
quick-cooking	½ cup	3.0	150	18%
(Ralston) 100% milled wheat cereal	½ cup	1.0	150	6%
(Roman Meal)				
cream of rye	1 serving	1.0	110	8%
oatmeal/instant				
oats/multi-bran/apple/cinnamon	1 serving	2.0	110	16%
oats/wheat/dates/raisins/almonds	1 serving	1.5	130	10%
oats/wheat/honey/coconut/almonds	1 serving	6.0	160	34%
oats/wheat/rye/bran/flax	1 serving	1.5	110	12%
wheat, rye, bran, flax	1 serving	0.5	90	5%
(Skinner's) oat bran	1 serving	2.0	110	16%
(Stone-Buhr)				
4 grain cereal mates	⅓ cup	1.5	140	10%
hot apple granola	⅓ cup	1.0	130	7%
oat bran	⅓ cup	2.0	90	20%
7-grain cereal	⅓ cup	2.0	140	13%
(Zoom) dry	⅓ cup	0.5	120	4%
CEREAL BAR (See GRANOLA/GRANOLA-TYPE BAR)				
CERVELAT (See SAUSAGE)				
CHAMPAGNE (See WINE)				
CHARD				
fresh				
cooked	½ cup	–	18	–
raw/chopped	½ cup	–	3	–
frozen				
(C&W) Swiss	3.3 oz	–	20	–

Food and Description	Amount	Fat Grams	Total Calories	% Fat Calories
CHARLOTTE RUSSE				
w/lady fingers & whipped cream filling	4 oz	16.6	326	46%
CHAYOTE/fresh				
boiled	½ cup	–	19	–
raw/whole	1 medium	–	56	–
CHEESE (*See also* CHEESE ALTERNATIVE/IMITATION; CHEESE SPREAD; COTTAGE CHEESE; CREAM CHEESE)				
■ **(Alouette)**				
baby Brie				
plain	1 oz	9.0	110	74%
w/herbs	1 oz	9.0	110	74%
■ **(Alpine Lace)**				
American				
fat-free	1 oz	–	45	–
regular	1 oz	6.0	80	68%
cheddar				
fat-free	1 oz	–	45	–
reduced fat	1 oz	4.5	80	51%
Colby/reduced fat	1 oz	5.0	80	56%
garlic & herb/fat-free	1 oz	–	40	–
Havarti/reduced fat	1 oz	8.0	90	80%
hot pepper	1 oz	6.0	80	68%
Mexican nacho/fat-free	1 oz	–	40	–
Monterey jack/reduced fat	1 oz	4.5	70	58%
mozzarella				
fat-free	1 oz	–	45	–
reduced sodium	1 oz	5.0	70	64%
Muenster/reduced sodium	1 oz	9.0	100	81%
Parmesan/fat-free	1 oz	–	60	–
provolone/reduced fat	1 oz	5.0	70	64%
Swiss/reduced fat				
baby	1 oz	6.0	90	60%
regular	1 oz	6.0	90	60%
■ **(Athenos)**				
feta/crumbled				
basil & tomato	1 oz	6.0	80	68%
traditional	1 oz	6.0	80	68%
■ **BONBEL** (*See* (Laughing Cow) in this section)				
■ **(Borden)**				
processed				
American				
original				
fat-free	⅔ oz	–	25	–
low-fat/light	⅔ oz	1.0	30	30%
regular	1 oz	9.0	110	74%
loaf	1 oz	9.0	110	74%
singles	1 oz	7.0	90	70%
sliced	1 slice	5.0	60	75%

Food and Description	Amount	Fat Grams	Total Calories	% Fat Calories
salad blend/shredded	1 oz	8.0	100	72%
sharp				
fat-free	⅔ oz	–	25	–
regular	1 oz	8.0	100	72%
very sharp	1 oz	9.0	110	74%
cheddar				
Lite Line	1 oz	2.0	50	36%
sharp/block	1 oz	9.0	100	74%
mozzarella/Lite Line	1 oz	2.0	50	36%
Swiss				
cheese food	⅔ oz	5.0	70	64%
fat-free	⅔ oz	–	25	–
Lite Line	1 oz	2.0	50	36%
sliced	1 oz	8.0	100	72%
■ (Breakstone)				
ricotta	¼ cup	8.0	110	65%
■ (Casino)				
natural				
Havarti	1 oz	11.0	120	83%
Romano				
chunk	1 oz	7.0	100	63%
grated	1 oz	9.0	130	62%
Swiss	1 oz	8.0	110	65%
■ (Churny)				
Maybud				
Edam/reduced fat	1 oz	5.0	80	56%
farmers	1 oz	8.0	100	72%
Gouda/reduced fat	1 oz	5.0	80	56%
Lite Line	1 oz	2.0	50	36%
regular				
cheddar/diet snack	1 oz	3.0	70	39%
port wine/diet snack	1 oz	3.0	70	39%
■ (Cornville)				
Brie	1 oz	7.0	90	70%
Camembert	1 oz	7.0	90	70%
■ (County Line)				
Crackerbackers				
Colby-jack	1 oz	9.0	110	74%
mild cheddar	1 oz	9.0	110	74%
Monterey jack	1 oz	9.0	110	74%
regular				
American/sliced	1 slice	5.0	70	64%
cheddar				
extra sharp	1 oz	10.0	120	75%
finely shredded	¼ cup	10.0	120	75%
medium sharp	1 oz	10.0	120	75%
mild	1 oz	10.0	120	75%

Food and Description	Amount	Fat Grams	Total Calories	% Fat Calories
sharp				
chunk	1 oz	10.0	120	75%
shredded	¼ cup	10.0	120	75%
Colby				
jack	1 oz	9.0	110	74%
medium sharp	1 oz	10.0	120	75%
mild				
chunk	1 oz	10.0	120	75%
sliced	1 slice	9.0	110	74%
sharp	1 oz	10.0	120	75%
Monterey jack	1 oz	9.0	110	74%
mozzarella				
part skim/low-moisture/finely shredded	¼ cup	5.0	80	56%
regular/chunk	1 oz	5.0	80	56%
Muenster	1 oz	9.0	110	74%
Swiss, Old World	1 oz	8.0	110	65%
taco/shredded	¼ cup	10.0	120	75%

■ **CRACKER BARREL** (*See* (Kraft) in this section)
■ **CRACKERBACKERS** (*See* (County Line) in this section)
■ **(Di Giorno)**

Parmesan				
chunk	2 tsp	1.0	20	45%
grated	2 tsp	1.5	20	68%
shredded	2 tsp	1.5	20	68%
Romano				
chunk	2 tsp	1.5	20	68%
grated	2 tsp	1.5	25	54%
shredded	2 tsp	1.5	20	68%

■ **(Dorman's)**

natural				
blue				
Castello/70%	1 oz	12.0	135	80%
Danablu				
40%	1 oz	8.0	100	72%
60%	1 oz	10.0	110	82%
brick	1 oz	9.0	110	74%
Brie	1 oz	6.5	80	73%
Camembert/50%	1 oz	7.0	90	70%
Cheda-Jack				
reduced fat/low-sodium	1 oz	5.0	80	56%
regular	1 oz	7.0	90	70%
cheddar				
reduced fat/low sodium	1 oz	5.0	80	56%
regular	1 oz	9.0	110	74%
Colby	1 oz	9.0	110	74%
Edam	1 oz	8.0	100	72%
feta/45%	1 oz	7.0	90	70%

Food and Description	Amount	Fat Grams	Total Calories	% Fat Calories
Gouda	1 oz	8.0	100	72%
Havarti				
45%	1 oz	7.0	90	70%
60%	1 oz	11.0	120	83%
Monterey jack				
reduced fat /low sodium	1 oz	5.0	80	56%
regular	1 oz	8.0	100	72%
mozzarella				
part skim/low-sodium	1 oz	5.0	80	56%
reduced fat/low-sodium	1 oz	4.0	80	45%
regular	1 oz	6.0	90	60%
Muenster				
low-sodium	1 oz	9.0	110	74%
reduced fat/low-sodium	1 oz	5.0	80	56%
regular	1 oz	9.0	100	81%
Parmesan	1 oz	9.0	130	62%
provolone				
reduced fat/low-sodium	1 oz	4.0	80	45%
regular	1 oz	7.0	100	63%
Romano	1 oz	7.0	100	63%
Slim Jack	1 oz	7.0	90	70%
Swiss				
no salt added	1 oz	8.0	100	72%
reduced fat/low-sodium	1 oz	5.0	90	50%
regular	1 oz	8.0	100	72%
tybo/45%	1 oz	7.5	100	68%
■ (Finlandia)				
Havarti	1 oz	10.0	115	78%
Muenster				
lite	1 oz	4.0	80	45%
regular	1 oz	9.0	110	74%
Swiss	1 oz	4.0	83	43%
■ (Friendship)				
farmer	2 Tbs	3.0	50	54%
hoop	2 Tbs	2.0	20	90%
■ (Frigo)				
natural				
asiago	1 oz	9.0	110	74%
cheddar	1 oz	9.0	110	74%
lite	1 oz	5.0	80	56%
feta	1 oz	8.0	100	72%
mozzarella				
all natural/shredded	¼ cup	6.0	80	45%
part skim/low-moisture	1 oz	5.0	80	56%
string				
light	1 oz	2.0	60	30%
regular	1 oz	6.0	80	45%
whole milk/lite	1 oz	2.0	60	30%

Food and Description	Amount	Fat Grams	Total Calories	% Fat Calories
Parmazest	1 oz	7.0	120	53%
Parmesan				
chunk	1 oz	7.0	110	57%
grated	1 oz	7.0	110	57%
Parmesan & Romano				
grated	1 oz	7.0	110	57%
grated/dry	1 oz	9.0	130	62%
pizza/shredded	1 oz	3.0	65	42%
provolone/lite	1 oz	4.0	70	51%
ricotta/low-fat				
low-salt	1 oz	1.0	30	30%
part skim	1 oz	3.0	40	68%
whole milk	1 oz	5.0	60	75%
Romano				
grated	1 oz	8.0	110	65%
grated/dry	1 oz	9.0	130	62%
whole	1 oz	8.0	110	65%
Swiss	1 oz	8.0	110	65%
taco/shredded	¼ cup	9.0	110	74%
■ GENERIC				
American				
chunk	1 oz	7.0	95	66%
sliced	1 oz	7.0	95	66%
blue	1 oz	8.0	100	72%
	1 cup	38.8	477	73%
Brie	1 oz	7.9	95	74%
Camembert	1 oz	7.0	85	74%
caraway	1 oz	8.0	107	67%
cheddar				
reduced fat	1.5 oz	6.0	105	51%
shredded	1 cup	37.0	455	73%
smoky/sharp	1 oz	9.0	110	74%
Cheshire				
reduced fat	1.5 oz	6.0	110	49%
regular	1 oz	9.0	110	74%
Colby	1 oz	9.0	110	74%
Edam				
reduced-fat	1.5 oz	6.0	110	49%
regular	1 oz	8.0	100	72%
feta	1 oz	6.0	75	72%
fontina	1 oz	9.0	110	74%
Gjetost	1 oz	8.0	130	55%
goat				
hard	1 oz	10.0	130	69%
semisoft	1 oz	8.0	105	69%
soft	1 oz	6.0	75	72%
Gouda	1 oz	9.0	110	74%
Gruyere	1 oz	9.0	120	68%

Food and Description	Amount	Fat Grams	Total Calories	% Fat Calories
Havarti	1 oz	10.6	121	79%
Lancashire	1.5 oz	12.0	150	72%
Limburger	1 oz	8.0	95	76%
Monterey	1 oz	8.5	105	73%
Monterey jack	1 oz	9.0	110	74%
mozzarella				
low-moisture	1 oz	7.0	90	70%
part skim	1 oz	5.0	80	56%
Muenster	1 oz	8.5	105	73%
Neufchatel	1 oz	7.0	80	79%
Parmesan				
grated	1 Tbs	1.5	23	59%
	1 oz	8.5	129	59%
hard	1 oz	7.0	110	57%
Port du Salut	1 oz	8.0	100	72%
provolone	1 oz	7.5	100	68%
ricotta/part skim	1 oz	3.0	42	64%
	½ cup	9.8	171	52%
Romano	1 oz	7.5	110	61%
Roquefort	1 oz	8.7	105	75%
Stilton				
blue	1.5 oz	15.0	175	77%
white	1.5 oz	14.0	155	81%
Swiss	1 oz	7.8	110	64%
Tilsit	1 oz	7.0	96	66%
yogurt	1 oz	–	20	–
■ HARVEST MOON (See (Kraft) in this section)				
■ (Healthy Choice)				
fat-free				
American				
white singles	⅗ oz	–	30	–
yellow singles	⅔ oz	–	25	–
	¾ oz	–	30	–
cheddar/shredded	¼ cup	–	45	–
Mexican/shredded	¼ cup	–	45	–
mozzarella				
ball	1" cube	–	45	–
shredded	¼ cup	–	45	–
string	1 stick	–	45	–
pizza				
shredded	¼ cup	–	45	–
string	1 stick	–	45	–
process cheese loaf	1" cube	–	35	–
■ (Heluva Good Cheese)				
cheese food/cold pack				
cheddar				
sharp	2 Tbs	7.0	90	70%
w/bacon	2 Tbs	7.0	90	70%

Food and Description	Amount	Fat Grams	Total Calories	% Fat Calories
w/horseradish	2 Tbs	7.0	90	70%
w/jalapeños	2 Tbs	7.0	90	70%
w/port wine	2 Tbs	7.0	90	70%
natural cheese				
cheddar				
curds snack	1 oz	9.0	115	39%
extra sharp/white or yellow	1 oz	9.0	110	74%
mild				
reduced fat/yellow	1 oz	6.0	80	68%
regular/white	1 oz	9.0	110	74%
sharp/white or yellow	1 oz	9.0	110	74%
shredded/white or yellow	¼ cup	9.0	110	74%
very low sodium/white or yellow	1 oz	9.0	110	74%
Colby	1 oz	9.0	110	74%
Colby jack	1 oz	9.0	110	74%
curd/washed	1 oz	9.0	110	74%
Monterey jack				
shredded	¼ cup	8.0	100	72%
w/jalapeños	1 oz	8.0	100	72%
mozzarella				
part skim/shredded	¼ cup	5.0	80	56%
whole milk	1 oz	6.0	80	68%
Swiss	1 oz	8.0	110	65%
■ (Hickory Farms)				
Neufchatel				
chocolate	1 oz	8.0	110	65%
orange	1 oz	8.0	100	72%
peach	1 oz	8.0	90	80%
pineapple	1 oz	8.0	90	80%
rum date nut	1 oz	8.0	100	72%
strawberry	1 oz	8.0	90	80%
■ (Hoffman)				
processed cheese food				
hot pepper	1 oz	7.0	90	70%
smoky sharp	1 oz	9.0	110	74%
super sharp	1 oz	9.0	110	74%
■ (Jarlsberg)				
Swiss/lite/reduced fat	1 oz	3.5	70	45%
■ (Kaukauna)				
cheese ball w/almonds/cheddar				
port wine	1 oz	7.0	100	63%
sharp	1 oz	7.0	100	63%
w/bacon	1 oz	7.0	100	63%
w/green onion	1 oz	7.0	100	63%
cheese log w/almonds				
cheddar				
port wine	1 oz	7.0	100	63%

Food and Description	Amount	Fat Grams	Total Calories	% Fat Calories
sharp				
white				
hickory smoke flavored	1 oz	7.0	100	63%
w/green onion	1 oz	7.0	100	63%
yellow	1 oz	7.0	100	63%
smoky bacon	1 oz	7.0	100	63%
Swiss	1 oz	7.0	100	63%
garden vegetable	2 Tbs	12.0	130	83%
garlic & herb	2 Tbs	12.0	130	83%
ranch	2 Tbs	12.0	130	83%
Edam	1 oz	8.0	100	72%
Gouda				
caraway seeds	1 oz	8.0	100	72%
hickory smoke	1 oz	8.0	100	72%
plain	1 oz	8.0	100	72%
Monterey jack	1 oz	9.0	110	74%
Muenster	1 oz	9.0	110	74%
Neufchatel				
garlic & herb	1 oz	7.0	80	79%
garden vegetable	1 oz	7.0	80	79%
■ (Kraft)				
natural cheese				
blue				
cold pack	1 oz	8.0	100	72%
crumbles	1 oz	8.0	100	72%
brick	1 oz	9.0	110	74%
cheddar				
Healthy Favorites	¼ cup	–	45	–
regular				
chunk	1 oz	9.0	110	74%
finely shredded	¼ cup	8.0	90	80%
shredded	¼ cup	10.0	120	75%
mild/⅓ less fat				
chunk	1 oz	5.0	80	56%
shredded	¼ cup	6.0	90	60%
sharp				
Cracker Barrel reduced fat				
chunk	1 oz	5.0	80	56%
shredded	¼ cup	5.0	80	56%
⅓ less fat	1 oz	5.0	80	56%
Colby				
chunk				
⅓ less fat	1 oz	5.0	80	56%
regular	1 oz	9.0	110	74%
shredded	¼ cup	10.0	120	75%
Colby & Monterey jack	1 oz	9.0	110	74%
farmers	1 oz	8.0	100	72%
Gouda	1 oz	9.0	110	74%

Food and Description	Amount	Fat Grams	Total Calories	% Fat Calories
Havarti	1 oz	11.0	120	83%
house Italian/reduced fat/grated	2 tsp	1.0	25	36%
Italian blend/grated	2 tsp	1.5	25	54%
Limburger	1 oz	8.0	90	80%
Monterey jack				
plain				
⅓ less fat	1 oz	5.0	80	56%
regular				
chunk	1 oz	9.0	110	74%
shredded	¼ cup	9.0	110	74%
w/jalapeño peppers	1 oz	9.0	110	74%
mozzarella				
fat-free	¼ cup	–	50	–
part skim/low-moisture				
chunk	1 oz	5.0	80	56%
finely shredded	¼ cup	4.5	70	58%
shredded	¼ cup	6.0	90	60%
string	1 stick	6.0	80	68%
⅓ less fat/shredded	¼ cup	5.0	80	56%
whole milk/shredded	¼ cup	7.0	90	70%
Muenster	1 oz	9.0	110	74%
nacho blend cheddar w/peppers	1 oz	9.0	110	74%
Neufchatel/Philadelphia brand	1 oz	6.0	70	77%
Parmesan				
fat-free/grated	2 tsp	–	15	–
regular				
grated	2 tsp	1.5	20	68%
shredded	2 tsp	1.5	20	68%
Parmesan & Romano/grated	2 tsp	1.5	25	54%
pizza cheese/shredded				
mild cheddar & whole milk/ low-moisture mozzarella	¼ cup	7.0	90	70%
four cheese	¼ cup	7.0	90	70%
low-moisture mozzarella & cheddar	¼ cup	8.0	100	72%
low-moisture mozzarella & provolone w/smoke flavor	¼ cup	7.0	90	70%
provolone w/smoke flavor added	1 oz	7.0	100	63%
Romano/grated	2 tsp	1.5	25	54%
Swiss				
chunk	1 oz	9.0	110	74%
shredded	¼ cup	9.0	110	74%
taco cheese/shredded				
cheddar & Monterey jack	¼ cup	8.0	100	72%
processed cheese foods & products				
American				
deluxe/white or yellow				
loaf	1 oz	9.0	100	81%

Food and Description	Amount	Fat Grams	Total Calories	% Fat Calories
sliced	¾ oz	7.0	80	79%
	1 oz	9.0	110	74%
Harvest Moon/sliced				
processed cheese	⅔ oz	6.0	70	77%
processed cheese product	⅔ oz	3.0	50	54%
grated	1 Tbs	1.5	25	54%
Light N' Lively processed cheese product/50% less fat				
white	¾ oz	2.5	50	45%
yellow	¾ oz	2.5	50	45%
Old English				
loaf	1 oz	9.0	100	81%
slice	1 oz	9.0	110	74%
shredded	¼ cup	9.0	110	74%
singles/sliced				
white				
Kraft Free	⅔ oz	–	30	–
	¾ oz	–	30	–
⅓ less fat	¾ oz	3.0	50	54%
regular	⅔ oz	4.5	60	68%
yellow/singles				
Kraft Free	⅔ oz	–	30	–
	¾ oz	–	30	–
⅓ less fat	¾ oz	3.0	50	54%
regular	¾ oz	5.0	70	64%
	1.2 oz	8.0	110	65%
25% less fat	¾ oz	5.0	70	64%
cheddar				
Cracker Barrel/cold pack				
extra sharp	2 Tbs	8.0	100	72%
sharp	2 Tbs	8.0	100	72%
singles/sharp				
Kraft Free	¾ oz	–	30	–
⅓ less fat	¾ oz	3.0	50	54%
regular	¾ oz	6.0	70	77%
cheese food				
w/garlic	1 oz	7.0	90	70%
w/jalapeno peppers	1 oz	7.0	90	70%
Mexican w/jalapeño peppers/singles	¾ oz	5.0	70	64%
Monterey/singles	¾ oz	5.0	70	64%
mozzarella string/Handi-Snacks	1 stick	6.0	80	68%
pimiento				
shredded	⅔ oz	4.5	60	68%
	¾ oz	5.0	70	64%
sliced	1 oz	8.0	100	72%
Swiss				
shredded				
regular	¾ oz	5.0	70	64%

Food and Description	Amount	Fat Grams	Total Calories	% Fat Calories
⅓ less fat	¾ oz	2.5	50	45%
singles/Kraft Free	¾ oz	–	30	–
sliced	¾ oz	5.0	70	64%
	1 oz	7.0	90	70%
Velveeta cheese product				
Mexican/shredded				
hot	¼ cup	9.0	130	62%
mild	¼ cup	9.0	130	62%
original				
light	1 oz	3.0	60	45%
regular				
shredded	¼ cup	9.0	130	62%
sliced	¾ oz	4.5	60	68%
	⅘ oz	4.5	70	58%
	1.2 oz	7.0	100	63%
■ (Land O'Lakes)				
natural cheese				
brick	1 oz	8.0	110	65%
cheddar				
Chedarella	1 oz	8.0	100	72%
regular	1 oz	9.0	110	74%
Colby	1 oz	9.0	110	74%
Edam	1 oz	8.0	100	72%
Gouda	1 oz	8.0	100	72%
Monterey jack				
hot pepper	1 oz	9.0	110	74%
plain	1 oz	9.0	110	74%
mozzarella/part skim/low-moisture	1 oz	5.0	80	56%
Muenster	1 oz	9.0	100	81%
provolone	1 oz	8.0	100	72%
Swiss	1 oz	8.0	110	65%
processed cheese food				
American				
regular	1 oz	9.0	110	74%
sharp	1 oz	9.0	100	81%
American & Swiss	1 oz	8.0	100	72%
cheddar				
& bacon	1 oz	9.0	110	74%
extra sharp	1 oz	9.0	100	81%
La Chedda	1 oz	7.0	90	70%
Italian herb	1 oz	7.0	90	70%
jalapeño	1 oz	7.0	90	70%
jalapeño jack onion	1 oz	8.0	90	80%
onion	1 oz	7.0	90	70%
pepperoni	1 oz	7.0	90	70%
salami	1 oz	7.0	90	70%
sliced	⅔ oz	4.0	60	60%
	¾ oz	5.0	70	64%

Food and Description	Amount	Fat Grams	Total Calories	% Fat Calories
■ **(Laughing Cow)**				
natural cheese				
Babybel				
mini	1 piece	6.0	70	77%
mini light	1 piece	3.0	45	60%
regular	1 oz	7.0	90	70%
Bonbel				
mini	1 piece	6.0	70	77%
regular	1 oz	8.0	100	72%
Bonbino	1 oz	9.0	100	81%
Edam	1 oz	8.0	100	72%
Gouda				
mini	1 piece	6.0	80	68%
regular	1 oz	9.0	110	74%
processed cheese food				
cheesebits	6 pieces	6.0	70	77%
wedges				
assorted	1 oz	6.0	70	77%
light	1 oz	3.0	50	54%
original	1 oz	6.0	70	77%
■ **(Lifetime)**				
fat-free				
cheddar	1 oz	–	40	–
Mexican/mild	1 oz	–	40	–
Swiss	1 oz	–	40	–
■ **LIGHT N' LIVELY** (*See* (Kraft) in this section)				
■ **MAYBUD** (*See* (Cherny) in this section)				
■ **(McCadam)**				
cheddar				
extra sharp	1 oz	9.0	110	74%
medium	1 oz	9.0	110	74%
mild	1 oz	9.0	110	74%
sharp	1 oz	9.0	110	74%
Monterey jack	1 oz	9.0	110	74%
pepper jack	1 oz	9.0	110	74%
■ **(Montrachet)**				
goat cheese				
bulk	1 oz	6.0	70	77%
chive	1 oz	6.0	70	77%
classic	1 oz	6.0	70	77%
herb	1 oz	6.0	70	77%
herbs & garlic	1 oz	6.0	70	77%
in oil/drained	1 oz	6.0	70	77%
plain	1 oz	6.0	70	77%
w/ash	1 oz	6.0	70	77%
■ **MOOTOWN SNACKERS** (*See* (Sargento) in this section)				
■ **(Nucoa)**				
Heart Beat sandwich slices	1 oz	2.0	50	36%

Food and Description	Amount	Fat Grams	Total Calories	% Fat Calories
■ **OLD ENGLISH** (*See* (Kraft) in this section)				
■ **(Precious)**				
mozzarella/part skim	1 oz	6.0	80	68%
ricotta				
part-skim				
fat-free	¼ cup	–	40	–
low-fat	¼ cup	3.0	60	45%
original	¼ cup	6.0	100	54%
whole milk	¼ cup	8.0	110	65%
string/part skim	1 oz	6.0	80	68%
■ **(Quaker)**				
pimiento loaf	2 Tbs	8.0	80	90%
relish loaf	2 Tbs	8.0	80	90%
scallion loaf	2 Tbs	9.0	90	90%
■ **(Sargento)**				
blue cheese/crumbled	¼ cup	8.0	100	72%
cheddar				
classic supreme/shredded				
mild	¼ cup	9.0	110	74%
mild white	¼ cup	9.0	110	74%
fancy supreme/shredded				
mild	¼ cup	9.0	110	74%
sharp	¼ cup	9.0	110	74%
Mootown Snackers				
mild/light	1 piece	4.0	60	60%
regular	1 piece	8.0	100	72%
preferred light/shredded	¼ cup	4.5	70	58%
regular/sharp/sliced	1 slice	9.0	110	74%
Colby/sliced	1 slice	9.0	110	74%
Colby-jack				
light/Mootown Snackers	1 piece	8.0	90	80%
regular/shredded	¼ cup	9.0	110	74%
Jarlsberg/sliced	1 slice	9.0	120	68%
Monterey jack				
shredded	¼ cup	9.0	100	81%
sliced	1 slice	9.0	100	81%
mozzarella				
classic supreme/shredded	¼ cup	6.0	80	68%
fancy supreme/shredded	¼ cup	6.0	80	68%
preferred light				
shredded	¼ cup	3.0	70	39%
sliced	1 slice	5.0	90	50%
regular/sliced	1 slice	9.0	130	62%
Muenster/sliced	1 slice	9.0	100	81%
nacho & taco/shredded	¼ cup	9.0	110	74%
Parmesan				
grated	1 Tbs	1.5	25	54%
shredded	¼ cup	7.0	110	57%

Food and Description	Amount	Fat Grams	Total Calories	% Fat Calories
Parmesan & Romano/grated	1 Tbs	1.5	25	54%
pizza cheese/shredded				
classic supreme	¼ cup	6.0	90	60%
fancy supreme double cheese	¼ cup	6.0	90	60%
provolone/sliced	1 slice	8.0	100	72%
recipe blend				
4 cheese Mexican	¼ cup	9.0	110	74%
6 cheese Italian	¼ cup	7.0	90	70%
ricotta				
light	¼ cup	2.5	60	38%
old fashioned	¼ cup	6.0	90	60%
part skim	¼ cup	5.0	80	56%
Romano/shredded	¼ cup	7.0	110	57%
string/Mootown Snackers				
light	1 piece	3.0	60	45%
regular	1 piece	5.0	70	64%
Swiss				
preferred light/sliced	1 slice	4.0	80	45%
regular				
shredded	¼ cup	8.0	110	65%
sliced	1 slice	6.0	80	68%
wafer thin sliced	2 slices	9.0	110	74%
taco/shredded				
preferred light	¼ cup	4.5	70	58%
regular	¼ cup	9.0	110	74%
■ (Schwan's)				
American	1 slice	6.0	70	77%
mozzarella				
nuggets/breaded	¼ cup	7.0	110	57%
sticks/breaded	2 sticks	6.0	100	54%
■ (Smart Beat)				
processed cheese food/sliced				
American	1 slice	2.0	35	51%
low-sodium	1 slice	2.0	35	51%
sharp	1 slice	2.0	35	51%
■ (Treasure Cave)				
blue cheese/crumbled	1 oz	9.0	110	74%
■ VELVEETA (See (Kraft) in this section)				
■ (Weight Watchers)				
fat-free				
American/fat-free/reduced sodium/ white or yellow	¾ oz	–	30	–
cheddar				
low-fat				
mild				
low-sodium	1 oz	5.0	80	56%
regular	1 oz	5.0	80	56%
sharp	1 oz	5.0	80	56%

Food and Description	Amount	Fat Grams	Total Calories	% Fat Calories
fat-free				
sharp	¾ oz	–	30	–
white or yellow/sliced	¾ oz	–	30	–
Parmesan/fat-free/grated	1 Tbs	–	15	–
Swiss/fat-free/sliced	¾ oz	–	30	–
■ (WisPride)				
chunk	1 oz	8.0	110	65%
cup				
garlic & herb	2 Tbs	7.0	100	63%
hickory smoked	2 Tbs	7.0	100	63%
port wine				
light	2 Tbs	3.0	80	34%
regular	2 Tbs	7.0	100	63%
sharp				
light	2 Tbs	3.0	80	34%
regular	2 Tbs	7.0	100	63%
mini cheese ball				
garden vegetable	2 pieces	5.0	60	75%
garlic & herb	2 pieces	5.0	60	75%
port wine	2 pieces	9.0	120	68%
sharp cheddar	2 pieces	7.0	90	70%
■ (Woody's)				
cup/cold pack				
bacon	2 Tbs	8.0	110	65%
port wine	2 Tbs	8.0	100	72%
sharp	2 Tbs	8.0	100	72%

CHEESE, COTTAGE (*See* COTTAGE CHEESE)
CHEESE, CREAM (*See* CREAM CHEESE)
CHEESE ALTERNATIVE/IMITATION

Food and Description	Amount	Fat Grams	Total Calories	% Fat Calories
(Borden)				
American	⅔ oz	5.0	60	75%
	1 oz	7.0	90	70%
cheddar/shredded	1 oz	8.0	100	72%
Cheeztwo	⅔ oz	5.0	60	75%
Monterey jack blend	1 oz	7.0	90	70%
mozzarella				
shredded	1 oz	7.0	90	70%
sliced	1 oz	8.0	100	72%
sandwich mate	⅔ oz	5.0	60	75%
Swiss	⅔ oz	5.0	60	75%
Taco Mate	1 oz	8.0	100	72%
(CEMAC) Nu Tofu				
fat-free				
cheddar	1 oz	–	40	–
Monterey jack	1 oz	–	40	–
mozzarella	1 oz	–	40	–
regular				
cheddar	1 oz	4.0	40	90%

Food and Description	Amount	Fat Grams	Total Calories	% Fat Calories
Monterey jack	1 oz	4.0	40	90%
mozzarella	1 oz	4.0	40	90%
(Dorman's) Lo-Chol				
cheddar	1 oz	7.0	100	63%
colby	1 oz	7.0	100	63%
mozzarella	1 oz	6.0	90	60%
Muenster	1 oz	7.0	100	63%
Swiss	1 oz	7.0	100	63%
(Fleischmann's)				
fat-free liquid spread/cheddar	1 Tbs	–	10	–
(Formagg)				
American/sliced				
fat-free	1 slice	–	25	–
white	1 slice	2.0	40	45%
yellow	1 slice	2.0	40	45%
cheddar				
shredded	1 oz	3.0	60	45%
sliced	1 slice	2.0	40	45%
Parmesan/grated	2 tsp	0.5	15	30%
mozzarella/shredded	1 oz	3.0	60	45%
ricotta/fat-free	½ cup	–	40	–
Swiss/sliced	1 slice	2.0	40	45%
(Frigo)				
cheddar	1 oz	7.0	90	70%
mozzarella	1 oz	7.0	90	70%
(Golden Image)				
American process cheese food	¾ oz	5.0	70	64%
(Harvest Moon) shredded				
American	¼ cup	9.0	120	68%
cheddar	¼ cup	9.0	120	68%
mozzarella	¼ cup	8.0	110	65%
(LunchWagon)				
American process cheese food	¾ oz	5.0	70	64%
(Sargento)				
cheddar/shredded	¼ cup	7.0	90	70%
mozzarella/shredded	¼ cup	6.0	80	68%
(Soya Kaas) tofu				
American cheddar/mild	1 oz	5.0	70	64%
garlic & herb	1 oz	5.0	70	64%
hickory smoked cheddar	1 oz	5.0	80	56%
mozzarella				
fat-free	1 oz	–	40	–
regular	1 oz	5.0	70	64%
(Soyco) tofu				
American/sliced				
mozzarella	1 slice	3.0	50	54%
Swiss				
regular	1 slice	3.0	50	54%

Food and Description	Amount	Fat Grams	Total Calories	% Fat Calories
veggie	1 slice	2.0	40	45%
yellow				
regular	1 slice	3.0	50	54%
veggie	1 slice	2.0	40	45%
Caesars Italian/grated	2 tsp	0.5	15	30%
Cajun/grated	2 tsp	0.5	15	30%
Cheddar				
baked potato/grated	2 tsp	0.5	15	30%
fat-free	1 oz	–	30	–
low-fat	1 oz	3.0	60	45%
jalapeño				
fat-free	1 oz	–	30	–
low-fat	1 oz	3.0	60	45%
Monterey/low-fat	1 oz	3.0	60	45%
mozzarella				
fat-free	1 oz	–	30	–
low-fat	1 oz	3.0	60	45%
veggie/sliced	1 slice	2.0	40	45%
Parmesan/grated	2 tsp	0.5	15	30%
pepper jack/veggie/sliced	1 slice	2.0	40	45%
provolone/veggie/sliced	1 slice	2.0	40	45%
Romano/grated	2 tsp	0.5	15	30%
(Soymage) tofu				
American/yellow/sliced	1 slice	–	20	–
cheddar	1 oz	–	40	–
grated cheese	2 tsp	0.5	15	30%
herb	1 oz	–	40	–
jalapeño	1 oz	–	40	–
mozzarella				
chunk	1 oz	–	40	–
sliced	1 slice	–	20	–
(Tofutti) Better Than Cream Cheese				
French onion	2 Tbs	8.0	80	90%
herbs & chives	2 Tbs	8.0	80	90%
plain	2 Tbs	8.0	80	90%

CHEESE DISH (*See* CHEESE SOUFFLÉ; FROZEN ENTRÉE/DINNER; VEGETARIAN FOODS; WELSH RAREBIT)
CHEESE SAUCE (*See* SAUCE)
CHEESE SEASONING (*See* SEASONINGS)
CHEESE SNACK (*See* SNACKS)
CHEESE SOUFFLÉ
Homemade/USDA Standard Home Recipe

8" square	~4 oz	19.0	240	71%

CHEESE SOUP (*See* SOUP)
CHEESE SPREAD (*See also* CHEESE ALTERNATIVE/IMITATION; CREAM CHEESE)
(Alouette)
creme de brie

herb	2 Tbs	8.0	90	80%

Food and Description	Amount	Fat Grams	Total Calories	% Fat Calories
original	2 Tbs	8.0	90	80%
cream cheese spread				
light				
herbs & garlic	2 Tbs	4.0	50	72%
spring vegetable	2 Tbs	4.0	50	72%
regular				
French onion melange	2 Tbs	7.0	80	79%
garlic & herbs	2 Tbs	7.0	70	90%
spinach Florentine	2 Tbs	6.0	60	90%
deli spread				
Cajun	2 Tbs	7.0	70	90%
French onion	2 Tbs	7.0	70	90%
French onion melange	2 Tbs	7.0	80	79%
garlic	2 Tbs	7.0	70	90%
salmon/fumé et capers	2 Tbs	7.0	70	90%
scallions	2 Tbs	7.0	70	90%
spinach	2 Tbs	6.0	60	90%
spinach Florentine	2 Tbs	6.0	60	90%
sun-dried tomatoes et basil	2 Tbs	7.0	70	90%
vegetable jardin	2 Tbs	6.0	60	90%
light/lite spread				
cucumber dill crudité	2 Tbs	4.0	50	72%
dill	2 Tbs	4.0	50	72%
garlic et herbs classique	2 Tbs	4.0	50	72%
herb	2 Tbs	4.0	50	72%
scalliion variete	2 Tbs	4.0	50	72%
spring vegetable	2 Tbs	4.0	50	72%
regular spread				
belle pepper trio	2 Tbs	7.0	70	90%
dijon moutarde et honey	2 Tbs	7.0	80	79%
ginger apple & spice	2 Tbs	6.0	80	68%
(Alpine Lace) cream cheese spread				
garden vegetable	2 Tbs	–	40	–
garlic & herb	2 Tbs	–	40	–
(Borden) processed American cheese spread	2 Tbs	6.0	80	68%
(Chavrie) goat cheese spread	2 Tbs	3.0	40	68%
Cheez Whiz (See (Kraft) in this section)				
(Churny)				
Rondele				
light				
French onion	2 Tbs	4.0	60	60%
garden vegetable	2 Tbs	4.0	60	60%
garlic & herb	2 Tbs	4.0	60	60%
regular				
garden vegetable	2 Tbs	9.0	90	90%
garlic & herb	2 Tbs	9.0	90	90%
savory herbs	2 Tbs	10.0	100	90%

Food and Description	Amount	Fat Grams	Total Calories	% Fat Calories
(Fleur de Lait)				
fresh-cut spread				
Bermuda onion & chives	2 Tbs	8.0	90	80%
date nut rum	2 Tbs	8.0	90	80%
garden vegetable	2 Tbs	8.0	80	90%
garlic & spice	2 Tbs	9.0	90	90%
herb & spice	2 Tbs	9.0	90	90%
lox/smoked salmon	2 Tbs	8.0	90	80%
peaches & cream	2 Tbs	7.0	90	70%
strawberry	2 Tbs	8.0	90	80%
Neufchatel spread				
Bermuda onion	2 Tbs	8.0	90	80%
date nut rum	2 Tbs	8.0	90	80%
garden vegetable	2 Tbs	8.0	80	90%
garlic & spice	2 Tbs	9.0	90	90%
herb & spice	2 Tbs	9.0	90	90%
lemon	2 Tbs	7.0	90	70%
lox/smoked salmon	2 Tbs	8.0	90	80%
mandarin orange	2 Tbs	7.0	90	70%
peach	2 Tbs	7.0	90	70%
pineapple	2 Tbs	8.0	90	80%
strawberry	2 Tbs	8.0	90	80%
toasted onion	2 Tbs	9.0	90	90%
wildberry	2 Tbs	7.0	90	70%
generic				
American cheese spread	2 Tbs	6.0	80	68%
Harvest Moon (*See* (Kraft) in this section)				
(Kaukauna) cold-pack cup				
lite 50				
port wine	2 Tbs	3.5	70	45%
sharp cheddar	2 Tbs	3.5	70	45%
smoky	2 Tbs	3.5	70	45%
Swiss w/almonds	2 Tbs	3.5	70	45%
original				
cheddar	2 Tbs	7.0	90	70%
bacon & horseradish	2 Tbs	7.0	100	63%
port wine	2 Tbs	7.0	90	70%
sharp	2 Tbs	7.0	90	70%
smoky sharp	2 Tbs	7.0	90	70%
(Kraft)				
Cheez Whiz				
jarred				
light	2 Tbs	3.0	80	34%
⅓ less fat	2 Tbs	7.0	90	70%
original	2 Tbs	8.0	100	72%
spread				
original	2 Tbs	7.0	90	70%

Food and Description	Amount	Fat Grams	Total Calories	% Fat Calories
salsa				
hot	2 Tbs	7.0	90	70%
mild	2 Tbs	7.0	90	70%
w/jalapeño peppers	2 Tbs	8.0	90	80%
Zap-a-Pack				
original	2 Tbs	8.0	90	80%
w/mild salsa	2 Tbs	8.0	90	80%
Harvest Moon				
American cheese spread	⅔ oz	4.0	60	60%
	¾ oz	4.5	60	68%
Mohawk Valley/limburger spread	2 Tbs	7.0	80	79%
Old English brand				
sharp spread	2 Tbs	8.0	90	80%
regular				
jalapeño pepper loaf	1 oz	6.0	80	68%
olive & pimiento	2 Tbs	6.0	70	77%
pimiento	2 Tbs	6.0	80	68%
pineapple	2 Tbs	5.0	70	64%
Roka/blue cheese spread				
plain	2 Tbs	7.0	80	79%
w/bacon	2 Tbs	8.0	90	80%
Spreadery cheese snack				
cheddar/cold pack				
medium	2 Tbs	4.5	80	51%
sharp	2 Tbs	4.5	80	51%
sharp white	2 Tbs	4.5	80	51%
Neufchatel spread				
classic ranch	2 Tbs	7.0	80	79%
garden vegetables	2 Tbs	6.0	70	77%
garlic & herb	2 Tbs	7.0	80	79%
pimento	2 Tbs	8.0	100	72%
Squeez-A-Snak/sharp	2 Tbs	8.0	90	80%
Velveeta spread				
Italian	1 oz	6.0	80	68%
Mexican				
hot	1 oz	6.0	80	68%
mild	1 oz	6.0	80	68%
original	1 oz	6.0	80	68%
(Land O'Lakes) Golden Velvet	1 oz	6.0	80	68%
(Merkts)				
almond Swiss	2 Tbs	8.0	100	72%
garlic herb	2 Tbs	8.0	100	72%
port wine	2 Tbs	8.0	100	72%
cheddar/sharp	2 Tbs	8.0	100	72%
Mohawk Valley (See (Kraft) in this section)				
(Nabisco) Easy Cheese spread				
cheddar				
regular	2 Tbs	7.0	100	63%

Food and Description	Amount	Fat Grams	Total Calories	% Fat Calories
sharp	2 Tbs	7.0	100	63%
cheddar 'n bacon	2 Tbs	7.0	100	63%
nacho	2 Tbs	7.0	100	63%
(New Holland)				
garlic	1 oz	7.0	90	70%
jalapeño	1 oz	6.0	80	68%
natural vegetable	1 oz	6.0	80	68%
plain	1 oz	7.0	90	70%
Old English (*See* (Kraft) in this section)				
Roka (*See* (Kraft) in this section)				
Rondele (*See* (Churny) in this section)				
Spreadery (*See* (Kraft) in this section)				
Velveeta (*See* (Kraft) in this section)				
CHEESE SUBSTITUTE (*See* CHEESE ALTERNATIVE/IMITATION)				
CHERIMOYA				
raw/whole/medium	2 lbs	2.0	515	3%
CHERRY				
candied				
generic				
sweet	1 oz	<1.0	96	5%
whole	10 medium	<1.0	119	4%
(S&W)				
glacé cherries/green or red	5 pieces	–	80	–
canned or jarred				
(Del Monte)				
dark/pitted/in heavy syrup	½ cup	–	100	–
generic				
maraschino				
drained	1 large	–	10	–
	10 large	–	97	–
w/liquid	1 oz	–	33	–
sour red				
in extra heavy syrup	1 cup	<1.0	296	2%
in heavy syrup	1 cup	<1.0	232	2%
in light syrup	1 cup	<1.0	188	2%
in water	1 cup	<1.0	87	5%
sweet				
in extra heavy syrup	1 cup	<1.0	266	2%
in heavy syrup	1 cup	<1.0	213	2%
in juice	1 cup	<1.0	136	3%
in light syrup	1 cup	<1.0	170	3%
in water	1 cup	<1.0	114	4%
(S&W)				
dark sweet/pitted/in heavy syrup	½ cup	–	140	–
maraschino/green or red	1 cherry	–	10	–
royal anne/light/sweet/pitted	½ cup	–	140	–
(World Classic) royal anne	½ cup	–	90	–

Food and Description	Amount	Fat Grams	Total Calories	% Fat Calories
dried				
(Chukar)				
Bing	2 oz	1.0	160	6%
Rainier	2 oz	1.0	160	6%
tart	2 oz	–	170	–
tart 'n sweet	2 oz	–	180	–
(Traverse Bay) cherry snax/red tart	1 oz	–	100	–
fresh				
sour red	1 cup	<1.0	51	9%
sweet	10 medium	0.7	49	13%
	1 cup	1.0	103	9%
(Dole)	1 cup	1.0	90	10%
frozen				
(Big Valley) dark sweet	½ cup	–	60	–
generic				
sour red				
sweetened	1 cup	0.7	224	3%
unsweetened	3.5 oz	<1.0	50	3%
	1 cup	0.7	72	9%
sweet				
sweetened	1 cup	<1.0	232	2%
unsweetened	3.5 oz	<1.0	60	8%
CHERRY DRINK (*See also* FRUIT PUNCH; SOFT DRINK MIX)				
bottled				
(Betty Crocker) Squeezit	6.76 fl oz	–	110	–
frozen				
(Welch's) Welchade	8 fl oz	–	130	–
CHERRY JUICE/JUICE BLEND/JUICE DRINK				
bottled, boxed, or canned				
(Capri Sun) wild cherry	6.75 oz	–	110	–
(Dole) mountain cherry	8 fl oz	–	120	–
(Hi-C)				
drink box	8.45 oz	–	130	–
pet	8 oz	–	130	–
(Libby's) Juicy Juice	4.23 oz	–	70	–
	8 oz	–	140	–
frozen/prepared				
(Dole) mountain cherry	8 oz	–	140	–
	10 oz	–	150	–
CHERVIL				
dried	1 tsp	–	1	–
raw	4 oz	–	65	–
CHESTNUT				
Chinese				
boiled or steamed	1 oz	–	44	–
dried	1 oz	0.5	103	4%
roasted	1 oz	–	68	–

Food and Description	Amount	Fat Grams	Total Calories	% Fat Calories
European				
boiled or steamed	1 oz	–	37	–
dried	1 oz	1.0	106	8%
roasted	1 oz	0.6	70	8%
Japanese				
boiled or steamed	1 oz	–	16	–
dried	1 oz	–	102	–
roasted	1 oz	–	57	–
CHESTNUT FLOUR (See FLOUR)				
CHEWING GUM (See GUM)				
CHICKEN (See also LUNCHEON MEAT; VEGETARIAN FOODS)				
■ **CHICKEN & CHICKEN PARTS/FRESH**				
broiler/fryer				
dark meat				
meat & skin				
batter-dipped & fried	~9.5 oz	51.8	828	56%
flour-coated & fried	~6.5 oz	31.0	523	53%
roasted	~6 oz	26.0	423	55%
stewed	~6.5 oz	27.0	428	57%
meat only				
fried	~5 oz	16.0	334	43%
roasted	~5 oz	13.6	286	43%
stewed	~5 oz	12.6	269	42%
giblets/organs				
giblets/chopped or diced				
flour-coated & fried	1 cup	19.5	402	44%
simmered	1 cup	6.9	228	27%
gizzard/simmered	1 oz	1.0	43	21%
	1 cup	5.0	222	20%
heart/simmered	3 oz	5.0	158	29%
	1 cup	11.5	268	39%
liver/simmered	~5 oz	7.6	219	31%
	1 cup	7.6	220	31%
half/meat & skin				
batter-dipped & fried	~1 lb	80.8	1347	54%
flour-coated & fried	~¾ lb	46.8	844	50%
roasted	~¾ lb	40.7	715	51%
stewed	~¾ lb	42.0	730	52%
light meat				
meat & skin				
batter-dipped & fried	~7 oz	29.0	520	50%
flour-coated & fried	~5 oz	15.7	320	44%
roasted	~5 oz	14.0	293	43%
stewed	~5 oz	15.0	302	45%
meat only				
fried	~5 oz	7.8	268	26%
roasted	~5 oz	6.0	242	22%
stewed	~5 oz	5.6	223	23%

Food and Description	Amount	Fat Grams	Total Calories	% Fat Calories
parts				
backs				
meat & skin				
batter-dipped & fried	~4 oz	26.0	397	59%
flour-coated & fried	~2.5 oz	14.9	238	56%
roasted	~2 oz	11.0	159	62%
stewed	~2 oz	11.0	158	63%
meat only				
fried	~2 oz	8.9	167	48%
roasted	~1.5 oz	5.0	96	47%
stewed	~1.5 oz	4.7	88	48%
breast				
meat & skin				
batter-dipped & fried	~5 oz	18.5	364	46%
flour-coated & fried	~3.5 oz	8.7	218	36%
roasted	~3.5 oz	7.6	193	35%
stewed	~4 oz	8.0	202	36%
meat only				
fried	~3 oz	4.0	161	22%
roasted	~3 oz	3.0	142	19%
stewed	~3 oz	2.9	144	18%
drumstick				
meat & skin				
batter-dipped & fried	~2.5 oz	11.0	193	51%
flour-coated & fried	~2 oz	6.7	120	50%
roasted	~2 oz	5.8	112	47%
stewed	~2 oz	6.0	116	47%
meat only				
fried	~1.5 oz	3.0	82	33%
roasted	~1.5 oz	2.0	76	24%
stewed	~1.5 oz	2.6	78	30%
leg				
meat & skin				
batter-dipped & fried	~5.5 oz	25.6	431	53%
flour-coated & fried	~4 oz	16.0	285	51%
roasted	~4 oz	15.0	265	51%
stewed	~4 oz	16.0	275	52%
meat only				
fried	~3 oz	8.8	195	40%
roasted	~3 oz	8.0	182	40%
stewed	~3.5 oz	8.0	187	39%
thigh				
meat & skin				
batter-dipped & fried	~3 oz	14.0	238	53%
flour-coated & fried	~2 oz	9.0	162	50%
roasted	~2 oz	9.6	153	56%
stewed	~2 oz	10.0	158	57%

Food and Description	Amount	Fat Grams	Total Calories	% Fat Calories
meat only				
fried	~2 oz	5.0	113	40%
roasted	~2 oz	5.7	109	47%
stewed	~2 oz	5.0	107	42%
wing				
meat & skin				
batter-dipped & fried	~2 oz	10.7	159	61%
flour-coated & fried	~1 oz	7.0	103	61%
roasted	~1.5 oz	6.6	99	60%
stewed	~1.5 oz	6.7	100	60%
meat only				
fried	~1 oz	1.8	42	39%
roasted	~1 oz	1.7	43	36%
stewed	~1 oz	1.7	43	36%
whole/including meat, skin, giblets, & neck				
batter-dipped & fried	~2¼ lb	180.0	2987	54%
flour-coated & fried	~1½ lb	108.0	1928	50%
roasted	~1½ lb	90.0	1598	51%
stewed	~1½ lb	92.9	1625	52%
roaster/roasted				
dark meat/meat only				
chopped or diced	1 cup	12.3	250	44%
sliced	4 oz	10.0	205	44%
half/w/bones	1 lb	64.0	1070	53%
light meat/meat only				
chopped or diced	1 cup	5.7	214	24%
sliced	4 oz	4.6	175	24%
whole/meat & skin	4 oz	15.0	253	53%
stewing chicken/stewed				
whole				
meat & skin	~9 oz	49.0	744	59%
meat only				
chopped or diced	1 cup	16.6	335	45%
sliced	4 oz	13.5	270	45%
meat, skin, & giblets	1½ lbs	107.0	1636	59%
dark meat/meat only				
chopped or diced	1 cup	21.0	360	53%
sliced	4 oz	17.0	295	52%
light meat/meat only				
chopped/diced	1 cup	11.2	300	34%
sliced	4 oz	9.0	240	34%
■ CHICKEN & CHICKEN PARTS/FRESH, FROZEN, OR CANNED/BRAND NAME				
(Butterball) fresh/raw				
best of the fryer	4 oz	14.0	200	63%
breast				
fillet				
seasoned				
Italian style	1 fillet	2.0	120	15%

Food and Description	Amount	Fat Grams	Total Calories	% Fat Calories
lemon butter	1 fillet	1.0	120	8%
mesquite	1 fillet	1.0	120	8%
teriyaki	1 fillet	1.0	120	8%
thin	1 fillet	0.5	110	4%
unseasoned	1 fillet	0.5	110	4%
split				
family pack	1 breast	18.0	300	54%
skinless	1 breast	0.5	110	4%
tenders	3 tenders	–	70	–
ground	4 oz	13.0	200	59%
roasting broiler	4 oz	16.0	220	65%
thighs/family pack	1 thigh	15.0	210	64%
wings				
drummettes	3 pieces	10.0	150	60%
regular	2 wings	16.0	210	69%
(Perdue)				
fresh/uncooked				
burgers				
cooked	3 oz	11.0	170	58%
raw	4 oz	11.0	180	55%
ground				
cooked	3 oz	11.0	180	55%
raw	4 oz	13.0	190	62%
parts				
Fit 'n Easy/skinless-boneless				
breast				
Oven Stuffer Roaster	3 oz	2.0	120	15%
regular	3 oz	2.5	120	19%
tenders	3 oz	0.5	100	5%
thin-sliced	3 oz	2.0	120	15%
breast & thighs				
dark meat	3 oz	8.0	158	46%
thighs				
Oven Stuffer Roaster	3 oz	8.0	160	45%
regular	3 oz	8.0	160	45%
white meat	3 oz	2.0	120	15%
young/roasted w/skin on				
breast quarters	3 oz	11.0	180	55%
breasts				
regular	3 oz	9.0	170	48%
skinless	3 oz	1.5	130	10%
drumsticks				
regular	3 oz	8.0	160	45%
skinless	3 oz	5.0	130	35%
leg quarters	3 oz	16.0	220	65%
legs	3 oz	14.0	200	63%
pick of the chicken/skinless				
dark meat	3 oz	8.0	160	45%

Food and Description	Amount	Fat Grams	Total Calories	% Fat Calories
white meat	3 oz	4.0	130	28%
thighs				
regular	3 oz	17.0	230	67%
skinless	3 oz	11.0	180	55%
wingettes	3 oz	14.0	200	63%
wings	3 oz	14.0	200	63%
whole/roasted w/skin on				
Oven Stuffer Roaster				
breast	3 oz	7.0	160	39%
dark meat	3 oz	14.0	200	63%
drumsticks	3 oz	9.0	170	48%
light meat	3 oz	8.0	160	45%
thighs	3 oz	15.0	220	61%
wing drumettes	3 oz	12.0	190	57%
wingettes	3 oz	13.0	200	59%
young				
dark meat	3 oz	16.0	220	65%
light meat	3 oz	10.0	170	53%
cooked				
BBQ chicken & chicken parts				
breast	5.5 oz	8.0	220	33%
dark meat	3 oz	10.0	160	56%
drumsticks	2 pieces	4.0	110	33%
light meat	3 oz	3.5	160	20%
thighs	1 thigh	12.0	180	60%
Perdue Done It! fully cooked chicken				
barbecued wings	3 oz	12.0	200	54%
chicken breast cutlets	3.5 oz	13.0	230	51%
chicken breast tenders	3 oz	7.0	160	39%
chicken & cheese nuggets	3 oz	15.0	220	61%
fun shapes	3 oz	12.0	200	54%
fun shapes chicken on a stick	3.5 oz	13.0	230	51%
hot & spicy wings	3 oz	12.0	200	54%
original chicken breast nuggets	3 oz	12.0	200	54%
oven-roasted chicken				
dark meat	3 oz	11.0	170	58%
white meat	3 oz	7.0	140	45%
roasted chicken				
breast	5 oz	6.0	190	28%
drumsticks	2.5 oz	4.0	100	36%
thighs	1 piece	12.0	170	64%
(Swanson) canned				
chunk white	2 oz	2.0	80	23%
mixin chicken in broth	¼ cup	8.0	110	65%
(TastyBird Foods) frozen/raw/ready to cook				
breast fillet patty				
hoagie-shaped	3.5 oz	10.8	211	46%
regular	3.5 oz	14.0	229	55%

Food and Description	Amount	Fat Grams	Total Calories	% Fat Calories
breast quarter/breaded	3.5 oz	11.0	192	52%
breast strip	1 oz	2.8	54	47%
breast tenderloin				
regular	3.5 oz	8.7	189	41%
spicy	3.5 oz	7.0	170	37%
chicken delites	3.5 oz	19.0	252	68%
hi-pro patty	3.5 oz	19.0	252	68%
leg quarter/breaded	3.5 oz	11.7	199	53%
nuggets	3.5 oz	13.8	215	58%
(TriFoods) ground	2 oz	8.0	110	65%
(Valley Fresh) canned				
premium white	2 oz	1.0	70	13%
white & dark	2 oz	2.0	80	23%

CHICKEN ENTRÉE/DINNER (*See also* ASIAN FOOD; FROZEN ENTRÉE/DINNER; MEXICAN FOOD; PASTA ENTRÉE/DINNER; RICE DISH)

Food and Description	Amount	Fat Grams	Total Calories	% Fat Calories
(Banquet) frozen				
bone-in				
breast/fried	4.45 oz	26.0	410	57%
drums & thighs/fried	3 oz	18.0	260	62%
fried chicken				
country fried	3 oz	18.0	270	60%
hot & spicy	3 oz	18.0	260	62%
original	3 oz	18.0	270	60%
skinless				
honey BBQ	3 oz	13.0	210	56%
regular	3 oz	13.0	210	56%
Southern	3 oz	18.0	270	60%
wings/hot & spicy	4 pieces	16.0	230	63%
boneless				
breast tenders/Southern-fried	~3 oz	16.0	260	55%
Drum-Snackers	2.25 oz	13.0	190	62%
hot popcorn chicken	3 oz	19.0	290	59%
nuggets				
hot 'n spicy	2.5 oz	17.0	230	67%
original	3 oz	15.0	240	56%
Southern-fried	6 pieces	20.0	340	53%
sweet & sour	6 pieces	18.0	320	51%
w/cheddar	2.86 oz	19.0	280	61%
patties				
original	2.5 oz	11.0	180	55%
Southern-fried	2.5 oz	12.0	190	57%
(Betty Crocker) Skillet Chicken Helper				
mix only	¼ cup	0.5	140	3%
prepared	1 cup	9.0	270	30%
(Country Pride) frozen				
chunks				
regular	3 oz	15.0	238	57%
Southern-fried	3 oz	20.0	276	65%

Food and Description	Amount	Fat Grams	Total Calories	% Fat Calories
patties				
regular	3 oz	16.0	245	59%
Southern-fried	3 oz	15.0	232	58%
sticks	3 oz	14.0	233	54%
(Country Skillet) frozen				
chunks				
regular	5 pieces	17.0	270	57%
Southern-fried	5 pieces	15.0	250	54%
nuggets	10 pieces	18.0	280	58%
patties				
regular	2.5 oz	12.0	190	57%
Southern-fried	2.5 oz	12.0	190	57%
(Delta Valley) frozen/white				
nuggets	4 pieces	14.0	230	55%
patties	1 patty	14.0	220	57%
(Dinty Moore)				
canned/chicken stew	1 cup	11.0	220	45%
microwaveable				
American classics				
chicken & noodles	1 bowl	8.0	260	21%
chicken w/mashed potatoes	1 bowl	4.0	220	16%
microwave cup				
chicken & dumpling	1 cup	6.0	190	28%
chicken stew	1 cup	8.0	180	40%
(Fall's) BBQ Chicken	3 oz	8.0	150	48%
generic/canned				
chicken à la king	~5 oz	11.7	182	58%
(Heinz) canned				
chicken stew w/dumplings	7.5 oz	9.0	210	39%
homemade/USDA Standard Home Recipe				
chicken à la king	1 cup	34.0	468	65%
chicken cacciatore	1 cup	32.0	525	55%
chicken cordon bleu	8 oz	13.0	335	35%
chicken fricassee	1 cup	22.0	386	51%
chicken hash	1 cup	11.0	239	41%
chicken pot pie/9" dia	⅓ pie	31.0	545	51%
chicken salad	½ cup	8.0	121	60%
chicken w/noodles	1 cup	18.0	365	44%
creamed chicken	½ cup	12.0	208	52%
creole chicken/w/o rice	¾ cup	3.0	137	20%
(Hormel)				
Chicken By George/refrigerated				
Cajun	~4 oz	4.0	120	30%
Caribbean grill	~4 oz	4.0	150	24%
garlic & herb	~4 oz	2.5	120	19%
Italian blue cheese	~4 oz	5.0	130	35%
lemon herb	~4 oz	3.0	120	23%
lemon oregano	~4 oz	4.0	130	28%

Food and Description	Amount	Fat Grams	Total Calories	% Fat Calories
mesquite barbeque	~4 oz	2.0	120	15%
mustard dill	~4 oz	5.0	140	32%
teriyaki	~4 oz	3.0	130	21%
tomato herb w/basil	~4 oz	5.0	140	32%
Top Shelf Two-Minute Entrées				
chicken à la king	1 bowl	12.0	380	28%
chicken cacciatore	1 bowl	2.5	210	11%
fiesta chicken	1 bowl	16.0	420	34%
glazed breast of chicken	1 bowl	5.0	200	23%
(Luck's)				
canned				
chicken & dumplings/traditional	1 cup	17.0	330	46%
microwaveable				
Brunswick stew	1 bowl	–	130	–
chicken & dumplings				
boneless	1 bowl	1.0	160	6%
regular	1 bowl	1.0	150	6%
chicken & rice	1 bowl	1.0	140	6%
(Lunch Bucket) microwaveable				
chicken fiesta	1 meal	2.0	160	11%
dumplings 'n chicken	1 meal	5.0	140	32%
(Micro Magic) microwaveable				
chicken sandwich	1 sandwich	16.0	360	40%
(Morton) frozen				
chicken pot pie	7 oz	18.0	320	51%
(Ozark Valley) frozen				
Mr. Dandy				
chix patty	1 patty	11.0	210	47%
nuggets	4 pieces	10.0	210	43%
tender	3 pieces	10.0	210	43%
regular				
nuggets	4 pieces	10.0	210	43%
patties	1 patty	11.0	210	47%
pie	7 oz	19.0	330	52%
(Passport Cuisine) frozen				
yakitori-skewered	3 oz	5.0	100	45%
(Schwan's) chicken/frozen/partially or fully cooked unless stated otherwise				
chicken breast				
fillet				
breaded	1 fillet	7.0	160	40%
Southern-style	1 fillet	15.0	240	56%
unbreaded/raw	3.25 oz	1.5	90	10%
meat for fajitas	½ cup	3.0	100	27%
patties	3 oz	14.0	220	60%
strips	3 pieces	–	170	–
stuffed	1 piece	14.0	290	43%
tenderloin/Southern-style	2 tenders	9.0	210	39%
chicken cordon bleu	5 oz	13.0	280	45%

Food and Description	Amount	Fat Grams	Total Calories	% Fat Calories
chicken Kiev	5 oz	21.0	350	60%
chicken Marco Polo	5.3 oz	12.0	260	37%
diced chicken	3 oz	4.0	130	30%
Drummies	3 pieces	17.0	240	52%
nuggets/breaded	6 nuggets	15.0	220	45%
popcorn chicken strips	3 oz	16.0	280	51%
wings				
BBQ	6 pieces	14.0	210	57%
hot	6 pieces	14.0	210	57%
(Sensible Chef) frozen				
fried chicken breast/32-oz pkg	3 oz	10.0	200	45%
(Swanson)				
canned				
chicken à la king	5.25 oz	12.0	190	57%
chicken salad lunch kit	1 kit	19.0	300	57%
chicken stew	7⅝ oz	7.0	160	39%
frozen				
chicken pot pie				
Hungry Man/14 oz	1 pie	35.0	650	48%
original/7 oz	1 pie	22.0	410	48%
Dipsters	3 oz	14.0	220	57%
Drumlets	3 oz	14.0	220	57%
fried chicken				
breast portion	4½ oz	20.0	360	50%
dark portions	11 oz	30.0	570	47%
takeout/prefried	3¼ oz	16.0	270	53%
white portions	11 oz	28.0	580	43%
Nibbles	3¼ oz	20.0	300	60%
nuggets	9.5 oz	21.0	450	42%
thighs & drumsticks	3¼ oz	19.0	280	61%
(Tyson)				
frozen				
breast/boneless				
chunks	6 pieces	14.0	220	57%
fillets	2 pieces	7.0	170	36%
fillets/Southern-fried	3 oz	11.0	220	45%
patties				
breaded	1 patty	12.0	190	57%
Southern-fried	2.6 oz	15.0	220	61%
thick & crispy	2.6 oz	14.0	220	57%
w/rib meat	1 patty	12.0	190	57%
tenders	5 pieces	14.0	210	60%
chick'n cheddar	2.6 oz	15.0	220	61%
chunks				
regular	2.6 oz	15.0	220	61%
Southern-fried	2.6 oz	15.0	220	61%
space shaped	4 pieces	18.0	260	62%
diced chicken	3 oz	3.0	130	21%

Food and Description	Amount	Fat Grams	Total Calories	% Fat Calories
pie				
light & dark meat	9 oz	20.0	390	46%
white meat	9 oz	20.0	400	45%
wings				
barbecue	4 wings	15.0	220	61%
hot & spicy	4 wings	15.0	220	61%
roasted	4 wings	15.0	220	61%
teriyaki	4 wings	15.0	220	61%
kit				
fajita/all white meat	1 fajita	1.5	120	11%
fried rice				
all white meat	1 cup	1.5	140	10%
breast tenders/fat-free	1 cup	–	180	–
stir-fry				
all white meat	1¼ cups	2.0	180	10%
breast tenders/fat-free	1 cup	–	100	–
marinated chicken breast				
barbecue	3.75 oz	3.0	120	23%
butter garlic	3.75 oz	7.0	160	39%
Italian	3.75 oz	2.0	130	14%
lemon pepper	3.75 oz	2.0	120	15%
microwaveable/frozen				
breast sandwich	1 sandwich	14.0	328	39%
chunks	4 oz	6.0	230	23%
corn dogs	3.5 oz	14.0	280	45%
mini sandwich	1 sandwich	5.0	230	20%
nuggets	4 oz	6.0	230	23%
tenders	3.5 oz	11.0	230	43%
ready to eat/roasted				
breast half	1 piece	13.0	220	53%
wings w/teriyaki sauce	2 wings	14.0	180	70%
wholesale club/frozen				
breast half				
bone-in	1 piece	11.0	210	47%
boneless				
skinless	1 piece	4.0	140	26%
w/skin	1 piece	16.0	240	60%
mesquite style	1 piece	6.0	110	49%
breast patties	1 patty	14.0	210	60%
breast tenders				
breaded	2 pieces	11.0	240	41%
unbreaded	4 pieces	0.5	120	4%
chicken cordon bleu	1 piece	21.0	410	46%
drumettes/wings of fire/Buffalo style	3 pieces	12.0	180	60%
drums & thighs	1 piece	20.0	260	69%
nuggets/breaded	6 pieces	16.0	260	55%
thighs/boneless-skinless	1 piece	10.0	170	53%
wings/honey BBQ	4 wings	12.0	200	54%

Food and Description	Amount	Fat Grams	Total Calories	% Fat Calories
(Weaver) frozen/boneless				
assorted parts				
batter-dipped	3.6 oz	18.0	290	56%
Crispy Dutch Frye	3.6 oz	18.0	290	56%
breast				
batter-dipped	4.4 oz	20.0	310	58%
Crispy Dutch Frye	4.5 oz	22.0	350	57%
breast fillet strips	3.3 oz	10.0	200	45%
breast fillets	4.5 oz	13.0	270	43%
breast patties	3 oz	11.0	205	48%
crispy light skinless chicken	2.9 oz	9.0	170	48%
croquettes				
w/½ cup gravy	½ cup	18.0	306	53%
w/o gravy	2 pieces	16.0	280	51%
drums & thighs				
batter-dipped	3 oz	14.0	210	60%
Crispy Dutch Frye	3.5 oz	19.0	290	59%
mini drums				
crispy	3 oz	12.0	210	51%
herb & spice	3 oz	11.0	200	50%
nuggets	2.6 oz	12.0	190	57%
rondelet				
cheese	2.6 oz	11.0	190	52%
Italian	2.6 oz	11.0	190	52%
original	3 oz	10.0	190	47%
tenders				
honey batter	3 oz	12.0	220	49%
premium	3 oz	9.0	170	48%
wings				
batter-dipped	4 oz	28.0	400	63%
Crispy Dutch Frye	4 oz	28.0	400	63%
hot	2.7 oz	11.0	170	48%
CHICKEN SALAD (*See* CHICKEN ENTRÉE/DINNER)				
CHICKEN SEASONING (*See* SEASONINGS)				
CHICKEN SOUP (*See* SOUP)				
CHICKPEA/GARBANZO BEAN				
canned				
(Bush's Best)	½ cup	–	80	–
(Eden) garbanzo	½ cup	1.5	110	12%
generic	½ cup	1.0	143	6%
(Goya) Spanish style	7.5 oz	2.0	150	12%
(Green Giant)	½ cup	1.5	110	12%
(Hain)	½ cup	2.5	120	19%
(Joan of Arc)	½ cup	1.5	110	12%
(Nutradiet)	½ cup	1.0	100	9%
(Old El Paso)	½ cup	<1.0	190	2%
(Progresso)	½ cup	2.5	130	17%

Food and Description	Amount	Fat Grams	Total Calories	% Fat Calories
(S&W)				
lite/50% less salt	½ cup	1.0	110	8%
marinated	½ cup	1.0	120	8%
premium	½ cup	1.0	110	8%
(Seneca) garbanzo beans	½ cup	0.5	110	4%
(Sun Vista)	½ cup	–	70	–
dry				
boiled	½ cup	1.0	134	13%
raw	½ cup	6.0	364	15%
(Arrowhead Mills)	¼ cup	2.0	170	11%
(Bean Cuisine)	½ cup	1.0	115	8%
CHICORY/raw	8 oz	–	15	–
CHILI (See MEXICAN FOOD)				
CHILI SAUCE (See SAUCE)				
CHINESE FOOD (See ASIAN FOOD)				
CHINESE PARSLEY (See CILANTRO)				
CHIVES				
freeze-dried	1 Tbs	–	1	–
raw	1 Tbs	–	1	–
	¼ cup	–	2	–
CHOCOLATE (See BAKING BITS, CHIPS, CHUNKS, & PIECES; CANDY)				
CHOCOLATE SYRUP (See ICE CREAM TOPPING; MILK MIX)				
CHUB (See CISCO)				
CHUTNEY				
generic				
apple	1 Tbs	–	30	–
apple-cranberry	1 Tbs	–	20	–
tomato	1 Tbs	–	23	–
(Major Grey's) mango	1 Tbs	–	60	–
CIDER				
bottled or boxed				
(Alpenglow) apple/sparkling				
mulled	8 fl oz	–	110	–
regular	8 fl oz	–	110	–
generic/apple/sweet	8 fl oz	–	124	–
(Indian Summer)				
apple	8 fl oz	–	110	–
apple-cherry	8 fl oz	–	130	–
apple-cinnamon	8 fl oz	–	100	–
apple-cranberry	8 fl oz	–	130	–
apple-raspberry	8 fl oz	–	100	–
cranberry	8 fl oz	–	130	–
(Knudsen) Thirst Quencher				
cherry	8 fl oz	–	130	–
cider & spice	8 fl oz	–	120	–
(Musselman's) apple				
Lucky Leaf	6 fl oz	–	90	–
(S. Martinelli) apple/sparkling	6 fl oz	–	100	–

Food and Description	Amount	Fat Grams	Total Calories	% Fat Calories
(TreeTop) apple	8 fl oz	–	120	–
mix				
(Alpine) apple cider drink/prepared				
original	8 fl oz	–	80	–
spiced	8 fl oz	–	80	–
sugar-free	8 fl oz	–	15	–
CILANTRO/CHINESE PARSLEY/CORIANDER LEAF				
dried	1 tsp	–	2	–
	1 Tbs	–	5	–
fresh	1 tsp	–	2	–
	1 Tbs	–	5	–
CINNAMON/ground	1 tsp	–	10	–
CISCO/CHUB				
meat only				
raw	3 oz	1.5	85	16%
smoked	2 oz	6.5	100	59%
CITRON/candied				
generic	1 oz	–	89	–
(S&W)	39 pieces	–	90	–
CITRUS JUICE/JUICE DRINK (*See also* FRUIT PUNCH)				
bottled, boxed, or canned				
(Ocean Spray) Refreshers				
citrus cranberry	6 fl oz	–	100	–
citrus peach	6 fl oz	–	90	–
(Season's Best) citrus medley	8 fl oz	–	120	–
frozen or refrigerated/prepared				
(Chiquita) Citrus Twist	8 fl oz	–	120	–
(Minute Maid) Five Alive				
citrus				
frozen	8 fl oz	–	120	–
refrigerated	8 fl oz	–	120	–
tropical citrus	8 fl oz	–	120	–
CLAM (*See also* SEAFOOD ENTRÉE/DINNER)				
canned				
(Crown Prince) baby	⅓ cup	2.0	60	30%
(Doxsee) solids & liquid				
chopped	6.5 oz	0.5	100	5%
minced	6.5 oz	0.5	100	5%
(Empress) baby/whole	4 oz	1.0	60	15%
generic	3 oz	1.7	125	12%
(Gorton's)				
chopped	¼ cup	–	20	–
minced	¼ cup	–	20	–
(Perla Picifica) baby	⅓ cup	–	50	–
(Progresso) minced	¼ cup	–	25	–
(S&W)				
baby				
smoked	2 oz	10.0	130	69%

Food and Description	Amount	Fat Grams	Total Calories	% Fat Calories
whole	¼ cup	1.5	50	27%
regular				
chopped	¼ cup	–	20	–
minced	¼ cup	–	20	–
fresh				
breaded & fried	3 oz	9.0	171	47%
	20 small	21.0	380	50%
raw	3 oz	0.8	63	11%
steamed	3 oz	1.7	126	12%
	20 small	1.8	133	12%
	1 cup	3.0	235	12%
frozen				
(Matlaw's) stuffed	1 clam	5.0	120	38%
(Mrs. Paul's) real	3 oz	15.0	280	48%
(Sea Pak) strips	5 oz	23.0	410	50%
(Singleton) strips	5 oz	13.0	300	39%
CLAM CHOWDER (See SOUP)				
CLAM JUICE				
(Doxsee)	3 fl oz	–	4	–
(Mott's) Clamato	6 fl oz	–	90	–
CLAM SAUCE (See SAUCE)				
CLOVES/ground	1 tsp	–	7	–
CLUB SODA (See COCKTAIL MIXER; SOFT DRINK)				
COBBLER (See PIE & COBBLER)				
COCKTAIL SAUCE (See SAUCE)				
COCKTAIL (See also LIQUEUR; LIQUOR, DISTILLED; WINE)				
general				
Alexander	2.5 fl oz	1.8	179	9%
Bacardi	2.5 fl oz	–	118	–
black Russian	3 fl oz	–	255	–
bloody Mary	5 fl oz	–	116	–
bourbon & soda	4 fl oz	–	105	–
brandy	1 fl oz	–	75	–
daiquiri	2 fl oz	–	111	–
Gibson	2.5 fl oz	–	158	–
gimlet	2.5 fl oz	–	132	–
gin rickey	7 fl oz	–	114	–
gin & tonic	7.5 fl oz	–	171	–
gold Cadillac	4.5 fl oz	3.6	394	8%
grasshopper	2.25 fl oz	3.6	164	20%
highball	8 fl oz	–	165	–
mai tai	4.5 fl oz	–	310	–
Manhattan	2.5 fl oz	–	128	–
margarita	~3 fl oz	–	170	–
martini	2.5 fl oz	–	156	–
mint julep	10 fl oz	–	215	–
old fashioned	4 fl oz	–	180	–

Food and Description	Amount	Fat Grams	Total Calories	% Fat Calories
piña colada				
canned	4.5 fl oz	11.0	347	29%
homemade/USDA Standard Home Recipe	4.5 fl oz	2.6	262	9%
rum/hot buttered	~9 fl oz	11.9	317	34%
screwdriver	7 fl oz	–	174	–
Singapore sling	8 fl oz	–	228	–
sloe gin fizz	8 fl oz	–	121	–
stinger	3 fl oz	–	282	–
tequila sunrise	5.5 fl oz	–	189	–
Tom Collins	7.5 fl oz	–	121	–
	10 fl oz	–	180	–
whiskey sour	3 fl oz	–	123	–
white Russian	3.5 fl oz	1.0	268	3%

COCKTAIL MIXER (*See also* SOFT DRINK; WATER; individual fruit juice listings)

Food and Description	Amount	Fat Grams	Total Calories	% Fat Calories
(Bacardi) frozen/prepared				
margarita	8 fl oz	–	100	–
piña colada	8 fl oz	6.0	190	28%
rum runner	8 fl oz	–	140	–
strawberry daiquiri	8 fl oz	–	140	–
(Canada Dry)				
club soda				
regular	8 fl oz	–	–	–
sodium-free	8 fl oz	–	–	–
Collins	8 fl oz	–	100	–
ginger ale				
diet	8 fl oz	–	–	–
regular	8 fl oz	–	90	–
half & half	8 fl oz	–	110	–
hi-spot	8 fl oz	–	110	–
island lime	8 fl oz	–	140	–
Jamaica cola	8 fl oz	–	110	–
lemon sour	8 fl oz	–	100	–
seltzer/sparkling water	8 fl oz	–	–	–
tonic water				
plain				
diet	8 fl oz	–	–	–
regular	8 fl oz	–	100	–
w/twist of lime				
diet	8 fl oz	–	–	–
regular	8 fl oz	–	100	–
Vichy water	8 fl oz	–	–	–
(Coco Lopez)				
cream of coconut	2 Tbs	5.0	110	41%
piña colada				
canned	3 fl oz	4.0	120	30%
jarred	3 fl oz	5.0	160	28%

Food and Description	Amount	Fat Grams	Total Calories	% Fat Calories
generic				
grenadine	1 fl oz	–	64	–
quinine water	12 fl oz	–	142	–
Tom Collins/bottled	1 fl oz	–	42	–
whisky sour				
bottled				
mix only	2 fl oz	–	55	–
prepared	3.5 fl oz	–	158	–
dry mix/mix only	1 pkg	–	64	–
(Health Valley) ginger ale	12 fl oz	1.0	153	6%
(Holland House)				
bloody Mary/bottled				
regular	4.5 fl oz	–	20	–
smooth n' spicy	1 fl oz	–	3	–
daiquiri				
raspberry/bottled	1 fl oz	–	30	–
regular/dry mix	1 pkg	–	65	–
strawberry/bottled	1 fl oz	–	31	–
mai tai				
bottled	1 fl oz	–	32	–
dry mix	1 pkg	–	64	–
Manhattan/bottled	1 fl oz	–	28	–
margarita				
regular				
bottled	1 fl oz	–	27	–
dry mix	1 pkg	–	57	–
strawberry				
bottled	1 fl oz	–	31	–
dry mix	1 pkg	–	66	–
old fashioned/bottled	1 fl oz	–	33	–
piña colada				
bottled	1 fl oz	–	33	–
dry mix	1 pkg	–	82	–
sweet & sour	1 fl oz	–	34	–
Tom Collins				
bottled	1 fl oz	–	47	–
dry mix	1 pkg	–	65	–
whisky sour				
bottled	1 fl oz	–	37	–
dry mix	1 pkg	–	64	–
(Mr. & Mrs. T) bottled				
bloody Mary				
regular	4.5 fl oz	–	20	–
rich & spicy	4.5 fl oz	–	30	–
margarita				
regular	3 fl oz	–	80	–
strawberry	3.5 fl oz	–	100	–
piña colada	4 fl oz	<1.0	150	3%

Food and Description	Amount	Fat Grams	Total Calories	% Fat Calories
sweet & sour	3 fl oz	–	70	–
(Nehi) ginger ale	8 fl oz	–	90	–
(Roses) grenadine syrup	1 fl oz	–	65	–
(Schweppes)				
bitter lemon	8 fl oz	–	110	–
club soda				
regular	8 fl oz	–	–	–
sodium-free	8 fl oz	–	–	–
Collins	8 fl oz	–	100	–
ginger ale				
diet	8 fl oz	–	–	–
regular	8 fl oz	–	90	–
lemon sour	8 fl oz	–	110	–
seltzer/sparkling water	8 fl oz	–	–	–
tonic water				
citrus	8 fl oz	–	90	–
cranberry	8 fl oz	–	90	–
plain				
diet	8 fl oz	–	–	–
regular	8 fl oz	–	90	–
raspberry	8 fl oz	–	90	–
(Tabasco) bloody Mary	8 fl oz	–	60	–
COCOA (*See also* MILK MIX)				
(Baker's)	3.5 oz	13.0	220	53%
generic	⅓ cup	4.0	120	30%
	½ cup	5.0	173	26%
(Ghirardelli)				
sweet ground chocolate & cocoa	2.5 Tbs	1.5	80	17%
unsweetened	1 Tbs	1.5	20	68%
(Hershey)				
European	½ cup	3.0	90	30%
original	⅓ cup	3.0	110	25%
(Nestle)	1 Tbs	1.0	15	60%
(Wonderslim) low-fat	1¼ tsp	–	15	–
COCONUT				
(Baker's) Angel Flake				
canned	2 Tbs	5.0	70	64%
packaged	2 Tbs	4.5	70	58%
premium shred	2 Tbs	4.0	60	60%
(Durkee) shredded	2 Tbs	6.0	80	68%
generic				
dried				
flaked/sweetened				
canned	4 oz	36.0	505	64%
packaged	1 cup	23.8	351	61%
	4 oz	36.1	539	61%
shredded				
sweetened	4 oz	40.0	570	63%

Food and Description	Amount	Fat Grams	Total Calories	% Fat Calories
unsweetened	1 oz	18.0	187	87%
raw/shredded	½ cup	13.4	141	86%
toasted	1 oz	13.0	168	70%
COCONUT CREAM				
canned/sweetened				
(Coco Lopez)	2 Tbs	5.0	110	41%
generic	1 Tbs	3.0	36	75%
	1 cup	52.0	568	82%
raw	1 Tbs	5.0	50	18%
	1 cup	83.0	795	94%
COCONUT MILK				
canned				
(A Taste of Thai) unsweetened				
lite	¼ cup	3.0	36	75%
original	¼ cup	11.0	110	90%
generic	1 Tbs	3.0	30	90%
	1 cup	48.0	445	97%
frozen	1 Tbs	3.0	30	90%
	1 cup	50.0	486	93%
raw	1 Tbs	3.6	35	92%
	1 cup	57.0	552	93%
COCONUT NECTAR				
(Kern's) coconut-pineapple	6 fl oz	4.0	140	26%
(Knudsen)	8 fl oz	5.0	140	32%
COCONUT WATER	1 Tbs	–	3	–
	1 cup	0.5	46	10%
COD (*See also* COD ROE; SEAFOOD ENTRÉE/DINNER)				
Atlantic & Pacific				
breaded & fried	3 oz	9.0	175	46%
canned	3 oz	0.7	89	7%
cooked-dry heat	3 oz	0.7	89	7%
dried	3 oz	2.0	246	7%
raw	3 oz	0.6	70	7%
COD ROE	3 oz	1.7	111	14%
COFFEE/COFFEE-LIKE BEVERAGE				
bottled				
(Maxwell House) iced cappuccino				
Coffee Cappio	8 fl oz	2.5	130	17%
Mocha Cappio	8 fl oz	2.5	140	16%
Vanilla Cappio	8 fl oz	2.5	140	16%
brewed				
decaffeinated				
(Brim)	6 fl oz	–	2	–
generic	6 fl oz	–	4	–
(Maxwell House)	6 fl oz	–	2	–
(Sanka)	6 fl oz	–	2	–
(Yuban)	6 fl oz	–	2	–
espresso	2 fl oz	–	1	–

Food and Description	Amount	Fat Grams	Total Calories	% Fat Calories
regular				
generic	6 fl oz	–	4	–
(Yuban)	6 fl oz	–	2	–
Turkish	4 fl oz		45	–
ground (Folger's)				
decaffeinated	1 Tbs	–	17	–
regular	1 Tbs	–	16	–
instant				
flavored				
generic/mix only				
w/cappuccino	2 round tsp	2.0	62	29%
w/chicory	1 round tsp	–	6	–
w/French flavor	2 round tsp	3.0	57	47%
(General Foods) International Coffees/ mix only				
Cafe Amaretto	1⅓ Tbs	3.0	60	45%
Cafe Francais	1⅓ Tbs	3.5	60	53%
Cafe Vienna				
regular	1⅓ Tbs	2.5	70	32%
sugar-free	1⅓ Tbs	1.5	30	45%
French vanilla cafe				
regular	1⅓ Tbs	2.5	60	38%
sugar-free	1⅓ Tbs	2.0	35	51%
hazelnut Belgian cafe	1⅓ Tbs	2.0	70	26%
Italian cappuccino	1⅓ Tbs	1.5	50	27%
kahlua cafe	1⅓ Tbs	2.0	60	30%
Viennese chocolate cafe	1⅓ Tbs	2.0	60	30%
orange cappuccino				
regular	1⅓ Tbs	2.0	70	26%
sugar-free	1⅓ Tbs	1.5	30	45%
Suisse Mocha				
regular				
decaffeinated	1⅓ Tbs	3.0	60	45%
regular	1⅓ Tbs	2.5	60	38%
sugar-free				
decaffeinated	1⅓ Tbs	1.5	30	45%
regular	1⅓ Tbs	2.0	30	60%
(Hills Bros) prepared				
Bavarian mint mocha				
regular	6 fl oz	1.0	50	18%
sugar-free	6 fl oz	1.0	35	26%
Cafe Vienna	6 fl oz	2.0	60	30%
Dutch Chocolate	6 fl oz	2.0	60	30%
Orange Capri	6 fl oz	2.0	60	30%
Swiss Mocha				
regular	6 fl oz	2.0	60	30%
sugar free	6 fl oz	2.0	40	45%

Food and Description	Amount	Fat Grams	Total Calories	% Fat Calories
(Maxwell House) cappuccino/mix only				
cinnamon	1 envelope	1.5	90	15%
coffee	1 envelope	1.0	90	10%
mocha				
decaffeinated	1 envelope	2.5	100	23%
regular	1 envelope	2.5	100	23%
vanilla				
decaffeinated	1 envelope	1.0	90	10%
regular	1 envelope	1.0	90	10%
(MJB) prepared				
banana nut mocha/sugar-free	6 fl oz	2.0	40	45%
cafe mocha	6 fl oz	1.0	50	18%
cherry mocha	6 fl oz	1.0	50	18%
fudge mocha/sugar-free	6 fl oz	2.0	40	45%
mint mocha				
regular	6 fl oz	1.0	50	18%
sugar-free	6 fl oz	1.0	35	26%
vanilla mocha/sugar-free	6 fl oz	2.0	40	45%
nonflavored				
(Brim) prepared	6 fl oz	–	4	–
(Kava) mix only	1 tsp	–	2	–
(Maxwell House) prepared	6 fl oz	–	2	–
(Nescafe) prepared				
Brava	6 fl oz	–	4	–
classic	6 fl oz	–	4	–
decaf	6 fl oz	–	4	–
Silka	6 fl oz	–	4	–
(Pero) hot beverage drink w/malt & barley/no caffeine/prepared	6 fl oz	–	4	–
(Postum) coffee-flavored grain beverage				
prepared w/water	6 fl oz	–	12	–
prepared w/whole milk	6 fl oz	6.0	121	44%
(Sanka) prepared	6 fl oz	–	2	–
(Taster's Choice) prepared				
decaffeinated	6 fl oz	–	4	–
regular	6 fl oz		4	–
(Worthington) Natural Touch				
Kaffree Roma/mix only	1 tsp	–	10	–
(Yuban) prepared	6 fl oz	–	4	–
COFFEE CREAMER (See CREAM; CREAMER, NONDAIRY)				
COLD CUTS (See LUNCHEON MEAT)				
COLESLAW (See CABBAGE DISH)				
COLLARDS				
canned				
(Glory Foods) collard greens	½ cup	1.0	50	18%
(Luck's) chopped greens seasoned w/pork	½ cup	3.0	60	45%

Food and Description	Amount	Fat Grams	Total Calories	% Fat Calories
fresh				
cooked	½ cup	–	13	–
raw/chopped	½ cup	–	18	–
frozen				
generic/cooked	½ cup	–	31	–
(Pictsweet)	3.3 oz	–	25	–
CONDIMENTS (*See* ASIAN FOOD; MEXICAN FOOD; SAUCE; SEASONINGS; individual listings)				
COOKIE (*See also* BROWNIE/BLONDIE; CRACKER; CAKE, SNACK)				
■ **(Andre Prost)**				
Olof ginger snaps	7 cookies	4.0	120	30%
■ **(Archway)**				
apple bar/fat-free	1 bar	–	60	–
apple 'n raisin	1 cookie	4.5	130	31%
apple-filled oatmeal	1 cookie	3.0	110	25%
apricot-filled	1 cookie	4.0	110	33%
Aunt Bea's pound cake	1 cookie	4.0	110	33%
black walnut ice box	1 cookie	6.0	120	45%
blueberry filled	1 cookie	4.0	110	33%
carrot cake	1 cookie	5.0	120	38%
cashew nougat	1 cookie	10.0	160	56%
cherry filled	1 cookie	4.0	110	33%
chocolate/fat-free	1 cookie	–	90	–
chocolate chip				
bag	1 cookie	7.0	130	48%
drop	1 cookie	10.0	140	64%
ice box	1 cookie	7.0	140	45%
supreme	1 cookie	5.0	120	38%
chocolate chip & toffee	1 cookie	7.0	140	51%
cinnamon honey hearts/fat-free	3 cookies	–	100	–
cinnamon snap	5 cookies	7.0	150	42%
coconut macaroon	1 cookie	5.0	90	50%
cookie jar hermit	1 cookie	3.0	110	25%
cranberry bar/fat-free	1 bar	–	70	–
dark molasses	1 cookie	4.0	110	33%
date-filled oatmeal	1 cookie	4.0	110	33%
Dutch cocoa	1 cookie	4.0	120	30%
fig bar/fat-free	1 bar	–	60	–
frosty lemon	1 cookie	5.0	120	38%
fruit bar/fat-free	1 bar	–	90	–
fruit & honey bar	1 bar	4.0	110	33%
ginger snap				
original	5 cookies	5.0	130	35%
reduced fat	5 cookies	3.5	130	24%
granola/fat-free	2 cookies	–	100	–
iced molasses	1 cookie	5.0	110	41%
iced oatmeal	1 cookie	5.0	120	38%
lemon drop	1 cookie	4.0	110	33%

Food and Description	Amount	Fat Grams	Total Calories	% Fat Calories
lemon nugget/fat-free	5 cookies	–	100	–
lemon snap	5 cookies	7.0	150	42%
molasses/old-fashioned	1 cookie	3.0	120	23%
mud pie	1 cookie	4.0	110	33%
New Orleans cake	1 cookie	4.0	110	33%
oatmeal	1 cookie	3.0	110	25%
oatmeal pecan	1 cookie	5.0	120	38%
oatmeal raisin				
fat-free	1 cookie	–	100	–
original				
bag	1 cookie	6.0	130	42%
packaged	1 cookie	4.0	110	33%
oatmeal raisin bran	1 cookie	4.0	110	33%
oatmeal raspberry/fat-free	1 cookie	–	100	–
party treats	1 cookie	7.0	140	45%
peanut butter				
old-fashioned	1 cookie	6.0	130	28%
regular	1 cookie	7.0	140	45%
peanut butter & chips	1 cookie	7.0	140	45%
peanut jumble	1 cookie	7.0	130	48%
pecan crunch	1 cookie	8.0	150	48%
pecan ice box	1 cookie	8.0	140	51%
raspberry filled	1 cookie	4.0	110	33%
rocky road	1 cookie	4.5	120	34%
Ruth's oatmeal	1 cookie	5.0	120	38%
soft molasses drop	1 cookie	4.0	110	33%
soft sugar	1 cookie	4.0	110	33%
soft sugar drop	1 cookie	4.0	110	33%
strawberry-filled	1 cookie	4.0	110	33%
sugar				
fat-free	1 cookie	–	100	–
original	1 cookie	4.0	120	30%
trees	1 cookie	8.0	150	48%
vanilla wafer	5 cookies	4.0	130	28%
windmill/old-fashioned	1 cookie	4.0	100	36%
■ (Auburn Farms)				
Jammers				
apple spice	2 cookies	–	80	–
chewy chocolate	2 cookies	0.5	80	6%
chocolate mint	2 cookies	–	90	–
oatmeal raisin	2 cookies	0.5	80	6%
peanut butter crisp	2 cookies	0.5	90	9%
■ (Austin)				
chocolate creme	1.8 oz	12.0	260	42%
lemon Ohs!	1.8 oz	11.0	260	38%
peanut butter & graham	1.8 oz	10.0	250	36%
vanilla creme	1.8 oz	11.0	260	38%
zoo animal cracker	16 cookies	2.0	130	14%

Food and Description	Amount	Fat Grams	Total Calories	% Fat Calories
■ **(Bakery Wagon)**				
cobbler/fat-free				
apple	1 cookie	–	70	–
boysenberry	1 cookie	–	70	–
cranberry apple	1 cookie	–	70	–
mixed fruit	1 cookie	–	70	–
peach/apricot	1 cookie	–	70	–
raspberry	1 cookie	–	70	–
strawberry	1 cookie	–	70	–
cookie/low-fat				
apple-filled oat	1 cookie	1.5	90	15%
date-filled oat	1 cookie	1.5	90	15%
iced molasses				
mini	3 cookies	2.0	130	14%
regular	1 cookie	2.0	90	20%
raspberry filled oat	1 cookie	1.5	90	15%
soft oatmeal				
iced	1 cookie	1.5	100	5%
plain	1 cookie	1.5	90	15%
ginger snap	5 cookies	7.0	160	37%
■ **(Barbara's Bakery)**				
regular cookies				
caramel apple/fat-free	6 cookies	–	110	–
cocoa mocha/fat-free	6 cookies	–	100	–
double chocolate mini/fat-free	6 cookies	–	90	–
fruit & nut	2 cookies	2.0	125	14%
fruit bar				
apricot	½ oz	1.0	50	18%
cherry	½ oz	1.0	50	18%
raspberry	½ oz	1.0	50	18%
oatmeal raisin				
fat-free	6 cookies	–	110	–
regular	2 cookies	2.0	100	18%
Small Indulgence				
butter pecan bites	6 cookies	8.0	140	51%
chocolate chip crisps	6 cookies	7.0	140	45%
coffee cake crunch	6 cookies	6.0	130	42%
lemon almond delights	6 cookies	6.0	140	39%
■ **(Betty Crocker)**				
mix/prepared				
gingerbread cake & cookie				
no-cholesterol recipe	⅛ pkg	6.0	220	25%
regular recipe	⅛ pkg	11.0	230	43%
M&M's cookie bar	1 bar	8.0	170	42%
ready to eat/Dunkaroos				
chocolate chip w/chocolate frosting	1 tray	7.0	120	48%
chocolate cookie w/vanilla frosting	1 tray	7.0	120	53%

Food and Description	Amount	Fat Grams	Total Calories	% Fat Calories
chocolate graham w/chocolate chip frosting	1 tray	7.0	130	48%
cinnamon graham w/vanilla frosting	1 tray	7.0	130	48%
■ (Break Cake)				
brownie creme/2-oz cookie	1 cookie	8.0	240	30%
chips & creme	1 cookie	6.0	140	39%
chocolate chip	1 oz	6.0	140	39%
chocolate sugar wafer	4 cookies	9.0	200	41%
coconut macaroon/2-oz cookie	2 cookies	14.0	270	47%
devil's food creme	1 cookie	5.0	130	35%
ginger snap	5 cookies	5.0	130	42%
hermit/2-oz cookie	1 cookie	7.0	230	27%
marshmallow pie				
banana	1.2 oz	5.0	150	30%
chocolate	1.2 oz	5.0	150	30%
devil's food	1.2 oz	4.0	140	26%
double decker chocolate	3 oz	11.0	360	28%
oatmeal	5 cookies	6.0	140	39%
peanut butter	1 cookie	7.0	140	45%
peanut butter wafer	1 cookie	9.0	180	45%
raisin creme	1 cookie	5.0	140	32%
shortbread	5 cookies	6.0	140	39%
strawberry wafer	4 cookies	11.0	220	45%
striper wafer	1 cookie	10.0	190	47%
vanilla sugar wafer	4 wafers	11.0	220	45%
■ BRETON (See (Dare) in this section)				
■ (Burns & Ricker)				
biscotti/~2 per oz				
almond	1 oz	4.5	130	31%
chocolate almond	1 oz	5.0	130	35%
■ CAMEO (See (Nabisco) in this section)				
■ (Carr's)				
butter				
all-butter shortbread	2 cookies	9.0	170	48%
dark chocolate	2 cookies	7.0	150	42%
milk chocolate	2 cookies	7.0	140	45%
Hob-Nobs	2 cookies	6.0	140	39%
home wheat				
dark chocolate	2 cookies	6.0	130	41%
graham cookies	2 cookies	6.0	140	39%
milk chocolate	2 cookies	6.0	130	41%
wafer/crispy milk chocolate	3 cookies	12.0	180	60%
■ CHIPS AHOY (See (Nabisco); (Pillsbury) in this section)				
■ CHIPS DELUXE (See (Keebler) in this section)				
■ (Dare)				
Breton				
Belmont				
Black Forest	1 cookie	3.0	81	33%

Food and Description	Amount	Fat Grams	Total Calories	% Fat Calories
mallow	1 cookie	2.4	78	28%
strawberry	1 cookie	3.0	81	33%
Breaktime				
chocolate chip	1 cookie	1.7	37	41%
coconut	1 cookie	1.4	35	36%
ginger	1 cookie	1.1	34	29%
oatmeal	1 cookie	1.3	29	40%
sprinkle	1 cookie	1.6	36	40%
butter creme	1 cookie	3.9	85	41%
butter shortbread	1 cookie	3.7	63	53%
chocolate chip	1 cookie	4.1	77	48%
chocolate fudge	1 cookie	4.8	97	45%
chocolate galore	1 cookie	4.0	80	45%
cinnamon Danish	1 cookie	1.6	47	31%
cinnamon snap	1 cookie	0.7	31	20%
coconut creme	1 cookie	5.2	99	47%
digestive	1 cookie	2.0	45	40%
Encore/low-fat	1 cookie	0.6	28	19%
French creme	1 cookie	5.3	80	60%
golden caramel	1 cookie	3.3	73	41%
graham/low-fat	1 cookie	0.8	31	23%
Harvest from the Rain Forest	1 cookie	4.0	68	53%
key lime creme	1 cookie	4.0	86	42%
lemon creme	1 cookie	4.5	95	43%
maple leaf creme	1 cookie	3.8	83	41%
maple walnut fudge	1 cookie	5.0	99	45%
midnight mint	1 cookie	4.0	75	48%
milk chocolate fudge	1 cookie	4.8	99	44%
oatmeal raisin	1 cookie	2.8	59	43%
Oats Up!	1 cookie	2.9	66	40%
Peanut Butter Delite	1 cookie	4.0	72	50%
social tea	1 cookie	1.0	26	35%
sugar	1 cookie	1.4	39	32%
Sun Maid				
chocolate & raisins	1 cookie	3.0	56	48%
raisin	1 cookie	2.5	52	43%
vanilla wafer	1 cookie	0.6	17	32%
■ (Delicious)				
almond windmill	1 cookie	3.0	80	34%
Betty Crocker brownie sandwich	2 cookies	6.0	150	36%
Chiquita Bananarama	2 cookies	5.0	120	38%
chocolate chip	2 cookies	8.0	140	51%
coconut bar	1 bar	3.0	70	39%
fig bar	2 bars	2.0	130	14%
ginger snap	0.5 oz	2.0	64	28%
Heath English toffee crunch	3 cookies	10.0	170	53%
honey graham				
cinnamon	2 whole	5.0	130	35%

Food and Description	Amount	Fat Grams	Total Calories	% Fat Calories
plain	2 whole	3.5	120	26%
iced oatmeal	2 cookies	6.0	130	42%
jelly top	0.8 oz	5.0	112	40%
Land O'Lakes butter	2 cookies	8.0	140	51%
macaroon	2 cookies	6.0	130	42%
Musselman's applesauce oatmeal	2 cookies	4.0	130	28%
oatmeal				
plain	2 cookies	5.0	130	35%
w/Raisinets	3 cookies	4.5	140	29%
peanut butter bits w/Butterfinger	3 cookies	6.0	130	42%
pecan	1 cookie	5.0	94	48%
Skippy peanut butter	3 cookies	10.0	150	60%
sugar cookie	2 cookies	6.0	130	42%
sugar wafer				
assorted	¼ oz	2.5	40	56%
chocolate	1 cookie	2.0	35	26%
chocolate/strawberry	1 cookie	2.0	35	26%
lemon	1 cookie	2.0	35	26%
mini creme	1 cookie	1.5	25	54%
strawberry	1 cookie	2.0	35	26%
strawberry/vanilla	1 cookie	2.0	35	26%
vanilla	1 cookie	2.0	35	26%
	¼ oz	2.5	40	56%
■ (Dolly Madison)				
chocolate chip	1 cookie	4.0	140	26%
molasses	1 cookie	3.5	110	29%
oatmeal	1 cookie	6.0	160	34%
■ (Drake's)				
chocolate chocolate chip	2 cookies	5.0	130	35%
coconut	2 cookies	5.0	130	35%
coconut macaroon	1 cookie	7.0	135	47%
hermit	1 cookie	7.0	230	27%
oatmeal	2 cookies	5.0	120	38%
oatmeal creme	1 cookies	9.0	240	34%
peanut butter wafer	1 cookie	16.0	325	44%
■ (Duncan Hines)				
mix				
chocolate chip				
mix only	½₄ pkg	5.0	140	32%
prepared	2 cookies	9.0	170	48%
fudge brownie cookie				
mix only	½₄ pkg	4.0	120	30%
prepared	2 cookies	7.0	140	45%
golden sugar				
mix only	½₄ pkg	4.0	120	30%
prepared	2 cookies	7.0	150	42%
peanut butter				
mix only	½₄ pkg	5.0	120	38%

Food and Description	Amount	Fat Grams	Total Calories	% Fat Calories
prepared	2 cookies	8.0	140	51%
■ DUNKAROOS (*See* (Betty Crocker) in this section)				
■ (Dunkin' Donuts)				
chocolate chocolate chunk	1 cookie	11.0	200	50%
chocolate chunk				
plain	1 cookie	10.0	200	45%
w/nuts	1 cookie	11.0	200	50%
chocolate white chocolate chunk	1 cookie	11.0	200	50%
oatmeal raisin pecan	1 cookie	9.0	190	43%
peanut butter chocolate chunk				
w/nuts	1 cookie	13.0	210	56%
w/peanuts	1 cookie	12.0	210	51%
■ (Eagle)				
gourmet cookies				
chocolate fudge brownie style	1 cookie	16.0	330	44%
ginger	1 cookie	3.5	240	13%
macadamia coconut	1 cookie	16.0	330	44%
oatmeal raisin	1 cookie	17.0	330	46%
peanut butter chocolate chip	1 cookie	20.0	360	50%
original cookies				
chocolate chip	1 cookie	8.0	190	38%
fudge stripe creme pie	1 cookie	12.0	310	35%
iced oatmeal	1 cookie	5.0	170	26%
lemon creme sandwich	6 cookies	11.0	260	38%
oatmeal creme pie	1 cookie	12.0	310	35%
peanut butter & graham sandwich	6 cookies	10.0	250	36%
peanut butter bar	1 bar	10.0	170	53%
vanilla creme sandwich	6 cookies	11.0	260	38%
■ ELFIN DELIGHTS (*See* (Keebler) in this section)				
▣ (Entenmann's)				
chocolate brownie/fat-free	2 cookies	–	80	–
chocolate chip	3 cookies	7.0	140	45%
oatmeal chocolatey chip/fat-free	2 cookies	–	80	–
oatmeal raisin/fat-free	2 cookies	–:	80	–
■ (Estee)				
chocolate chip				
mix/mix only	3 Tbs	2.0	90	20%
ready to eat	4 cookies	7.0	150	42%
chocolate sandwich	3 cookies	6.0	160	34%
coconut	4 cookies	6.0	140	39%
fig bar/low-fat				
apple	2 bars	1.0	100	9%
cranberry	2 bars	1.0	100	9%
original	2 bars	1.0	100	9%
fudge	4 cookies	7.0	150	42%
lemon	4 cookies	6.0	140	39%
oatmeal raisin	4 cookies	5.0	130	35%
original sandwich	3 cookies	6.0	160	34%

Food and Description	Amount	Fat Grams	Total Calories	% Fat Calories
peanut butter sandwich	3 cookies	7.0	160	39%
shortbread	4 cookies	4.0	130	28%
sugar wafer				
chocolate creme	7 cookies	8.0	160	45%
double decker lemon creme	5 cookies	8.0	170	42%
triple decker banana, chocolate, strawberry creme	3 cookies	7.0	140	45%
vanilla creme	7 cookies	7.0	160	37%
vanilla & strawberry creme	5 cookies	8.0	170	42%
vanilla	4 cookies	6.0	140	39%
vanilla sandwich	3 cookies	5.0	160	28%
■ (Famous Amos)				
apple fruit bar/fat-free	2 bars	–	90	–
chocolate chip & pecans	4 cookies	7.0	150	42%
chocolate sandwich	3 cookies	8.0	150	48%
coconut caramel	2 cookies	8.0	140	51%
fig bar/fat-free	2 bars	–	100	–
iced ginger snap/low-fat	7 cookies	1.0	120	8%
iced lemon/low-fat	7 cookies	2.0	130	14%
iced oatmeal/low-fat	7 cookies	1.5	130	10%
oatmeal cinnamon raisin	4 cookies	5.0	130	35%
oatmeal macaroon	3 cookies	7.0	150	18%
peanut butter sandwich	3 cookies	7.0	150	42%
pecan caramel	2 cookies	9.0	150	54%
strawberry fruit bar/fat-free	2 bars	–	90	–
vanilla sandwich	3 cookies	7.0	150	42%
■ (Featherweight)				
chocolate chip	4 cookies	5.0	140	32%
creme wafer				
chocolate	7 cookies	8.0	160	45%
vanilla	7 cookies	7.0	160	39%
double chocolate chip	4 cookies	5.0	140	32%
lemon	4 cookies	5.0	140	32%
oatmeal raisin	4 cookies	5.0	140	32%
peanut butter	4 cookies	5.0	140	32%
vanilla	4 cookies	5.0	140	32%
■ (FFV)				
animal	9 cookies	3.0	110	28%
caramel patty	2 cookies	7.0	160	42%
fig bar				
vanilla	1 bar	1.0	60	15%
whole wheat	1 bar	1.0	60	15%
ginger boy	6 cookies	3.0	120	30%
jelly tart	2 cookies	4.0	110	33%
mint sandwich	2 cookies	7.0	160	39%
oatmeal w/calcium	5 cookies	5.0	130	35%
peanut butter sandwich	2 cookies	8.0	170	42%
regal graham	2 cookies	7.0	140	45%

Food and Description	Amount	Fat Grams	Total Calories	% Fat Calories
Royal Dainty	1 cookie	6.0	120	45%
T.C. Round	2 cookies	8.0	160	45%
Tango	2 cookies	5.0	160	28%
Trolley Cake/devil's food	2 cookies	2.0	120	15%
vanilla wafer	8 cookies	5.0	120	38%
■ FIG NEWTON (*See* (Nabisco) in this section)				
■ (Formagg)				
chocolate chip cheesecake	1 cookie	2.0	49	37%
■ (Frookie)				
American banana/fat-free	2 cookies	–	90	–
American chocolate delight/fat-free	2 cookies	–	100	–
American cran-orange/fat-free	2 cookies	–	90	–
apple cinnamon oat bran	3 cookies	5.0	130	35%
apple spice/fat-free	2 cookies	–	90	–
chocolate chip	3 cookies	7.0	140	45%
Dream Cream				
strawberry	2 cookies	4.0	70	51%
vanilla	2 cookies	4.0	70	51%
Frookaroon/fat-free	2 cookies	–	80	–
Frookwich				
chocolate	2 cookies	4.0	100	36%
chocolate & vanilla	2 cookies	4.0	100	36%
duplex power	2 cookies	6.0	140	39%
lemon	2 cookies	4.0	100	36%
peanut butter	2 cookies	4.0	100	36%
vanilla	2 cookies	4.0	100	36%
vanilla power	2 cookies	6.0	140	39%
Fruitin				
apple	2 cookies	2.0	110	16%
fig				
fat free	2 cookies	–	90	–
regular	2 cookies	2.0	110	16%
raspberry/fat free	2 cookies	–	90	–
Funky Monkey				
chocolate	16 cookies	4.0	120	30%
vanilla	16 cookies	4.0	120	30%
ginger spice	3 cookies	5.0	130	35%
graham				
cinnamon power	10 pieces	4.0	120	30%
honey	2 cookies	2.0	130	14%
vanilla power	10 pieces	4.0	120	30%
Mandarin orange chocolate chip	3 cookies	7.0	130	49%
mint chocolate chip	3 cookies	7.0	140	45%
oatmeal raisin				
fat-free	2 cookies	–	90	–
original	3 cookies	5.0	130	35%
7-grain	3 cookies	5.0	130	35%

Food and Description	Amount	Fat Grams	Total Calories	% Fat Calories
■ GENERIC				
animal crackers	1 cookie	<1.0	11	30%
	11 cookies	4.0	126	30%
arrowroot	1 cookie	1.0	25	36%
butter	1 cookie	1.0	23	39%
chocolate chip				
refrigerated dough/¼" thick/2¼" dia	4 cookies	11.0	225	44%
soft style	1 cookie	4.0	70	51%
chocolate w/creme filling	1 cookie	5.0	80	56%
chocolate sandwich/1¾" dia	4 cookies	8.0	195	37%
chocolate wafer	1 cookie	1.0	25	36%
coconut bar	1 bar	5.0	110	41%
coconut macaroon	2 cookies	5.0	100	45%
fig bar	4 bars	4.0	210	17%
fortune	1 cookie	–	30	–
fudge	1 cookie	1.0	75	13%
ginger snap	1 cookie	1.0	30	30%
lady finger	1 cookie	1.0	40	23%
marshmallow/chocolate-coated	1 cookie	2.0	55	33%
marshmallow pie/chocolate-coated	1 cookie	7.0	165	38%
molasses	1 cookie	2.0	65	28%
oatmeal				
refrigerated	1 cookie	3.0	60	45%
soft style	1 cookie	2.0	60	30%
traditional	1 cookie	4.0	70	51%
oatmeal raisin	1 cookie	3.0	80	34%
peanut butter				
refrigerated	1 cookie	3.0	60	45%
soft style	1 cookie	4.0	70	51%
peanut butter sandwich	1 cookie	3.0	70	39%
shortbread	1 cookie	2.0	40	45%
shortbread pecan	1 cookie	5.0	80	56%
sugar/refrigerated dough/¼" thick/2½" dia	1 cookie	3.0	60	45%
sugar wafer w/creme filling	1 cookie	1.0	20	45%
vanilla sandwich/1¾" dia	4 cookies	8.0	190	37%
vanilla wafer/1¾" dia	10 cookies	7.0	185	34%
zwieback	1 oz	1.0	107	8%
■ (Grandma's)				
big cookies				
chocolate chip	1 cookie	9.0	190	43%
fudge chocolate chip	1 cookie	6.0	170	32%
molasses	1 cookie	4.0	160	23%
nutty fudge	1 cookie	8.0	190	38%
oatmeal apple spice	1 cookie	6.0	170	32%
peanut butter	1 cookie	9.0	190	43%
peanut butter chocolate chip	1 cookie	10.0	190	47%
cookie bits				
chocolate	9 cookies	8.0	170	42%

Food and Description	Amount	Fat Grams	Total Calories	% Fat Calories
lemon	9 cookies	6.0	150	36%
peanut butter	9 cookies	6.0	150	36%
vanilla	9 cookies	7.0	150	42%
regular cookies				
apple oatmeal spice bar	1 bar	5.0	170	26%
chocolate fudge bar	1 bar	7.0	190	33%
chocolate sandwich/value line	3 cookies	5.0	180	25%
combination sandwich/value line	3 cookies	4.0	150	24%
peanut butter sandwich	5 cookies	9.0	210	39%
sandwich wafer/value line				
strawberry	1 pkg	8.0	230	31%
vanilla	1 pkg	8.0	230	31%
soft granola bar	1 bar	6.0	180	30%
vanilla sandwich				
regular	5 cookies	9.0	210	39%
value line	3 cookies	5.0	180	25%
■ (Greenfield)				
Healthy Foods/fat free				
double chocolate lace	1 cookie	–	60	–
Dutch apple	1 cookie	–	60	–
iced oatmeal raisin	1 cookie	–	60	–
■ (Hain)				
animal graham				
chocolate	15 cookies	3.0	120	23%
original	15 cookies	3.0	80	34%
graham cracker				
chocolate	2 cookies	3.0	120	23%
cinnamon	2 cookies	3.0	80	34%
honey	2 cookies	3.0	80	34%
■ (Health Valley)				
fat-free cookies				
chocolate				
caramel centers	2 cookies	–	70	–
fudge centers	2 cookies	–	70	–
mint fudge centers	2 cookies	–	70	–
fruit bake				
apple spice	3 cookies	–	100	–
apricot delight	3 cookies	–	100	–
banana spice	3 cookies	–	100	–
date delight	3 cookies	–	100	–
Hawaiian fruit	3 cookies	–	100	–
raisin oatmeal	3 cookies	–	100	–
raspberry apple	3 cookies	–	100	–
fruit bar				
apple	1 bar	–	140	–
apricot	1 bar	–	140	–
date	1 bar	–	140	–
raisin	1 bar	–	140	–

Food and Description	Amount	Fat Grams	Total Calories	% Fat Calories
fruit center				
mini				
peach-apricot	2 cookies	–	70	–
raspberry-apple	2 cookies	–	70	–
strawberry	2 cookies	–	70	–
regular/raspberry	3 cookies	–	70	–
graham cracker				
amaranth	8 cookies	–	100	–
oat bran	8 cookies	–	100	–
healthy chips				
double chocolate	3 cookies	–	100	–
old-fashioned	3 cookies	–	100	–
original flavor	3 cookies	–	100	–
jumbo				
apple raisin	1 cookie	–	80	–
raisin raisin	1 cookie	–	80	–
raspberry	1 cookie	–	80	–
The Great Tofu Cookie	2 cookies	3.0	90	30%
The Great Wheat-Free Cookie	2 cookies	3.0	80	34%
■ HOMEMADE				
USDA Standard Home Recipe (Note: All homemade cookies were made with margarine.)				
chocolate chip/2½" dia	4 cookies	12.0	206	52%
macaroons/¼" thick/2¾" dia	2 cookies	8.8	181	44%
oatmeal				
traditional	1 cookie	3.0	65	42%
w/raisins/¼" thick/2⅝" dia	4 cookies	10.0	245	37%
oatmeal chocolate chip	1 cookie	3.0	60	45%
peanut butter/2⅝" dia	4 cookies	14.0	245	51%
pumpkin bar	1.5 oz	11.0	190	52%
shortbread	1 cookie	4.0	60	60%
sugar/¼" thick/2½" dia	1 cookie	3.0	90	30%
■ HONEY MAID (See (Nabisco) in this section)				
■ HYDROX (See (Sunshine) in this section)				
■ JAMMERS (See (Auburn Farms) in this section)				
■ (Kashi)				
graham cracker				
amaranth graham	8 cookies	–	100	–
oat bran honey	6 cookies	3.0	110	25%
great tofu cookie	2 cookies	3.0	90	30%
oat bran fruit & nut	2-3 cookies	4.0	110	33%
■ (Keebler)				
Classic Collection				
fudge creme	1 cookie	3.5	80	39%
oatmeal	2 cookies	8.0	150	48%
peanut butter	2 cookies	9.0	150	54%
sugar	2 cookies	7.0	140	45%
vanilla creme	1 cookie	3.5	80	39%

Food and Description	Amount	Fat Grams	Total Calories	% Fat Calories
Elfin Delights				
fat-free devil's food				
chocolate middle	1 cookie	–	70	–
vanilla middle	1 cookie	–	70	–
50% reduced fat				
plain	2 cookies	2.5	110	20%
w/fudge creme	2 cookies	2.5	110	20%
w/vanilla creme	2 cookies	2.5	110	20%
Fantastic Delights fruit bar/fat-free				
apple	1 bar	–	40	–
blueberry	1 bar	–	40	–
raspberry	1 bar	–	40	–
Fudge Shoppe cookies				
fudge-covered grahams/deluxe	1 cookie	2.0	40	45%
fudge n caramel	2 cookies	6.0	120	45%
fudge sticks	3 cookies	8.0	150	48%
fudge stripes	3 cookies	8.0	160	45%
grasshoppers	4 cookies	7.0	150	42%
peanut butter fudgebutters	2 cookies	7.0	130	48%
Graham Select				
apple cinnamon	8 cookies	4.0	130	28%
cinnamon crisp/low-fat	8 cookies	1.5	110	12%
honey graham				
low-fat	9 cookies	1.5	120	11%
regular	8 cookies	6.0	150	36%
original	8 cookies	3.0	130	21%
original cookies				
Chips Deluxe				
bakery crisp crispy chocolate chip	3 cookies	9.0	180	45%
chocolate chip				
bite-size	8 cookies	9.0	160	51%
regular	1 cookie	4.5	80	51%
chocolate lovers	1 cookie	5.0	90	50%
rainbow				
bite-size	7 cookies	7.0	140	45%
regular	1 cookie	4.0	80	45%
25% reduced fat	1 cookie	3.0	70	39%
chocolate wafer/reduced fat	8 cookies	3.5	130	24%
Danish wedding	4 cookies	5.0	120	38%
E.L. Fudge/sandwich w/creme filling				
butter w/fudge filling	3 cookies	8.0	170	42%
chocolate w/vanilla filling	3 cookies	8.0	170	42%
fudge w/fudge filling	3 cookies	7.0	160	37%
French vanilla creme	1 cookie	3.5	80	39%
iced animal	6 cookies	4.5	140	29%
Krisp Kreem sugar wafer	5 pieces	7.0	140	45%
Opera Creme	1 cookie	3.5	80	30%

Food and Description	Amount	Fat Grams	Total Calories	% Fat Calories
Pecan Sandies				
original				
bite-size	8 cookies	10.0	170	53%
regular	1 cookie	5.0	80	56%
sandwich w/praline creme	1 cookie	6.0	80	68%
25% reduced fat	1 cookie	3.0	70	39%
Pitter Patter peanut butter creme	1 cookie	4.0	90	40%
Sweet Spots/shortbread w/chocolate-flavored centers	1 pkg	6.0	120	45%
Toffee Sandies	1 cookie	3.0	70	39%
vanilla wafer/golden	8 cookies	7.0	150	42%
Soft Batch cookies				
chocolate chip	1 cookie	3.5	80	45%
oatmeal raisin	1 cookie	3.0	70	34%
■ (Laguna Cookie Co.)				
cookie				
Endangered Species/low-fat	11 cookies	2.0	110	16%
oat bran/fat-free	2 cookies	–	100	–
white chocolate chip/bite-size	10 cookies	7.0	140	45%
filled cookie bar/fat-free				
apple	1 bar	–	150	–
mixed berry	1 bar	–	150	–
strawberry	1 bar	–	150	–
■ (Lance)				
bars				
apple/fat-free	1 bar	–	160	–
apple-oatmeal	2 bars	6.0	190	28%
cranberry/fat-free	1 bar	–	160	–
fig	1 bar	3.5	180	18%
peanut butter creme wafer				
1½-oz bar	1 bar	12.0	230	47%
2¼-oz bar	½ bar	9.0	170	45%
cookies				
Big Town/2-oz cookie				
banana	1 cookie	10.0	250	36%
chocolate	1 cookie	8.0	250	29%
vanilla	1 cookie	11.0	250	40%
Bonnie sandwich	1 pkg	7.0	160	39%
chocolate chip/2-oz cookie				
fudge	1 cookie	5.0	130	35%
gourmet	1 cookie	6.0	130	42%
Choc-O-Lunch sandwich				
regular	1 pkg	8.0	200	36%
value pack	7 cookies	9.0	230	35%
Choc-O-Mint sandwich	1 pkg	9.0	190	43%
coated graham sandwich	1 pkg	8.0	190	38%
Lem-O-Lunch sandwich/value pack	7 cookies	11.0	240	41%
malt sandwich	1 pkg	10.0	190	47%

Food and Description	Amount	Fat Grams	Total Calories	% Fat Calories
nekot				
lemon	1 pkg	10.0	210	43%
original	1 pkg	10.0	210	43%
Nut-O-Lunch sandwich/value pack	7 cookies	11.0	240	41%
oatmeal creme/2-oz cookie	1 cookie	10.0	240	38%
oatmeal/2-oz cookie	1 cookie	6.0	130	42%
toasty sandwich	1 pkg	11.0	190	52%
Van-O-Lunch sandwich				
regular	1 pkg	8.0	210	34%
value pack	7 cookies	9.0	230	35%
■ (Little Debbie)				
bars				
caramel cookie bar	1 bar	8.0	160	45%
nutty bar				
boxed	1 pkg	17.0	290	53%
individual pkg	1.2 oz	11.0	180	55%
	1.9 oz	16.0	270	53%
peanut butter bar				
boxed	1 pkg	15.0	270	50%
individual pkg	1 pkg	14.0	250	50%
creme pies				
oatmeal				
boxed	1 pkg	8.0	170	42%
individual pkg	2.5 oz	12.0	300	36%
	3 oz	14.0	360	35%
raisin				
boxed	1 pkg	5.0	140	32%
individual pkg	1 pkg	12.0	290	37%
cookies				
animal cookie	1 pkg	5.0	190	24%
apple delight	1 pkg	4.5	130	31%
Back-To-School	1 pkg	7.0	200	32%
chocolate chip cookie/individual pkg	1 cookie	9.0	180	45%
coconut round	1 pkg	7.0	140	45%
cookie wreaths	1 pkg	6.0	100	54%
Easter puffs	1 pkg	6.0	150	36%
Figaroos				
fat-free/individual pkg	1 pkg	–	180	–
regular	1 pkg	2.5	150	15%
fudge creme wafer	1 pkg	8.0	130	55%
fudge round				
boxed	1 pkg	6.0	140	39%
individual pkg	2.5 oz	12.0	290	37%
	3 oz	14.0	350	36%
ginger	1 pkg	3.0	90	30%
lemon creme wafer	1 pkg	5.0	100	45%
marshmallow supreme	1 pkg	5.0	130	35%
mint creme wafer	1 pkg	9.0	150	54%

Food and Description	Amount	Fat Grams	Total Calories	% Fat Calories
oatmeal lights snack	1 pkg	2.5	130	17%
oatmeal raisin/individual pkg	1 cookie	6.0	160	34%
peanut butter & jelly	1 pkg	5.0	130	35%
peanut cluster	1 pkg	11.0	190	52%
pumpkin delight	1 pkg	5.0	140	32%
pumpkin shaped smiley face mini cookie	1 pkg	5.0	130	35%
star crunch snack				
boxed	1 pkg	6.0	140	39%
individual pkg	1 pkg	12.0	280	39%
strawberry fruit/fat-free	1 pkg	–	130	–
marshmallow pies				
banana				
boxed	1 pkg	5.0	160	28%
individual pkg	1 pkg	11.0	320	31%
chocolate				
boxed	1 pkg	5.0	160	28%
individual pkg	1 pkg	11.0	320	31%
■ (LU)				
Aloha	1 cookie	5.0	75	60%
barre chocolat	1 cookie	3.0	65	42%
chips chocolat				
fudge	1 cookie	4.0	75	48%
regular	1 cookie	5.0	85	53%
chocolatiers	3 cookies	11.0	170	42%
craquelin	1 cookie	3.0	55	49%
crokine	2 cookies	–	20	–
Euphrates	2 cookies	2.0	40	45%
fondant	4 cookies	8.0	170	37%
gaufrettes	2 cookies	4.0	85	42%
Marie LU				
mini	12 cookies	5.0	130	35%
original	3 cookies	6.0	170	32%
whole wheat	3 cookies	4.0	140	26%
milk lunch	4 cookies	4.0	140	26%
palmito	1 cookie	3.0	50	54%
petit-beurre	4 cookies	4.0	150	26%
petit-ecolier/little schoolboy				
dark chocolat	2 cookies	7.0	130	48%
milk chocolat	2 cookies	7.0	130	48%
pims				
orange	2 cookies	4.0	100	35%
raspberry	2 cookies	3.0	100	27%
truffe	4 cookies	11.0	180	55%
■ (M&M ★ Mars)				
Twix cookie bars				
caramel				
family size	1 cookie	7.0	140	45%

Food and Description	Amount	Fat Grams	Total Calories	% Fat Calories
fun size	1 cookie	4.0	80	45%
king size	1 cookie	6.0	120	45%
single	2 cookies	14.0	280	45%
peanut butter	1 cookie	8.0	130	55%
■ (Manischewitz)				
chocolate chip	3 cookies	7.0	150	42%
macaroon				
chocolate	2 cookies	6.0	100	54%
chocolate chip	2 cookies	5.0	100	45%
■ (Mother's)				
almond shortbread	3 cookies	11.0	180	55%
butter-flavored	5 cookies	6.0	140	39%
checkerboard wafer	8 cookies	8.0	150	48%
chocolate chip				
bag	5 cookies	5.0	140	32%
package	2 cookies	8.0	160	45%
chocolate chip angel	3 cookies	9.0	180	45%
chocolate chip parade	4 cookies	5.0	130	35%
chocolate sandwich/reduced fat	3 cookies	5.0	170	26%
circus animal	6 cookies	6.0	140	39%
classic assortment	2 cookies	7.0	140	45%
cocadas coconut	5 cookies	7.0	150	42%
cookie parade	4 cookies	7.0	140	45%
Dinosaur Grrrahams	2 cookies	3.0	130	21%
double fudge sandwich	2 cookies	9.0	180	45%
duplex sandwich/reduced fat	3 cookies	5.0	160	28%
English tea sandwich	2 cookies	7.0	180	35%
fig bar				
regular				
fat-free	1 bar	–	70	–
regular	1 bar	2.0	80	23%
whole wheat				
fat-free	1 bar	–	70	–
regular	1 bar	3.0	80	34%
Flaky Flix fudge wafer	2 cookies	7.0	140	45%
Flaky Flix vanilla wafer	2 cookies	8.0	140	51%
Gaucho peanut butter sandwich	2 cookies	10.0	190	47%
iced oatmeal				
bag	4 cookies	4.0	120	30%
package	2 cookies	4.0	130	28%
iced raisin	2 cookies	8.0	180	40%
MLB double header duplex	3 cookies	8.0	170	42%
macaroon	2 cookies	8.0	150	48%
Marias	3 cookies	6.0	170	32%
oatmeal	2 cookies	5.0	110	41%
oatmeal chocolate chip	2 cookies	5.0	120	38%
oatmeal raisin	5 cookies	7.0	150	42%
oatmeal walnut chocolate chip	2 cookies	6.0	130	28%

Food and Description	Amount	Fat Grams	Total Calories	% Fat Calories
rainbow wafer	8 wafers	8.0	150	48%
striped shortbread	3 cookies	8.0	170	42%
sugar	2 cookies	6.0	140	39%
taffy sandwich	2 cookies	8.0	180	40%
triplet assortment	2 cookies	7.0	140	45%
vanilla sandwich/reduced fat	3 cookies	5.0	170	26%
vanilla wafer	6 cookies	6.0	150	36%
walnut fudge	2 cookies	7.0	130	48%
zoo pals	14 cookies	5.0	140	32%
■ (Murray)				
assortment	5 cookies	5.0	120	38%
butter pecan	4 cookies	6.0	160	34%
choco chips	6 cookies	5.0	140	32%
chocolate chip	2 cookies	6.0	130	42%
chocolate creme	3 cookies	6.0	150	36%
coconut	2 cookies	6.0	130	42%
creme/assorted	3 cookies	5.0	150	30%
creme wafer/sugar-free				
strawberry	6 cookies	8.0	160	45%
vanilla	6 cookies	9.0	160	51%
duplex creme	3 cookies	5.0	150	30%
fig bar	2 cookies	2.0	90	20%
ginger snap/old-fashioned	6 cookies	2.5	130	17%
lemon creme	3 cookies	6.0	150	36%
oatmeal				
frosted	2 cookies	4.0	120	30%
plain	2 cookies	4.0	120	30%
peanut butter creme	3 cookies	6.0	150	36%
6 in 1 assortment	5 cookies	6.0	140	39%
sugar wafer/duplex	5 cookies	10.0	150	60%
vanilla creme	3 cookies	6.0	150	36%
vanilla wafer	8 cookies	3.0	120	23%
windmill	3 cookies	5.0	150	30%
■ (Nabisco)				
Family Favorites				
fudge-covered graham cracker	3 cookies	7.0	140	45%
fudge-striped graham cracker	3 cookies	8.0	160	45%
oatmeal	1 cookie	5.0	80	56%
vanilla sandwich	3 cookies	8.0	170	42%
Honey Maid/graham cracker				
cinnamon	10 cookies	3.0	140	19%
oatmeal crunch	8 cookies	2.5	120	19%
original	8 cookies	3.0	120	23%
pure chocolate	3 cookies	8.0	160	45%
Nabisco				
Barnum's animal crackers	12 cookies	4.0	140	26%
Biscos sugar wafer	8 cookies	6.0	140	39%
Biscos waffle creme	4 cookies	9.0	180	45%

Food and Description	Amount	Fat Grams	Total Calories	% Fat Calories
brown edge wafer	5 cookies	6.0	140	39%
Bugs Bunny graham cookies				
chocolate	13 cookies	5.0	140	32%
cinnamon	13 cookies	4.5	140	29%
plain	10 cookies	5.0	140	32%
Cameo creme sandwich	2 cookies	5.0	130	35%
Chips Ahoy				
chewy chocolate chip	3 cookies	8.0	170	42%
chunky	1 cookie	4.0	80	45%
mini chocolate chip	14 cookies	7.0	150	42%
real chocolate chip	3 cookies	8.0	160	45%
reduced fat	3 cookies	1.5	150	9%
sprinkled	3 cookies	8.0	170	42%
striped	1 cookie	4.0	80	45%
chocolate chip snaps	7 cookies	5.0	150	30%
chocolate snap	7 cookies	5.0	140	32%
Cookie Break vanilla creme sandwich	3 cookies	6.0	160	34%
Danish/imported	5 cookies	8.0	170	42%
Famous chocolate wafer	5 cookies	4.0	140	26%
Fig Newton				
fat-free	2 cookies	–	100	–
original	2 cookies	2.5	110	20%
Fruit Newton/fat-free				
apple	2 cookies	–	100	–
cranberry	2 cookies	–	100	–
raspberry	2 cookies	–	100	–
strawberry	2 cookies	–	100	–
ginger snap/old-fashioned	4 cookies	2.5	120	19%
graham cracker	8 cookies	3.0	120	23%
Heyday bar	1 bar	5.0	110	41%
Lorna Doone shortbread	4 cookies	7.0	140	45%
Mallomars chocolate cakes	2 cookies	5.0	120	38%
marshmallow puffs	1 cookie	4.0	90	40%
marshmallow twirls	1 piece	6.0	130	42%
Mystic Mint sandwich	1 cookie	4.0	90	40%
National arrowroot biscuit	1 cookie	0.5	20	23%
Nilla vanilla wafer	8 cookies	5.0	140	32%
Nutter Butter				
bites	10 cookies	7.0	150	42%
peanut butter creme patty	5 cookies	9.0	160	51%
peanut butter sandwich	2 cookies	6.0	130	42%
Oreo				
double stuff	2 cookies	7.0	140	45%
fudge covered	1 cookie	6.0	110	50%
Halloween treats	2 cookies	7.0	140	45%
original	3 cookies	7.0	160	39%
reduced fat	3 cookies	5.0	140	32%
white fudge-covered	1 cookie	6.0	110	49%

Food and Description	Amount	Fat Grams	Total Calories	% Fat Calories
Pecan Passion	1 cookie	5.0	90	50%
Pinwheels chocolate-marshmallow cake	1 cookie	5.0	130	35%
Social Tea biscuits	6 cookies	4.0	120	30%
Teddy Grahams				
chocolate	24 pieces	5.0	140	32%
cinnamon	24 pieces	4.0	140	26%
honey	24 pieces	4.0	140	26%
zwieback	1 piece	1.0	35	26%
SnackWell's				
fat-free				
chocolate truffle	1 cookie	–	60	–
cinnamon graham	20 pieces	–	110	–
devil's food cookie cakes	1 cookie	–	50	–
double fudge cookie cakes	1 cookie	–	50	–
reduced fat				
chocolate chip	13 cookies	3.5	130	24%
chocolate sandwich w/chocolate creme	2 cookies	2.5	100	23%
oatmeal raisin	2 cookies	2.5	110	20%
vanilla sandwich w/vanilla creme	2 cookies	2.5	110	23%
■ (Nature's Warehouse)				
almond butter	2 cookies	4.0	120	30%
banana/wheat-free	1 oz	1.0	90	10%
caramel crisp/wheat-free	1 oz	1.0	90	10%
cherry/wheat-free	1 oz	1.0	90	10%
chocolate chocolate chip	2 cookies	6.0	140	39%
cinnamon graham	1 cookie	3.5	115	27%
fig bar				
wheat-free				
apple cinnamon	1 oz	2.0	100	18%
original	1 oz	2.0	100	–
raspberry	1 oz	2.0	100	18%
whole wheat	1 oz	2.0	100	18%
oat bran/wheat-free	2 cookies	6.0	130	42%
oat bran chocolate chip	2 cookies	6.0	140	39%
peanut butter chocolate chip	2 cookies	8.5	140	55%
raspberry/wheat-free	1 oz	1.0	90	10%
■ (Nestle)				
Toll House				
refrigerated/ready to bake				
chocolate chip				
original	1⅔ Tbs	5.0	130	35%
reduced-fat	1⅔ Tbs	4.0	125	29%
sugar	2¼" square	5.0	130	35%
■ (Obie's)				
mix				
chewy chocolate chip	1 cookie	1.0	90	10%
chewy oatmeal raisin	1 cookie	1.0	90	10%

Food and Description	Amount	Fat Grams	Total Calories	% Fat Calories
double chocolate fudge	1 cookie	1.0	90	10%
■ OREO (*See* (Nabisco) in this section)				
■ (Peak Frean)				
arrowroot	5 cookies	5.1	179	26%
Bourbon creme	3 cookies	8.0	196	37%
bran crunch	4 cookies	7.3	190	35%
coffee creme	3 cookies	9.1	201	41%
dark chocolate biscuits	3 cookies	10.1	206	44%
delectable	2 cookies	8.1	193	38%
French vanilla creme	3 cookies	10.3	207	45%
fruit creme	3 cookies	8.6	194	40%
fruit shortcake	3 cookies	8.5	197	39%
garden creme	3 cookies	9.8	203	43%
ginger crisp	5 cookies	4.5	178	23%
milk chocolate biscuits	3 cookies	10.4	206	45%
Nice	5 cookies	6.6	189	31%
oatmeal/traditional	2 cookies	6.2	184	30%
petit beurre	6 cookies	5.0	180	25%
rich tea	5 cookies	6.2	187	30%
Sable shortcake	3 cookies	9.6	204	42%
Sweetmeal	5 cookies	8.5	197	39%
■ PECAN SANDIES (*See* (Keebler) in this section)				
■ (Pepperidge Farm)				
American Collection				
Beacon Hill brownie nut	1 cookie	7.0	130	48%
Charleston milk chocolate toffee	1 cookie	7.0	130	48%
Chesapeake chocolate chunk pecan	1 cookie	8.0	140	51%
Nantucket chocolate chunk	1 cookie	7.0	130	48%
Santa Fe oatmeal raisin	1 cookie	4.5	120	34%
Sausalito milk chocolate macadamia	1 cookie	7.0	140	45%
Tahoe white chunk macadamia	1 cookie	7.0	130	48%
biscotti				
almond				
chocolate-dipped				
3.5" cookie	1 cookie	4.0	110	33%
5.5" cookie	1 cookie	10.0	210	43%
plain				
3.5" cookie	1 cookie	3.5	90	35%
5.5" cookie	1 cookie	6.0	160	34%
anise	1 cookie	3.0	90	30%
chocolate hazelnut				
3.5" cookie	1 cookie	5.0	90	50%
5.5" cookie	1 cookie	9.0	160	51%
cinnamon chip				
3.5" cookie	1 cookie	3.5	90	35%
5.5" cookie	1 cookie	6.0	160	34%
cranberry pistachio				
3.5" cookie	1 cookie	3.0	90	30%

Food and Description	Amount	Fat Grams	Total Calories	% Fat Calories
5.5" cookie	1 cookie	6.0	160	34%
orange/chocolate-dipped				
3.5" cookie	1 cookie	4.5	110	37%
5.5" cookie	1 cookie	8.0	200	36%
Distinctive Assortment				
cafe favorites	4 cookies	7.0	140	45%
chocolate laced pirouettes	5 cookies	10.0	180	50%
dessert favorites	3 cookies	9.0	170	48%
party favorites	3 cookies	8.0	170	42%
personal favorites	4 cookies	9.0	170	48%
toy chest butter assortment	3 cookies	5.0	120	38%
Distinctive cookies				
Bordeaux				
milk chocolate	3 cookies	9.0	160	51%
original	4 cookies	5.0	130	35%
Brussels				
individual pkg	2 cookies	4.0	100	36%
regular pkg	3 cookies	7.0	150	42%
Brussels mint	3 cookies	10.0	190	47%
butter chessmen				
individual pkg	3 cookies	4.0	100	36%
regular pkg	3 cookies	5.0	120	38%
Chantilly hazelnut	1 cookie	3.0	80	34%
Geneva	3 cookies	9.0	160	51%
Lido	1 cookie	4.5	90	45%
Linzer				
original	1 cookie	4.0	100	36%
raspberry-filled	1 cookie	4.0	100	36%
Milano				
double chocolate	2 cookies	8.0	150	48%
milk chocolate	3 cookies	10.0	180	50%
mint	2 cookies	8.0	140	51%
orange	2 cookies	8.0	140	51%
original				
individual pkg	2 cookies	6.0	110	49%
regular pkg	3 cookies	10.0	180	50%
Nantucket/individual pkg	2 cookies	11.0	220	45%
fat-free cookies				
double chocolate fudge	1 cookie	–	60	–
milk chocolate ripple	1 cookie	–	60	–
fruit cookies				
apricot-raspberry	3 cookies	6.0	140	39%
cherry cobbler	1 cookie	2.5	70	32%
peach tart	2 cookies	3.0	120	23%
strawberry	3 cookies	5.0	140	32%
Goldfish cookies				
chocolate	19 pieces	5.0	140	53%
chocolate chunk	19 pieces	7.0	150	42%

Food and Description	Amount	Fat Grams	Total Calories	% Fat Calories
cinnamon graham	19 pieces	7.0	150	42%
goldfish cookies on the go	1 pouch	7.0	200	32%
graham goldfish	19 pieces	7.0	150	42%
vanilla	19 pieces	7.0	150	42%
International Collection				
Biarritz	6 cookies	8.0	160	45%
chocolat a l'orange	2 cookies	6.0	150	36%
deli choc dark chocolate	2 cookies	4.0	110	33%
espirit blanc	1 cookie	4.5	80	51%
esprits-noir/dark chocolate	1 cookie	5.0	90	50%
Highland shortbread	2 cookies	7.0	140	45%
madallon au beurre	4 cookies	5.0	150	30%
selection de choix	5 cookies	7.0	150	42%
large cookies				
brownie	2 cookies	13.0	260	45%
chocolate chip	2 cookies	11.0	240	41%
chocolate chocolate chip	2 cookies	12.0	250	43%
cinnamon chip	2 cookies	10.0	230	39%
oatmeal	2 cookies	9.0	240	34%
sugar	2 cookies	10.0	240	38%
mini cookies				
almond shortbread	9 cookies	17.0	300	51%
chocolate chip	9 cookies	14.0	260	48%
lemon nut	9 cookies	18.0	300	54%
oatmeal raisin	9 cookies	10.0	270	33%
peanut butter milk chocolate	9 cookies	15.0	280	48%
pecan Scotties	9 cookies	17.0	300	51%
toffee milk chocolate chunk	9 cookies	14.0	260	48%
old-fashioned cookies				
brownie chocolate nut	3 cookies	9.0	160	51%
butterscotch oatmeal	3 cookies	9.0	170	48%
chocolate chip	3 cookies	7.0	140	45%
ginger man				
individual pkg	3 cookies	3.0	90	30%
regular pkg	4 cookies	3.5	120	26%
hazelnut	3 cookies	8.0	160	45%
Irish oatmeal	3 cookies	6.0	130	42%
lemon nut crunch	3 cookies	9.0	170	48%
molasses crisp	5 cookies	6.0	150	36%
oatmeal raisin	3 cookies	6.0	160	34%
pecan shortbread	2 cookies	9.0	140	58%
shortbread	2 cookies	7.0	140	45%
sugar	3 cookies	6.0	140	39%
reduced-fat cookies				
chocolate chunk	1 cookie	4.5	120	34%
oatmeal raisin	1 cookie	3.0	110	25%
vanilla creme Chantilly	1 cookie	2.0	70	26%

Food and Description	Amount	Fat Grams	Total Calories	% Fat Calories
soft-baked cookies				
caramel pecan	1 cookie	7.0	130	37%
chocolate chocolate walnut	1 cookie	6.0	130	42%
chocolate chunk	1 cookie	6.0	130	42%
milk chocolate macadamia	1 cookie	6.0	130	42%
oatmeal raisin	1 cookie	4.0	110	33%
Wholesome Choice				
vanilla raspberry tart	2 cookies	3.0	120	23%
■ (Pillsbury)				
mix/prepared				
Chips Ahoy	1 bar	7.0	180	35%
Fudge Swirl	1 bar	8.0	180	40%
Nutter Butter	1 bar	7.0	180	35%
Oreo	1 bar	6.0	150	36%
refrigerated				
candy	1 oz	6.0	130	42%
chocolate chip	1 oz	6.0	130	42%
chocolate chocolate chip	1 oz	6.0	130	42%
dinosaurs	2 cookies	5.0	120	38%
holiday	2 cookies	7.0	130	48%
oatmeal chocolate chip	1 oz	6.0	120	45%
peanut butter	1 oz	5.0	110	41%
sugar	2 cookies	5.0	130	35%
teddy bears	2 cookies	5.0	120	38%
■ (Planters)				
Mr. Peanut peanut butter crisps/graham				
0.5-oz pkg	2 pkgs	7.0	140	45%
1.5-oz pkg	12 pieces	8.0	150	48%
	1 pkg	16.0	210	69%
1-oz pkg	1 pouch	7.0	140	45%
■ (Rippin' Good)				
carousel	6 cookies	6.0	140	39%
chocolate chip creme	2 cookies	6.0	160	34%
cookie jar	3 cookies	6.0	150	36%
creme wafers/assorted	3 cookies	7.0	140	45%
duplex creme	2 cookies	4.0	100	36%
fudge stripe oatmeal	2 cookies	8.0	140	51%
ginger snap	5 cookies	4.0	130	26%
granola & peanut butter sandwich	2 cookies	6.0	140	39%
iced oatmeal	2 cookies	2.0	90	30%
iced spice	3 cookies	3.0	130	21%
lemon crisp	3 cookies	8.0	160	45%
macaroon cremes	2 cookies	8.0	160	45%
marshmallow blossoms	2 cookies	2.0	90	30%
marshmallow daisies	2 cookies	2.0	90	30%
marshmallow fudge stripes	2 cookies	4.0	100	36%
peanut butter	2 cookies	4.0	100	36%
Rippie Cremes vanilla sandwich	3 cookies	6.0	160	34%

Food and Description	Amount	Fat Grams	Total Calories	% Fat Calories
spice wafer	3 cookies	4.0	140	26%
striped dainties	1 cookie	3.0	50	54%
■ (Sara Lee)				
chocolate brownie/fat-free	2 cookies	–	80	–
peanut butter	2 cookies	7.0	140	45%
white chocolate macadamia	2 cookies	7.0	130	48%
■ (Savoir Faire)				
Galettes butter	1 oz	5.0	130	35%
petit butter biscuit	1 oz	5.0	170	26%
■ (Schwan's)				
frozen	1 cookie	5.0	120	38%
■ SMALL INDULGENCE (See (Barbara's Bakery) in this section)				
■ SMART SNACKERS (See (Weight Watchers) in this section)				
■ SNACKWELL'S (See (Nabisco) in this section)				
■ (Spaans Cookie Co.)				
banana/low-fat	2 cookies	3.0	100	27%
butter melt	2 cookies	6.0	130	42%
cherry crisp/sugar-free	4 cookies	5.0	110	41%
chocolate chip				
low-fat	2 cookies	3.0	110	25%
plain	2 cookies	6.0	120	45%
w/walnuts	1 cookie	7.0	130	48%
cinnamon bears	1 cookie	4.0	100	36%
cocoa bears	1 cookie	4.0	100	36%
coconut krispies	2 cookies	5.0	120	38%
crunchy vanilla/sugar-free	4 cookies	5.0	120	38%
date oatmeal	2 cookies	4.5	120	34%
Dutch chocolate/sugar-free	3 cookies	5.0	110	41%
fruit 'n honey	2 cookies	3.5	110	29%
fudge brownie	2 cookies	4.5	120	34%
fudge 'n chips				
low-fat	2 cookies	2.5	100	23%
w/walnuts	1 cookie	6.0	120	45%
harvest	2 cookies	6.0	130	42%
holiday	2 cookies	7.0	130	48%
lemon coconut/sugar-free	3 cookies	6.0	120	45%
oat bran 'n chips/low-fat	2 cookies	3.0	100	27%
oat bran 'n raisin				
fat-free	2 cookies	–	80	–
regular	2 cookies	4.5	110	37%
peanut butter	2 cookies	7.0	130	48%
shortbread	2 cookies	5.0	120	38%
soft oatmeal	2 cookies	3.5	110	29%
speculaas/windmills	2 cookies	6.0	130	42%
spiced windmill/sugar-free	2 cookies	5.0	110	41%
sugar bear	1 cookie	4.0	100	36%
toasted almond	2 cookies	7.0	130	48%

Food and Description	Amount	Fat Grams	Total Calories	% Fat Calories
■ **(Stella D'Oro)**				
almond toast	1 piece	1.0	60	15%
angel bars	1 cookie	5.0	80	56%
angel wings	1 cookie	5.0	70	64%
Angelica goodies	1 cookie	4.0	110	33%
anginetti	1 cookie	1.0	30	30%
anisette sponge	1 cookie	1.0	50	18%
anisette toast				
jumbo	1 cookie	1.0	110	8%
regular	1 cookie	1.0	50	18%
apple pastry	1 piece	3.0	80	34%
biscottini cashews	1 cookie	6.0	110	4%
breakfast treat	1 piece	4.0	100	36%
castelets				
chocolate	1 piece	3.0	60	45%
vanilla	1 piece	3.0	70	39%
Chinese dessert	1 cookie	9.0	170	48%
coconut macaroon	1 cookie	3.0	60	45%
Como delight	1 cookie	7.0	150	42%
deep night fudge	1 cookie	4.0	65	55%
Dutch apple bar	1 piece	3.0	110	25%
egg biscuit				
low-sodium	3 pieces	3.0	120	23%
Roman	1 piece	5.0	140	32%
sugared	1 piece	1.0	80	11%
egg jumbo	1 piece	1.0	50	18%
fruit delight				
apple-cinnamon/fat-free	1 cookie	–	70	–
peach-apricot/fat-free	1 cookie	–	70	–
fruit slice				
fat-free	1 cookie	–	50	–
original	1 cookie	2.0	60	30%
golden bar	1 cookie	4.0	110	33%
holiday rings & stars	1 cookie	1.0	45	20%
holiday trinkets	1 cookie	2.0	40	45%
hostess assortment	1 cookie	2.0	40	45%
kichel/low-sodium	21 pieces	9.0	150	54%
Lady Stella assortment	1 cookie	2.0	40	45%
Margherite				
chocolate	1 cookie	3.0	70	39%
vanilla	1 cookie	3.0	70	39%
peach-apricot pastry	1 piece	3.0	80	34%
pfeffernusse/spice drops	1 cookie	1.0	40	23%
prune pastry	1 piece	3.0	90	30%
royal nugget	1 piece	–	2	–
sesame Regina	1 piece	2.0	50	36%
Swiss fudge	1 piece	3.0	70	39%

Food and Description	Amount	Fat Grams	Total Calories	% Fat Calories
■ (Sugar Kake)				
sandwich cookies				
assorted	3 cookies	6.0	150	36%
chocolate	3 cookies	6.0	150	36%
duplex	3 cookies	6.0	150	36%
lemon	3 cookies	6.0	150	36%
strawberry	3 cookies	6.0	150	36%
vanilla	3 cookies	6.0	150	36%
■ (Sunshine)				
almond crescents	4 cookies	6.0	150	36%
animal crackers	14 cookies	4.0	140	26%
butter-flavored	5 cookies	6.0	140	39%
Chip-A-Roos	3 cookies	10.0	190	47%
chocolate chip/mini	5 cookies	8.0	160	39%
fig bar	2 cookies	2.5	110	20%
fudge mint patties	2 cookies	7.0	130	48%
fudge-dipped grahams	4 cookies	9.0	170	48%
fudge-striped shortbread	3 cookies	9.0	160	51%
ginger snap	7 cookies	4.5	130	31%
golden fruit				
apple/low-fat	1 cookie	1.5	80	17%
apple bar/fat-free	1 cookie	–	60	–
apple-cinnamon bar/fat-free	1 cookie	–	60	–
cranberry/low-fat	1 cookie	1.0	70	13%
raisin/low-fat	1 cookie	1.5	80	17%
graham cracker				
cinnamon	2 cookies	6.0	140	39%
honey	2 cookies	4.0	120	30%
Hydrox				
original	3 cookies	7.0	150	42%
reduced fat	3 cookies	4.0	130	28%
iced gingerbread	5 cookies	6.0	130	42%
lemon coolers	5 cookies	6.0	140	39%
oatmeal				
chocolate chip	3 cookies	8.0	170	42%
country style	3 cookies	7.0	170	37%
iced	2 cookies	5.0	120	38%
Oh Berry wafer				
fat-free	8 cookies	–	100	–
fudge dipped	3 cookies	4.5	120	34%
sugar wafer				
chocolate	3 cookies	7.0	130	48%
peanut butter	4 cookies	9.0	170	48%
vanilla	3 cookies	6.0	130	42%
Sunshine Jingles	6 cookies	5.0	150	30%
vanilla wafer	7 cookies	7.0	150	42%
Vienna Fingers				
chocolate/reduced fat	2 cookies	3.5	120	26%

Food and Description	Amount	Fat Grams	Total Calories	% Fat Calories
original				
low-fat	2 cookies	3.5	130	24%
regular	2 cookies	6.0	140	39%
■ (Sweet Pretenders)				
chocolate flavored chip	1 cookie	2.0	45	40%
lemon	1 cookie	2.0	45	40%
oatmeal raisin	1 cookie	2.0	45	40%
peanut butter	1 cookie	2.0	40	45%
vanilla	1 cookie	2.0	45	40%
■ (Tastykake)				
bars				
apple cinnamon	1 bar	7	180	35%
chocolate chip	1 bar	8	200	36%
chunky peanut butter	1 bar	11	240	41%
fudge	1 bar	7	190	33%
oatmeal raisin	1 bar	7	190	33%
peanut butter krunch	1 bar	8	140	45%
cookies				
chocolate chip/soft & chewy	2 cookies	14	350	36%
chocolate chocolate chip/soft & chewy	2 cookies	13	350	33%
holiday tub	4 cookies	8	160	45%
oatmeal raisin/soft & chewy	2 cookies	14	350	36%
sugar vanilla wafer	5 cookies	10	170	53%
■ TOLL HOUSE (See (Nestle) in this section)				
■ TWIX (See (M&M★Mars) in this section)				
■ (Twookies)				
creamy chocolate	1 oz	6.0	130	42%
creamy peanut butter	1 oz	5.0	130	35%
strawberry	1 oz	6.0	140	39%
vanilla creme	1 oz	6.0	140	39%
■ (Ultra Slim Fast)				
chocolate sandwich	3 cookies	3.0	130	21%
cinnamon graham	4 cookies	1.5	120	11%
fig	1 cookie	0.5	60	8%
vanilla sandwich	3 cookies	3.0	130	21%
■ (Umeya)				
fortune cookie	4 cookies	<1.0	120	4%
■ (Vermont Country Maple)				
mix/prepared				
hearty oatmeal	2 cookies	0.5	110	4%
■ (Vicenzi)				
butter cookie				
w/dark chocolate	2 cookies	7.0	140	45%
w/milk chocolate	2 cookies	7.0	140	45%
crispy wafer/milk chocolate	2 cookies	8.0	120	60%
■ VIENNA FINGERS (See (Sunshine) in this section)				
■ (Voortman)				
almonette	1 cookie	5.0	90	50%

Food and Description	Amount	Fat Grams	Total Calories	% Fat Calories
chocolate chip	1 cookie	5.0	100	45%
chocolate wafer	3 cookies	9.0	160	51%
coconut delight	1 cookie	5.0	90	50%
Dutch creme	1 cookie	5.0	110	41%
oatmeal apple	1 cookie	3.0	80	34%
shortbread swirl	2 cookies	6.0	110	49%
strawberry wafer	3 cookies	9.0	170	43%
vanilla wafer	3 cookies	9.0	170	43%
■ (Weight Watchers)				
Smart Snackers				
apple raisin bar	0.75 oz	2.0	70	26%
chocolate chip	1.06 oz	5.0	140	32%
chocolate sandwich	1.06 oz	3.5	140	32%
fruit-filled bar				
fig	1 bar	–	70	–
raspberry	1 bar	–	70	–
oatmeal spice	1.06 oz	2.0	120	15%
vanilla sandwich	1.06 oz	3.0	140	19%
■ (Westbrae)				
Cookie Jar Classics				
Dutch apple cinnamon	1 cookie	4.0	110	32%
honey almond	1 cookie	4.0	110	32%
raspberry vanilla	1 cookie	4.0	110	32%
regular cookies				
crispy chocolate chip	1 cookie	4.0	110	32%
Dinosnaps animal oatmeal raisin	8 cookies	5.0	130	35%
soft chocolate chip				
coconut	1 cookie	4.5	110	37%
pecan	1 cookie	4.5	110	37%
walnut	1 cookie	5.0	110	41%
soft chocolate chocolate chip	1 cookie	3.0	90	30%
rice malt cookies				
ginger snap	3 cookies	5.0	130	35%
oatmeal	3 cookies	6.0	140	39%
COOKIE CRUMBS (See also CRACKER CRUMBS & MEAL)				
(Nabisco)				
Honey Maid graham cracker	1 serving	1.5	70	19%
Nilla	2 Tbs	2.5	70	32%
Oreo	2 Tbs	3.0	80	34%
COOKING SPRAY				
(Mazola)	2-sec spray	0.8	6	100%
(Pam)				
butter flavor	⅓ of 10" skillet	1.0	2	100%
olive oil	⅓ of 10" skillet	1	2	100%
original	¼-sec spray	1	7	100%

Food and Description	Amount	Fat Grams	Total Calories	% Fat Calories
(Tryson House) flavor spray				
buttery delite	1-sec spray	0.8	8	100%
garlic mist	1-sec spray	0.8	8	100%
Italian mist	1-sec spray	0.8	8	100%
mesquite mist	1-sec spray	0.8	8	100%
olive mist	1-sec spray	0.8	8	100%
Oriental mist	1-sec spray	0.8	8	100%
(Weight Watchers)				
butter	0.28 gm	–	–	–
cooking	0.33 gm	–	–	–
(Wesson)	0.27 gm	<1.0	<1	100%
CORIANDER LEAF (See CILANTRO)				
CORIANDER SEED				
whole	1 tsp	<1.0	5	53%
	1 Tbs	0.9	15	53%
	1 oz	5.0	85	53%
CORN				
canned				
(Bristol) baby corn on cob	4 ears	–	12	–
(Del Monte)				
cream style				
golden				
no salt added	½ cup	0.5	90	5%
regular	½ cup	0.5	90	5%
supersweet	½ cup	0.5	60	8%
white	½ cup	1.0	100	9%
whole kernel				
golden				
regular	½ cup	1.0	90	10%
supersweet				
no salt added	½ cup	1.0	60	15%
no sugar added	½ cup	1.0	60	15%
vacuum packed	½ cup	1.0	70	13%
white	½ cup	–	80	–
(Fancifood) baby	6 pieces	–	25	–
(Freshlike)				
cream style/golden				
no salt added	½ cup	1.0	110	8%
regular	½ cup	1.0	110	8%
crisp 'n sweet	½ cup	1.0	80	11%
whole kernel				
vacuum packed	½ cup	1.0	100	9%
water packed				
no salt added	½ cup	1.0	80	11%
no sugar or salt added	½ cup	1.0	80	11%
generic/cream style	½ cup	0.5	93	5%
(Green Giant)				
cream style	½ cup	0.5	100	5%

Food and Description	Amount	Fat Grams	Total Calories	% Fat Calories
Mexicorn	⅓ cup	–	60	–
Niblets				
white shoepeg	⅓ cup	0.5	80	6%
yellow				
extra sweet	⅓ cup	0.5	50	9%
50% less sodium	⅓ cup	–	60	–
no salt or sugar added	⅓ cup	–	60	–
regular	⅓ cup	–	70	–
whole kernel/sweet				
50% less sodium	½ cup	0.5	80	6%
regular	½ cup	0.5	80	6%
(S&W)				
cream style				
regular	½ cup	1.0	100	9%
w/starch	½ cup	1.0	100	9%
whole kernel				
regular	½ cup	1.0	90	10%
sweet 'n crisp	⅓ cup	1.5	70	19%
(Seneca)				
cream style	½ cup	–	80	–
whole kernel	½ cup	0.5	80	6%
(Stokely)				
cream style				
golden	½ cup	–	100	–
white	½ cup	–	100	–
whole kernel				
golden	½ cup	–	90	–
white	½ cup	–	90	–
(Veg-All) golden				
cream style	½ cup	1.0	110	8%
whole kernel				
regular	½ cup	1.0	80	11%
vacuum packed	½ cup	1.0	100	9%
fresh/sweet/white or yellow				
kernels/cooked	½ cup	1.0	89	10%
whole ear	1 medium	1.0	89	10%
frozen				
(Birds Eye)				
big ears	1 ear	1.0	160	6%
kernels	½ cup	1.0	80	11%
little ears	2 ears	1.0	130	7%
sweet corn on cob	2 ears	1.0	110	8%
tender deluxe	½ cup	1.0	80	11%
(C&W) early harvest petite				
petite white	⅔ cup	1.0	80	11%
sweet corn	⅔ cup	1.0	80	11%
generic				
corn on the cob	1 ear	1.0	150	6%

Food and Description	Amount	Fat Grams	Total Calories	% Fat Calories
cream style	½ cup	0.6	120	5%
kernels/white shoepeg	½ cup	1.0	70	13%
(Green Giant)				
corn on the cob				
extra sweet	1 ear	2.0	120	15%
Nibblers/6-ear pkg	1 ear	0.5	70	6%
Niblets/4-ear pkg	1 ear	1.5	160	8%
kernels				
Harvest Fresh				
white shoepeg	½ cup	0.5	70	6%
yellow	⅔ cup	0.5	80	6%
Niblets				
extra sweet	⅔ cup	1.0	70	13%
regular	⅔ cup	0.5	80	6%
regular/white				
extra sweet	⅔ cup	0.5	50	9%
shoepeg	¾ cup	1.0	100	9%
(Ore-Ida) corn on the cob				
mini gold	1 ear	1.0	80	11%
regular	1 ear	1.5	140	10%
(Pictsweet)				
corn on the cob				
3" ear	1 ear	<1.0	50	8%
6" ear	1 ear	1.0	110	8%
kernels/cut	½ cup	1.0	80	11%
(Seneca)				
corn on the cob	1 ear	–	140	–
kernels	⅔ cup	0.5	90	5%
CORN CAKE (See RICE CAKES)				
CORN CHIPS (See TORTILLA CHIPS)				
CORN CHOWDER (See SOUP)				
CORN DISH (See also FROZEN ENTRÉE/DINNER; VEGETABLES, MIXED)				
canned				
(Green Giant) corn relish	1 Tbs	–	20	–
frozen				
(Green Giant)				
cream style corn in cheese & cream sauce	½ cup	1.0	110	8%
Niblets in butter sauce	⅔ cup	3.0	130	21%
white shoepeg in butter sauce	¾ cup	2.5	120	19%
(Mrs. Paul's) corn fritter	2 fritters	9.0	240	34%
homemade/USDA Standard Home Recipe				
corn fritter	1 oz	2.0	62	29%
corn pudding	½ cup	6.6	136	44%
scalloped corn	½ cup	7.0	250	25%
CORN FLAKE CRUMBS				
(Kellogg's)	2 Tbs	–	40	

Food and Description	Amount	Fat Grams	Total Calories	% Fat Calories
CORN GRITS				
(Albers) quick hominy	¼ cup	0.5	140	3%
(Arrowhead Mills) dry				
white	¼ cup	–	140	–
yellow	¼ cup	–	130	–
generic				
canned				
white	1 cup	1.5	115	11%
yellow	1 cup	1.5	115	11%
dry				
cooked	4 oz	<1.0	68	3%
	1 cup	0.5	146	3%
uncooked	1 Tbs	<1.0	36	3%
	1 oz	<1.0	105	3%
	1 cup	1.8	579	3%
(Quaker) dry				
instant				
original	1 pkt	–	100	–
real butter flavor	1 pkt	1.5	100	14%
white hominy	1 pkt	–	80	–
w/imitation bacon bits	1 pkt	0.5	100	5%
w/imitation ham bits	1 pkt	0.5	100	5%
w/real cheddar cheese	1 pkt	1.5	100	14%
w/sausage bits	1 pkt	1.0	100	9%
zesty cheddar	1 pkt	1.5	100	14%
quick				
white hominy	¼ cup	0.5	130	3%
yellow hominy	¼ cup	0.5	120	4%
regular/white hominy	¼ cup	0.5	140	4%
CORN NUT (*See* SNACKS)				
CORN PONE (*See* BREAD)				
CORN PUDDING (*See* PUDDING & MOUSSE)				
CORN SYRUP (*See also* PANCAKE/WAFFLE SYRUP)				
generic	1 Tbs	–	59	–
(Karo)				
dark	2 Tbs	–	120	–
	½ cup	–	495	–
light	2 Tbs	–	120	–
	½ cup	–	500	–
CORNBREAD (*See* BREAD)				
CORNED BEEF (*See also* BEEF; LUNCHEON MEAT)				
generic				
canned	1 oz	4.0	71	51%
jellied loaf	1 oz	1.9	46	37%
(Hormel)	2 oz	7.0	120	53%
(Morton's) fresh	4 oz	8.0	150	48%
CORNED BEEF HASH (*See* BEEF DISH/ENTRÉE)				

Food and Description	Amount	Fat Grams	Total Calories	% Fat Calories
CORNISH GAME HEN				
fresh & frozen				
(Perdue) whole				
dark meat	3 oz	15.0	210	64%
white meat	3 oz	10.0	170	53%
(Tyson)	3.5 oz	14.0	240	57%
fully cooked				
(Perdue) oven roasted				
dark meat	3 oz	9.0	140	58%
white meat	3 oz	7.0	130	48%
CORNMEAL				
(Albers) yellow or white	3 Tbs	–	110	–
(Arrowhead Mills) blue	2 oz	3.0	210	13%
(Aunt Jemima) self-rising				
white/enriched				
bolted	3 Tbs	0.5	90	5%
degermed	3 Tbs	0.5	90	5%
CORNMEAL MIX				
(Aunt Jemima) self-rising				
buttermilk white	3 Tbs	0.5	80	6%
white/bolted	3 Tbs	0.5	80	6%
yellow	3 Tbs	0.5	80	6%
CORNSTARCH	1 Tbs	–	30	–
	1 cup	–	463	–
COTTAGE CHEESE (*See also* CHEESE)				
(Alta Dena)				
low-fat	½ cup	2.0	90	20%
(Borden)				
creamed				
4% fat	½ cup	5.0	120	38%
2% fat	½ cup	2.0	90	20%
dry curd/5% fat	½ cup	1.0	80	11%
(Breakstone)				
creamed				
4% fat				
large curd	½ cup	5.0	120	38%
small curd	½ cup	5.0	120	38%
2% fat				
large curd	½ cup	4.0	90	40%
small curd	½ cup	4.0	90	40%
dry curd/<0.5% fat	¼ cup	–	45	–
(Carnation)				
creamed				
4% fat				
large curd	½ cup	5.0	115	38%
small curd	½ cup	5.0	115	38%
w/pineapple	½ cup	5.0	130	35%
1.5% fat/Slender	½ cup	2.0	90	20%

Food and Description	Amount	Fat Grams	Total Calories	% Fat Calories
(Crowley) creamed				
4% fat				
plain	½ cup	5.0	120	38%
w/peaches	½ cup	3.0	140	19%
w/pineapple	½ cup	4.0	140	26%
1% fat				
calcium-fortified	½ cup	1.0	90	10%
plain	½ cup	1.0	90	10%
w/pineapple	½ cup	1.0	110	8%
(Darigold) creamed				
4% fat	½ cup	4.0	120	30%
2% fat/trim	½ cup	3.0	100	27%
(Friendship) creamed				
4% fat				
California style	½ cup	5.0	120	38%
w/pineapple	½ cup	4.0	140	26%
1% fat				
plain	½ cup	1.0	90	10%
lactose reduced	½ cup	1.0	90	10%
no salt added	½ cup	1.0	90	10%
w/pineapple	½ cup	1.0	110	8%
2% fat/large curd pot-style	½ cup	2.0	100	18%
generic				
creamed				
4% fat				
large curd	½ cup	5.0	117	39%
small curd	½ cup	5.0	117	39%
1% fat	½ cup	1.0	80	11%
2% fat	½ cup	2.0	100	18%
dry curd				
large curd	½ cup	0.5	95	5%
small curd	½ cup	0.5	95	5%
(Kemps)				
creamed				
nonfat	4 oz	<1.0	80	3%
1% fat/lite	4 oz	1.0	90	10%
2% fat/low-fat	4 oz	2.0	100	18%
whole milk	4 oz	5.0	120	38%
dry curd	4 oz	1.0	80	11%
(Knudsen) creamed				
4% fat				
large curd	½ cup	5.0	130	35%
small curd	½ cup	5.0	120	38%
nonfat/free	½ cup	–	80	–
1.5% fat				
peach	½ cup	1.5	110	12%
pineapple	½ cup	1.5	110	12%
strawberry	½ cup	1.5	110	12%

Food and Description	Amount	Fat Grams	Total Calories	% Fat Calories
tropical fruit	½ cup	2.0	120	15%
2% fat/small curd	½ cup	2.5	100	23%
(Land O'Lakes) creamed				
4% fat	½ cup	5.0	120	38%
1% fat	½ cup	1.0	90	10%
2% fat	½ cup	2.0	100	18%
(Light N' Lively) creamed				
1% fat				
plain	½ cup	1.5	80	17%
w/garden salad	½ cup	1.5	90	15%
w/peach & pineapple	½ cup	1.0	120	8%
nonfat	½ cup	–	80	–
(Lite-Line) creamed/1.5% Fat	½ cup	2.0	90	20%
(Sealtest) creamed				
4% fat				
large curd	½ cup	5.0	120	38%
small curd	½ cup	5.0	120	38%
2% fat/small curd	½ cup	2.5	90	25%
(Weight Watchers) creamed				
1% fat	½ cup	1.0	90	10%
2% fat	½ cup	2.0	90	20%
COUSCOUS (See PASTA, SOUP/DEHYDRATED)				
COWPEA (See BLACK-EYED PEA)				
CRAB (See also CRAB, IMITATION; CRAB DISH; SEAFOOD ENTRÉE/DINNER)				
canned/meat only				
(Crown Prince) drained	½ cup	–	50	–
generic/blue	3 oz	1.0	84	11%
(S&W) Dungeness	⅓ cup	1.0	80	11%
fresh/meat only				
Alaska/Alaskan king				
cooked-moist heat	3 oz	1.0	82	11%
	1 leg	2.0	129	14%
raw	3 oz	1.0	71	13%
	1 leg	1.0	145	6%
blue				
cooked-moist heat	3 oz	1.5	90	15%
raw	3 oz	1.0	75	12%
Dungeness				
cooked-moist heat	3 oz	1.0	95	9%
raw	3 oz	1.0	75	12%
queen/raw	3 oz	1.0	76	12%
soft shell				
cooked-moist heat	3 oz	1.5	90	15%
fried	1 medium	13.0	213	55%
frozen				
(Wakefield) snow	3 oz	1.0	60	15%
CRAB, IMITATION				
generic/from surimi	3 oz	1.0	87	10%

Food and Description	Amount	Fat Grams	Total Calories	% Fat Calories
(Icicle Seafood)	⅔ cup	–	90	–
(Louis Kemp) crab delights				
chunk style	½ cup	–	80	–
flake style	½ cup	–	80	–
leg style	½ cup	–	80	–
salad style	½ cup	–	80	–
CRAB DISH (*See also* SEAFOOD ENTRÉE/DINNER)				
frozen				
(Carnival) crab cake/low-fat	1 cake	1.0	110	8%
(King & Prince)				
crab crisp	4 oz	19.0	310	55%
crab del ray	3 oz	9.0	155	52%
(Mrs. Paul's) deviled crab cake				
miniatures	3.5 oz	12.0	240	45%
regular	1 cake	9.0	180	45%
homemade/USDA Standard Home Recipe				
crab cake/fried	4 oz	8.5	180	43%
crab salad	5.5 oz	10.7	205	47%
CRAB SOUP (*See* SOUP)				
CRABAPPLE				
canned				
(Lucky Leaf) spiced	½ cup	–	110	–
fresh/raw/w/skin				
sliced	½ cup	–	40	–
whole	3 oz	–	60	–
CRACKER (*See also* COOKIE; MATZO; SNACKS)				
■ **(Adrienne's)**				
Appeteazers				
double cheddar	1 oz	5.0	130	35%
garlic & herb	1 oz	4.0	130	28%
original	1 oz	4.0	130	28%
Crunch Wells/low-fat crumpet chips				
apple cinnamon	1 oz	1.0	110	8%
Parmesan garlic	1 oz	1.0	100	9%
spicy barbecue	1 oz	1.0	100	9%
very raspberry	1 oz	1.0	110	8%
Gourmet Lavosh Hawaii flatbread				
caraway & rye	1 oz	3.0	115	23%
classic island	1 oz	3.0	120	23%
peppercorn	1 oz	3.0	115	23%
rosemary-garlic	1 oz	3.0	125	22%
slightly onion	1 oz	3.0	120	23%
ten grain	1 oz	3.0	110	25%
■ **(AK-MAK)**				
cracker bread	5 pieces	2.3	116	18%
■ **(Andre Prost)**				
Olof crispbread/Sweden crisp				
four grain	2 pieces	2.0	90	29%

Food and Description	Amount	Fat Grams	Total Calories	% Fat Calories
whole-grain	2 pieces	1.5	60	23%

■ APPETEAZERS (*See* (Adrienne's) in this section)
■ **(Auburn Farms)**
spicy snack

pesto & dill	20 crackers	–	110	–
pizza	20 crackers	–	110	–

■ **(Austin)**
snack pack
cheese 'n peanut butter

50% more	6 crackers	14.0	260	49%
regular	4 crackers	8.0	140	51%
	6 crackers	11.0	200	50%
cheese 'n cheese filling	4 crackers	8.0	140	51%
	6 crackers	11.0	200	50%

Smackers crackers

cheese	25 crackers	7.0	150	42%
	33 crackers	9.0	200	9%
wheat	25 crackers	9.0	160	51%
	33 crackers	11.0	210	47%

toast crackers

w/cheese filling	6 crackers	11.0	200	50%
w/peanut butter	4 crackers	7.0	140	45%
	6 crackers	10.0	190	47%

wafers

w/cheddar cheese filling	6 crackers	11.0	200	50%
w/creme cheese filling	6 crackers	10.0	190	47%
w/honey roasted peanut butter filling	6 crackers	11.0	230	43%

wheat crackers

reduced fat/w/cheese	6 crackers	7.0	170	37%
regular/w/cheese filling	4 crackers	8.0	140	51%
	6 crackers	11.0	200	50%

■ **(Barbara's Bakery)**
Wheatines/all natural

cracked pepper	4 crackers	1.5	50	27%
lightly salted tops	4 cracers	1.5	50	27%
original	4 crackers	1.5	50	27%
sesame	4 crackers	1.5	50	27%
unsalted tops	4 crackers	1.5	50	27%

■ BITELIFE (*See* (McCormicks) in this section)
■ BRETON (*See* (Dare) in this section)
■ **(Burns & Ricker)**
Crispini

fat-free	½ cup	–	110	–
seeds & spice	5 pieces	3.0	110	25%
sesame	5 pieces	3.0	110	25%
sesame garlic	5 pieces	3.0	110	25%
S.F. stone-ground wheat	5 pieces	<0.5	110	4%

Food and Description	Amount	Fat Grams	Total Calories	% Fat Calories
Pita Crisps/~5 per oz				
pesto	1 oz	5.0	130	35%
tomato & onion	1 oz	6.0	130	42%
Tuscany toast				
pesto	10 pieces	5.0	120	38%
tomato & onion	10 pieces	6.0	130	42%
■ (Campbell's)				
soup & oyster	32 pieces	3.0	70	39%
■ (Carr's)				
cheddar cheese biscuits	4 pieces	5.0	90	50%
croissant crackers				
mini snacks				
plain	24 pieces	6.0	140	39%
w/sesame & onion	21 pieces	7.0	150	42%
original	3 pieces	3.0	70	39%
poppy & sesame seed	4 pieces	4.0	80	45%
table water				
bite-size	5 pieces	1.5	70	19%
king size	2 pieces	1.0	60	15%
w/cracked pepper	5 pieces	1.5	70	19%
w/sesame seeds	5 pieces	1.5	70	19%
wheatmeal/bite-size	2 pieces	3.5	80	39%
Wheatolo	1 piece	3.0	70	39%
whole wheat	2 pieces	3.5	80	39%
■ CHRISTIE BROWN (See (Nabisco) in this section)				
■ COMBOS (See (M&M★Mars) in this section)				
■ CRISPINI (See (Burns & Ricker) in this section)				
■ CRUNCH WELLS (See (Adrienne's) in this section)				
■ (Dare)				
Breton				
50% less salt	1 cracker	1.1	22	45%
	4 crackers	4.0	84	43%
light	1 cracker	0.6	20	27%
	4 crackers	2.4	80	27%
original	1 cracker	0.9	21	39%
	4 crackers	3.6	84	39%
sesame	1 cracker	1.1	22	45%
	4 crackers	4.4	88	45%
Cabaret	1 cracker	1.1	23	43%
	4 crackers	4.4	92	43%
	4 crackers	2.4	80	27%
Vivant	1 cracker	1.0	21	43%
	4 crackers	4.0	84	43%
■ (Delicious)				
cheddar cheese/low-fat	22 crackers	1.5	110	12%
cracked pepper/fat-free	17 crackers	–	110	–
crispy bacon	11 crackers	7.0	150	42%

Food and Description	Amount	Fat Grams	Total Calories	% Fat Calories
garden vegetable				
low-fat	14 crackers	1.5	120	11%
original	13 crackers	7.0	150	42%
real cheese	28 crackers	7.0	150	42%
sesame wheat	13 crackers	7.0	150	42%
smoked bacon/low-fat	14 crackers	2.0	120	15%
snack crackers	9 crackers	8.0	150	48%
▣ (Devonsheer)				
Melba Rounds				
garlic	5 pieces	1.5	60	23%
honey bran	5 pieces	–	50	–
onion	5 pieces	–	50	–
plain				
regular	5 pieces	–	50	–
unsalted	3 pieces	–	50	–
rye	3 pieces	–	50	–
savory herb	5 pieces	0.5	50	9%
sesame				
regular	5 pieces	2.5	60	38%
unsalted	3 pieces	1.5	50	27%
twelve grain	5 pieces	–	50	–
vegetable	5 pieces	–	50	–
wheat				
regular	3 pieces	–	50	–
unsalted	3 pieces	–	50	–
▣ (Eagle)				
cheese on cheese	6 crackers	11.0	210	47%
peanut butter & cheese	6 crackers	12.0	230	47%
peanut butter on toast	6 crackers	10.0	210	43%
wheat & cheddar cheese	6 crackers	10.0	200	45%
▣ (Estee) unsalted	1 cracker	2.0	70	26%
▣ (Featherweight)				
cheddar cheese snack	24 crackers	2.0	120	15%
onion poppy snack	15 crackers	2.0	120	15%
sesame wheat snack	18 crackers	2.0	120	15%
unsalted	1 serving	2.0	70	26%
▣ (Finn)				
crispbread/dark				
plain	2 pieces	–	40	–
w/caraway seeds	2 pieces	–	40	–
▣ (Frito Lay)				
bacon cheddar	1 pkg	10.0	200	45%
cheese peanut butter	1 pkg	10.0	200	45%
golden toast & cheddar	1 pkg	13.0	230	51%
jalapeño & cheddar	1 pkg	10.0	200	45%
original cracker snacks	1 pkg	12.0	220	49%
toast peanut butter	1 pkg	9.0	190	43%
wheat cheese	1 pkg	9.0	200	41%

Food and Description	Amount	Fat Grams	Total Calories	% Fat Calories
■ (Frookie)				
Frisps				
apple cinnamon	½ oz	–	60	–
honey crunch	½ oz	–	60	–
Frookitas				
chili	10 crackers	3.0	110	25%
salsa	10 crackers	3.0	110	25%
Frookwheats				
onion-poppy	10 crackers	–	60	–
original	10 crackers	–	60	–
Frookwich crackers				
cracked pepper	4 crackers	–	35	–
garlic & herb	4 crackers	–	35	–
water	4 crackers	–	35	–
whole wheat	4 crackers	–	35	–
Froysters				
vegetable & herb	60 crackers	–	110	–
■ GENERIC				
cracker				
cheese				
plain	1 cracker	<1.0	5	51%
	14 crackers	4.0	70	51%
w/peanut butter	1 cracker	2.0	35	51%
oyster	10 crackers	1.0	44	21%
peanut butter sandwich	1 cracker	2.0	35	51%
rye				
wafers				
plain	8 crackers	2.0	90	20%
seasoned	8 crackers	2.0	90	20%
w/cheese	1 cracker	2.0	35	51%
saltine square	1 square	<1.0	13	18%
	4 squares	1.0	50	18%
soup	1 cracker	–	4	–
wafer/plain	13 crackers	3.0	130	21%
water biscuit	3 pieces	3.0	90	30%
wheat				
thin	2 crackers	<1.0	10	39%
	7 crackers	3.0	70	39%
w/cheese filling	1 cracker	2.0	35	51%
w/peanut butter filling	1 cracker	2.0	35	51%
whole wheat	1 cracker	1.0	20	45%
crispbread				
plain	3 pieces	2.0	60	30%
rusk/½" thick/3⅜" dia	1 piece	0.8	38	19
rye	3 pieces	1.0	75	12%
■ (Hain)				
cheese bites				
golden cheddar	22 crackers	1.5	120	11%

Food and Description	Amount	Fat Grams	Total Calories	% Fat Calories
white cheddar	22 crackers	1.5	120	11%
oyster/fat-free	35 crackers	–	80	–
saltine/fat-free	5 crackers	–	60	–
■ (Health Valley)				
cheese wheels	1 oz	9.0	140	48%
fire crackers/fat-free				
hot 3 chilis & cheese	6 crackers	–	50	–
medium jalapeño & cheese	6 crackers	–	50	–
mild chili & cheese	6 crackers	–	50	–
garden vegetable	1 oz	5.0	120	38%
healthy pizza crackers/fat-free				
garlic & herb	6 crackers	–	50	–
pizza Italiano	6 crackers	–	50	–
zesty cheese	6 crackers	–	50	–
herb	1 oz	6.0	120	45%
rice bran	1 oz	3.0	100	27%
sesame	1 oz	6.0	130	42%
7 grain & vegetable	1 oz	5.0	130	35%
stoned wheat				
herb/no salt	½ oz	2.0	55	33%
original	½ oz	2.0	55	33%
sesame/no salt	½ oz	2.0	55	33%
7 grain & vegetable/no salt	½ oz	2.0	55	33%
whole wheat/fat-free				
cheese	5 crackers	–	50	–
herb	5 crackers	–	50	–
onion	5 crackers	–	50	–
original	5 crackers	–	50	–
vegetable				
no salt	5 crackers	–	50	–
regular	5 crackers	–	50	–
■ (Hopi)				
seaweed wrap	18 pieces	–	110	–
sesame bits	½ cup	–	120	–
■ (Ideal)				
crispbread				
extra thins	3 slices	–	48	–
fiber thins	2 slices	–	40	–
oat bran thins	2 slices	–	50	–
flatbread				
fiber w/sesame seeds	2 slices	–	40	–
whole grain/no salt	2 slices	–	43	–
■ (J.J. Flats)				
flatbread				
flavorall	1 piece	1.0	50	18%
garlic	1 piece	1.0	50	18%
italian herb	1 piece	1.5	50	27%

Food and Description	Amount	Fat Grams	Total Calories	% Fat Calories
multigrain	1 piece	1.5	50	27%
oat bran	1 piece	0.5	50	9%
onion	1 piece	1.0	50	18%
poppy	1 piece	1.0	50	18%
sesame	1 piece	1.0	50	18%
■ (Kavli)				
Norwegian crispbread				
crispy thin	2 slices	<1.0	15	10%
hearty thick	1 slice	<1.0	35	10%
rye-bran	2 slices	–	30	–
■ (Keebler)				
cracker sandwiches				
cheese & peanut butter	1 pkg	9.0	190	43%
Club & cheddar	1 pkg	11.0	190	52%
toast & peanut butter	1 pkg	9.0	190	43%
Town House & cheddar	1 pkg	13.0	200	59%
Munch 'Ems				
cheddar	30 crackers	4.0	130	28%
chili cheese	23 crackers	4.0	130	28%
original/savory	30 crackers	5.0	130	35%
ranch	33 crackers	4.0	130	28%
salsa	8 crackers	4.0	130	28%
sour cream & onion	28 crackers	6.0	140	39%
Southwestern style	23 crackers	4.0	130	28%
regular crackers				
Club partners				
50% reduced sodium	4 crackers	3.0	70	39%
garlic bread flavored	4 crackers	3.0	70	39%
original	4 crackers	3.0	70	39%
onion toast	9 crackers	6.0	140	39%
toasted sesame	9 crackers	6.0	140	39%
toasted wheat	9 crackers	6.0	140	39%
touch of cheddar	4 crackers	2.5	70	32%
Town House				
original	5 crackers	4.5	80	51%
reduced sodium	5 crackers	4.5	80	51%
wheat	5 crackers	4.0	80	45%
Wheatables				
French onion				
reduced fat	27 crackers	4.0	130	28%
regular	25 crackers	7.0	150	42%
original/savory				
reduced fat	29 crackers	3.5	130	24%
reduced sodium	25 crackers	7.0	150	42%
regular	26 crackers	7.0	150	42%
ranch				
reduced fat	29 crackers	3.5	130	24%

```
ATLANTIC BOOKS          #607
01/21/01    15:51    J    19      11500
    1@   1.98  A089529738      $      1.98
              COMP UP-TO-DATE
    1@   5.98  A006018281      $      5.98
              UNIDENTIFIED    T
    1@   3.98  A031217102      $      3.98
              FAT BLOCKER DIET
    1@   3.98  A039572860      $      3.98
              ULTIMATE CONSUME
    1@   6.98  A087596480      $      6.98
              FIGHT FAT
    1@   4.98  A087596412      $      4.98
              FAT TO FIRM AT A
SUBTOTAL                       $     27.88
SALES TAX @ 6.000%             $      1.67
TOTAL                          $     29.55
TENDER CASH                    $     30.00
CHANGE                         $      0.45

10 DAYS FOR REFUND - 1 MONTH TO EXCHANGE
NJ SALES TX 3% ELIZABETH FRANCHISE TX 3%
```

```
ATLANTIC BOOKS #607
01/21/01    15:51    1  19   11500
     10   1.98 A0895297389    $    1.98
            COMP UP-TO-DATE
     10   5.98 A0060188281    $    5.98
            UNIDENTIFIED     ?
     10   3.98 A0121271105    $    3.98
            FAT BLOCKER DIET
     10   3.98 A0895972860    $    3.98
            ULTIMATE CONSUME
     10   6.98 A0875966480    $    6.98
            FIGHT FAT
     10   4.98 A0875966416    $    4.98
            FAT TO FIRM AT A

SUBTOTAL                      $   27.88
SALES TAX @ 6.000X            $    1.67
TOTAL                         $   29.55
TENDER CASH                   $   30.00
CHANGE                        $    0.45

10 DAYS FOR REFUND - 1 MONTH TO EXCHANGE
NJ SALES TX 3X ELIZABETH FRANCHISE TX 2X
```

Food and Description	Amount	Fat Grams	Total Calories	% Fat Calories
regular	25 crackers	7.0	150	42%
white cheddar				
reduced fat	27 crackers	4.0	130	28%
regular	25 crackers	7.0	150	42%
Zesta saltines				
fat-free	5 crackers	–	50	–
original	5 crackers	2.0	60	30%
reduced sodium	5 crackers	2.0	60	30%
soup	42 crackers	2.5	70	32%
unsalted tops	5 crackers	2.0	70	26%
▧ (Lance)				
Melba Toast				
plain				
oblong	4 slices	0.5	70	6%
round	6 pieces	0.5	60	8%
garlic/round	6 pieces	1.0	60	15%
onion/round	6 pieces	0.5	60	6%
sesame/oblong	6 slices	1.5	60	23%
regular crackers				
captain's wafer	6 crackers	9.0	190	43%
cheese-on-wheat	6 crackers	10.0	190	47%
Lanchee	6 crackers	11.0	190	52%
Nip-Chee	6 crackers	10.0	190	47%
oyster	1 pkg	2.0	60	30%
peanut butter wheat	6 crackers	11.0	190	52%
Rye-Chee	6 crackers	11.0	210	47%
sourdough w/cheddar & sour cream	6 crackers	15.0	240	56%
Toastchee	6 crackers	12.0	200	54%
snack crackers				
Gold-N-Chees	½ cup	5.0	130	35%
	¾ cup	7.0	180	35%
Italian herb wheat snack cracker	¾ cup	11.0	200	50%
multigrain snack cracker	4 crackers	2.5	70	32%
pizza flavored wheat snack cracker	¾ cup	10.0	200	45%
saltines	4 crackers	1.5	50	27%
sour dough wafer	4 crackers	3.0	70	39%
wheatswafer	4 crackers	2.5	60	38%
▧ (Little Debbie)				
toasty crackers w/peanut butter				
boxed	1 pkg	7.0	140	45%
individual pkg	1 pkg	10.0	210	43%
wheat crackers w/cheddar cheese	1 pkg	7.0	140	45%
▧ (Log House Foods)				
Snack Toast				
blueberry swirl	1 slice	–	45	–
cinnamon	1 slice	–	40	–
cinnamon raisin	1 slice	–	45	–

Food and Description	Amount	Fat Grams	Total Calories	% Fat Calories
original	1 slice	–	35	–
raspberry swirl	1 slice	–	45	–
■ (LU)				
Crokine crispbread	2 slices	–	37	–
■ (M&M ★ Mars)				
Combos snack crackers				
cheddar cheese				
family	1 oz	8.0	140	51%
singles	1.7 oz	13.0	250	47%
peanut butter/family	1 oz	8.0	140	51%
■ (Manischewitz)				
Tam Tams				
garlic	10 pieces	8.0	153	47%
no salt	10 pieces	7.0	138	46%
onion	10 pieces	8.0	150	48%
regular	10 pieces	8.0	147	49%
wheat	10 pieces	8.0	150	48%
■ (McCormicks)				
Bitelife				
potato crisps				
BBQ	23 pieces	4.0	130	28%
regular	23 pieces	5.0	130	35%
triangles/5 vegetables	37 pieces	4.0	130	28%
wheat bubbles	24 pieces	4.0	130	28%
■ MUNCH 'EMS (See (Keebler) in this section)				
■ (Nabisco)				
Christie Brown & Co.				
Today's Choice/reduced fat				
classic wheat	4 crackers	1.5	70	19%
cracked pepper	4 crackers	1.5	70	19%
garden vegetable	4 crackers	1.5	70	19%
Red Oval Farms				
Club	3½ crackers	4.6	117	35%
Entertainers				
golden crisp	6 crackers	5.7	124	41%
poppy	6 crackers	3.2	112	26%
sesame	6 crackers	3.9	103	34%
sesame & onion	3½ crackers	4.0	114	32%
stoned rye	3½ crackers	2.5	105	21%
stoned wheat thins				
low-salt	3½ crackers	2.6	108	22%
mini	16 crackers	2.5	105	21%
original	3½ crackers	2.6	107	22%
Nabisco				
cracker sandwich				
NABS				
cheese peanut butter	6 pieces	10.0	190	47%
cheese peanut butter toast	6 pieces	10.0	190	47%

Food and Description	Amount	Fat Grams	Total Calories	% Fat Calories
Ritz Bits				
peanut butter	13 pieces	8.0	150	48%
w/real cheese	14 pieces	10.0	160	56%
crackers				
bacon-flavored thins	15 crackers	8.0	160	45%
Better Cheddars				
low-sodium	22 crackers	7.0	150	42%
reduced fat	24 crackers	6.0	140	39%
regular	22 crackers	8.0	150	48%
Cheese Nips				
air crisps	32 crackers	4.0	130	28%
regular	29 crackers	6.0	150	36%
Cheese Tid-Bits	32 crackers	8.0	150	48%
Chicken In a Biskit	14 crackers	9.0	160	51%
Crown Pilot	1 cracker	1.5	70	19%
Garden Crisps	15 pieces	3.5	130	24%
Harvest Crisps				
5-grain	13 crackers	3.5	130	24%
oat	13 crackers	4.5	140	29%
oat thins	18 crackers	6.0	140	39%
Oysterettes soup & oyster	19 crackers	2.5	60	38%
Premium saltine				
bits	34 crackers	7.0	150	42%
fat-free	5 crackers	–	50	–
low-sodium	5 crackers	1.0	60	15%
original	5 crackers	1.5	60	23%
soup & oyster	23 crackers	1.5	60	23%
unsalted tops	5 crackers	1.5	60	23%
Ritz				
air crisps	24 crackers	5.0	140	32%
bits	48 crackers	9.0	160	51%
chocolate-covered	3 crackers	9.0	150	54%
low-sodium	54 crackers	4.0	80	45%
regular	54 crackers	4.0	80	45%
w/real cheese	1 pkg	12.0	210	51%
Royal Lunch	1 cracker	2.0	50	36%
Snorkels	56 crackers	5.0	140	32%
Sociable	7 crackers	4.0	80	45%
Swiss cheese snack	15 crackers	7.0	140	45%
Triscuit				
deli-style rye	7 crackers	5.0	140	32%
garden herb	6 crackers	7.0	130	48%
low-sodium	7 crackers	6.0	150	36%
original	7 crackers	5.0	140	32%
reduced fat	8 crackers	3.0	130	21%
wheat 'n bran	7 crackers	5.0	140	32%
Twigs/sesame & cheese	15 pieces	7.0	150	42%
Uneeda biscuit/unsalted tops	2 crackers	1.5	60	23%

Food and Description	Amount	Fat Grams	Total Calories	% Fat Calories
vegetable thin	14 crackers	9.0	160	51%
Waverly	5 crackers	3.5	70	45%
wheat thin				
low-salt	16 crackers	6.0	140	39%
multigrain	17 crackers	4.0	130	28%
original	16 crackers	6.0	140	39%
reduced fat	18 crackers	4.0	120	30%
Wheatsworth	5 crackers	3.5	80	39%
SnackWell's				
fat-free				
cracked pepper	7 crackers	–	60	–
wheat	5 crackers	–	60	–
reduced fat				
classic golden	6 crackers	1.0	60	15%
French onion snack	32 crackers	2.0	120	15%
Italian ranch	32 crackers	2.0	120	15%
salsa cheese	32 crackers	2.0	120	15%
zesty cheese snack	32 crackers	2.0	120	15%
■ (North Castle) Jarlsberg Cheese Crisps				
cheese pizza	11 pieces	6.0	140	39%
cheese & garlic	11 pieces	7.0	150	42%
■ (Old London)				
melba snacks				
bacon flavor	5 pieces	1.5	60	23%
cheese	5 pieces	1.0	60	15%
garlic	5 pieces	1.5	60	23%
Mexicali corn	5 pieces	1.5	60	23%
onion	5 pieces	1.5	60	23%
rye	5 pieces	1.5	60	23%
sesame	5 pieces	3.0	60	45%
white	5 pieces	1.5	60	23%
whole-grain	5 pieces	1.5	60	23%
melba toast				
onion	3 pieces	0.5	50	18%
rye	3 pieces	0.5	50	18%
sesame				
regular	3 pieces	1.5	50	27%
unsalted	3 pieces	1.5	50	27%
wheat	3 pieces	0.5	50	9%
whole wheat/unsalted	3 pieces	0.5	50	9%
■ (O.T.C.)				
chowder & oyster	3 pieces	2.0	70	26%
wine	11 pieces	3.0	130	21%
■ (Pacific Grain)				
No Fries/fat-free				
potato crackers				
BBQ	30 pieces	–	110	–
augratin	30 pieces	–	110	–

Food and Description	Amount	Fat Grams	Total Calories	% Fat Calories
tortilla crackers				
cheddar	30 pieces	–	110	–
ranch	30 pieces	–	110	–
salsa	30 pieces	–	110	–
sour cream	30 pieces	–	110	–
■ (Pepperidge Farm)				
International Collection				
cracked pepper water biscuit	5 crackers	1.0	60	15%
original water biscuit	5 crackers	1.0	60	15%
Distinctive crackers				
butter thins	4 crackers	3.0	70	39%
cracked wheat	4 crackers	2.5	70	32%
English water biscuits	4 crackers	1.5	70	19%
hearty wheat	3 crackers	3.5	80	39%
quartet assortment	3 crackers	2.5	60	38%
sesame	3 crackers	2.5	70	32%
three-cracker assortment	3 crackers	2.5	60	38%
Goldfish/tiny				
cheddar cheese				
low-salt	55 pieces	6.0	140	39%
reduced sodium	60 pieces	6.0	150	36%
regular				
on-the-go or variety pack	1 pouch	5.0	130	35%
regular pkg	55 pieces	6.0	140	39%
Halloween pack	1 pouch	2.5	70	32%
original				
on-the-go or variety pack	1 pouch	6.0	130	42%
regular or warehouse club pkg	55 pieces	6.0	140	39%
Parmesan cheese	60 pieces	5.0	140	32%
pizza-flavored	55 pieces	6.0	140	39%
pretzel				
on-the-go or variety pack	1 pouch	2.5	110	20%
regular or warehouse club pkg	45 pieces	2.5	120	19%
■ (Planters)				
cracker sandwich				
cheese peanut butter	1 pkg	10.0	190	47%
toast peanut butter	1 pkg	10.0	190	47%
■ RED OVAL FARMS (See (Nabisco) in this section)				
■ RITZ (See (Nabisco) in this section)				
■ (Ry-Krisp)				
fat-free	2 crackers	–	60	–
fiber plus	1 slice	1.0	35	–
golden rye	1 slice	–	30	–
hearty rye	1 slice	–	50	–
lite rye	2 slices	–	50	–
natural	2 crackers	–	40	–
seasoned	2 crackers	1.0	45	20%
sesame	2 crackers	2.0	50	36%

Food and Description	Amount	Fat Grams	Total Calories	% Fat Calories
■ **(Ryvita)**				
crispbread				
dark	2 pieces	–	38	–
dark rye				
plain	2 pieces	1.0	50	18%
w/caraway seeds	2 pieces	1.0	50	18%
high-fiber	2 pieces	1.0	45	20%
light rye/high-fiber	2 pieces	1.0	50	18%
original wheat	2 pieces	1.0	45	20%
toasted sesame rye	2 pieces	1.0	60	15%
■ **(Savoir Faire)**				
cracker bread	1 oz	1.0	110	8%
■ **(Sesmark)**				
cheese thins	15 crackers	3.0	130	21%
rice thins				
original	15 crackers	3.0	130	21%
teriyaki	13 crackers	3.0	130	21%
sesame thins				
garlic	9 crackers	8.0	150	48%
original	9 crackers	8.0	150	48%
unsalted	9 crackers	8.0	150	48%
■ **SNACKWELL'S** (*See* (Nabisco) in this section)				
■ **(Sunshine)**				
American Heritage				
cheddar	5 crackers	4.0	80	45%
Parmesan	4 crackers	4.0	70	51%
sesame	4 crackers	4.0	70	51%
wheat	4 crackers	3.0	60	45%
Cheez-It				
hot & spicy	26 crackers	8.0	160	39%
low-sodium	27 crackers	8.0	160	39%
original				
reduced fat	30 crackers	4.5	130	31%
white cheddar	26 crackers	9.0	160	51%
Hi-Ho				
butter-flavored	9 crackers	9.0	160	51%
cracked pepper	9 crackers	9.0	160	51%
multgrain	9 crackers	9.0	160	51%
original	9 crackers	9.0	160	51%
reduced fat	10 crackers	5.0	140	32%
whole wheat	9 crackers	8.0	150	48%
Krispy saltine				
cracked pepper	5 crackers	1.5	60	23%
fat-free	5 crackers	–	60	–
mild cheddar	5 crackers	2.0	60	30%
original	5 crackers	1.5	60	23%
soup & oyster	17 crackers	1.5	60	23%
whole wheat	5 crackers	1.5	60	23%

Food and Description	Amount	Fat Grams	Total Calories	% Fat Calories
wheat snack	8 crackers	4.0	70	51%
wheat wafers	8 crackers	4.0	80	45%
■ TODAY'S CHOICE (*See* (Nabisco) in this section)				
■ TRISCUIT (*See* (Nabisco) in this section)				
■ TUSCANY TOAST (*See* (Burns & Ricker) in this section)				
■ UNEEDA (*See* (Nabisco) in this section)				
■ (Valley Lahvosh)				
cracker bread				
hearts	9 crackers	1.0	110	8%
rounds				
15" dia	1.8 oz	2.0	190	9%
5" dia	1 cracker	0.5	70	6%
3" dia	4 crackers	1.0	110	8%
2" dia	7 crackers	1.0	110	8%
wheat rounds				
15" dia	1.8 oz	2.0	190	9%
5" dia	1 cracker	0.5	60	8%
3" dia	4 crackers	1.0	110	8%
sweetheart crispies	7 crackers	2.0	120	15%
■ (Venus)				
bran wafers	5 crackers	1.0	60	15%
cracked wheat wafers	5 crackers	1.0	60	15%
cracker bread				
Armenian thin	2 pieces	1.0	100	9%
original	5 pieces	1.0	60	15%
lavosh wafer bread				
crisp original	2 pieces	1.0	60	15%
crisp sesame	2 pieces	1.0	60	15%
oat bran wafers				
regular	5 crackers	1.0	60	15%
salt free	5 crackers	1.0	60	15%
Old Brussells Waferettes				
cheddar	5 pieces	5.0	80	56%
jalapeño	5 pieces	5.0	80	56%
stoned wheat wafers/bite-size	7 crackers	1.0	60	15%
water crackers/fat-free	5 crackers	–	55	
wheat wafers	8 crackers	2.0	100	18%
■ (Wasa)				
cracker bread/extra crisp	1 piece	1.0	25	33%
crispbread				
breakfast	1 slice	1.0	50	18%
dark	2 slices	<1.0	38	12%
extra crisp	1 slice	–	25	–
falu rye	1 slice	–	30	–
royal	½ slice	–	25	–
savory sesame	1 slice	1.0	30	30%
sesame rye	1 slice	1.0	30	30%

Food and Description	Amount	Fat Grams	Total Calories	% Fat Calories
sesame wheat	1 slice	–	60	–
toasted wheat	1 slice	1.0	50	18%
flatbread/extra thin	3 slices	–	48	–
◼ (Westbrae)				
wafers				
5-piece	4½ crackers	–	40	–
no salt	4½ crackers	–	40	–
onion garlic	4½ crackers	–	40	–
sesame	4½ crackers	–	40	–
◼ (Wheat-Krisp)				
crispbread/whole wheat	2 pieces	1.0	50	18%
CRACKER CRUMBS/MEAL (*See also* MATZO MEAL & MIX)				
(Golden Dipt) cracker meal	¼ cup	0.5	140	3%
(Keebler)	1 cup	3.0	100	27%
(Nabisco) crumbs				
Honey Maid graham	1 serving	1.5	70	19%
Premium/fat-free	¼ cup	–	100	–
Ritz	⅓ cup	7.0	140	45%
(Sunshine)	3 Tbs	2.0	80	23%
CRANBERRY				
canned				
(Ocean Spray)	2 oz	–	25	–
dried				
(Ocean Spray) Craisins	⅓ cup	–	130	–
(Traverse Bay)	⅓ cup	0.5	140	3%
fresh				
chopped	½ cup	–	27	–
	1 cup	–	54	–
whole/w/o stems	½ cup	–	23	–
	1 cup	–	46	–
CRANBERRY BEAN				
canned/generic				
w/liquid	½ cup	<1.0	110	4%
dried				
(Bean Cuisine)	½ cup	1.0	115	8%
fresh				
boiled	½ cup	<1.0	120	4%
raw	½ cup	1.0	330	3%
CRANBERRY DRINK (*See also* LEMONADE/LEMONADE-FLAVORED DRINK; FRUIT PUNCH; SOFT DRINK MIX)				
(Ocean Spray)				
cran-apple				
low-calorie	6 fl oz	–	35	–
regular	6 fl oz	–	120	–
cran-blueberry	6 fl oz	–	120	–
cran-grape	6 fl oz	–	120	–
cran-raspberry				
low-calorie	6 fl oz	–	40	–

Food and Description	Amount	Fat Grams	Total Calories	% Fat Calories
regular	6 fl oz	–	110	–
cran-strawberry	6 fl oz	–	110	–
CRANBERRY JUICE/JUICE BLEND/JUICE BLEND DRINK				
bottled, boxed, or canned				
(Chiquita) cranberry seabreeze	8 fl oz	–	120	–
(Hain) concentrate	1 oz	–	40	–
(Knudsen) Thirst Quencher				
Cape Cod cranberry	8 fl oz	–	100	–
cranberry nectar	8 fl oz	–	150	–
Just Cranberry	8 fl oz	–	60	–
(Ocean Spray)				
cranberry juice cocktail				
low calorie	6 fl oz	–	40	–
regular	6 fl oz	–	100	–
Cranicot	6 fl oz	–	120	–
Crantastic	6 fl oz	–	100	–
(Season's Best) cranberry medley	8 fl oz	–	120	–
(Smucker's)	8 fl oz	–	130	–
(Snapple) cranberry royal	10 fl oz	–	150	–
(Tropicana) Twister/cranberry, raspberry, strawberry				
light	8 fl oz	–	45	–
	10 fl oz	–	60	–
regular	8 fl oz	–	120	–
	10 fl oz	–	160	–
(Welch's) cocktail	10 fl oz	–	180	–
frozen/prepared				
(Seneca) juice cocktail				
cranberry	8 fl oz	–	140	–
cranberry-apple	8 fl oz	–	130	–
	10 fl oz	–	140	–
(Welch's) juice cocktail				
cranberry				
light	8 fl oz	–	50	–
regular	8 fl oz	–	140	–
cranberry-apple	8 fl oz	–	160	–
cranberry-cherry	8 fl oz	–	150	–
cranberry-orange	8 fl oz	–	140	–
cranberry-raspberry				
light	8 fl oz	–	50	–
regular	8 fl oz	–	150	–
CRANBERRY SAUCE/canned				
generic/sweetened	½ cup	–	210	–
(Ocean Spray)				
Cran-Fruit cranberry crushed fruit				
orange	2 oz	–	90	–
raspberry	2 oz	–	90	–
strawberry	2 oz	–	90	–

Food and Description	Amount	Fat Grams	Total Calories	% Fat Calories
jellied	2 oz	–	80	–
whole berry	2 oz	–	80	–
(S&W)				
jellied	¼ cup	–	100	–
whole berry	¼ cup	–	100	–
CRANBERRY-ORANGE RELISH				
canned	½ cup	–	246	–
uncooked	½ cup	–	245	–
CRAYFISH/mixed species				
cooked-moist heat	3 oz	1.0	97	9%
raw	3 medium	<1.0	24	19%
	3 oz	0.9	76	11%
CREAM (See also CREAMER, NONDAIRY; SOUR CREAM; SOUR CREAM SUBSTITUTE; WHIPPED TOPPING)				
(Farmland)				
half & half	2 Tbs	3.0	40	68%
light cream	2 Tbs	3.0	30	90%
generic				
coffee/table cream				
light	1 Tbs	3.0	30	90%
	1 cup	46.0	470	88%
medium/25% fat	1 Tbs	4.0	40	90%
	1 cup	60.0	585	92%
half & half	1 Tbs	2.0	20	90%
	1 cup	28.0	315	80%
whipping cream				
heavy				
unwhipped	1 cup	88.0	820	96%
whipped	2 cups	88.0	820	97%
light				
unwhipped	1 cup	74.0	700	95%
whipped	2 cups	74.0	700	95%
(Land O' Lakes)				
half & half	1 Tbs	2.0	20	90%
whipping cream				
heavy/gourmet				
unwhipped	1 Tbs	6.0	60	90%
whipped	1 cup	73.9	704	94%
regular				
unwhipped	1 Tbs	5.0	45	90%
whipped	2 cups	73.9	704	94%
CREAM CHEESE (See also CHEESE ALTERNATIVE/IMITATION; CHEESE SPREAD)				
(Breakstone) Temp-Tee/whipped	3 Tbs	10.0	110	82%
(Darigold)	2 Tbs	10.0	100	90%
(Dorman's)				
70% fat	2 Tbs	10.0	100	90%
65% fat	2 Tbs	8.0	90	80%

Food and Description	Amount	Fat Grams	Total Calories	% Fat Calories
(Formagg)				
fat-free	2 Tbs	–	25	–
original	2 Tbs	7.0	80	79%
(Friendship)				
New York style/reduced fat	2 Tbs	3.0	50	54%
soft	2 Tbs	10.0	100	90%
(Healthy Choice) fat-free				
herbs & garlic	2 Tbs	–	25	–
plain	2 Tbs	–	25	–
strawberry	2 Tbs	–	35	–
(Heluva Good Cheese)	2 Tbs	10.0	100	90%
(Fleur de Lait) light				
blueberries & cream	2 Tbs	4.0	70	51%
chive & onion	2 Tbs	4.0	60	60%
fresh garden delight	2 Tbs	6.0	60	90%
garden vegetable	2 Tbs	4.0	50	72%
garlic	2 Tbs	4.0	60	60%
nacho	2 Tbs	4.0	60	60%
salsa	2 Tbs	4.0	60	60%
strawberry	2 Tbs	4.0	60	60%
(Kraft) Philadelphia brand				
plain				
fat-free				
brick	2 Tbs	–	25	–
soft	2 Tbs	–	30	–
light/soft	2 Tbs	5.0	70	64%
original				
brick	2 Tbs	10.0	100	90%
soft	2 Tbs	10.0	100	90%
whipped	3 Tbs	11.0	110	90%
Philly for toast	3 Tbs	12.0	120	90%
w/chives/brick	2 Tbs	9.0	90	90%
w/chives & onion/soft	2 Tbs	10.0	110	82%
w/herb & garlic/soft	2 Tbs	10.0	110	82%
w/olive & pimento/soft	2 Tbs	9.0	100	81%
w/pimientos/brick	1 oz	9.0	90	90%
w/pineapple/soft	2 Tbs	9.0	100	81%
w/smoked salmon				
soft	2 Tbs	9.0	100	81%
whipped	3 Tbs	9.0	100	81%
w/strawberries/soft	2 Tbs	9.0	100	81%
(Weight Watchers) light	2 Tbs	2.5	45	50%
CREAM OF TARTAR	1 tsp	–	7	–
	1 Tbs	–	23	–
CREAMER, NONDAIRY (See also CREAM)				
liquid				
(Carnation) Coffee Mate				
amaretto	1 Tbs	2.0	40	45%

Food and Description	Amount	Fat Grams	Total Calories	% Fat Calories
butter rum	1 Tbs	2.0	40	45%
cinnamon	1 Tbs	2.0	40	45%
French vanilla	1 Tbs	2.0	40	45%
hazelnut	1 Tbs	2.0	40	45%
Irish creme	1 Tbs	2.0	40	45%
original				
fat-free	1 Tbs	–	10	–
light	1 Tbs	0.5	10	45%
regular	1 Tbs	1.0	20	45%
(Coffee Delight)	1 Tbs	2.0	20	90%
(International Delight)				
amaretto				
fat-free	1 Tbs	–	30	–
original	1 Tbs	1.5	45	34%
cappuccino fat-free	1 Tbs	–	25	–
French vanilla				
fat-free	1 Tbs	–	30	–
original	1 Tbs	1.5	45	34%
Hawaiian macadamia/fat-free	1 Tbs	–	25	–
hazelnut	1 Tbs	1.5	45	34%
Irish creme				
fat-free	1 Tbs	–	30	–
original	1 Tbs	1.5	45	34%
raspberry/fat-free	1 Tbs	–	25	–
Suisse chocolate mocha	1 Tbs	1.5	45	34%
(Kemp's) frozen	1 Tbs	2.0	20	90%
(Mocha Mix)				
amaretto	1 Tbs	1.0	35	20%
Irish creme	1 Tbs	1.0	35	20%
Kahlua/fat-free	1 Tbs	–	35	–
original				
lite/fat-free	1 Tbs	–	10	–
regular	1 Tbs	2.0	20	90%
(Real) half & half				
almond roca	2 Tbs	1.0	80	11%
French vanilla	2 Tbs	2.0	80	23%
Irish cream	2 Tbs	3.5	80	39%
(Rich's) frozen				
Coffee Rich				
light	1 Tbs	1.0	10	90%
original	1 Tbs	1.5	25	54%
Farm Rich				
fat-free	1 Tbs	–	10	–
light	1 Tbs	1.0	10	90%
original	1 Tbs	1.5	20	68%
Poly Rich	1 Tbs	1.0	20	68%
(Westbrae)	1 Tbs	<1.0	10	45%

Food and Description	Amount	Fat Grams	Total Calories	% Fat Calories
powdered				
(Borden) Cremora				
fat-free	1 tsp	–	10	–
lite	1 tsp	–	10	–
original	1 tsp	1.0	10	90%
(Carnation) Coffee Mate				
amaretto	1⅓ Tbs	2.5	60	38%
cinnamon	1⅓ Tbs	3.0	60	45%
French vanilla	1⅓ Tbs	3.0	60	45%
hazelnut	1⅓ Tbs	3.0	60	45%
Irish creme	1⅓ Tbs	3.0	60	45%
mocha almond	1⅓ Tbs	3.0	60	45%
original				
fat-free	1 tsp	–	10	–
lite	1 tsp	–	10	–
regular	1 tsp	0.5	10	45%
(Hershey) Great American Cafe				
chocolate amaretto	1⅓ Tbs	2.5	60	38%
French vanilla	1⅓ Tbs	2.5	60	38%
(N-Rich)	1 tsp	–	10	–
CREPE				
frozen				
(Chef Francois)	1 crepe	3.0	80	34%
mix				
(Krusteaz)				
mix only	2 Tbs	1.0	80	11%
prepared	2 crepes	3.0	100	27%
ready to serve				
(Table de France) 9" dia	1 crepe	1.0	45	20%
CRISPBREAD (See CRACKER)				
CROAKER				
breaded & fried	3 oz	10.0	188	48%
raw	3 oz	2.7	89	27%
CROISSANT				
frozen				
(Chef Pierre) prebaked/all-butter				
1-oz croissant	1 croissant	5.0	110	41%
2-oz croissant	1 croissant	9.0	210	39%
3-oz croissant	1 croissant	22.0	360	55%
(Sara Lee) all-butter/petite	2 croissants	11.0	230	43%
homemade/USDA Standard Home Recipe				
~2-oz croissant	1 croissant	12.0	235	46%
ready to serve				
(Awrey's)				
butter	2 oz	11.0	200	50%
	3 oz	17.0	300	51%
margarine	1.25 oz	7.0	120	53%
	2.5 oz	14.0	250	50%

Food and Description	Amount	Fat Grams	Total Calories	% Fat Calories
wheat	2.5 oz	14.0	240	53%
(Dunkin' Donuts)				
almond	1 croissant	21.0	360	53%
cheese	1 croissant	15.0	240	56%
chocolate	1 croissant	23.0	370	56%
plain	1 croissant	17.0	270	57%
(Pepperidge Farm) all-butter				
petite	1 croissant	8.0	130	55%
regular	1 croissant	14.0	240	53%
(Rainbo) wheat	1 croissant	19.0	300	57%
(Sara Lee) food service				
1⅛-oz croissant	1 croissant	6.0	130	42%
1½-oz croissant	1 croissant	8.0	170	43%
2-oz croissant	1 croissant	10.0	220	41%
3-oz sandwich croissant	1 croissant	15.0	320	42%
sandwich croissant/sliced	1 croissant	11.0	220	45%
CROUTONS				
(Arnold) crispy				
cheese garlic	2 Tbs	1.0	30	30%
fine herb	2 Tbs	1.0	30	30%
Italian	2 Tbs	1.0	30	30%
onion & garlic	2 Tbs	1.0	30	30%
ranch	2 Tbs	1.0	30	30%
seasoned	2 Tbs	1.0	30	30%
(Brownberry)				
Caesar salad	2 Tbs	1.5	30	39%
cheddar cheese	2 Tbs	1.5	30	39%
cheese & garlic	2 Tbs	1.0	30	30%
onion & garlic	2 Tbs	1.0	30	30%
ranch	2 Tbs	2.0	30	30%
seasoned	2 Tbs	1.0	30	30%
toasted	2 Tbs	1.0	30	30%
(Mrs. Cubberson's) restaurant style				
Caesar salad	5 croutons	1.0	30	30%
cheese & garlic	5 croutons	1.0	30	30%
onion & garlic	5 croutons	1.0	30	30%
ranch	5 croutons	1.0	30	30%
seasoned	5 croutons	1.0	30	30%
(Old London) restaurant style				
garlic	2 Tbs	1.5	30	39%
Italian	2 Tbs	1.5	30	39%
sourdough	2 Tbs	1.5	30	39%
(Pepperidge Farm)				
homestyle				
Caesar	6 croutons	1.5	35	39%
olive oil & garlic	6 croutons	1.0	30	30%
sourdough cheese	6 croutons	1.0	30	30%
zesty Italian	6 croutons	1.5	35	39%

Food and Description	Amount	Fat Grams	Total Calories	% Fat Calories
regular				
cheddar & Romano cheese	9 croutons	1.0	30	30%
cheese & garlic	6 croutons	1.5	35	39%
cracked pepper & Parmesan	6 croutons	1.5	35	39%
onion & garlic	9 croutons	1.0	30	30%
ranch	9 croutons	1.5	35	39%
seasoned	9 croutons	1.5	35	39%
(Rothberry Farms) fat-free				
French style	8 pieces	–	25	–
seasoned	11 pieces	–	25	–
CROWDER PEA/canned				
(Luck's) seasoned w/pork	7.5 oz	7.0	200	32%
CRUMPET				
(Sara Lee) fresh				
brown sugar-cinnamon	1 crumpet	1.5	100	14%
classic	1 crumpet	0.5	90	5%
raspberry	1 crumpet	–	100	–
(Wolferman's)				
blueberry	1 crumpet	0.5	100	5%
brown sugar-cinnamon	1 crumpet	1.5	100	14%
lemon-poppy seed	1 crumpet	0.5	90	5%
original	1 crumpet	0.5	90	5%
raspberry	1 crumpet	1.5	100	5%
whole-grain	1 crumpet	1.0	100	9%
CUCUMBER (*See also* PICKLE)				
raw				
sliced	½ cup	–	7	–
whole	1 medium	–	29	–
CUCUMBER DISH (*See also* PICKLE; PICKLE RELISH)				
(Rosoff's) cucumber salad	1 oz	–	12	–
(Schorr's) cucumber garden salad	1 oz	–	12	–
CUMIN SEED/whole	1 tsp	0.5	8	56%
CUPCAKE (*See* CAKE, SNACK)				
CURRANT				
black				
dried	½ cup	–	204	–
raw	½ cup	–	36	–
	½ lb	–	140	–
red or white/raw	½ cup	–	31	–
	½ lb	–	125	–
Zante/dried				
(Del Monte) dried	½ cup	–	200	–
(S&W) canned	¼ cup	–	130	–
(Sun Maid)	½ cup	–	210	–
CURRANT JUICE/black	8 fl oz	–	138	–
CURRY POWDER/ground	1 tsp	–	6	–
CURRY SAUCE (*See* SAUCE)				

Food and Description	Amount	Fat Grams	Total Calories	% Fat Calories
CUSK				
raw	3 oz	1.0	74	12%
steamed	1 oz	<1.0	30	15%
	1 lb	3.0	481	6%
CUSTARD (*See also* BABY FOOD; PUDDING & MOUSSE)				
Homemade/USDA Standard Home Recipe				
baked	1 cup	14.6	305	43%
boiled	½ cup	7.0	164	38%
zabaglione	¼ cup	4.0	80	45%
mix (Note: 1 serving of mix = the amount in ½ cup prepared)				
(Goya) flan/prepared	½ cup	0.5	60	8%
(Jell-O)				
custard dessert				
mix only	1 serving	–	80	–
prepared w/2% milk	½ cup	2.5	140	16%
flan				
mix only	1 serving	–	80	0
prepared w/2% milk	½ cup	2.5	140	16%
(Knorr) Alsa international dessert				
creme caramel flan/mix only	¼ pkg	–	110	–
(Royal) flan-caramel custard/prepared	½ cup	–	60	–
CUTTLEFISH/				
cooked-moist heat	3 oz	1.0	135	6%
raw	3 oz	0.6	67	8%

D

Food and Description	Amount	Fat Grams	Total Calories	% Fat Calories
DANDELION GREENS/fresh				
cooked	½ cup	–	17	–
raw/chopped	½ cup	–	13	–
DANISH (*See* PASTRY)				
DATE				
(Del Monte)				
chopped	¼ cup	–	120	–
pitted	5-6 medium	–	120	–
(Dole)				
chopped	½ cup	–	230	–
dried/ground	1 oz	–	110	–
pitted	½ cup	<1.0	280	2%

Food and Description	Amount	Fat Grams	Total Calories	% Fat Calories
(Dromedary)				
chopped	¼ cup	–	130	–
whole/pitted	5 medium	–	100	–
generic				
chopped	1 cup	0.8	489	2%
natural/dried	10 medium	–	228	–
(Sun Giant)				
chopped	1 cup	1.0	490	2%
whole/pitted	10 medium	1.0	220	4%
DATE FILLING (Solo)	2 Tbs	1.0	100	9%
DEER (See VENISON)				
DESSERT TOPPING (See CREAM; ICE CREAM TOPPING; WHIPPED TOPPING)				
DIETING AID (See BREAKFAST DRINK; GRANOLA/GRANOLA-TYPE BAR; NUTRITIONAL SUPPLEMENT)				
DILL LEAVES/fresh	1 cup	–	5	–
DILL SAUCE (See SAUCE)				
DILL SEED				
dried	1 tsp	–	3	–
whole	1 tsp	–	6	–
DINNER (See ASIAN FOOD; BEEF DISH/ENTRÉE; EGG DISH/MEAL; FAST FOOD; FROZEN ENTRÉE/DINNER; MEXICAN FOOD; PASTA ENTRÉE/DINNER; PIZZA; PORK ENTRÉE/DINNER; RICE DISH; SEAFOOD ENTRÉE/DINNER; VEGETARIAN FOODS; individual listings)				
DIP (See also SALAD DRESSING; SAUCE; SEASONINGS)				
▣ **FROZEN**				
(AVO King) Southwestern guacamole	2 Tbs	5.0	57	79%
(Calavo) Mexican-style avocado guacamole	2 Tbs	4.5	50	81%
▣ **MIX**				
(Note: Unless otherwise stated, data are for dry mix only)				
(Casbah) hummus	2 oz	10.0	220	41%
(Fantastic Foods) hummus	2 Tbs	2.0	60	30%
(Golden Dipt)				
clam seafood	½ tsp	–	5	–
dill seafood	½ tsp	–	5	–
horseradish	½ tsp	–	–	–
Louis	1 tsp	–	10	–
pesto	1 tsp	–	10	–
(Hain)				
hot bean	4 Tbs	1.0	70	13%
Mexican bean	4 Tbs	1.0	60	15%
(Hidden Valley)				
(Note: 1 serving of mix = the amount in 2 Tbs prepared.)				
Fiesta				
mix only	1 serving	–	5	–
prepared	2 Tbs	6.0	70	77%
French onion				
mix only	1 serving	–	5	–

Food and Description	Amount	Fat Grams	Total Calories	% Fat Calories
prepared	2 Tbs	6.0	70	77%
garden vegetable				
mix only	1 serving	–	5	–
prepared	2 Tbs	6.0	70	77%
original				
reduced calorie				
mix only	1 serving	–	5	–
prepared	2 Tbs	3.0	40	68%
regular recipe				
mix only	1 serving	–	5	–
prepared	2 Tbs	6.0	70	77%
(Knorr)				
black bean	¹⁄₁₆ pkg	–	10	–
chili caliente	¹⁄₂₀ pkg	–	5	–
cracked pepper ranch	¹⁄₂₀ pkg	–	5	–
garden dill	¹⁄₂₀ pkg	–	2	–
Mexican bean	¹⁄₁₆ pkg	–	10	–
nacho cheese	¹⁄₁₅ pkg	–	10	–
onion chive	¹⁄₂₀ pkg	–	5	–
(McCormick/Schilling)				
Dip Classics				
country herb	1 tsp	–	10	–
French onion	¾ tsp	–	5	–
garlic & pepper	¾ tsp	–	5	–
ranch	¾ tsp	–	5	–
spring onion	½ tsp	–	5	–
vegetable	½ tsp	–	–	–
McCormick Collection				
black bean	1 Tbs	–	35	–
jalapeño bean	1 Tbs	–	40	–
pinto bean	1 Tbs	–	40	–
poppy seed	2 tsp	–	25	–
spinach	1 tsp	–	5	–
spring vegetable	2 tsp	–	10	–
toasted onion	1 tsp	–	5	–
(Produce Partners)				
garden vegetable	2 tsp	–	10	–
guacamole				
mild	2 tsp	–	15	–
spicy	2 tsp	–	15	–
jalapeño	¾ tsp	–	5	–
outrageous onion	1 tsp	–	5	–
salsa				
mild	¼ tsp	–	5	–
spicy	¼ tsp	–	5	–
(The Spice Hunter)				
Cajun fire	½ tsp	–	–	–

Food and Description	Amount	Fat Grams	Total Calories	% Fat Calories
California salsa	¾ tsp	–	–	–
5 onion & herb	¾ tsp	–	–	–
■ READY TO SERVE				
(Birds Eye) Veggie Dips				
dill				
fat-free	2 Tbs	–	30	–
original	2 Tbs	7.0	80	79%
herb & garlic				
fat-free	2 Tbs	–	30	–
original	2 Tbs	7.0	80	79%
ranch	2 Tbs	7.0	80	78%
(Breakstone) sour cream dip				
bacon & onion	2 Tbs	5.0	60	75%
Chesapeake clam	2 Tbs	4.0	50	72%
French onion	2 Tbs	4.0	50	72%
jalapeño cheddar	2 Tbs	4.0	60	60%
toasted onion	2 Tbs	4.0	50	72%
(Calavo) guacamole				
Mexican avocado	2 Tbs	3.0	45	60%
mild	2 Tbs	4.0	45	80%
original avocado	2 Tbs	3.0	45	60%
zesty	2 Tbs	4.0	45	80%
(Chi-Chi's)				
fiesta bean	2 Tbs	1.5	35	39%
fiesta cheese	2 Tbs	3.0	40	68%
(Dean's)				
French onion				
extra light	2 Tbs	2.0	30	60%
original	2 Tbs	4.0	50	72%
w/bacon bits	2 Tbs	4.0	50	72%
ranch	2 Tbs	4.0	50	72%
(Doritos) cheese n' salsa	2 Tbs	2.0	40	45%
(Eagle)				
black bean	2 Tbs	1.0	35	26%
cheese & salsa	2 Tbs	3.0	40	68%
mild bean	2 Tbs	1.5	40	34
salsa				
medium	2 Tbs	–	10	–
mild	2 Tbs	–	10	–
(Enrico's) fat-free				
black spicy bean	2 Tbs	–	32	–
nacho cheese/mild	2 Tbs	–	20	–
(Frito-Lay)				
cheddar cheese/mild	2 Tbs	3.0	50	54%
French onion	2 Tbs	5.0	60	75%
hot bean	2 Tbs	1.0	35	26%
jalapeño & cheese	2 Tbs	3.0	50	54%
jalapeño bean	2 Tbs	1.0	40	23%

Food and Description	Amount	Fat Grams	Total Calories	% Fat Calories
(Guiltless Gourmet) spicy				
black bean				
BBQ	2 Tbs	–	35	–
regular	2 Tbs	–	30	–
nacho	2 Tbs	–	25	–
pinto bean				
BBQ	2 Tbs	–	40	–
regular	2 Tbs	–	35	–
(Hannah) Mediterranean-style hummus	2 Tbs	4.0	50	72%
(Heluva Good Cheese)				
bacon horseradish	2 Tbs	5.0	60	75%
clam	2 Tbs	5.0	50	90%
French onion				
light	2 Tbs	2.0	35	51%
original	2 Tbs	5.0	50	90%
homestyle onion	2 Tbs	5.0	60	75%
jalapeño cheddar/light	2 Tbs	2.0	40	45%
ranch	2 Tbs	5.0	60	75%
(Knudsen)				
bacon & onion/premium	2 Tbs	5.0	60	75%
creamy ranch/free	2 Tbs	–	25	–
creamy salsa/free	2 Tbs	–	20	–
French onion				
free	2 Tbs	–	25	–
premium	2 Tbs	4.0	50	72%
nacho cheese/premium	2 Tbs	4.0	60	60%
(Kraft)				
avocado/guacamole	2 Tbs	4.0	60	60%
bacon horseradish				
premium	2 Tbs	5.0	50	72%
regular	2 Tbs	5.0	60	75%
bacon onion/premium	2 Tbs	5.0	60	60%
cheese				
blue/premium	2 Tbs	4.0	45	60%
jalapeño/premium	2 Tbs	5.0	60	75%
nacho/premium	2 Tbs	5.0	60	75%
clam				
premium	2 Tbs	4.0	45	80%
regular	2 Tbs	4.0	60	60%
creamy cucumber/premium	2 Tbs	4.0	50	72%
creamy onion/premium	2 Tbs	4.0	45	80%
French onion				
premium	2 Tbs	4.0	50	72%
regular	2 Tbs	4.0	60	60%
green onion	2 Tbs	4.0	60	60%
jalapeño pepper	2 Tbs	4.0	60	60%
ranch	2 Tbs	4.0	60	60%

Food and Description	Amount	Fat Grams	Total Calories	% Fat Calories
(La Famous)				
mild bean	2 Tbs	–	25	–
spicy bean	2 Tbs	–	25	–
(Louise's) fat-free				
honey mustard	1 oz	–	40	–
sour cream & onion	1 oz	–	25	–
white cheese peppercorn	1 oz	–	25	–
(Marzetti)				
for fruit				
caramel apple				
fat-free	2 Tbs	–	110	–
original	2 Tbs	7.0	160	39%
reduced fat	2 Tbs	3.0	130	21%
chocolate-flavored				
fat-free	2 Tbs	–	100	–
original	2 Tbs	4.0	120	30%
peanut butter caramel	2 Tbs	6.0	150	36%
for vegetables				
blue cheese	2 Tbs	19.0	180	95%
cheese veggie topping	2 Tbs	7.0	90	70%
dill/fat-free	2 Tbs	–	35	–
lemon-dill	2 Tbs	14.0	140	90%
ranch				
regular				
fat-free	2 Tbs	–	35	–
light	2 Tbs	7.0	80	79%
original	2 Tbs	14.0	140	90%
Southwestern				
fat-free	2 Tbs	–	35	–
original	2 Tbs	14.0	140	90%
salsa con queso	2 Tbs	12.0	120	90%
sour cream & onion	2 Tbs	14.0	140	90%
spinach	2 Tbs	14.0	140	90%
(Nasoya) Vegi-Dip				
French onion	2 Tbs	3.0	50	54%
garlic & herb	2 Tbs	2.0	50	36%
(Old El Paso)				
black bean	2 Tbs	–	20	–
cheese 'n salsa				
medium	2 Tbs	3.0	40	68%
mild	2 Tbs	3.0	40	68%
jalapeño	2 Tbs	1.0	30	30%
(Poore Brothers)				
bean	2 Tbs	1.5	40	34%
sour cream & onion	2 Tbs	5.0	60	75%
(Robert Rothchild Berry Farm)				
raspberry honey mustard	5 gm	–	10	–

Food and Description	Amount	Fat Grams	Total Calories	% Fat Calories
(Rod's)				
dip				
French onion				
regular	2 Tbs	6.0	70	77%
w/bacon	2 Tbs	6.0	70	77%
green onion	2 Tbs	6.0	70	77%
ranch	2 Tbs	6.0	70	77%
dip & dressing				
avocado	2 Tbs	11.0	110	90%
French onion/fat-free	2 Tbs	–	25	–
guacamole				
regular	2 Tbs	11.0	110	90%
zesty	2 Tbs	8.0	80	90%
ranch				
regular	2 Tbs	11.0	110	90%
fat-free	2 Tbs	–	25	–
w/bacon	2 Tbs	11.0	110	90%
(Santa Barbara) seafood	2 Tbs	4.5	60	68%
(Sealtest) sour cream dip				
bacon & horseradish	2 Tbs	6.0	70	77%
French onion	2 Tbs	4.0	50	72%
(Slender Choice)				
French onion	1 Tbs	1.0	15	60%
green onion	1 Tbs	1.0	20	45%
jalapeño	1 Tbs	1.0	20	45%
ranch style	1 Tbs	1.0	20	45%
(Smucker's) fat-free				
caramel fruit	2 Tbs	–	130	–
chocolate fruit	2 Tbs	–	130	–
(Taco Bell)				
wild black bean	2 Tbs	–	25	–
wild salsa	2 Tbs	–	15	–
(Thank You)				
creamy ranch	2 Tbs	5.0	60	75%
French onion	2 Tbs	5.0	60	75%
nacho cheese	2 Tbs	5.0	50	90%
(Tostitos)				
black bean/fat-free	2 Tbs	–	25	–
salsa con queso	2 Tbs	2.0	40	45%
(Wise)				
bean	2 Tbs	–	12	–
jalapeño bean	2 Tbs	–	25	–
DISTILLED LIQUOR (*See* LIQUOR, DISTILLED)				
DOCK				
cooked-drained	3 oz	0.5	17	26%
raw/chopped	3 oz	0.5	15	30%
DOGFISH (*See also* SHARK)				
raw	3 oz	8.0	135	53%

Food and Description	Amount	Fat Grams	Total Calories	% Fat Calories
DOLPHIN FISH (*See also* MAHI MAHI)				
raw	3 oz	0.6	73	7%
DONUT (*See also* PASTRY)				
(Break Cake)				
chocolate	1 donut	8.0	130	55%
cinnamon	1 donut	6.0	115	47%
powdered	1 donut	5.0	115	39%
(Dolly Madison)				
chocolate				
gems	4 gems	15.0	260	52%
iced/old-fashioned	1 donut	14.0	300	42%
cinnamon stix	1 stix	9.0	170	48%
cinnamon sugar				
gems	6 gems	17.0	360	43%
stix	2 stix	12.0	230	47%
crunch				
gems	6 gems	18.0	390	42%
regular	1 donut	6.0	140	39%
dunkin stix	2 stix	19.0	360	48%
frosted	1 donut	6.0	130	42%
glazed/old-fashioned	1 donut	14.0	300	42%
iced/jumbo	1 donut	12.0	230	47%
plain				
jumbo	1 donut	11.0	190	52%
regular	2 donuts	10.0	170	53%
powdered sugar/gems	6 gems	17.0	360	43%
sugar				
jumbo	1 donut	12.0	230	47%
regular	1 donut	6.0	130	42%
white iced/old-fashioned	1 donut	14.0	230	55%
yeast glazed	1 donut	8.0	180	40%
(Drake's)				
old fashioned	1 pkg	8.0	180	40%
powdered sugar	1 pkg	15.0	300	45%
(Dunkin' Donuts)				
crullers/sticks				
chocolate/glazed	1 donut	24.0	410	53%
Dunkin' donut	1 donut	14.0	240	53%
glazed	1 donut	14.0	340	37%
jelly stick	1 donut	14.0	330	38%
plain	1 donut	14.0	260	48%
powdered	1 donut	15.0	290	47%
sugar	1 donut	14.0	270	47%
donuts				
cake				
blueberry	1 donut	10.0	230	39%
blueberry crumb	1 donut	11.0	260	38%
butternut	1 donut	20.0	340	53%

Food and Description	Amount	Fat Grams	Total Calories	% Fat Calories
chocolate				
double chocolate	1 donut	14.0	260	48%
glazed	1 donut	14.0	240	50%
regular	1 donut	14.0	210	60%
chocolate coconut	1 donut	15.0	250	54%
cinnamon	1 donut	19.0	300	57%
coconut				
regular	1 donut	20.0	320	56%
toasted	1 donut	19.0	320	53%
old-fashioned	1 donut	19.0	280	61%
peanut	1 donut	22.0	340	58%
powdered	1 donut	19.0	310	55%
sugared	1 donut	20.0	310	58%
whole-wheat/glazed	1 donut	11.0	230	43%
yeast				
apple crumb	1 donut	11.0	250	40%
apple n' spice	1 donut	10.0	230	39%
Bavarian kreme	1 donut	11.0	250	40%
black raspberry	1 donut	10.0	240	38%
Boston kreme	1 donut	11.0	270	37%
chocolate frosted	1 donut	8.0	210	34%
chocolate kreme filled	1 donut	16.0	320	45%
glazed	1 donut	7.0	160	39%
French cruller	1 donut	8.0	150	48%
jelly filled	1 donut	10.0	240	38%
lemon	1 donut	11.0	240	41%
maple frosted	1 donut	8.0	210	34%
raised/sugar	1 donut	7.0	170	37%
strawberry	1 donut	10.0	240	38%
strawberry frosted	1 donut	8.0	220	33%
vanilla frosted	1 donut	8.0	220	33%
Munchkins				
cake				
butternut	1 Munchkin	4.0	70	51%
cake/glazed	1 Munchkin	3.0	70	39%
chocolate/glazed	1 Munchkin	3.0	60	45%
cinnamon	1 Munchkin	3.0	60	45%
coconut				
regular	1 Munchkin	4.0	70	51%
toasted coconut	1 Munchkin	4.0	70	51%
plain	1 Munchkin	3.0	50	54%
powdered sugar	1 Munchkin	3.0	60	45%
yeast				
raised				
glazed	1 Munchkin	1.5	50	27%
sugar	1 Munchkin	1.5	35	39%
jelly	1 Munchkin	1.5	60	23%

Food and Description	Amount	Fat Grams	Total Calories	% Fat Calories
lemon	1 Munchkin	2.0	50	36%
(Earth Grains)				
cinnamon-apple	1 donut	17.0	310	49%
devil's food	1 donut	21.0	330	57%
glazed/old-fashioned	1 donut	18.0	310	52%
powdered/old-fashioned	1 donut	19.0	290	59%
(Entenmann's)				
donuts				
buttermilk/glazed	1 donut	13.0	270	43%
crumb-topped				
regular	1 donut	13.0	260	45%
variety donuts	1 donut	22.0	420	47%
devil's food crumb	1 donut	12.0	250	43%
frosted mini	2 donuts	20.0	270	67%
cinnamon sugar/variety donuts	1 donut	19.0	310	55%
rich frosted				
regular	1 donut	19.0	280	61%
variety donuts	1 donut	27.0	400	61%
Popems				
glazed	6 pieces	11.0	240	41%
chocolate/glazed	4 pieces	10.0	200	45%
generic/1" high/3¼" dia				
cake type	1 donut	7.8	164	43%
yeast-leavened/glazed				
jelly-filled	1 donut	9.0	225	36%
plain	1 donut	13.0	235	50%
(Hostess)				
Donettes bite-size donuts				
chocolate frosted	3 donettes	14.0	230	55%
crumb gem	6 donettes	11.0	320	31%
frosted gem	6 donettes	23.0	390	53%
powdered gem	6 donettes	16.0	350	41%
donuts				
bakery assorted	1 donut	11.0	200	50%
glazed whirl	1 donut	7.0	180	35%
low-fat	4 donuts	3.0	170	16%
powdered	1 donut	6.0	110	49%
raspberry O's	1 donut	6.0	160	34%
(Lance) Dunking Sticks	1 piece	10.0	180	50%
(Little Debbie) donut sticks				
box	1 pkg	13.0	210	56%
individual pkg	2 oz	15.0	250	54%
(Rich's) frozen/glazed	1 donut	7.0	130	48%
(Sara Lee) reduced fat/assorted	1 donut	9.0	220	4%
(TastyKake)				
Mini Donuts				
honey wheat	6 donuts	13.0	280	42%

Food and Description	Amount	Fat Grams	Total Calories	% Fat Calories
powdered sugar	6 donuts	12.0	290	37%
rich frosted	6 donuts	23.0	400	52%
regular donuts				
assortment pkg				
cinnamon	1 donut	12.0	210	51%
plain	1 donut	11.0	180	55%
powdered sugar	1 donut	11.0	210	47%
dunkin stix	1 piece	11.0	190	52%
honey wheat	1 donut	10.0	230	39%
orange glazed	1 donut	9.0	220	37%
rich frosted	1 donut	16.0	270	53%
(Winchell's)				
apple fritter	1 donut	37.0	580	57%
chocolate				
bar/iced	1 donut	11.0	220	45%
cake/iced	1 donut	10.0	230	39%
devil's/iced	1 donut	12.0	240	45%
French/iced	1 donut	13.0	220	53%
raised/iced	1 donut	10.0	210	43%
cinnamon crumb	1 donut	11.0	240	41%
cinnamon roll	1 donut	21.0	360	53%
donut hole/plain	1 donut	3.0	50	54%
jelly/glazed	1 donut	13.0	300	39%
glazed				
round	1 donut	12.0	210	51%
twist	1 donut	11.0	210	47%
plain	1 donut	11.0	200	50%

DRESSING (*See* MAYONNAISE/MAYONNAISE-TYPE DRESSING; SALAD DRESSING; STUFFING/DRESSING)

DRUM/ freshwater

baked	3 oz	5.0	130	35%
raw	3 oz	4.0	100	36%

DUCK

domesticated

liver/raw	1.5 oz	2.0	60	30%
(Maple Leaf Farms) fully cooked duckling w/orange sauce packet/ chilled/frozen	6 oz	27.0	390	62%
meat & skin/roasted	~¾ lb	108.0	1287	76%
meat only/roasted	8 oz	25.0	456	49%
wild/raw	3 oz	9.0	170	48%
breast meat only	3 oz	3.5	105	30%
meat & skin	9.5 oz	41.0	570	65%

DUMPLING MIX (*See also* FROZEN ENTRÉE/DINNER; PASTRY)

(Maggi)

tiny Swiss style spaetzle mix	¼ cup	1.5	180	8%
(Panni)				
Bavarian potato dumpling mix	½ pkg	–	80	–

E

Food and Description	Amount	Fat Grams	Total Calories	% Fat Calories
ECLAIR (*See* PASTRY)				
EEL				
cooked-dry heat	3 oz	12.7	200	57%
raw	3 oz	10.0	156	58%
smoked	~2 oz	16.0	188	77%
EGG (*See also* EGG SUBSTITUTE; VEGETARIAN FOODS)				
chicken				
boiled, hard or soft	1 medium	4.0	70	51%
	1 large	5.6	79	64%
fried in butter	1 large	7.0	95	66%
pickled	1 large	5.0	80	56%
poached	1 large	5.6	79	64%
raw				
white only	1 medium	–	14	–
	1 large	–	16	–
	1 cup	–	120	–
whole	1 medium	4.0	70	51%
	1 large	5.6	79	64%
yolk only	1 medium	4.0	56	64%
	1 large	5.6	63	64%
duck/raw	1 egg	9.6	130	67%
goose/raw	1 egg	19.0	276	62%
quail/raw	1 egg	1.0	14	64%
turkey/raw	1 egg	9.0	135	60%
EGG DISH/MEAL (*See also* BREAKFAST SANDWICH; EGG; EGG SUBSTITUTE)				
frozen or refrigerated				
(Chef Pierre) quiche				
bacon	⅛ quiche	25.0	340	66%
broccoli	⅛ quiche	26.0	340	69%
spinach	⅛ quiche	23.0	320	65%
(La Terra Fina) broccoli-cheddar quiche	6 oz	15.0	292	46%
(Nabisco) Easy Omelet/microwaveable				
cheddar				
regular	1 container	8.0	160	45%
w/bell pepper & onion	1 container	8.0	150	48%
w/real ham bits	1 container	8.0	150	48%
Monterey Jack	1 container	8.0	150	48%
(Nancy's) quiche/microwaveable				
broccoli cheddar	1 quiche	33.0	490	61%

Food and Description	Amount	Fat Grams	Total Calories	% Fat Calories
classic French				
French baked	1 quiche	33.0	470	63%
petite	6 quiche	22.0	370	54%
Florentine				
French baked	1 quiche	32.0	480	60%
petite	6 quiche	22.0	370	54%
Italian	1 quiche	30.0	460	59%
Monterey				
French baked	1 quiche	36.0	510	64%
petite	6 quiche	22.0	370	54%
Southwestern	1 quiche	29.0	440	59%
spring vegetable	1 quiche	30.0	450	60%
(Quelle) quiche				
broccoli	⅕ quiche	28.0	360	70%
Lorraine	⅕ quiche	28.0	360	70%
spinach	⅕ quiche	28.0	360	70%
(Swanson)				
budget meal				
eggs & silver dollar pancakes	1 meal	14.0	250	50%
sausage, eggs, & home fries	1 meal	12.0	200	54%
Great Starts omelet				
Spanish style	7.75 oz	16.0	240	60%
w/bacon & home fries	1 meal	19.0	290	59%
w/sausage & hash browns	1 meal	26.0	360	65%
(Weight Watchers) Handy Omelet				
ham & cheese	4 oz	6.0	230	23%
homemade/USDA Standard Home Recipe				
deviled egg	2 halves	13.0	145	81%
egg foo young	~5 oz	10.0	150	60%
egg salad	⅓ cup	19.0	205	83%
omelet/made w/1 egg & 1 Tbs whole milk/cooked in butter	1 omelet	7.0	95	66%
quiche				
cheese	5 oz	33.0	470	63%
Lorraine/8" dia	⅛ quiche	48.0	600	72%
mushroom	5 oz	30.0	430	63%
spinach	5 oz	26.0	337	69%
scrambled egg/made w/whole milk/cooked in butter	1 egg	7.0	95	66%

EGG ROLL (*See* ASIAN FOOD; FROZEN ENTRÉE/DINNER; SEAFOOD ENTRÉE/DINNER)

EGG SALAD (*See* EGG DISH/MEAL)

EGG SUBSTITUTE

Food and Description	Amount	Fat Grams	Total Calories	% Fat Calories
generic				
frozen	¼ cup	6.7	96	64%
liquid	1½ oz	1.6	39	37%
powder	0.35 oz	1.0	44	21%
(Featherweight) Egg Magic	1 pouch	8.0	110	65%

Food and Description	Amount	Fat Grams	Total Calories	% Fat Calories
(Fleischmann's) Egg Beaters				
cheese omelet mix	½ cup	5.0	110	41%
plain	¼ cup	–	25	–
vegetable omelet mix	½ pkg	–	50	–
(Healthy Choice)	¼ cup	–	25	–
(Just Whites) dried egg whites	2 tsp	–	14	–
(Morningstar Farms)				
Better 'n Eggs	¼ cup	–	20	–
Scramblers	¼ cup	–	35	–
(Nulaid) no cholesterol/no fat				
cheese	¼ cup	–	40	–
original	¼ cup	–	30	–
(Second Nature)	2 oz	2.0	60	30%
(Tofutti) Egg Watchers	¼ cup	–	30	–
(Wonderslim) fat & egg substitute	¼ cup	–	35	–
EGGNOG				
canned				
(Borden)				
light	4 fl oz	2.0	130	14%
original	4 fl oz	9.0	160	51%
mix				
generic				
mix only	2 tsp	–	110	–
prepared				
w/skim milk	8 fl oz	1.0	200	5%
w/1% low-fat milk	8 fl oz	3.0	215	13%
w/2% low-fat milk	8 fl oz	5.0	230	20%
w/whole milk	8 fl oz	8.0	260	28%
(PDQ) prepared w/whole milk	8 fl oz	5.0	230	20%
refrigerated				
(Darigold)	8 fl oz	17.0	350	44%
classic	8 fl oz	17.0	390	39%
(Farm Rich) nondairy	8 fl oz	18.0	380	43%
generic				
light	4 fl oz	1.0	60	15%
regular	8 fl oz	19.0	342	50%
(Kemp's)				
Holly Nog	4 fl oz	2.0	110	16%
lite	4 fl oz	3.0	120	23%
original	4 fl oz	9.0	175	46%
premium	4 fl oz	9.0	180	45%
(Land O'Lakes)	8 fl oz	15.0	300	45%
EGGPLANT/fresh				
boiled	½ cup	–	13	–
raw/sliced	½ cup	–	11	–
EGGPLANT DISH (See also FROZEN ENTRÉE/DINNER)				
(Michael Angelo's) eggplant Parmesan	1 cup	21.0	300	63%
(Progresso) appetizer	2 Tbs	2.0	30	60%

Food and Description	Amount	Fat Grams	Total Calories	% Fat Calories
ELDERBERRY/raw	1 cup	0.8	105	7%
	½ lb	1.0	154	6%
ELK/meat only				
raw	1 oz	0.4	31	17%
	1 pound	6.6	504	12%
roasted	3 oz	1.6	124	12%
ENCHILADA (See FROZEN ENTRÉE/DINNER; MEXICAN FOOD)				
ENCHILADA SAUCE (See MEXICAN FOOD; SAUCE)				
ENDIVE/raw	½ cup	–	4	–
ENGLISH MUFFIN (See MUFFIN)				
ESCARGOT (See SNAIL)				
ESCAROLE/raw	4 oz	–	20	–
ESCAROLE SOUP (See SOUP)				
EXTRACTS & FLAVORINGS				
(Durkee)				
almond extract	1 tsp	–	13	–
anise extract	1 tsp	–	16	–
banana flavor	1 tsp	–	15	–
black walnut flavor	1 tsp	–	4	–
brandy flavor	1 tsp	–	15	–
butter flavor	1 tsp	–	3	–
cherry extract	1 tsp	–	3	–
chocolate flavor	1 tsp	–	7	–
coconut flavor	1 tsp	–	8	–
creme de menthe extract	1 tsp	–	9	–
lemon extract	1 tsp	–	17	–
maple extract	1 tsp	–	6	–
orange extract	1 tsp	–	14	–
peppermint extract	1 tsp	–	15	–
pineapple flavor	1 tsp	–	6	–
raspberry extract	1 tsp	–	10	–
rum flavor	1 tsp	–	14	–
strawberry extract	1 tsp	–	12	–
vanilla butter & nut extract	1 tsp	–	5	–
vanilla extract	1 tsp	–	8	–
vanilla flavor	1 tsp	–	3	–
(McCormick/Schilling)				
almond extract	1 tsp	–	10	–
anise extract	1 tsp	–	23	–
banana imitation extract	1 tsp	–	11	–
black walnut extract				
cold	1 tsp	–	12	–
heated	1 tsp	–	<1	–
brandy imitation extract	1 tsp	–	20	–
butter flavor	1 tsp	–	<1	–
chocolate extract				
cold	1 tsp	–	8	–
heated	1 tsp	–	2	–

Food and Description	Amount	Fat Grams	Total Calories	% Fat Calories
coconut imitation extract	1 tsp	–	7	–
lemon extract				
cold	1 tsp	–	35	–
heated	1 tsp	–	<1	–
maple imitation flavor	1 tsp	–	8	–
mint & peppermint extract	1 tsp	–	20	–
orange extract	1 tsp	–	23	–
pineapple imitation extract	1 tsp	–	12	–
root beer concentrate	1 tsp	–	13	–
rum imitation extract	1 tsp	–	19	–
sherry extract	1 tsp	–	14	–
strawberry imitation extract	1 tsp	–	7	–
vanilla				
cold	1 tsp	–	12	–
heated	1 tsp	–	<1	–

F

Food and Description	Amount	Fat Grams	Total Calories	% Fat Calories
FAJITA (*See* MEXICAN FOOD; FROZEN ENTRÉE/DINNER)				
FALAFEL				
homemade/USDA Standard Home Recipe				
pattied or balled	1 oz	6.0	115	47%
mix				
(Casbah) prepared	5 balls	3.0	130	21%
(Fantastic Foods) Fantastic Falafil				
mix only	½ cup	4.0	250	14%
prepared	1 cup	4.0	250	14%
(Near East) vegetable burger mix				
broiled	1½ patties	1.5	110	12%
fried	2½ patties	15.0	230	59%
FAST FOOD (*See* separate section at end of book)				
FAT (*See also* BEEF TALLOW; BUTTER; COOKING SPRAY; LARD; MARGARINE, MARGARINE SPREAD, & SPRAY; OIL; PORK FAT; SHORTENING)				
bacon fat	1 Tbs	14.0	126	100%
beef fat/separable/raw	1 Tbs	12.0	108	100%
chicken fat	1 Tbs	12.0	115	100%
duck fat	1 Tbs	12.0	115	100%
pork backfat/raw	2 oz	50.0	464	100%

Food and Description	Amount	Fat Grams	Total Calories	% Fat Calories
FAT SUBSTITUTE (*See also* OIL/SHORTENING ALTERNATIVE)				
(Wonderslim) fat & egg substitute	¼ cup	–	35	–
FAVA BEAN/canned				
(Progresso)	½ cup	0.5	110	4%
FENNEL LEAVES/raw	2 oz	–	15	–
FENNEL SEED	1 tsp	–	7	–
FENUGREEK SEED	1 tsp	–	12	–
FIELD PEA				
(Allen's)				
fresh	½ cup	0.5	100	5%
tiny	½ cup	0.5	100	5%
w/snaps	½ cup	0.5	100	5%
(Bush's Best)	½ cup	–	80	–
(Glory Foods)	½ cup	0.5	120	4%
FIG				
canned				
generic/solids & liquid				
In extra heavy syrup	1 cup	–	280	–
In heavy syrup	1 cup	–	228	–
In light syrup	1 cup	–	175	–
In water	1 cup	–	130	–
(Oregon) Kadota/In heavy syrup	½ cup	1.0	130	7%
(S&W) Kadota/in heavy syrup	5 pieces	1.0	140	6%
dried				
generic				
cooked	1 large	–	55	–
	½ cup	–	140	–
uncooked	½ cup	1.0	250	4%
(Mariani) Calimyrna	½ cup	2.0	250	7%
(Sun Maid)				
Calimyrna	¼ cup	–	110	–
Mission	¼ cup	–	110	–
fresh	1 medium	–	37	–
	1 large	–	47	–
FILBERT/HAZELNUT (*See also* HAZELNUT SPREAD)				
(Diamond)				
in the shell	1 oz	19.0	190	90%
shelled	1 oz	19.0	190	90%
generic				
dried				
blanched	1 oz	17.8	179	90%
unblanched	1 oz	18.5	190	88%
dry-roasted	1 oz	18.8	188	90%
oil-roasted	1 oz	18.0	187	87%
FISH (*See* GEFILTE FISH; SEAFOOD ENTRÉE/DINER; individual listings)				
FISH CHOWDER (*See* SOUP)				
FISH SEASONING (*See* SEASONINGS)				
FIVE SPICE SEASONING (*See* SEASONINGS)				

Food and Description	Amount	Fat Grams	Total Calories	% Fat Calories
FLAN (*See* CUSTARD)				
FLATBREAD (*See* CRACKER)				
FLATFISH (*See also* FLOUNDER)				
cooked	3 oz	1.0	100	9%
raw	3 oz	1.0	80	11%
FLAVORINGS (*See* EXTRACTS & FLAVORINGS)				
FLAXSEED (Arrowhead Mills)	3 Tbs	10.0	140	64%
FLOUNDER (*See also* SEAFOOD ENTRÉE/DINNER)				
baked				
w/butter	3 oz	7.0	171	37%
w/o butter	3 oz	1.0	80	11%
frozen				
breaded	5 oz	15.0	300	45%
(Van de Kamp's) raw	1 fillet	2.0	110	16%
FLOUR				
acorn	1 oz	9.0	142	57%
amaranth				
(Arrowhead Mills)	¼ cup	1.5	110	13%
generic	1 oz	<1.0	95	3%
	1 cup	2.0	698	3%
arrowroot	1 Tbs	–	29	–
barley				
(Arrowhead Mills)	¼ cup	0.5	75	6%
generic	1 Tbs	<1.0	28	16%
bread				
(Betty Crocker) Gold Medal/Better for Bread	¼ cup	–	100	–
generic	1 cup	3.0	401	7%
(Hodgson Mill) Best for Bread	¼ cup	–	100	–
(Pillsbury)	¼ cup	–	100	–
buckwheat				
(Arrowhead Mills)	¼ cup	1.0	100	9%
generic				
dark	1 cup	2.0	326	6%
light	1 cup	1.0	340	3%
whole-grain	1 cup	2.0	335	5%
(Hodgson Mill)	⅓ cup	1.0	160	6%
cake or pastry				
(Arrowhead Mills) soft pastry	¼ cup	0.5	100	5%
(Betty Crocker) Softasilk velvet cake	¼ cup	–	100	–
generic	1 cup	1.0	430	2%
(Swan's Down) cake	¼ cup	–	100	–
carob				
(St. John's Bread)	1 cup	3.0	420	6%
chestnut	4 oz	4.0	410	9%
corn	1 oz	0.7	102	6%
	1 cup	3.0	430	6%

Food and Description	Amount	Fat Grams	Total Calories	% Fat Calories
cottonseed				
low-fat	1 oz	–	95	–
partially defatted	1 oz	–	40	–
	1 cup	6.0	335	16%
garbanzo/toasted				
(Arrowhead Mills)	¼ cup	1.0	90	10%
gluten				
(Arrowhead Mills) Vital wheat gluten	3 Tbs	–	35	–
(Betty Crocker) Supreme Hygluten	¼ cup	–	100	–
generic	1 cup	3.0	530	5%
kamut				
(Arrowhead Mills)	¼ cup	0.5	110	4%
millet				
(Arrowhead Mills)	¼ cup	1.0	110	8%
multigrain				
(Arrowhead Mills) multi-blend	¼ cup	0.5	120	4%
oat				
(Arrowhead Mills)	⅓ cup	2.0	120	15%
(Hodgson Mill) oat bran blend	¼ cup	1.0	110	8%
peanut				
defatted	1 oz	–	92	–
	1 cup	–	200	–
low-fat	1 oz	6.0	120	45%
	1 cup	13.0	260	45%
pecan	1 oz	–	93	–
potato	1 cup	1.5	632	2%
quinoa				
(Quinoa) gluten-free, whole-grain	¼ cup	2.0	130	14%
rice				
(Arrowhead Mills)				
brown	¼ cup	1.0	120	8%
white	¼ cup	0.5	130	3%
generic				
brown	1 oz	<1.0	100	5%
white	1 oz	<1.0	100	2%
	1 cup	1.0	398	2%
(Tres Estrellas)	¼ cup	1.0	150	6%
rye				
(Arrowhead Mills)	¼ cup	1.0	100	9%
generic				
dark	1 cup	3.0	419	6%
light	1 cup	1.0	364	3%
(Hodgson Mill)	¼ cup	1.0	90	10%
(Krusteaz) medium	⅓ cup	0.5	110	4%
(Pillsbury)				
Bohemian style rye-wheat	¼ cup	–	100	–
medium	¼ cup	–	100	–

Food and Description	Amount	Fat Grams	Total Calories	% Fat Calories
sesame				
high-fat	4 oz	42.0	595	64%
low-fat	1 cup	–	95	–
	4 oz	2.0	380	5%
partially defatted	4 oz	14.0	440	29%
soy				
(Arrowhead Mills)	½ cup	9.0	200	41%
generic				
defatted	1 cup	1.0	327	3%
full-fat				
not stirred	1 cup	17.6	358	44%
stirred	1 cup	14.0	295	43%
gluten-free	½ cup	<1.0	180	3%
low-fat	1 cup	6.0	326	17%
spelt				
(Arrowhead Mills)	¼ cup	0.5	100	5%
sunflower seed	1 Tbs	<1.0	16	4%
	1 cup	1.3	261	4%
triticale	1 oz	0.5	95	5%
	1 cup	2.5	440	5%
white				
(Arrowhead Mills)				
semolina mix	½ cup	1.0	240	4%
unbleached	⅓ cup	0.5	160	3%
(Betty Crocker)				
All Trump	¼ cup	–	100	–
Gold Medal				
all-purpose	¼ cup	–	100	–
self-rising	¼ cup	–	100	–
unbleached	¼ cup	–	100	–
Wondra	¼ cup	–	100	–
La Pina	¼ cup	–	100	–
Red Band				
all-purpose	¼ cup	–	100	–
self-rising	¼ cup	–	100	–
Robin Hood				
all-purpose	¼ cup	–	100	–
self-rising	¼ cup	–	100	–
unbleached	¼ cup	–	100	–
generic				
all-purpose	1 cup	1.0	401	2%
self-rising	1 cup	1.0	440	2%
(Hodgson Mill)				
regular	¼ cup	–	100	–
seasoned	¼ cup	–	90	–
(Pillsbury)				
all-purpose				
bleached	¼ cup	–	100	–

Food and Description	Amount	Fat Grams	Total Calories	% Fat Calories
unbleached	¼ cup	–	100	–
self-rising				
bleached	¼ cup	–	100	–
unbleached	¼ cup	–	100	–
shake & blend	¼ cup	–	100	–
(Quaker) Aunt Jemima self-rising/ enriched	3 Tbs	–	90	–
whole wheat				
(Alma)				
coarse wheat	¼ cup	–	100	–
fine wheat	¼ cup	–	100	–
(Arrowhead Mills)				
stone-ground	¼ cup	0.5	130	3%
whole-grain	¼ cup	0.5	110	4%
(Betty Crocker) Gold Medal				
whole wheat	¼ cup	0.5	90	5%
whole wheat blend	¼ cup	0.5	100	5%
generic				
regular	1 cup	2.0	400	5%
stone-ground	2 oz	1.0	200	5%
(Hodgson Mill)				
50/50	¼ cup	1.0	100	9%
whole wheat	¼ cup	1.0	100	9%
(Pillsbury)	¼ cup	1.0	120	8%

FRANKFURTER (*See also* FRANKFURTER, VEGETARIAN; SAUSAGE; VEGETARIAN FOODS; individual FAST FOOD listings)

Food and Description	Amount	Fat Grams	Total Calories	% Fat Calories
(Armour) beef & turkey	2 oz	6.0	90	60%
(Ball Park)				
beef				
bun size	1 frank	16.0	180	80%
regular	1 frank	16.0	180	80%
Fun Franks/microwave	2 pkgs	21.0	230	54%
lite	1 frank	8.0	110	65%
meat				
bun size	1 frank	16.0	180	80%
regular	1 frank	16.0	180	80%
(Best's) kosher/lower fat	1 frank	8.0	110	66%
(Butterball) turkey	1 frank	11.0	130	76%
(Denver Buffalo Co.) Buffalo Will's Western hot dogs w/buffalo & beef	1 frank	8.0	110	65%
(Don Lee Farms) beef corn dogs	1 corn dog	9.0	200	9%
(Eckrich) jumbo				
cheese	1 frank	17.0	180	85%
regular	1 frank	17.0	190	80%
generic				
Cheesefurter	1.5 oz	12.5	141	80%

Food and Description	Amount	Fat Grams	Total Calories	% Fat Calories
(Healthy Choice)				
beef	1 frank	1.0	60	26%
bun size	1 frank	2.0	70	26%
regular	1 frank	1.0	50	18%
(Hebrew National)				
cocktail franks				
2-oz link/4 per pkg	1 link	16.0	180	80%
1.8-oz link/6 per pkg	1 link	15.0	160	84%
dinner franks/beef	4 oz	34.0	350	87%
Dr. Stein's kosher beef bagel dog	1 frank	17.0	400	38%
franks				
beef	1.7 oz	14.0	150	84%
lite	1.7 oz	10.0	120	75%
(Hillshire Farm)				
franks				
bun size				
beef	2 oz	16.0	180	80%
cheese	2 oz	16.0	180	80%
regular	2 oz	16.0	180	80%
light & mild/jumbo	1 frank	8.0	110	65%
Lit'l Beef	2 oz	16.0	180	80%
wieners				
bun size	2 oz	17.0	180	85%
light & mild	1 wiener	7.0	90	70%
Lit'l	2 oz	16.0	180	80%
natural casing	2 oz	17.0	180	85%
(Hormel)				
cocktail franks				
smokies	5 smokies	16.0	180	80%
wieners	5 wieners	14.0	160	79%
corn dogs	2.75 oz	11.0	220	45%
franks				
beef/10 per pkg	1 frank	12.0	140	77%
Big 8	1 frank	17.0	180	85%
(Light & Lean 97)				
beef	1 frank	1.0	45	20%
jumbo	1 frank	1.5	60	23%
regular	1 frank	1.0	45	20%
meat/10 per pkg	1 frank	13.0	140	84%
(Wranglers)				
beef	1 frank	15.0	170	79%
cheese	1 frank	15.0	170	79%
smoked	1 frank	15.0	170	79%
(Jimmy Dean) mini hot dogs	2 hot dogs	13.0	210	56%
(Kahn's)				
franks				
beef				
bun size	1 frank	17.0	190	81%

Food and Description	Amount	Fat Grams	Total Calories	% Fat Calories
jumbo	2 oz	18.0	190	85%
regular	1 frank	13.0	140	84%
beef 'n cheddar	1 frank	16.0	180	80%
fat-free/jumbo	1 frank	–	40	–
pork & beef				
bun size	1 frank	17.0	190	81%
jumbo	2 oz	16.0	170	85%
smoky				
Big Red	1 frank	14.0	170	74%
bun size	1 frank	15.0	180	75%
wieners				
bun size	2 oz	16.0	180	80%
cheese	1 wiener	13.0	150	78%
regular	1 wiener	13.0	140	84%
(Louis Rich)				
bun-length/8 per 16-oz pkg	1 frank	8.0	110	65%
cheese/10 per 16-oz pkg	1 frank	7.0	90	70%
turkey & chicken				
10 per 16-oz pkg	1 frank	6.0	80	68%
8 per 12-oz pkg	1 frank	6.0	80	68%
(Oscar Mayer)				
franks				
big & juicy/beef				
deli style	1 frank	22.0	230	86%
original	1 frank	22.0	240	83%
quarter pound	1 frank	33.0	350	85%
bun-length	1 frank	17.0	180	85%
light	1 frank	8.0	110	65%
regular				
beef	1 frank	13.0	140	77%
cheese	1 frank	13.0	140	77%
hot dogs/Free/fat-free	1 hot dog	–	40	–
wieners				
big & juicy				
hot 'n spicy	1 wiener	20.0	220	82%
original beef	1 wiener	22.0	240	83%
Smokie Links	1 wiener	19.0	220	78%
bun-length/pork & turkey	1 wiener	17.0	180	85%
light/pork, turkey, & beef	1 wiener	9.0	110	74%
regular				
little				
hot & spicy	6 links	15.0	160	84%
original	6 links	17.0	180	85%
pork & turkey	1 link	13.0	150	78%
regular/pork & turkey	1 wiener	13.0	150	78%
(Perdue)				
chicken franks	1 frank	11.0	140	71%
turkey franks	1 frank	8.0	106	68%

Food and Description	Amount	Fat Grams	Total Calories	% Fat Calories
(Schwan's)				
franks/skinless	1 link	13.0	140	84%
wieners/old-fashioned	1 link	15.0	170	79%
(State Fair) beef corn dogs	1 corn dog	10.0	210	43%
(Tyson)				
cheese	1 frank	11.0	145	68%
chicken	1 frank	10.0	115	78%
chicken corn dogs	1 frank	14.0	280	45%
(Woody's) Corny Dogs	1 corn dog	11.0	210	47%
FRANKFURTER, VEGETARIAN (*See also* VEGETARIAN FOODS)				
(Loma Linda)				
Big Franks	1 frank	7.0	110	57%
corn dogs	1 corn dog	9.0	200	41%
Linketts	1 link	4.5	70	58%
Little Links	2 links	6.0	90	69%
(Lightlife)				
Smart Dogs	1.5 oz	–	45	–
Tofu Pups	1.5 oz	2.5	60	38%
Wonderdogs	1.5 oz	1.0	55	16%
(Morningstar Farms) deli franks	1 frank	7.0	110	57%
(Worthington)				
Leanies/frozen	1.4 oz	6.0	100	54%
Super-Links	1.7 oz	7.0	100	63%
Veja-Links/canned	2.2 oz	10.0	140	64%
(Yves) Veggie Cuisine				
chili dogs	1 chili dog	–	70	–
tofu wieners	1 wiener	0.5	57	8%
veggie wieners	1 wiener	–	60	–
FRANKFURTER WRAP				
(Wiener Wrap) refrigerated	1 wrap	2.0	60	30%
FRENCH FRIES (*See* FROZEN ENTRÉE/DINNER; POTATO; individual FAST FOOD listings)				
FRENCH ONION SOUP (*See* SOUP)				
FRENCH TOAST				
(Aunt Jemima)				
cinnamon swirl	2 slices	6.0	240	23%
original	2 slices	6.0	240	23%
(Downyflake)				
cinnamon swirl	2 slices	6.0	260	21%
plain	2 slices	6.0	260	21%
(Farm Rich) sticks				
apple-cinnamon	1 serving	15.0	310	44%
blueberry	1 serving	14.0	310	41%
original	1 serving	15.0	300	45%
(Hain) homestyle	1 slice	3.5	130	24%
homemade/USDA Standard Home Recipe	1 slice	7.0	155	41%
(Krusteaz)				
cinnamon swirl	2 slices	5.0	230	20%

Food and Description	Amount	Fat Grams	Total Calories	% Fat Calories
classic style	2 slices	5.0	230	20%
sourdough	1 slice	2.0	140	13%
(Morningstar Farms) vegetarian				
cinnamon swirl w/patties	6.5 oz	15.0	380	36%
(Nulaid) liquid mix	¼ cup	–	40	–
(Schwan's) apple-cinnamon sticks	5 sticks	22.0	450	44%
(Swanson)				
French stix w/syrup	1 meal	10.0	320	28%
Great Starts				
cinnamon swirl w/sausages	5½ oz	21.0	390	48%
mini w/sausage	2.5 oz	9.0	190	43%
regular w/sausage	5.5 oz	21.0	380	50%
oatmeal w/lite links	4.65 oz	13.0	310	38%
Kid's Breakfast Blast				
mini French stix w/syrup	1 meal	14.0	310	41%
FRITTER (See also CORN DISHES; PASTRY)				
USDA Standard Home Recipe	1 fritter	7.5	132	51%
FROG/legs				
floured & fried	1 oz	4.8	70	61%
	3 oz	17.0	250	61%
raw	3 oz	<1.0	63	7%
FROSTING (See CAKE ICING/FROSTING)				
FROZEN ENTRÉE/DINNER (See also ASIAN FOOD; BEEF DISH/ENTRÉE; CHICKEN ENTRÉE/DINNER; MEXICAN FOOD; PASTA DISH; PIZZA; POTATO DISH; RICE DISH; VEGETARIAN FOODS)				
▨ (Armour)				
Classics				
beef pepper/lite	11 oz	4.0	210	17%
chicken & noodles	11 oz	9.0	280	29%
chicken Burgundy/lite	10 oz	5.0	210	21%
chicken fettuccini	10 oz	8.0	230	36%
chicken mesquite	9.5 oz	13.0	280	42%
chicken Parmigiana	10.75 oz	18.0	360	45%
chicken w/wine & mushroom sauce	10 oz	11.0	260	38%
glazed chicken	10.75 oz	14.0	280	45%
meat loaf	11.25 oz	10.0	300	30%
Salisbury steak				
lite	11.5 oz	7.0	260	24%
regular	11.25 oz	18.0	330	49%
shrimp Creole/lite	10 oz	5.0	220	20%
Swedish meatballs	10 oz	17.0	300	51%
sweet & sour chicken/lite	11 oz	1.0	220	4%
turkey & dressing w/gravy	11.25 oz	7.0	270	23%
veal Parmigiana	11.25 oz	22.0	400	50%
▨ (Award)				
entrées				
beef pie	7 oz	18.0	350	46%
chicken pie	7 oz	19.0	350	49%

Food and Description	Amount	Fat Grams	Total Calories	% Fat Calories
■ **(Banquet)**				
casseroles & pot pies				
macaroni & cheese	7 oz	3.0	200	14%
vegetable pie				
w/beef	7 oz	15.0	330	41%
w/chicken	7 oz	18.0	350	46%
w/turkey	7 oz	20.0	370	49%
vegetables & cheese	7 oz	18.0	390	42%
dinners				
BBQ style chicken	9 oz	12.0	320	34%
beef	9 oz	7.0	240	26%
beef enchilada	11 oz	12.0	320	34%
cheese enchilada	11 oz	6.0	350	15%
chicken & dumpling	10 oz	8.0	260	28%
chicken chow mein	9 oz	7.0	400	16%
chicken enchilada	11 oz	10.0	360	25%
chicken nuggets	6.75 oz	21.0	420	45%
chicken Parmigiana	9.5 oz	15.0	290	47%
chicken-fried steak	10 oz	20.0	400	45%
chimichanga meal	9.5 oz	23.0	470	44%
fried chicken	9 oz	27.0	470	52%
gravy & beef patty	9.5 oz	20.0	300	60%
meat loaf	9.5 oz	17.0	280	55%
Mexican style	11 oz	13.0	340	34%
Mexican style combination	11 oz	11.0	380	26%
Oriental style chicken	9 oz	9.0	260	31%
Salisbury steak	9.5 oz	16.0	310	46%
Southern fried meal	8.75 oz	30.0	260	36%
turkey & gravy w/dressing	9.25 oz	10.0	270	33%
veal Parmigiana	9 oz	14.0	530	24%
Western style meal	9.5 oz	20.0	210	86%
white meat meal	8.75 oz	28.0	470	54%
Extra Helping Dinners				
all white chicken	18 oz	41.0	820	45%
chicken Parmigiana	19 oz	33.0	650	46%
chicken-fried steak	18.5 oz	44.0	800	50%
fried chicken	18 oz	39.0	790	44%
meat loaf	19 oz	38.0	650	53%
Mexican style	22 oz	34.0	820	37%
Salisbury steak	19 oz	45.0	740	55%
Southern-fried chicken	17.5 oz	37.0	750	44%
turkey	18.8 oz	20.0	560	32%
Family Entrées				
beef enchilada w/cheese	4.67 oz	4.0	130	28%
beef stew	8.13 oz	4.0	160	23%
chicken & dumplings	7.47 oz	14.0	290	43%
chicken Parmigiana	4.67 oz	13.0	240	49%
chicken pie	8 oz	30.0	450	60%

Food and Description	Amount	Fat Grams	Total Calories	% Fat Calories
gravy & sliced beef	5.6 oz	3.0	100	27%
gravy & sliced turkey	4.8 oz	5.0	100	45%
gravy w/charbroiled beef	4.67 oz	13.0	180	65%
lasagna w/meat sauce	8 oz	7.0	240	26%
macaroni & beef	8 oz	7.0	230	27%
macaroni & cheese	8 oz	10.0	300	30%
noodles & beef w/gravy	7.47 oz	4.0	140	26%
noodles & chicken	8 oz	9.0	210	39%
onion gravy & beef patties	4.67 oz	14.0	180	70%
Salisbury steak	4.67 oz	14.0	200	63%
veal Parmagiana	4.67 oz	14.0	230	55%
Hot Sandwich Toppers				
chicken à la king	4.5 oz	4.0	100	36%
creamed chipped beef	4 oz	3.0	100	27%
gravy & sliced beef	4 oz	2.0	70	26%
gravy & sliced turkey	5 oz	4.0	90	40%
Salisbury steak	5 oz	16.0	220	65%
sloppy joe	4 oz	7.0	140	45%
■ (Budget Gourmet)				
dinners/Light & Healthy				
beef sirloin meatballs & gravy	11 oz	8.0	310	23%
beef sirloin Salisbury steak w/red potatoes	11 oz	8.0	260	28%
chicken in mesquite barbecue sauce	11 oz	6.0	280	19%
chicken Parmigiana	11 oz	10.0	300	30%
herbed chicken	11 oz	8.0	300	24%
honey mustard chicken breast	11 oz	6.0	310	17%
roast chicken breast w/herb gravy	11 oz	7.0	240	26%
shrimp mariner	11 oz	6.0	260	21%
sliced sirloin in wine	11 oz	6.0	270	20%
special recipe sirloin beef	11 oz	7.0	310	20%
stuffed turkey breast	11 oz	6.0	260	21%
teriyaki beef	10.75 oz	6.0	310	17%
teriyaki chicken breast	11 oz	6.0	290	16%
Yankee pot roast	10.5 oz	7.0	270	23%
entrées				
Light & Healthy				
baked potato w/broccoli & cheese	10.5 oz	8.0	270	27%
beef sirloin Salisbury steak	9 oz	5.0	240	19%
beef stroganoff	8.75 oz	7.0	290	22%
cheese ravioli	9.5 oz	13.0	310	38%
chicken au gratin	9.1 oz	8.0	250	29%
chicken Oriental	9 oz	6.0	300	18%
French recipe chicken & vegetables	10 oz	8.0	240	30%
glazed turkey	9 oz	4.0	250	25%
ham & asparagus au gratin	8.7 oz	13.0	290	40%
lasagna w/meat sauce	9.4 oz	7.0	250	25%
linguine w/shrimp & clams	9.5 oz	8.0	280	26%

Food and Description	Amount	Fat Grams	Total Calories	% Fat Calories
Mandarin chicken	10 oz	5.0	250	18%
orange glazed chicken breast	9 oz	2.0	300	6%
Oriental beef	10 oz	8.0	270	27%
sirloin beef in herb sauce	9.5 oz	7.0	260	24%
vegetable lasagna	10.5 oz	10.0	290	31%
original				
beef Cantonese	9.1 oz	8.0	280	26%
cheese manicotti w/meat sauce	10 oz	22.0	420	47%
chicken & egg noodles w/broccoli	10 oz	23.0	410	50%
chicken Marsala	9 oz	7.0	270	23%
chicken w/fettuccini	10 oz	19.0	380	45%
Italian sausage lasagna	10.5 oz	21.0	430	40%
linguine w/shrimp	10 oz	11.0	300	33%
Mandarin vegetable	5.5 oz	13.0	180	65%
open-faced roast beef w/mashed potatoes & gravy	8 oz	17.0	340	45%
open-faced turkey & gravy w/mashed potatoes	8 oz	15.0	330	41%
pepper steak w/rice	10 oz	8.0	290	25%
roast sirloin supreme	9.5 oz	13.0	300	39%
sirloin cheddar melt	9.4 oz	21.0	370	51%
sirloin tips w/country style vegetables	10 oz	13.0	250	47%
Swedish meatballs	10 oz	34.0	550	56%
sweet & sour chicken w/rice	10 oz	5.0	330	14%
three cheese lasagna	10.5 oz	16.0	370	39%
side dishes				
cheddared potatoes	5.5 oz	17.0	260	59%
cheddared potatoes & broccoli	5.25 oz	8.0	170	42%
cheese tortellini	6.25 oz	8.0	190	40%
macaroni & cheese	6 oz	13.0	270	43%
Mandarin vegetables	5.5 oz	13.0	180	65%
New England recipe vegetables	5.5 oz	16.0	240	60%
Oriental rice & vegetables	5.75 oz	12.0	220	49%
pasta Alfredo w/broccoli	5.8 oz	11.0	230	47%
rice pilaf w/green beans	5.62 oz	12.0	230	47%
spinach au gratin	5.5 oz	11.0	150	66%
spring vegetables in cheese sauce	5.5 oz	10.0	150	60%
three cheese potatoes	6.125 oz	12.0	230	47%
ziti in Marinara sauce	6.25 oz	10.0	220	41%
Special Selections				
Light & Healthy				
Chinese style vegetables & chicken	10 oz	9.0	290	28%
Italian style vegetables & chicken	10 oz	7.0	280	23%
macaroni & cheese w/cheddar & Parmesan	10 oz	8.0	340	21%
penne pasta w/chunky tomato sauce & Italian sausage	10.8 oz	6.0	330	16%

Food and Description	Amount	Fat Grams	Total Calories	% Fat Calories
rigatoni in cream sauce w/broccoli & chicken	10.8 oz	6.0	310	17%
spaghetti w/chunky tomato & meat sauce	10 oz	7.0	320	20%
original				
escalloped noodles & turkey	10.75 oz	20.0	440	41%
fettuccini Alfredo w/four cheeses	11.5 oz	24.0	480	45%
homestyle macaroni & cheese	10 oz	20.0	400	45%
linguine w/tomato sauce & Italian sausage	10.25 oz	14.0	360	35%
spicy Szechwan style vegetables & chicken	10 oz	9.0	300	27%
wide ribbon pasta w/ricotta & tomato sauce	10.25 oz	22.0	420	47%
■ **(Campbell's)** food service				
meat lasagna	8 oz	15.0	360	38%
■ **(Celentano)**				
entrées				
baked pasta & cheese	6 oz	7.0	280	23%
broccoli stuffed shells	6.75 oz	14.0	270	47%
cannelloni Florentine	12 oz	8.0	350	21%
cavatelli	3.2 oz	1.0	250	4%
chicken Parmigiana	9 oz	21.0	400	47%
chicken primavera	11.5 oz	7.0	260	24%
eggplant Parmigiana				
16-oz pkg	8 oz	15.0	280	48%
10-oz pkg	7 oz	21.0	320	59%
25-oz pkg	6.25 oz	10.0	260	35%
eggplant rollettes	11 oz	14.0	320	39%
lasagna				
low-fat	10 oz	2.5	260	9%
regular				
14-oz pkg	7 oz	10.0	280	32%
16-oz pkg	8 oz	19.0	370	46%
25-oz pkg	6.25 oz	16.0	300	48%
lasagna primavera	10 oz	7.0	240	38%
manicotti				
14-oz pkg	7 oz	15.0	310	44%
16-oz pkg	8 oz	11.0	300	33%
10-oz pkg	10 oz	14.0	380	37%
ravioli				
low-fat	10 oz	2.5	260	9%
mini	4 oz	5.0	250	18%
regular	6.5 oz	11.0	380	26%
stuffed shells				
low-fat	3 shells	2.5	250	9%
regular				
16-oz pkg	8 oz	11.0	330	30%

Food and Description	Amount	Fat Grams	Total Calories	% Fat Calories
10-oz pkg	10 oz	14.0	410	31%
12.5-oz pkg	6.25 oz	16.0	340	42%
■ **(Chef America)** stuffed sandwiches				
Hot Pockets				
barbecue	1 sandwich	12.0	340	32%
beef & cheddar	1 sandwich	18.0	360	45%
beef fajita	1 sandwich	17.0	360	43%
chicken & cheddar w/broccoli	1 sandwich	12.0	300	36%
ham & cheese	1 sandwich	15.0	340	40%
pepperoni pizza	1 sandwich	17.0	350	44%
pepperoni & sausage	1 sandwich	16.0	340	42%
sausage pizza	1 sandwich	16.0	350	42%
turkey & ham w/cheese	1 sandwich	13.0	320	37%
Lean Pockets				
beef & broccoli	1 sandwich	7.0	250	25%
chicken fajita	1 sandwich	8.0	260	28%
chicken Parmesan	1 sandwich	8.0	260	28%
glazed chicken	1 sandwich	7.0	240	26%
pizza deluxe	1 sandwich	8.0	270	27%
turkey, broccoli, & cheese	1 sandwich	7.0	260	24%
turkey & ham w/cheese	1 sandwich	7.0	260	24%
■ **(Farm Rich)**				
frozen snacks				
grilled cheese sticks	2 pieces	9.0	150	54%
jalapeño cheese snacks	2 pieces	6.0	100	54%
■ **(Freezer Queen)**				
Family Supper				
gravy & Salisbury steak	10 oz	22.0	380	52%
mushroom gravy & charbroiled beef patties	10 oz	17.0	300	51%
onion gravy & beef patties	10 oz	18.0	320	51%
Salisbury steak	10 oz	22.0	380	52%
■ **(Golden)**				
blintzes				
apple-raisin	2.25 oz	2.0	80	23%
blueberry	2.25 oz	1.0	90	10%
cheese	2.25 oz	2.0	80	23%
cherry	2.25 oz	1.0	95	9%
potato	2.25 oz	4.0	90	40%
pierogies				
potato-cheese	3 pierogies	8.0	250	29%
potato-onion	3 pierogies	6.0	210	17%
potato pancakes				
Mexican	1 pancake	2.0	70	26%
regular	1 pancake	3.0	71	34%
■ **(Great Value)**				
entrées				
beef pie	7 oz	19.0	390	44%

Food and Description	Amount	Fat Grams	Total Calories	% Fat Calories
chicken pie	7 oz	20.0	380	47%
turkey pie	7 oz	22.0	400	50%
■ (Growing Healthy Baby Food) (See BABY FOOD)				
■ (Hain)				
Vegetarian Classics				
Hawaiian nuggets	10 oz	5.0	310	15%
Mexican style taco	10 oz	9.0	420	19%
pepper steak	10 oz	6.0	310	17%
radiatore Bolognese	10 oz	2.5	290	8%
■ (Healthy Choice)				
classics				
beef broccoli Beijing	1 meal	3.0	330	8%
cacciatore chicken	1 meal	3.0	260	10%
chicken Francesca	1 meal	5.0	360	13%
country inn roast turkey	1 meal	4.0	250	14%
ginger chicken Hunan	1 meal	2.5	350	5%
mesquite beef w/BBQ sauce	1 meal	4.0	310	12%
pasta Salisbury steak	1 meal	6.0	260	21%
pasta shells marinara	1 meal	4.0	370	10%
sesame chicken	1 meal	5.0	310	15%
shrimp & vegetables Maria	1 meal	3.0	270	10%
traditional Swedish meatballs	1 meal	9.0	320	25%
turkey fettuccini	1 meal	4.0	350	10%
dinners				
beef & pepper Cantonese	1 meal	5.0	270	17%
beef enchilada Rio Grande	1 meal	8.0	410	18%
beef stroganoff	1 meal	6.0	310	17%
beef tips w/BBQ	1 meal	6.0	290	19%
cacciatore chicken	1 meal	4.0	300	12%
chicken broccoli Alfredo	1 meal	8.0	370	19%
chicken Cantonese	1 meal	0.5	210	2%
chicken Dijon	1 meal	4.0	280	13%
chicken enchilada	1 meal	6.0	320	17%
chicken Parmigiana	1 meal	4.0	240	15%
chicken picante	1 meal	2.0	220	8%
country breaded chicken	1 meal	7.0	350	18%
country herb chicken	1 meal	4.0	270	13%
lemon pepper fish	1 meal	5.0	290	16%
mesquite chicken BBQ	1 meal	2.0	320	6%
shrimp marinara	1 meal	0.5	220	2%
smoky chicken BBQ	1 meal	5.0	380	12%
Southwest glazed chicken	1 meal	3.0	300	9%
sweet & sour chicken	1 meal	5.0	310	15%
teriyaki chicken	1 meal	2.0	270	7%
traditional beef tips	1 meal	5.0	260	17%
traditional breast of turkey	1 meal	3.0	280	10%
traditional meat loaf	1 meal	5.0	320	14%

Food and Description	Amount	Fat Grams	Total Calories	% Fat Calories
traditional Salisbury steak	1 meal	6.0	320	17%
Yankee pot roast	1 meal	5.0	280	16%
entrées & quick meals				
beef macaroni	1 meal	1.0	200	5%
beef pepper steak Oriental	1 meal	4.0	250	14%
beef tips Francais	1 meal	5.0	280	16%
broccoli & cheese potato casserole	1 meal	5.0	310	15%
cheese ravioli Parmigiana	1 meal	4.0	250	14%
chicken enchilada suiza	1 meal	7.0	300	21%
chicken fettuccini Alfredo	1 meal	3.0	250	11%
chicken imperial	1 meal	4.0	230	16%
chicken & vegetables Marsala	1 meal	1.0	220	4%
country glazed chicken	1 meal	1.5	200	7%
country roast turkey w/mushrooms	1 meal	4.0	220	16%
fettuccini Alfredo	1 meal	5.0	240	19%
fiesta chicken fajitas	1 meal	4.0	260	14%
garden potato casserole	1 meal	4.0	200	18%
garlic chicken Milano	1 meal	4.0	240	15%
honey mustard chicken	1 meal	2.0	260	7%
lasagna Roma	1 meal	5.0	390	12%
macaroni & cheese	1 meal	5.0	290	16%
manicotti w/3 cheeses	1 meal	9.0	310	26%
Mandarin chicken	1 meal	2.5	280	8%
pepperoni French bread pizza	1 pizza	9.0	360	23%
sausage French bread pizza	1 pizza	4.0	330	11%
sesame chicken	1 meal	3.0	240	11%
spaghetti Bolognese	1 meal	3.0	260	10%
vegetable pasta Italiano	1 meal	1.0	220	4%
zucchini lasagna	1 meal	1.5	330	4%
Handfuls				
chicken & broccoli	1 Handful	5.0	320	14%
chicken & mushroom	1 Handful	4.0	300	12%
garlic chicken	1 Handful	5.0	330	14%
Philly beef steak	1 Handful	5.0	290	16%
roast beef	1 Handful	4.5	310	13%
turkey & vegetables	1 Handful	4.5	310	13%
■ (Heinz)				
Bagel Bites				
cheese & sausage	4 Bites	7.0	200	32%
cheeseburger	4 Bites	7.0	210	30%
supreme	4 Bites	5.0	180	25%
Cheese Bites				
Monterey jack	2 Bites	7.0	100	63%
Dyna Bites				
broccoli & cheese	2 Bites	5.0	90	50%
cheese & pepperoni	3 Bites	15.0	210	64%
Monterey jack & jalapeño	2 Bites	6.0	100	54%

Food and Description	Amount	Fat Grams	Total Calories	% Fat Calories
■ (Hormel)				
Mrs. Patterson's Aussie Pie				
chicken	1 pie	25.0	460	49%
steak & mushroom	1 pie	24.0	420	51%
turkey w/broccoli	1 pie	26.0	470	50%
quick meal				
BBQ beef sandwich	1 sandwich	16.0	360	40%
BBQ pork sandwich	1 sandwich	15.0	350	39%
Cheesy Dog	1 "dog"	17.0	310	49%
chicken Sandwich	1 sandwich	12.0	340	32%
chili dog w/cheese	1 "dog"	20.0	350	51%
corn dog				
mini	5 "dogs"	15.0	250	54%
regular	1 "dog"	11.0	220	45%
fish fillet sandwich	1 sandwich	16.0	400	36%
grilled chicken sandwich	1 sandwich	9.0	300	27%
ham & Swiss	1 sandwich	8.0	330	22%
jumbo dog	1 "dog"	21.0	350	54%
pepperoni bagel	1 bagel	15.0	350	39%
■ HOT POCKETS (*See* (Chef America) in this section.				
■ (Kibun Gold)				
chicken Oriental	8 oz	3.0	230	12%
Ellen's homestyle chicken	10 oz	4.0	300	12%
honey garlic chicken	10 oz	4.0	290	12%
lemon ginger beef	8 oz	4.0	230	16%
pasta & chicken				
w/dressing	½ pkg	9.0	220	37%
w/o dressing	½ pkg	2.0	150	12%
pasta & turkey ham				
w/dressing	½ pkg	12.0	250	43%
w/o dressing	½ pkg	2.0	140	13%
sweet & sour chicken	10 oz	1.0	310	3%
■ (Kid Cuisine)				
beef patty sandwich w/cheese	1 meal	15.0	410	33%
cheese pizza	1 meal	11.0	430	23%
chicken nuggets	1 meal	16.0	440	33%
chicken sandwich	1 meal	15.0	480	28%
fish sticks	1 meal	12.0	370	29%
fried chicken	1 meal	19.0	440	39%
hamburger pizza	1 meal	11.0	400	25%
macaroni & beef	1 meal	9.0	370	22%
macaroni & cheese	1 meal	12.0	420	26%
mini cheese ravioli	1 meal	4.5	320	13%
■ LEAN CUISINE (*See* (Stouffer's) in this section)				
■ LEAN POCKETS (*See* (Chef America) in this section)				
■ (Life Choice)				
entrées				
black bean burrito	1 meal	1.5	410	3%

Food and Description	Amount	Fat Grams	Total Calories	% Fat Calories
garden potato casserole	1 meal	0.5	160	3%
linguine Roma	1 meal	0.5	230	2%
sun-dried tomato manicotti	1 meal	2.5	220	10%
vegetable enchiladas Sonora	1 meal	1.5	420	3%
vegetable lasagna primavera	1 meal	1.0	170	5%
▆ **(Marie Callender's)**				
dinners				
chicken Parmigiana	1 dinner	27.0	620	39%
chicken-fried steak	1 dinner	31.0	650	43%
country fried chicken	1 dinner	27.0	610	40%
herb roasted chicken	1 dinner	42.0	670	56%
meat loaf w/mashed potatoes & vegetable	1 dinner	30.0	540	50%
turkey & dressing	1 dinner	17.0	530	29%
entrées				
angel hair pasta w/sausage & 2 breadsticks	1 cup + breadstick	15.0	370	36%
beef stroganoff w/noodles	1 cup	27.0	440	55%
breaded shrimp over angel hair pasta	1 cup	12.0	300	36%
Callender's deluxe pasta	1 cup	23.0	350	59%
chili & cornbread	1 cup + cornbread	13.0	350	33%
escalloped noodles & chicken				
40-oz pkg	1 cup	16.0	270	53%
13-oz pkg	1 cup	16.0	270	53%
extra cheese lasagna	1 cup	16.0	330	44%
fettuccini Alfredo	1 cup	21.0	350	54%
fettuccini primavera tortellini	1 cup	19.0	310	55%
fettuccini w/broccoli & chicken	1 cup	26.0	420	56%
lasagna w/meat sauce	1 cup	18.0	370	44%
macaroni & beef	1 cup + breadstick	11.0	310	32%
Marie's special macaroni & cheese	1 cup	17.0	420	36%
old-fashioned pot roast	1 cup	5.0	180	25%
pasta primavera w/chicken	1 cup	19.0	310	55%
ravioli marinara w/garlic bread	1 cup + garlic bread	14.0	370	34%
rigatoni Parmigiana				
40-oz pkg	1 cup	14.0	320	39%
13-oz pkg	1 cup + 1 breadstick	14.0	300	42%
spaghetti & meat sauce w/garlic bread	1 cup + garlic bread	10.0	260	35%
spaghetti w/marinara w/cheese & garlic bread	1 cup + garlic bread	10.0	270	33%
pot pies				
chicken				
17-oz pkg	1 cup	31.0	620	45%

Food and Description	Amount	Fat Grams	Total Calories	% Fat Calories
10-oz pkg	1 cup	34.0	520	59%
chicken & broccoli				
17-oz pkg	1 cup	49.0	800	55%
10-oz pkg	1 cup	38.0	620	55%
chicken au gratin				
17-oz pkg	1 cup	53.0	740	64%
10-oz pkg	1 cup	41.0	610	60%
turkey				
17-oz pkg	1 cup	47.0	740	57%
10-oz pkg	1 cup	37.0	570	58%
Yankee				
17-oz pkg	1 cup	39.0	640	54%
10-oz pkg	1 cup	31.0	490	57%
■ **(Michelina's)**				
entrées				
Alfredo w/broccoli & chicken	1 pkg	13.0	350	33%
cheese ravioli w/Alfredo & broccoli sauce	1 pkg	24.0	420	51%
cheese tortellini	1 pkg	13.0	360	33%
chicken à la king	1 pkg	7.0	260	24%
chili mac	1 pkg	8.0	290	25%
creamed sauce, croutons, & shaved cured beef	1 pkg	20.0	360	50%
egg noodles & Swedish meatballs w/gravy	1 pkg	12.0	320	34%
fettuccine Alfredo	1 pkg	18.0	430	38%
double-serving pkg	1 cup	16.0	350	41%
fettuccine carbonara	1 pkg	13.0	370	32%
lasagna Alfredo	1 pkg	18.0	390	42%
double-serving pkg	1 cup	16.0	350	41%
lasagna pollo	1 pkg	12.0	330	33%
lasagna w/meat sauce	1 pkg	10.0	320	28%
double-serving pkg	1 cup	8.0	290	25%
lasagna w/vegetables	1 pkg	6.0	270	20%
linguine w/clams	1 pkg	4.5	310	13%
linguine w/seafood	1 pkg	5.0	270	17%
macaroni & cheese	1 pkg	13.0	380	31%
double-serving pkg	1 cup	12.0	360	30%
marinara sauce, penne pasta, Italian sausages & peppers/ double-serving pkg	1 cup	7.0	240	26%
meat ravioli w/pomodoro sauce	1 pkg	12.0	300	36%
mostaccioli Parmesano	1 pkg	6.0	280	19%
noodles stroganoff	1 pkg	13.0	290	40%
noodles w/chicken, peas & carrots	1 pkg	10.0	280	32%
penne pasta w/marinara sauce & Italian sausage	1 pkg	8.0	270	27%

Food and Description	Amount	Fat Grams	Total Calories	% Fat Calories
penne pollo	1 pkg	11.0	330	30%
double-serving pkg	1 cup	10.0	300	30%
penne primavera	1 pkg	12.0	340	32%
rigatoni pomodoro	1 pkg	3.0	230	12%
risotto Parmesano	1 pkg	20.0	360	50%
shells & cheese w/jalapeño peppers	1 pkg	13.0	350	33%
spaghetti & pomodoro sauce				
w/6 meatballs/double-serving pkg	1 cup	5.0	230	20%
w/3 meatballs	1 pkg	6.0	290	19%
spaghetti Bolognese	1 pkg	6.0	270	20%
double-serving pkg	1 cup	5.0	240	19%
spaghetti marinara	1 pkg	3.0	250	11%
spinach ravioli w/primavera sauce	1 pkg	18.0	370	44%
turkey & dressing w/gravy	1 pkg	14.0	260	48%

■ MRS. PATTERSON'S AUSSIE PIE (*See* (Hormel) in this section)
■ **(Morton)**
casseroles & pot pies
macaroni & cheese

6-oz pkg	6 oz	3.0	160	17%
16-oz pkg	8 oz	6.0	220	25%
28-oz pkg	8 oz	4.0	230	16%
vegetable pie				
w/beef	7 oz	17.0	310	49%
w/chicken	7 oz	18.0	320	51%
w/turkey	7 oz	18.0	300	54%

dinners

breaded chicken patty	6.75 oz	15.0	280	48%
chicken nuggets	7 oz	17.0	320	48%
fried chicken	9 oz	25.0	420	54%
meat loaf	9 oz	13.0	250	47%
Mexican	10 oz	7.0	260	24%
Salisbury steak	9 oz	9.0	210	39%
turkey	9 oz	8.0	230	31%
Western meal	9 oz	16.0	290	50%

■ **(Pasta Favorites)**

chicken lo mein	10.5 oz	6.0	270	20%
chicken pasta prima	10.5 oz	13.0	330	35%
fettuccini Alfredo	10.5 oz	18.0	370	44%
Italian sausage & peppers	10.5 oz	13.0	340	34%
lasagna	10.5 oz	9.0	290	28%
macaroni & cheese	10.5 oz	12.0	350	31%
pasta primavera	10.5 oz	14.0	320	39%
spaghetti w/meatballs	10.5 oz	16.0	370	39%
vegetable lasagna	10.5 oz	6.0	260	21%
white cheddar & rotini	10.5 oz	12.0	350	31%

■ **(Patio)**
dinners

beef enchilada	12 oz	8.0	320	23%

Food and Description	Amount	Fat Grams	Total Calories	% Fat Calories
cheese enchilada	12 oz	8.0	330	22%
chicken enchilada	12 oz	9.0	380	21%
Fiesta	12 oz	9.0	340	24%
Mexican	13.25 oz	15.0	440	31%
Ranchera	13 oz	15.0	410	33%
salis con queso	11 oz	20.0	390	46%
Family Entrées				
beef & cheese enchilada	2 pieces w/sauce	6.0	250	22%
beef enchilada				
15.5-oz pkg	2 pieces w/sauce	7.0	250	25%
17-oz pkg	2 pieces w/sauce	4.0	170	21%
cheese enchilada	2 pieces w/sauce	4.0	170	21%
■ (Pepperidge Farm)				
Meal Kit				
beef stroganoff	1 filled	29.0	420	62%
chicken à la king	1 filled	26.0	400	59%
hors d'oeuvres	7 filled	28.0	470	54%
shrimp Newburg	1 filled	20.0	340	53%
vegetables in pastry				
broccoli w/cheese	1 pastry	14.0	240	53%
■ (Pitaria)				
Pita Stuffs				
gyros	6 oz	29.0	520	50%
ham 'n Swiss	6 oz	17.0	420	36%
pizza	6 oz	18.0	430	38%
taco	6 oz	16.0	390	37%
■ (Prego)				
beef Marsala w/noodles	11.3 oz	15.0	384	35%
■ (Sara Lee)				
croissants				
chicken & broccoli	1 croissant	13.0	280	42%
ham & Swiss cheese	1 croissant	16.0	300	48%
■ (Schwan's)				
Ethnic Choices				
Barquito meat trio	1 piece	22.0	390	51%
crab Rangoon	7 pieces	22.0	430	46%
Family Entrées				
beef casserole	1 cup	17.0	340	45%
beef shepherd's pie	1 cup	12.0	250	43%
California style vegetable lasagna	1 cup	10.0	210	43%
cheese ravioli	5 ravioli	13.0	320	37%
cheese tortellini	1 cup	6.0	240	23%
chicken Alfredo lasagna	1 cup	12.0	280	39%
chicken casserole	1 cup	17.0	360	43%

Food and Description	Amount	Fat Grams	Total Calories	% Fat Calories
chicken ravioli	5 ravioli	11.0	310	32%
chicken tortellini	1 cup	4.0	230	16%
homestyle beef goulash	1 cup	13.0	280	42%
lasagna w/beef sauce	1 cup	11.0	320	31%
macaroni & cheese	1 cup	20.0	340	53%
stuffed pasta shells	3 shells	15.0	330	41%
vegetable lasagna	1 cup	10.0	280	32%
sandwiches				
bagel dog w/cheese	1 sandwich	18.0	350	46%
chicken breast, unbreaded	1 sandwich	6.0	200	27%
club croissant	1 sandwich	19.0	310	55%
corn dog	1 sandwich	11.0	190	52%
French bread stuffed w/chicken & cheese	1 sandwich	8.0	270	27%
Ranchero	1 sandwich	18.0	400	41%
■ (Shanghai) stir-fry shrimp & Oriental vegetables	10.3 oz	2.0	140	13%
■ (Stouffer's)				
entrées				
beef pie	10 oz	26.0	450	52%
beef stroganoff w/parsley noodles	9.75 oz	20.0	390	46%
cheese enchilada & Mexican rice	9.75 oz	14.0	370	36%
cheese manicotti	9 oz	16.0	340	42%
chicken à la king w/rice	9.5 oz	10.0	320	28%
chicken enchilada & Mexican rice	10 oz	14.0	370	34%
chicken pie				
16-oz pkg	8 oz	35.0	540	58%
10-oz pkg	10 oz	36.0	560	58%
chili w/beans	8.75 oz	10.0	270	33%
creamed chicken	6.5 oz	20.0	280	64%
creamed chipped beef	½ cup	11.0	160	62%
creamy chicken & broccoli	8⅞ oz	15.0	320	42%
escalloped chicken & noodles	10 oz	28.0	450	56%
fettuccini Alfredo	10 oz	39.0	580	61%
four cheese lasagna	10.75 oz	19.0	410	42%
green pepper steak w/rice	10.5 oz	9.0	330	25%
ham & asparagus bake	9.5 oz	36.0	520	62%
lasagna w/meat sauce				
40-oz pkg	1 cup	10.0	260	35%
96-oz pkg	1 cup	12.0	290	37%
10½-oz pkg	10.5 oz	13.0	360	33%
21-oz pkg	1 cup	10.0	260	35%
macaroni & beef w/tomatoes	11.5 oz	20.0	420	43%
macaroni & cheese				
76-oz pkg	8.4 oz	14.0	340	37%
12-oz pkg	6 oz	17.0	330	46%
20-oz pkg	8 oz	16.0	310	46%
spaghetti w/meatballs	12⅝ oz	15.0	420	32%

Food and Description	Amount	Fat Grams	Total Calories	% Fat Calories
stuffed green peppers w/beef in tomato sauce	7.75 oz	7.0	180	35%
stuffed pepper/single serving	10 oz	8.0	200	36%
Swedish meatballs	11 oz	23.0	440	47%
tuna noodle casserole	10 oz	10.0	320	28%
turkey pie	10 oz	33.0	530	56%
turkey tetrazzini	10 oz	17.0	360	43%
vegetable lasagna				
96-oz pkg	1 cup	17.0	340	45%
10½-oz pkg	10.5 oz	23.0	450	46%
Homestyle Dinners				
baked chicken & gravy w/whipped potatoes	8⅞ oz	12.0	270	40%
beef pot roast & browned potatoes	8⅞ oz	10.0	270	33%
chicken & noodles	10 oz	13.0	300	39%
chicken fettuccini	10½ oz	15.0	390	35%
chicken Monterey w/Mexican-style rice	9⅜ oz	20.0	410	44%
chicken Parmigiana w/spaghetti	10⅞ oz	10.0	320	28%
fish fillet w/macaroni & cheese	9 oz	21.0	430	44%
fried chicken & whipped potatoes	7⅛ oz	16.0	330	44%
meat loaf & whipped potatoes	9⅞ oz	24.0	390	55%
roast turkey & homestyle stuffing	7⅞ oz	11.0	280	35%
Salisbury steak, gravy & macaroni & cheese	9⅝ oz	19.0	370	46%
veal Parmigiana w/spaghetti	11⅞ oz	19.0	420	41%
Lean Cuisine				
Cafe Classics				
bow tie pasta & chicken	9.5 oz	6.0	270	20%
calypso chicken	8.5 oz	6.0	280	19%
cheese lasagna w/chicken scaloppini	10 oz	8.0	290	25%
chicken breast in wine sauce	8⅛ oz	6.0	220	25%
chicken carbonara	9 oz	8.0	290	25%
chicken Mediterranean	10⅛ oz	4.0	250	14%
chicken Parmesan	10⅞ oz	7.0	240	26%
chicken piccata	9 oz	6.0	290	19%
glazed turkey	9 oz	6.0	250	22%
grilled chicken salsa	8⅞ oz	6.0	240	23%
grilled fish w/vegetables	8⅞ oz	5.0	170	26%
herb roasted chicken	8 oz	5.0	210	21%
honey mustard chicken	8 oz	5.0	270	17%
mesquite beef w/rice	9 oz	7.0	280	23%
sirloin beef peppercorn	8¾ oz	7.0	210	30%
entrées				
angel hair pasta	10 oz	4.0	210	17%
baked cheese ravioli w/tomato sauce	8.5 oz	8.0	240	30%
baked chicken & whipped potatoes & stuffing	8⅝ oz	6.0	250	22%

Food and Description	Amount	Fat Grams	Total Calories	% Fat Calories
baked fish w/cheddar shells	9 oz	8.0	260	28%
beef pot roast & whipped potatoes	9 oz	7.0	210	30%
cheddar bake w/pasta	9 oz	6.0	220	25%
cheese cannelloni	9⅛ oz	5.0	240	19%
chicken a l'orange	9 oz	2.5	260	9%
chicken & vegetables pie	9.5 oz	10.0	320	28%
	10.5 oz	5.0	240	19%
chicken cacciatore	10⅞ oz	7.0	280	23%
chicken chow mein w/rice	9 oz	7.0	210	30%
chicken enchiladas suiza	9 oz	5.0	290	15%
chicken fettuccini	9 oz	6.0	270	26%
chicken in peanut sauce	9 oz	6.0	280	19%
chicken Italiano w/fettuccini	9 oz	6.0	270	26%
chicken Oriental w/vegetables	9 oz	6.0	260	23%
classic cheese lasagna	11.5 oz	6.0	290	19%
country vegetables & beef	9 oz	4.0	220	16%
deluxe cheddar potato	10⅜ oz	6.0	230	23%
fettuccini Alfredo	9 oz	7.0	270	23%
fettuccini primavera	10 oz	8.0	260	28%
fiesta chicken w/rice	8.5 oz	5.0	260	17%
glazed chicken w/vegetable rice	8.5 oz	6.0	240	23%
homestyle turkey	9⅜ oz	6.0	230	23%
lasagna w/meat sauce	10½ oz	8.0	290	25%
macaroni & beef in tomato sauce	10 oz	8.0	280	26%
macaroni & cheese	9 oz	7.0	270	23%
marinara twist	10 oz	3.0	240	11%
meat loaf & whipped potatoes	9⅜ oz	7.0	250	25%
Oriental beef w/vegetables	9 oz	8.0	250	29%
rigatoni	9 oz	4.0	180	20%
rigatoni bake w/meat sauce	9 oz	4.0	180	20%
roasted turkey breast & stuffing & cinnamon apples	9.75 oz	4.0	290	12%
Salisbury steak w/macaroni & cheese	9.5 oz	8.0	270	27%
spaghetti & meat sauce	11.5 oz	6.0	290	19%
spaghetti w/meatballs	9.5 oz	7.0	220	29%
stuffed cabbage w/whipped potatoes	9.5 oz	7.0	220	29%
Swedish meatballs in gravy w/pasta	9⅛ oz	8.0	290	25%
three bean chili w/rice	9 oz	6.0	210	26%
turkey pie	9.5 oz	9.0	300	27%
vegetable lasagna	10.5 oz	7.0	270	23%
lunch entrées				
broccoli & cheddar cheese sauce over baked potato	10 oz	6.0	220	25%
cheese lasagna casserole	9.5 oz	7.0	270	23%
chicken fettuccini w/broccoli	10.25 oz	8.0	290	25%
macaroni & cheese & broccoli	9.75 oz	6.0	240	23%
Mandarin chicken	9.75 oz	6.0	270	20%
Mexican-style rice w/chicken	9 oz	8.0	270	27%

Food and Description	Amount	Fat Grams	Total Calories	% Fat Calories
pasta & chicken marinara	9⅛ oz	6.0	270	20%
pasta & tuna casserole	9⅝ oz	6.0	280	19%
rice & chicken stir-fry	9 oz	9.0	280	28%
teriyaki stir-fry	9 oz	5.0	260	17%
turkey Dijon	9⅞ oz	6.0	270	20%
Lunch Express entrées				
cheese ravioli	9.75 oz	14.0	360	35%
chicken Alfredo	9⅝ oz	17.0	360	43%
chicken chow mein w/rice	10⅝ oz	4.0	260	14%
chicken Oriental	9.75 oz	12.0	370	29%
chicken w/garden vegetables & rice	9⅞ oz	11.0	340	29%
chicken w/linguine	9⅝ oz	11.0	300	33%
fettuccini primavera	10.25 oz	25.0	420	54%
grilled chicken & angel hair pasta	9⅞ oz	13.0	340	34%
lasagna w/meat sauce	10.25 oz	10.0	330	27%
macaroni & cheese w/broccoli	10⅜ oz	19.0	360	48%
Mexican-style chicken w/rice	9⅛ oz	8.0	280	26%
Oriental beef	9.5 oz	8.0	290	25%
spaghetti w/meat sauce	9⅝ oz	10.0	320	28%
Swedish meatballs w/pasta	10.25 oz	32.0	530	54%
side dishes				
corn soufflé/12-oz pkg	½ cup	7.0	170	37%
creamed spinach/9-oz pkg	½ cup	12.0	160	68%
escalloped apples/12-oz pkg	⅔ cup	3.0	180	15%
green bean-mushroom casserole/9.5-oz pkg	½ cup	8.0	140	51%
potatoes au gratin/11.5-oz pkg	½ cup	6.0	130	42%
scalloped potatoes/11.5-oz pkg	½ cup	6.0	140	41%
spinach soufflé/12-oz pkg	½ cup	10.0	150	60%
Welsh rarebit/10-oz pkg	¼ cup	9.0	120	68%
■ (Swanson)				
dinners				
Hungry Man				
beef & broccoli	1 dinner	16.0	500	29%
beef pot pie	14 oz	32.0	670	43%
boneless pork rib	1 dinner	38.0	770	44%
chicken pot pie	14 oz	35.0	650	48%
chopped beef steak	1 dinner	37.0	640	52%
fried chicken	1 dinner	43.0	820	47%
grilled chicken patties	1 dinner	19.0	580	29%
Mexican style	1 dinner	27.0	691	35%
Salisbury steak	1 dinner	34.0	610	50%
sirloin beef tips	1 dinner	16.0	450	32%
turkey/mostly white meat	1 dinner	17.0	530	29%
turkey pot pie	14 oz	36.0	650	50%
Yankee pot roast	1 dinner	11.0	400	25%
4-compartment				
beef & broccoli	1 dinner	10.0	340	26%

Food and Description	Amount	Fat Grams	Total Calories	% Fat Calories
beef enchiladas	1 dinner	21.0	480	39%
beef in barbecue sauce	1 dinner	17.0	460	33%
boneless pork ribs	1 dinner	23.0	510	41%
chicken nuggets	1 dinner	35.0	470	67%
chopped sirloin beef	1 dinner	17.0	350	44%
fish 'n' chips	1 dinner	20.0	500	36%
fried chicken				
BBQ flavored	1 dinner	22.0	540	37%
dark meat	1 dinner	30.0	570	47%
white meat	1 dinner	28.0	580	43%
meat loaf	1 dinner	18.0	410	40%
Mexican style combination	1 dinner	19.0	481	36%
Salisbury steak	1 dinner	20.0	420	43%
Swiss steak	1 dinner	11.0	350	28%
turkey/mostly white meat	1 dinner	8.0	320	23%
veal Parmigiana	1 dinner	18.0	400	41%
Western style	1 dinner	19.0	430	40%
Yankee pot roast	1 dinner	7.0	270	23%
3-compartment				
beans & franks	1 dinner	19.0	440	39%
macaroni & beef	1 dinner	15.0	370	37%
macaroni & cheese	1 dinner	15.0	380	36%
noodles & chicken	1 dinner	8.0	280	26%
entrées				
chicken				
chicken nibbles	3.25 oz	19.0	300	57%
chicken nuggets	3 oz	14.0	230	55%
fried chicken breast	4.5 oz	20.0	360	50%
fried chicken parts/1-lb pkg	3.25 oz	16.0	270	53%
thighs & drumsticks	3.25 oz	18.0	290	56%
Homestyle Recipe				
chicken nibbles	4.25 oz	20.0	340	53%
fish 'n' fries	6.5 oz	16.0	340	42%
fried chicken	7 oz	21.0	390	48%
lasagna w/meat sauce	10 oz	23.0	410	51%
macaroni & cheese	12¼ oz	18.0	340	48%
Salisbury steak	10 oz	16.0	320	45%
scalloped potatoes & ham	9 oz	13.0	300	39%
seafood Creole w/rice	9 oz	6.0	240	23%
sirloin tips in Burgundy sauce	7 oz	5.0	160	28%
turkey w/dressing & potatoes	9 oz	11.0	290	34%
veal Parmigiana	10 oz	13.0	330	36%
pot pies				
beef	7 oz	19.0	370	46%
chicken	7 oz	22.0	380	52%
macaroni & cheese	7 oz	8.0	200	36%
turkey	7 oz	21.0	380	50%

Food and Description	Amount	Fat Grams	Total Calories	% Fat Calories
Kid's Fun Feast				
Chillin Cheese Pizza	1 pkg	9.0	350	23%
Chompin Chicken Drumlets	1 pkg	25.0	490	46%
Frenzied Fish Sticks	1 pkg	14.0	360	35%
Munchin Mini Tacos	1 pkg	15.0	380	36%
Rollin Rib Fingers	1 pkg	24.0	450	48%
Wobblin Wheels & Cheese	1 pkg	11.0	380	26%
Lunch & More				
breaded chicken patty strips	1 meal	19.0	340	50%
breaded fish & macaroni & cheese	1 meal	15.0	350	39%
cheesy vegetable lasagna casserole	1 meal	13.0	350	33%
chicken & noodle casserole	1 meal	9.0	290	28%
chicken & rice stir-fry	1 meal	3.0	240	11%
lasagna w/meat sauce casserole	1 meal	9.0	330	25%
macaroni & beef	1 meal	5.0	270	17%
meat loaf & tomato sauce	1 meal	13.0	270	43%
pork rib shaped patty	1 meal	22.0	460	43%
Salisbury steak in gravy	1 meal	19.0	330	52%
3 cheese macaroni bake casserole	1 meal	14.0	400	32%
tuna noodle casserole	1 meal	11.0	320	31%
turkey/mostly white meat	1 meal	7.0	250	25%
■ **(Tyson)**				
Healthy Portion meals				
BBQ chicken	1 meal	8.0	370	19%
chicken marinara	1 meal	5.0	420	11%
herb chicken	1 meal	3.0	450	6%
honey mustard chicken	1 meal	2.5	400	6%
Italian style chicken	1 meal	4.0	390	9%
mesquite chicken	1 meal	10.0	430	21%
premium dinners				
blackened chicken	1 meal	5.0	270	17%
chicken Francais	1 meal	10.0	260	35%
chicken Kiev	1 meal	24.0	430	50%
chicken Marsala	1 meal	4.0	180	20%
chicken mesquite	1 meal	8.0	310	23%
chicken Parmigiana	1 meal	11.0	290	34%
chicken picante	1 meal	5.0	250	18%
chicken piccata	1 meal	3.0	190	14%
chicken supreme	1 meal	9.0	260	31%
chicken w/broccoli & cheese	1 meal	6.0	230	23%
glazed chicken w/sauce	1 meal	6.0	270	20%
grilled chicken	1 meal	3.0	220	12%
grilled chicken Italian style	1 meal	4.0	210	17%
honey roasted chicken	1 meal	4.0	220	16%
roasted chicken	1 meal	3.0	240	11%
■ **(Weight Watchers)**				
regular entrées				
barbecue glazed chicken	7.5 oz	3.5	190	18%

Food and Description	Amount	Fat Grams	Total Calories	% Fat Calories
broccoli & cheese baked potato	10 oz	7.0	230	27%
cheese manicotti	9.25 oz	9.0	290	28%
chicken cordon bleu	9 oz	6.0	220	25%
chicken enchiladas suiza	9 oz	8.0	250	29%
chicken fettuccini	8.25 oz	9.0	280	29%
chicken Parmigiana	9.1 oz	6.0	230	23%
fettuccini Alfredo w/broccoli	8.5 oz	6.0	220	25%
fried fillet of fish	7.7 oz	8.0	230	31%
garden lasagna	11 oz	5.0	230	20%
grilled Salisbury steak	8.5 oz	9.0	250	32%
Italian cheese lasagna	11 oz	8.0	300	24%
lasagna w/meat sauce	10.25 oz	7.0	290	22%
macaroni & beef	9.5 oz	4.5	220	18%
macaroni & cheese	9 oz	6.0	260	21%
nacho grande chicken enchiladas	9 oz	8.0	290	25%
penne pasta w/sun-dried tomatoes	10 oz	9.0	290	28%
roast glazed chicken	8.9 oz	5.0	200	23%
Southern fried chicken	8 oz	11.0	280	35%
spaghetti w/meat sauce	10 oz	6.0	250	22%
stuffed turkey breast	8.75 oz	8.0	240	30%
Swedish meatballs	9 oz	8.0	280	26%
Tex-Mex chicken	8.3 oz	4.0	260	14%
tuna noodle casserole	9.5 oz	7.0	240	26%
Smart Ones				
angel hair pasta	9 oz	2.0	180	10%
chicken chow mein	9 oz	2.0	200	9%
chicken Marsala	9 oz	2.0	150	12%
chicken Mirabella	9.2 oz	2.0	170	11%
fiesta chicken	8.5 oz	2.0	220	8%
honey mustard chicken	8.5 oz	2.0	200	9%
lasagna curls w/Italian vegetables	9.5 oz	2.0	170	11%
lasagna Florentine	10 oz	2.0	210	9%
lemon herb chicken piccata	8.5 oz	2.0	190	9%
ravioli Florentine	8.5 oz	2.0	200	9%
roast turkey medallions	8.5 oz	2.0	190	9%
shrimp marinara	9 oz	2.0	190	9%
Sandwiches On-The-Go!				
pocket sandwiches				
chicken, broccoli, & cheddar	5 oz	6.0	250	22%
deluxe pizza	5 oz	7.0	300	21%
ham & cheese	5 oz	7.0	240	26%
Reuben	5 oz	6.0	250	22%
pretzel sandwiches				
hickory smoked ham & cheddar	4 oz	8.0	260	28%
honey Dijon turkey	4 oz	4.0	230	16%
sandwich/grilled chicken	4 oz	5.0	210	21%

Food and Description	Amount	Fat Grams	Total Calories	% Fat Calories
FROZEN NONDAIRY DESSERT (See FRUIT ICES, BARS, & POPS; ICE CREAM & ICE CREAM-LIKE FROZEN DESSERTS; RICE FROZEN DESSERT; SHERBET; TOFU FROZEN DESSERT)				
FRUCTOSE (See SUGAR SUBSTITUTE)				
FRUIT (See FRUIT, MIXED; FRUIT COCKTAIL; individual listings)				
FRUIT, MIXED (See also FRUIT COCKTAIL; SNACK MIX)				
candied				
(S&W) glace cake mix/orange peel, grapefruit peel, cherries, pineapple, citron, lemon peel	2 Tbs	–	90	–
canned				
(Del Monte)				
chunky mixed				
in extra light syrup	½ cup	–	60	–
in heavy syrup	½ cup	–	100	–
naturals/in fruit juices	½ cup	–	60	–
fruit cups				
in extra light syrup	4¼ oz	–	60	–
in heavy syrup	4¼ oz	–	90	–
in light syrup	3½ oz	–	70	–
naturals/in fruit juices	4¼ oz	–	60	–
tropical fruit salad/in light syrup	½ cup	–	80	–
(Dole) tropical fruit salad/in light syrup	½ cup	–	80	–
generic				
fruit salad				
in extra heavy syrup	½ cup	<1.0	114	4%
in heavy syrup	½ cup	<1.0	94	15%
in juice	½ cup	<1.0	62	7%
in water	½ cup	<1.0	37	12%
tropical fruit	½ cup	–	110	–
(Kraft)	½ cup	–	50	–
(S&W) natural style/chunky	½ cup	–	70	–
dried				
(Del Monte)	⅓ cup	–	110	–
(Mariani)				
fruit medley	¼ cup	1.0	150	5%
tropical	1 oz	1.0	90	10%
(Sun Giant)	1.5 oz	–	100	–
(Sun Maid)				
fruit bits	¼ cup	–	120	–
mixed fruit	¼ cup	–	110	–
frozen				
(Birds Eye)	½ cup	–	120	–
(C&W)				
berry medley	1 cup	–	60	–
mixed melon balls	⅔ cup	–	40	–
generic				
sweetened	1 cup	0.5	245	2%

Food and Description	Amount	Fat Grams	Total Calories	% Fat Calories
unsweetened	3.5 oz	<1.0	45	10%
FRUIT & NUT MIX (*See* SNACKS)				
FRUIT COCKTAIL (*See also* FRUIT, MIXED)				
canned				
generic				
in extra heavy syrup	½ cup	–	115	–
in extra light syrup	½ cup	–	55	–
in heavy syrup	½ cup	–	93	–
in juice	½ cup	–	56	–
in light syrup	½ cup	–	70	–
in water	½ cup	–	40	–
(Del Monte)				
in heavy syrup	½ cup	–	100	–
in light/extra light syrup	½ cup	–	60	–
naturals/in fruit juices	½ cup	–	60	–
(Hunt's)	½ cup	–	90	–
(Libby's) Lite	½ cup	–	50	–
(Nutradiet)	½ cup	–	40	–
(S&W)				
in heavy syrup	½ cup	–	90	–
natural style	½ cup	–	80	–
FRUIT DRINK (*See also* LEMONADE/LEMONADE-FLAVORED DRINK; TEA; FRUIT PUNCH; SOFT DRINK; SOFT DRINK MIX; individual listings)				
bottled, boxed, or canned				
(Fruitopia)				
Fruit Integration	8 fl oz	–	125	–
Tropical Consideration	8 fl oz	–	75	–
(Hi-C)				
Double Fruit Cooler	6 fl oz	–	93	–
Ecto Cooler	6 fl oz	–	95	–
Hula	6 fl oz	–	97	–
(Libby's) Fruit Medley	8 fl oz	–	80	–
(Powerade) Mountain Blast	8 fl oz	–	73	–
(Welch's)				
Sparkling Red Cocktail	8 fl oz*	–	160	–
Sparkling White Cocktail	8 fl oz	–	160	–
Tropical Cocktail	10 fl oz	–	180	–
	11.5 fl oz	–	210	–
frozen/prepared				
(Mott's) Fruit Basket Tropical Blend	8 fl oz	–	120	–
(Welch's)				
orange-pineapple-apple	8 fl oz	–	140	–
	8.45 fl oz	–	150	–
Orchard Fruit Harvest	8 fl oz	–	140	–
FRUIT ICES, BARS, & POPS (*See also* SHERBET)				
(Baskin-Robbins)				
daiquiri ice	½ cup	–	110	–
	reg scoop	–	130	–

Food and Description	Amount	Fat Grams	Total Calories	% Fat Calories
grape ice	½ cup	–	110	–
margarita ice	½ cup	–	110	–
red raspberry sorbet	½ cup	–	120	–
	reg scoop	–	140	–
(Chiquita) fruit & juice				
cherry	1 bar	–	50	–
raspberry	1 bar	–	50	–
strawberry	1 bar	–	50	–
strawberry-banana	1 bar	–	50	–
(Dole)				
Fruit Juice Bars				
grape				
no sugar added	1.75 oz	–	25	–
regular	1.75 oz	–	45	–
raspberry				
no sugar added	1.75 oz	–	25	–
regular	1.75 oz	–	45	–
strawberry				
no sugar added	1.75 oz	–	25	–
regular	1.75 oz	–	45	–
Fruit 'N Juice Bars				
coconut	4 oz	7.0	210	30%
lemonade	4 oz	–	120	–
lime	4 oz	–	110	–
peach passion	2.5 oz	–	70	–
pine-coconut	4 oz	4.0	140	26%
pine-orange-banana	2.5 oz	–	70	–
	4 oz	–	110	–
raspberry	1 bar	<1.0	70	6%
strawberry	1 bar	<1.0	70	6%
(Dreyer's) Tropical Fruit Bars				
Calypso Coconut	1 bar	8.0	190	38%
Loco Lime	1 bar	–	90	–
pineapple orange	1 bar	–	90	–
Savage Strawberry	1 bar	–	90	–
(Edy's) Tropical Fruit Bars				
Calypso Coconut	1 bar	8.0	190	38%
Loco Lime	1 bar	–	90	–
pineapple orange	1 bar	–	90	–
Savage Strawberry	1 bar	–	90	–
(Eskimo) Rainbow Twin Pops	1 pop	–	60	–
(Frookie) Cool Fruits				
Fruit Juice Freezers				
cranberry	2 pops	–	70	–
pink lemonade	2 pops	–	70	–
raspberry-apple	2 pops	–	70	–
strawberry-banana	2 pops	–	70	–
watermelon berry	2 pops	–	70	–

Food and Description	Amount	Fat Grams	Total Calories	% Fat Calories
(Good Humor)				
Bubble Play Sports	1 bar	1.0	110	8%
Calippo				
cherry	1 bar	–	100	–
grape	1 bar	–	90	–
lemon	1 bar	–	90	–
Dinosaur Bar	1 bar	2.0	110	16%
First 'N' Goal Sports	1 bar	–	90	–
Freeza Pizza	1 bar	5.0	140	32%
Free Kick Sports	1 bar	–	90	–
Hyper Stripe	1 bar	–	80	–
Jumbo Jet Star	1 bar	<1.0	85	5%
Shoot Hoops Sports	1 bar	–	90	–
Snowfruit				
coconut	1 bar	4.0	150	24%
orange	1 bar	–	140	–
strawberry	1 bar	–	120	–
tropical fruit	1 bar	–	110	–
watermelon	1 bar	–	80	–
(Jell-O) gelatin pops				
all flavors/averaged data	1 bar	–	35	–
(Kool-Aid) Kool-pops/all flavors	1 bar	–	40	–
(M&M★Mars) Starburst fruit juice bars				
12 per pkg	1 bar	–	50	–
Out-of-Home				
orange	1 bar	–	80	–
strawberry	1 bar	–	80	–
(Minute Maid) Fruit Juice Bars				
cherry	1 bar	0.5	60	7%
grape	1 bar	0.5	60	7%
orange	1 bar	0.5	60	7%
(Mr. Freeze) freezer bars				
assorted flavors				
1-oz bars				
regular	3 bars	–	50	–
sugar-free	3 bars	–	20	–
1.5-oz bars				
regular	2 bars	–	50	–
sugar-free	2 bars	–	20	–
2-oz bars/regular	1 bar	–	35	–
tropical				
1-oz bars	3 bars	–	50	–
1.5-oz bars	2 bars	–	50	–
(Nabisco) Life Saver pops				
all flavors	1 bar	–	40	–
(Natural Nectar)				
lemony-lime	1 bar	<1.0	70	6%
tropical delite	1 bar	<1.0	70	6%

Food and Description	Amount	Fat Grams	Total Calories	% Fat Calories
(Planter's) Life Savers				
regular	1 bar	–	35	–
sugar-free	1 bar	–	12	–
(Popsicle)				
cotton candy	1 bar	–	55	–
Big Stick				
cherry/pineapple	1 bar	–	50	–
bubble gum swirl	1 bar	–	55	–
Firecracker Jr.	1 bar	–	40	–
Laser Blazer	1 bar	–	70	–
Lick-A-Color	1 bar	–	90	–
rainbow	1 bar	–	90	–
Super Twin				
cello	1 bar	–	70	–
paper	1 bar	–	70	–
Supersicle				
Neon Traffic Signal	1 bar	–	80	–
Sour Tower	1 bar	–	80	–
Razzle Dazzle	1 bar	–	80	–
(Schwan's)				
Schwan's Pops	1 pop	–	15	–
Twin Pops/assorted	1 pop	–	60	–
specialty items				
Garfield	1 bar	–	90	–
Screwball Cup	1 cup	1.0	100	9%
Snow Cone	1 cone	–	60	–
Super Mario	1 bar	1.0	120	8%
The Great White Bar	1 bar	–	70	–
(Sunkist) bars				
coconut	1 bar	10.0	170	52%
lemonade	1 bar	–	90	–
orange juice	1 bar	–	100	–
wild berry fruit & juice	4 oz	–	140	–
(Trix) pops/all flavors	1 bar	–	40	–
(Welch's) fruit juice bars				
grape				
light	1 bar	–	25	–
regular				
1.75-oz bar	1 bar	–	45	–
3-oz bar	1 bar	–	80	–
orange-pineapple-banana	1 bar	–	45	–
pineapple	1 bar	–	45	–
raspberry				
light	1 bar	–	25	–
regular	1 bar	–	45	–
strawberry				
light	1 bar	–	25	–
regular	1 bar	–	45	–

Food and Description	Amount	Fat Grams	Total Calories	% Fat Calories
strawberry-banana				
1.75-oz bar	1 bar	–	45	–
3 oz-bar	1 bar	–	80	–
(Wyler's) Fruit Slush/freeze & eat				
cherry	4 oz	–	157	–
fruit punch	4 oz	–	157	–
grape	4 oz	–	157	–
orange	4 oz	–	157	–
pink lemonade	4 oz	–	157	–
strawberry	4 oz	–	157	–
tropical punch fruit	4 oz	–	157	–
FRUIT JUICE/JUICE DRINK, MIXED (*See also* FRUIT PUNCH; individual listings)				
bottled, boxed, or canned				
(Capri Sun) juice drink				
Mountain Cooler	6.75 fl oz	–	100	–
Pacific Cooler	6.75 fl oz	–	110	–
Surfer Cooler	6.75 fl oz	–	100	–
(Chiquita)				
Caribbean Splash	8 fl oz	–	120	–
	8.45 fl oz	–	130	–
Hawaiian Sunrise	8 fl oz	–	120	–
Tropical Paradise	8 fl oz	–	120	–
	8.45 fl oz	–	130	–
(Dole)				
Fruit Fiesta	8 fl oz	–	140	–
	16 fl oz	–	270	–
Lanai Breeze	8 fl oz	–	120	–
	16 fl oz	–	240	–
mixed fruit	8.45 fl oz	–	130	–
Tropical Breeze blend	8 fl oz	–	140	–
	10 fl oz	–	180	–
Tropical Breeze drink	8 fl oz	–	120	–
	10 fl oz	–	130	–
	16 fl oz	–	240	–
(Knudsen)				
Morning Blend	8 fl oz	–	120	–
Natural Breakfast	8 fl oz	–	110	–
Thirst Quencher/Hibiscus Cooler	8 fl oz	–	90	–
(Libby's) Juicy Juice	8 fl oz	–	130	–
	8.45 fl oz	–	140	–
(Mott's) In-A-Minute unfrozen concentrate/tropical blend	2 fl oz	–	130	–
(Season's Best) fruit medley	8 fl oz	–	130	–
(Snapple) Passion Supreme	10 fl oz	–	160	–
(TreeTop) apple-grape	11.5 fl oz	–	190	–
(Welch's) juice cocktail				
harvest blend	8 fl oz	–	140	–
orange, pineapple, apple	8 fl oz	–	140	–

Food and Description	Amount	Fat Grams	Total Calories	% Fat Calories
Tropical Orange Passion frozen/prepared	8 fl oz	–	140	–
(Dole)				
Fruit Fiesta	8 fl oz	–	140	–
Lanai Breeze	8 fl oz	–	120	–
Tropical Breeze	8 fl oz	–	120	–
tropical fruit blend	8 fl oz	–	140	–
(Mott's) Fruit Basket juice cocktail/ tropical blend	8 fl oz	–	120	–
(Welch's) Orchard Harvest juice blend	8 fl oz	–	140	–
FRUIT PECTIN				
(Certo)	1 Tbs	–	2	–
(Sure-Jell)				
light	¼ tsp	–	5	–
sweetened	¼ tsp	–	5	–
FRUIT PROTECTOR (*See also* FRUIT PECTIN)				
(Ever-Fresh)	¼ tsp	–	5	–
FRUIT PUNCH (*See also* SOFT DRINK; SOFT DRINK MIX; SPORTS DRINK)				
bottled, boxed, or canned				
(Betty Crocker)				
Squeezit				
green	6.75 fl oz	–	110	–
red	6.76 fl oz	–	110	–
tropical	6.76 fl oz	–	110	–
Squeezit 100/Pilot Punch	6.76 fl oz	–	90	–
(Capri Sun)				
fruit	6.75 fl oz	–	100	–
Maui	6.75 fl oz	–	110	–
safari	6.75 fl oz	–	100	–
(Dole) Paradise Punch	10 fl oz	–	150	–
(Hawaiian Punch)				
Fruit Juicy Red				
lite	6 fl oz	–	60	–
regular	6 fl oz	–	90	–
Island Fruit Cocktail	6 fl oz	–	90	–
Tropical Fruits	6 fl oz	–	90	–
Very Berry	6 fl oz	–	90	–
Wild Fruit	6 fl oz	–	90	–
(Hi-C)				
fruit	8 fl oz	–	120	–
	8.45 fl oz	–	130	–
Hula	8 fl oz	–	110	–
	8.45 fl oz	–	120	–
(Knudsen) Rain Forest Punch	8 fl oz	–	120	–
(Libby's) Juicy Juice				
orange	4.23 fl oz	–	80	–
	8 fl oz	–	100	–
	8.45 fl oz	–	100	–

Food and Description	Amount	Fat Grams	Total Calories	% Fat Calories
(Minute Maid)				
berry	8.45 fl oz	–	120	–
Concord	8 fl oz	–	127	–
fruit	8 fl oz	–	120	–
	8.45 fl oz	–	125	–
orange	8.45 fl oz	–	120	–
tropical	8.45 fl oz	–	120	–
(Mondo) Fruit Squeezers				
Adventure Quencher	8 fl oz	–	130	–
Chillin' Cherry	8 fl oz	–	130	–
Legendary Berry	8 fl oz	–	130	–
Primo Punch	8 fl oz	–	130	–
(Mott's)				
In-A-Minute unfrozen concentrate	2 fl oz	–	140	–
ready to drink	8.45 fl oz	–	120	–
	10 fl oz	–	170	–
(Powerade) fruit	8 fl oz	–	72	–
(Seneca) fruit				
100% Juice	8 fl oz	–	130	–
10% Juice	8 fl oz	–	120	–
(TreeTop)				
fruit punch				
100% Juice	8.45 fl oz	–	130	–
	10 fl oz	–	150	–
	11.5 fl oz	–	170	–
25% Juice	8 fl oz	–	130	–
	10 fl oz	–	160	–
	11.5 fl oz	–	180	–
Juice Rivers				
citrus	8.45 fl oz	–	130	–
fruit	8.45 fl oz	–	130	–
grape	8.45 fl oz	–	140	–
red	8.45 fl oz	–	130	–
(Tropicana)				
berry	8 fl oz	–	130	–
citrus	8 fl oz	–	140	–
	10 fl oz	–	180	–
cranberry	8 fl oz	–	140	–
	10 fl oz	–	170	–
	11.5 fl oz	–	200	–
fruit	8 fl oz	–	130	–
	10 fl oz	–	160	–
	11.5 fl oz	–	180	–
pineapple	8 fl oz	–	130	–
	10 fl oz	–	160	–
(Welch's)				
fruit	11.5 fl oz	–	200	–
Fruit Harvest	8.45 fl oz	–	140	–

Food and Description	Amount	Fat Grams	Total Calories	% Fat Calories
fruit juice cocktail	10 fl oz	–	170	–
10% fruit	11.5 fl oz	–	180	–
10% fruit juice cocktail	8 fl oz	–	130	–
	10 fl oz	–	160	–
frozen or refrigerated/prepared (Minute Maid)				
berry	8 fl oz	–	120	–
citrus	8 fl oz	–	120	–
fruit	8 fl oz	–	120	–
grape	8 fl oz	–.	120	–
tropical	8 fl oz	–	120	–
mix				
(Country Time) lemonade punch/ mix only	⅛ cap	–	70	–

FRUIT SALAD (*See* BERRIES, MIXED; FRUIT, MIXED; FRUIT COCKTAIL)
FRUIT SNACK (*See also* individual fruit listings)

(Betty Crocker)				
Color-By-The-Foot	1 roll	1.5	80	17%
Fruit-By-The-Foot				
cherry	1 roll	1.5	80	17%
grape	1 roll	1.5	80	17%
strawberry	1 roll	1.5	80	17%
Fruit Roll-Ups				
cherry	2 rolls	1.0	110	8%
pouch	1 roll	0.5	50	9%
Crazy Colors	2 rolls	1.0	110	8%
green/pouch	1 roll	0.5	50	9%
grape	2 rolls	1.0	110	8%
pouch	1 roll	0.5	50	9%
hot colors	2 rolls	1.0	110	8%
pouch	1 roll	0.5	50	9%
raspberry	2 rolls	1.0	110	8%
pouch	1 roll	0.5	50	9%
Secret Pictures	2 rolls	1.0	110	8%
pouch	1 roll	0.5	50	9%
strawberry	2 rolls	1.0	110	8%
pouch	1 roll	0.5	50	9%
Fruit String Thing				
berry 'n blue	1 pouch	1.0	80	11%
cherry	1 pouch	1.0	80	11%
strawberry	1 pouch	1.0	80	11%
Fun Snacks				
Friends/assorted fruit	1 pouch	1.0	90	10%
Rollerblade/assorted fruit	1 pouch	1.0	90	10%
Shark Bites/assorted fruit	1 pouch	1.0	90	10%
Tasmanian Devil/assorted fruit	1 pouch	1.0	90	10%
X Men	1 pouch	1.0	90	10%

Food and Description	Amount	Fat Grams	Total Calories	% Fat Calories
Gushers				
Fruitomic Punch	1 pouch	1.0	90	10%
sour berry	1 pouch	1.0	90	10%
sour cherry	1 pouch	1.0	90	10%
sour grape	1 pouch	1.0	90	10%
sour punch	1 pouch	1.5	90	15%
sour strawberry	1 pouch	1.0	90	10%
(Del Monte) yogurt raisins				
strawberry	0.9 oz	3.0	110	25%
vanilla	0.9 oz	3.0	110	25%
(Farley)				
Funnies/Trolls				
cherry	1 pouch	2.0	80	23%
strawberry	1 pouch	2.0	80	23%
turtles	1 pouch	–	80	–
Snacks				
cherry	1 pouch	–	80	–
Creepy Crawlers	1 pouch	–	80	–
dinosaurs	1 pouch	–	80	–
strawberry	1 pouch	–	80	–
Troll	1 pouch	–	80	–
The Roll/strawberry	1 pouch	2.0	80	23%
(Flavor Tree)				
Fruit Bears/assorted	1.05 oz	1.6	117	12%
Fruit Circus/assorted	1.05 oz	1.6	117	12%
Fruit Roll				
apple	1 roll	–	75	–
apricot	1 roll	0.5	75	6%
cherry	1 roll	–	75	–
grape	1 roll	–	75	–
raspberry	1 roll	–	75	–
strawberry	1 roll	–	75	–
(Fruit Wrinkles) all flavors	1 pouch	1.0	100	9%
(Hanna Barbera)				
Flintstones	1 pkg	–	100	–
Jetsons	1 pkg	–	100	–
Yo Yogi	1 pkg	–	100	–
(Nintendo)				
Link	1 pouch	–	100	–
Super Mario Bros	1 pouch	–	100	–
(Sunkist) Fruit Roll/prepared				
apple/21-gm roll	1 roll	–	70	–
apricot/21-gm roll	1 roll	–	70	–
cherry				
14-gm roll	1 roll	–	50	–
21-gm roll	1 roll	–	70	–
fruit punch/21-gm roll	1 roll	–	70	–

Food and Description	Amount	Fat Grams	Total Calories	% Fat Calories
grape				
14-gm roll	1 roll	–	50	–
21-gm roll	1 roll	–	80	–
raspberry				
14-gm roll	1 roll	–	45	–
21-gm roll	1 roll	–	70	–
strawberry				
14-gm roll	1 roll	–	45	–
21-gm roll	1 roll	–	70	–
(Weight Watchers) fruit snack				
apple	0.5 oz	–	50	–
cinnamon	0.5 oz	–	50	–
peach	0.5 oz	–	50	–
strawberry	0.5 oz	–	50	–

FRUIT SPREAD (*See* JAM/JELLY/PRESERVES)

G

Food and Description	Amount	Fat Grams	Total Calories	% Fat Calories
GARBANZO BEAN (*See* CHICKPEA)				
GARLIC (*See also* SEASONINGS)				
fresh/raw				
minced	1 clove	–	4	–
whole	1 clove	–	5	–
jar (Christopher Ranch) chopped	1 tsp	1.0	10	90%
powdered				
generic	1 tsp	–	9	–
(Spice Island)	1 tsp	–	5	–
GARLIC SALT (*See also* SEASONINGS)				
(Lawry's)	1 tsp	–	4	–
GAZPACHO (*See* SOUP)				
GEFILTE FISH				
generic/sweet	~ 1.5 oz	0.7	35	18%
(Manischewitz)				
gefilte fish & pike				
regular	1 piece	4.0	100	36%
sweet	1 piece	4.0	130	28%
homestyle				
regular	1 piece	4.0	111	32%
sweet	1 piece	4.0	132	27%

Food and Description	Amount	Fat Grams	Total Calories	% Fat Calories
(Mother's)				
old-fashioned				
12-oz jar	1 ball	1.0	55	16%
24-oz jar	1 ball	1.0	70	13%
Old World				
regular	1 ball	1.0	70	13%
sweet	1 ball	1.0	55	16%
unsalted	1 ball	1.0	45	20%
whitefish				
jellied				
31-oz jar	1 ball	1.0	60	15%
12-oz jar	1 ball	<1.0	50	14%
24-oz jar	1 ball	1.0	60	15%
regular				
31-oz jar	1 ball	1.0	70	13%
12-oz jar	1 ball	<1.0	55	13%
24-oz jar	1 ball	1.0	70	13%
whitefish & pike				
jellied				
31-oz jar	1 ball	1.0	60	15%
12-oz jar	1 ball	<1.0	50	14%
24-oz jar	1 ball	1.0	60	15%
regular	1 ball	1.0	70	13%
(Rokeach)				
natural broth	2 oz	1.0	46	20%
Old Vienna	2 oz	1.0	54	17%
	2.6 oz	2.0	68	27%
redi-jelled	2 oz	1.0	46	20%
whitefish & pike/jellied	1 oz	1.0	46	20%
GELATIN				
■ **DRINKING POWDER**				
generic/1 packet + water	4 fl oz	–	67	–
(Knox) w/NutraSweet	1 envelope	–	39	–
■ **DRY**	1 pkt	–	23	–
■ **MIX**				
(D-Zerta) low-calorie/strawberry	½ cup	–	8	–
(Estee) Low-Cal Gelatin Desserts	½ cup	–	8	–
(Hain) SuperFruits dessert mix				
cherry				
mix only	2 Tbs	–	90	–
prepared	½ cup	–	90	–
kiwi-pineapple				
mix only	2 Tbs	–	90	–
prepared	½ cup	–	90	–
orange-pineapple				
mix only	2 Tbs	–	90	–
prepared	½ cup	–	90	–

Food and Description	Amount	Fat Grams	Total Calories	% Fat Calories
strawberry				
mix only	2 Tbs	–	90	–
prepared	½ cup	–	90	–
tropical fruit punch				
mix only	2 Tbs	–	90	–
prepared	½ cup	–	90	–
(Jell-O)				
apricot	½ cup	–	80	–
berry blue				
regular	½ cup	–	80	–
sugar-free	½ cup	–	10	–
black cherry	½ cup	–	80	–
black raspberry	½ cup	–	80	–
blackberry	½ cup	–	80	–
cherry				
regular	½ cup	–	80	–
sugar-free	½ cup	–	10	–
cranberry	½ cup	–	80	–
grape	½ cup	–	80	–
lemon				
regular	½ cup	–	80	–
sugar-free	½ cup	–	8	–
lime				
regular	½ cup	–	80	–
sugar-free	½ cup	–	8	–
mango	½ cup	–	80	–
mixed fruit				
regular	½ cup	–	80	–
sugar-free	½ cup	–	8	–
orange				
regular	½ cup	–	80	–
sugar-free	½ cup	–	8	–
orange-pineapple	½ cup	–	80	–
peach	½ cup	–	80	–
pineapple				
Hawaiian/sugar-free	½ cup	–	8	–
regular	½ cup	–	80	–
raspberry				
regular	½ cup	–	80	–
sugar-free	½ cup	–	8	–
strawberry				
1-2-3	⅔ cup	1.5	130	10%
regular	½ cup	–	80	–
sugar-free	½ cup	–	8	–
strawberry-banana				
regular	½ cup	–	80	–
sugar-free	½ cup	–	8	–

Food and Description	Amount	Fat Grams	Total Calories	% Fat Calories
triple berry/sugar-free	½ cup	–	8	–
tropical punch	½ cup	–	80	–
watermelon				
regular	½ cup	–	80	–
sugar-free	½ cup	–	10	–
wild strawberry	½ cup	–	80	–
(Jell-Well)				
cherry	½ cup	–	80	–
lemon	½ cup	–	80	–
lime	½ cup	–	80	–
mixed fruit	½ cup	–	80	–
orange				
regular	½ cup	–	80	–
sugar-free	½ cup	–	8	–
raspberry				
regular	½ cup	–	80	–
sugar-free	½ cup	–	8	–
strawberry				
regular	½ cup	–	80	–
sugar-free	½ cup	–	8	–
strawberry-banana				
regular	½ cup	–	80	–
sugar-free	½ cup	–	8	–
(Royal)				
apple	½ cup	–	80	–
blackberry	½ cup	–	80	–
cherry				
regular	½ cup	–	80	–
sugar-free	½ cup	–	6	–
Concord grape	½ cup	–	80	–
lemon	½ cup	–	80	–
lemon-lime	½ cup	–	80	–
lime				
regular	½ cup	–	80	–
sugar-free	½ cup	–	6	–
mixed berry	½ cup	–	80	–
orange				
regular	½ cup	–	80	–
sugar-free	½ cup	–	6	–
peach	½ cup	–	80	–
pineapple	½ cup	–	80	–
raspberry				
regular	½ cup	–	80	–
sugar-free	½ cup	–	6	–
strawberry				
regular	½ cup	–	80	–
sugar-free	½ cup	–	6	–

Food and Description	Amount	Fat Grams	Total Calories	% Fat Calories
strawberry-banana	½ cup	–	80	–
tropical fruit	½ cup	–	80	–
(SnackWell's)				
cherry	½ cup	–	80	–
lime	½ cup	–	80	–
orange	½ cup	–	80	–
strawberry	½ cup	–	80	–
■ READY TO SERVE				
(Del Monte) snack cups				
blueberry	3.5 oz cup	–	70	–
cherry	3.5 oz cup	–	70	–
grape	3.5 oz cup	–	70	–
strawberry	3.5 oz cup	–	70	–
(Jell-O)				
gelatin				
berry blue	1 snack	–	80	–
cherry				
regular	1 snack	–	80	–
sugar-free	1 snack	–	10	–
grape	1 snack	–	80	–
orange				
regular	1 snack	–	80	–
sugar-free	1 snack	–	10	–
raspberry				
regular	1 snack	–	80	–
sugar-free	1 snack	–	10	–
strawberry				
regular	1 snack	–	80	–
sugar-free	1 snack	–	10	–
strawberry-banana	1 snack	–	80	–
Jigglers Bits & Yogurt				
berry blue	6 oz	1.5	230	6%
cherry	6 oz	1.5	220	6%
orange	6 oz	1.5	220	6%
strawberry	6 oz	1.5	220	6%
(Hunt's) Snack Pack Juicy Gels				
cherry	1 snack	–	100	–
lemon	1 snack	–	100	–
mixed fruit	1 snack	–	100	–
orange	1 snack	–	100	–
strawberry	1 snack	–	100	–
(Kraft) Handi-Snacks				
blue raspberry	1 snack	–	80	–
cherry	1 snack	–	80	–
orange	1 snack	–	80	–
strawberry	1 snack	–	80	–

GIN (See LIQUOR, DISTILLED)
GINGER ALE (See SOFT DRINK)

Food and Description	Amount	Fat Grams	Total Calories	% Fat Calories
GINGER ROOT				
candied	1 oz	–	95	–
fresh/raw/sliced	5 slices	–	8	–
	¼ cup	–	17	–
powdered-ground	1 tsp	–	6	–
GINGERBREAD (*See* BREAD; CAKE)				
GINKGO				
canned	1 oz	0.5	32	14%
dried	1 oz	0.6	99	5%
raw	1 oz	–	52	–
GIZZARD (*See* CHICKEN; GOOSE; TURKEY)				
GOAT/boneless				
raw	4 oz	3.0	125	22%
roasted	3 oz	3.0	122	22%
roasted/diced	1 cup	4.0	200	18%
GOOSE (*See also* PÂTÉ)				
domesticated/roasted				
gizzard, raw	3 oz	4.5	119	34%
liver				
raw	3 oz	3.6	114	28%
meat & skin	~2 lb	170.0	2362	65%
meat only	4 oz	14.5	270	48%
	1¼ lbs	75.0	1406	48%
GOOSEBERRY				
canned/in light syrup	½ cup	–	93	–
raw	1 cup	0.9	67	12%
GOULASH (*See* BEEF DISH/ENTREÉ; FROZEN ENTRÉE/DINNER)				
GOURD				
dishcloth				
boiled-drained	½ cup	0.5	65	7%
boiled-drained/sliced	½ cup	0.3	50	5%
raw	~ 8.5 oz	0.5	40	11%
raw/sliced	½ cup	–	10	–
wax				
boiled-drained	½ cup	–	15	–
boiled-drained/chopped	½ cup	–	11	–
raw	~1 lb	<1.0	45	10%
raw/chopped	½ cup	–	8	–
white				
boiled-drained	½ cup	–	17	–
boiled-drained/chopped	½ cup	–	11	–
raw	~1 lb	<1.0	45	10%
raw/chopped	½ cup	–	8	–
GRAHAM CRACKER (*See* COOKIE)				
GRAHAM CRACKER CRUMBS (*See* CRACKER CRUMBS/MEAL)				
GRANADILLA (*See* PASSION FRUIT)				
GRANOLA (*See* CEREAL)				

Food and Description	Amount	Fat Grams	Total Calories	% Fat Calories
GRANOLA/GRANOLA-TYPE BAR				
(Barbara's)				
Fi-Bar				
fruit & nut bar				
apple oatmeal & spice	1 bar	3.5	130	24%
banana nut	1 bar	3.5	130	24%
strawberry oatmeal almond	1 bar	3.0	130	21%
nectar bar				
almond crunch	1 bar	4.5	140	30%
apple oatmeal spice	1 bar	3.5	130	24%
peanut butter crunch	1 bar	4.5	140	30%
vanilla chocolate cranberry	1 bar	4.5	140	30%
vanilla chocolate raspberry	1 bar	4.5	140	30%
vanilla chocolate strawberry	1 bar	4.5	140	30%
Nature's Choice				
cereal bar				
blueberry/fat free	1 bar	–	110	–
raspberry/fat free	1 bar	–	110	–
granola bar				
carob chip	1 bar	2.0	80	23%
cinnamon & raisin	1 bar	2.0	80	23%
oats 'n honey	1 bar	2.0	80	23%
peanut butter	1 bar	3.0	80	34%
(Carnation) breakfast bar				
chocolate chip/chewy	1 bar	6.0	150	36%
chocolate chunk granola	1 bar	5.0	140	32%
honey & oats granola	1 bar	4.0	130	28%
peanut butter chocolate chip/chewy	1 bar	5.0	150	30%
Fi-Bar (See (Barbara's); (Natural Nectar) in this section)				
(Glenny's) brown rice treat				
carob mint w/oat bran	1 bar	2.0	180	10%
cinnamon & raisin	1 bar	1.0	170	5%
peanut & raisin	1 bar	5.0	210	21%
plain & fancy	1 bar	1.0	120	8%
raisin bran	1 bar	1.0	170	5%
toasted almond w/oat bran	1 bar	5.0	200	23%
(Grist Mill)				
chocolate granola bar snack				
chocolate chip	1 bar	10.0	180	50%
nutty fudge	1 bar	11.0	190	52%
granola bar				
chewy				
apple-cinnamon	1 bar	4.0	120	30%
chocolate chip	1 bar	4.0	130	28%
chunky nut & raisin	1 bar	6.0	130	42%
peanut butter	1 bar	5.0	130	35%
peanut butter chocolate	1 bar	4.0	130	28%

Food and Description	Amount	Fat Grams	Total Calories	% Fat Calories
crunchy				
cinnamon	1 bar	5.0	110	41%
oats 'n honey	1 bar	5.0	110	41%
(Hain) Mini-Munchies bar/low-fat				
banana split	1 bar	1.5	90	15%
chewy caramel	1 bar	1.5	90	15%
double chocolate	1 bar	1.5	90	15%
peanut butter crunch	1 bar	1.5	90	15%
strawberry marshmallow	1 bar	1.5	90	15%
(Health Valley) fat-free				
Bakes				
apple	1 bar	–	70	–
date	1 bar	–	70	–
raisin	1 bar	–	70	–
cereal bar/healthy				
fiber 7 flakes w/strawberry filling	1 bar	–	110	–
oat bran flakes w/blueberry filling	1 bar	–	110	–
raisin bran flakes w/raisin-apple filling	1 bar	–	110	–
chocolate flavor sandwich/healthy				
Bavarian creme	1 bar	–	150	–
caramel creme	1 bar	–	150	–
peanut creme	1 bar	–	150	–
vanilla creme	1 bar	–	150	–
crisp rice bar/healthy				
apple raisin	1 bar	–	110	–
orange date	1 bar	–	110	–
tropical fruit	1 bar	–	110	–
fruit bar				
apricot	1 bar	–	140	–
date fruit	1 bar	–	140	–
raisin	1 bar	–	140	–
granola bar				
blueberry	1 bar	–	140	–
chocolate flavor chip	1 bar	–	140	–
date almond	1 bar	–	140	–
raisin	1 bar	–	140	–
raspberry	1 bar	–	140	–
strawberry	1 bar	–	140	–
Healthy Breakfast Break				
apple cinnamon	1 bar	–	110	–
California strawberry	1 bar	–	110	–
mountain blueberry	1 bar	–	110	–
red raspberry	1 bar	–	110	–
marshmallow bar/healthy				
chocolate flavor chips	1 bar	–	90	–
old fashioned	1 bar	–	90	–
tropical fruit	1 bar	–	90	–

Food and Description	Amount	Fat Grams	Total Calories	% Fat Calories
(Jack La Lanne) chewy fruit & nut bar				
apple	1 bar	2.0	90	20%
banana	1 bar	2.0	90	20%
date	1 bar	2.0	90	20%
orange	1 bar	3.0	100	27%
(Kellogg's)				
cereal bar				
chocolate chip Rice Krispies	1 bar	4.0	120	30%
Rice Krispies Treats squares	1 bar	2.0	90	20%
crunchy granola bar/low-fat				
almond & brown sugar	1 bar	1.5	80	17%
apple spice	1 bar	1.5	80	17%
cinnamon raisin	1 bar	1.5	80	17%
Nutri-Grain cereal bar				
apple-cinnamon	1 bar	3.0	140	19%
blueberry	1 bar	3.0	140	19%
peach	1 bar	3.0	140	19%
raspberry	1 bar	3.0	140	19%
strawberry	1 bar	3.0	140	19%
(Kudos) whole-grain bar				
blueberry/low-fat	1 bar	1.5	90	15%
chocolate chip	1 bar	5.0	120	38%
chocolate chunk	1 bar	3.0	90	30%
M&M's milk chocolate mini's	1 bar	2.5	90	25%
milk & cookies	1 bar	5.0	130	35%
nutty fudge	1 bar	5.0	130	35%
peanut butter	1 bar	5.0	130	35%
strawberry/low-fat	1 bar	1.5	80	17%
(Nabisco)				
Chips Ahoy	1 bar	4.0	120	30%
Nutter Butter	1 bar	4.0	120	30%
Oreo	1 bar	4.0	120	30%
(Natural Nectar)				
Fi-Bar A.M.				
apple-oatmeal spice	1 bar	3.0	150	18%
banana nut	1 bar	4.0	150	24%
raisin nut bran	1 bar	4.0	150	24%
strawberry-oatmeal w/almonds	1 bar	4.0	150	24%
Fi-Bar chewy & nutty				
cocoa almond	1 bar	4.0	130	28%
cocoa peanut	1 bar	4.0	130	28%
vanilla almond	1 bar	4.0	130	28%
vanilla peanut butter	1 bar	4.0	130	28%
granola bar				
coconut	1 bar	4.0	120	30%
peanut butter	1 bar	4.0	130	28%
original fruit bar				
cranberry & wild berries	1 bar	2.0	120	15%

Food and Description	Amount	Fat Grams	Total Calories	% Fat Calories
lemon	1 bar	3.0	100	27%
Mandarin orange	1 bar	3.0	100	27%
raspberry	1 bar	2.0	120	15%
strawberry	1 bar	2.0	120	15%
(Nature Valley)				
granola bar				
chewy/low-fat				
apple brown sugar	1 bar	2.0	110	16%
chocolate chip	1 bar	2.0	110	16%
honey nut	1 bar	2.0	110	16%
oatmeal raisin	1 bar	2.0	110	16%
orchard blend	1 bar	2.0	110	16%
triple berry	1 bar	2.0	110	16%
regular				
chocolate chip	2 bars	9.0	110	37%
cinnamon	2 bars	8.0	120	34%
oat bran-honey graham	2 bars	8.0	110	34%
oats 'n honey	2 bars	8.0	120	34%
peanut butter	2 bars	10.0	120	41%
Granola Bites/chewy/low-fat				
apple cinnamon	1 pouch	2.0	120	15%
chocolate chip	1 pouch	2.0	120	15%
oats & honey	1 pouch	2.0	120	15%
Nature's Choice (See (Barbara's) in this section)				
(Nature's Wafers)				
oat bran bar				
chocolate creme	1 bar	2.0	80	23%
peanut butter	1 bar	2.0	80	23%
vanilla	1 bar	3.0	80	34%
yogurt bar				
chocolate creme	1 bar	2.0	80	23%
strawberry	1 bar	2.0	80	23%
vanilla	1 bar	2.0	80	23%
(Nestle) Sweet Success bar				
chewy				
chocolate brownie	1 bar	4.0	120	30%
chocolate chip	1 bar	4.0	120	30%
chocolate raspberry	1 bar	4.0	120	30%
chocolate peanut butter	1 bar	4.0	120	30%
oatmeal raisin	1 bar	4.0	120	30%
oatmeal raisin & almond	1 bar	4.0	120	30%
regular/apple cinnamon	1 bar	4.0	120	30%
Nutri-Grain (See (Kellogg's) in this section)				
(Obie's) mix/prepared				
apple cinnamon	1 bar	–	100	–
oats & honey	1 bar	–	110	–
(Pillsbury) Figurine bar				
chocolate	2 bars	11.0	220	45%

Food and Description	Amount	Fat Grams	Total Calories	% Fat Calories
chocolate caramel	2 bars	11.0	220	45%
chocolate peanut butter	2 bars	11.0	220	45%
s'mores	2 bars	11.0	220	45%
vanilla	2 bars	11.0	220	45%
(Quaker) chewy granola bar				
apple berry/low-fat	1 bar	2.0	110	16%
chocolate chip	1 bar	3.5	120	26%
chocolate chunk/low-fat	1 bar	2.0	110	16%
chocolate mint/low-fat	1 bar	2.0	110	16%
cookies 'n cream/low-fat	1 bar	2.0	110	16%
peanut butter chocolate chip	1 bar	4.5	120	34%
s'mores/low-fat	1 bar	2.0	110	16%
(Slim Fast) (See also (Ultra Slim Fast) in this section)				
breakfast & lunch bar/				
peanut butter	1 bar	5.0	150	30%
(SnackWell's) cereal bar				
apple cinnamon	1 bar	–	120	–
blueberry	1 bar	–	120	–
strawberry	1 bar	–	120	–
(Sunbelt)				
chewy granola bar				
almond				
1-oz bar	1 bar	7.0	130	48%
1.5-oz bar	1 bar	10.0	190	47%
apple cinnamon/low-fat	1 bar	2.5	130	17%
chocolate chip				
fudge-dipped/1.5-oz bar	1 bar	10.0	200	45%
regular				
1.2-oz bar	1 bar	7.0	160	37%
1.76-oz bar	1 bar	10.0	220	41%
macaroon/fudge-dipped				
1.37-oz bar	1 bar	12.0	200	54%
2-oz bar	1 bar	17.0	280	55%
oatmeal raisin/low-fat	1 bar	2.5	130	17%
oats & honey				
1-oz bar	1 bar	5.0	120	38%
1.69-oz bar	1 bar	9.0	210	39%
w/peanuts/fudge-dipped				
1.5-oz bar	1 bar	9.0	200	41%
2-oz bar	1 bar	15.0	270	50%
Fruit Boosters snack bar				
apple	1.3 oz	2.0	130	14%
blueberry	1.3 oz	2.0	130	14%
strawberry				
low-fat	2 oz	3.0	190	14%
original	1.3 oz	2.0	130	14%
(Tiger's Milk) energy bar				
peanut butter	1 bar	8.0	170	42%

Food and Description	Amount	Fat Grams	Total Calories	% Fat Calories
peanut butter & honey	1 bar	5.0	160	28%
protein rich	1 bar	6.0	160	34%
raisin nut crunch	1 bar	9.0	170	48%
(Ultra Slim Fast) (*See also* (Slim Fast) in this section) nutrition bar				
chewy caramel	1 bar	3.5	120	26%
chocolate chip	1 bar	4.0	120	30%
cocoa almond	1 bar	4.0	120	30%
peanut butter	1 bar	4.0	120	30%
peanut caramel	1 bar	4.0	120	30%
snack bar/vanilla almond crunch	1 bar	4.0	120	30%
GRAPE				
canned				
generic/Thompson seedless				
in heavy syrup	½ cup	–	94	–
in water	½ cup	–	48	–
(S&W)				
fancy jubilee/in heavy syrup	½ cup	–	130	–
Thompson/in heavy syrup	½ cup	–	100	–
fresh/with or without seeds				
Concord	10 grapes	<1.0	15	15%
	½ cup	<1.0	30	15%
(Dole)	1⅓ cups	–	85	–
muscat	10 grapes	<1.0	40	8%
	½ cup	<1.0	55	8%
Thompson	10 grapes	<1.0	40	8%
	½ cup	<1.0	55	8%
Tokay	10 grapes	<1.0	40	8%
	½ cup	<1.0	55	8%
GRAPE JUICE/JUICE BLEND				
bottled, boxed, or canned				
generic/bottled				
purple grape	6 fl oz	–	120	–
white grape	6 fl oz	–	110	–
(Libby's) Juicy Juice/grape	4.23 fl oz	–	70	–
	8 fl oz	–	130	–
	8.45 fl oz	–	140	–
(Minute Maid) grape juice blend	8.45 fl oz	–	130	–
(Mott's)				
grape/In-a-Minute unfrozen concentrate	2 fl oz	–	140	–
grape-apple blend	10 fl oz	–	170	–
(Season's Best) grape	8 fl oz	–	160	–
	10 fl oz	–	190	–
(Seneca)				
purple grape	8 fl oz	–	160	–
white grape	8 fl oz	–	160	–
(Sippin' Pak) grape	8.45 fl oz	–	130	–

Food and Description	Amount	Fat Grams	Total Calories	% Fat Calories
(TreeTop) grape	5.5 fl oz	–	110	–
(Welch's)				
Concord grape cocktail/Juicemakers unfrozen concentrate/prepared	8 fl oz	–	130	–
grape	10 fl oz	–	210	–
	11.5 fl oz	–	240	–
grape-apple	8 fl oz	–	150	–
grape-cranberry	8 fl oz	–	160	–
grape-peach	8 fl oz	–	160	–
grape-raspberry	8 fl oz	–	140	–
purple grape	8 fl oz	–	170	–
red grape	8 fl oz	–	170	–
	8.45 fl oz	–	170	–
USDA grape	8 fl oz	–	170	–
white grape	8 fl oz	–	160	–
	8.45 fl oz	–	160	–
frozen				
generic/grape/concentrate				
prepared	8 fl oz	–	130	–
undiluted	6 oz	–	385	–
(Seneca) prepared				
blush grape	8 fl oz	–	160	–
purple grape	8 fl oz	–	160	–
white grape	8 fl oz	–	140	–
(Sunkist)	6 fl oz	–	70	–
(Welch's) prepared				
100% grape	8 fl oz	–	160	–
purple grape				
regular	8 fl oz	–	170	–
sweetened	8 fl oz	–	130	–
red grape	8 fl oz	–	170	–
white grape				
regular	8 fl oz	–	170	–
sweetened	8 fl oz	–	140	–
white grape-cranberry	8 fl oz	–	150	–
white grape-peach	8 fl oz	–	160	–
white grape-raspberry	8 fl oz	–	140	–

GRAPE JUICE DRINK (*See also* FRUIT PUNCH; SOFT DRINK, SOFT DRINK MIX)

Food and Description	Amount	Fat Grams	Total Calories	% Fat Calories
bottled, boxed, or canned				
(Bama)	8.45 fl oz	–	120	–
(Betty Crocker)				
Squeezit grape	6.76 fl oz	–	110	–
Squeezit 100 Caped Grape	6.76 fl oz	–	100	–
(Capri Sun)	6.75 fl oz	–	100	–
(Chiquita) grape-apple-raspberry liquid concentrate	1.6 fl oz	–	130	–
(Dole)	10 fl oz	–	150	–
(Fruitopia) The Grape Beyond	8 fl oz	–	127	–

Food and Description	Amount	Fat Grams	Total Calories	% Fat Calories
(Hi-C)				
box	8.45 fl oz	–	130	–
can	7.7 fl oz	–	110	–
pet	8 fl oz	–	120	–
(Juicy Juice)	6 fl oz	–	90	–
	8.45 fl oz	–	130	–
(Minute Maid) grape juice beverage	8 fl oz	–	120	–
(Mott's) drink	10 fl oz	–	170	–
(Powerade)	8 fl oz	–	73	–
(Snapple) Grapeade	8 fl oz	–	120	–
(TreeTop) Juice Rivers grape punch	1 box	–	130	–
(Welch's)				
grape juice beverage	8 fl oz	–	150	–
grape juice cocktail	8 fl oz	–	150	–
	10 fl oz	–	170	–
grape juice drink	8 fl oz	–	150	–
	8.45 fl oz	–	150	–
	10 fl oz	–	170	–
	11.5 fl oz	–	200	–
grape-apple juice cocktail	8 fl oz	–	150	–
grape-apple juice drink	8.45 fl oz	–	150	–
	10 fl oz	–	160	–
	11.5 fl oz	–	210	–
grape-peach juice cocktail	8 fl oz	–	130	–
	10 fl oz	–	160	–
	11.5 fl oz	–	180	–
sparkling red grape juice drink	8 fl oz	–	160	–
sparkling white grape juice drink	8 fl oz	–	160	–
white grape juice cocktail	8.45 fl oz	–	160	–
frozen/prepared				
(Mott's) fruit basket cocktail	8 fl oz	–	130	–
(Seneca) cocktail	10 fl oz	–	130	–
(Welch's)				
juice cocktail/light	8 fl oz	–	50	–
orchard grape apple	8 fl oz	–	150	–
Welchade	8 fl oz	–	130	–
GRAPE LEAVES				
(Alma)				
California	2 leaves	–	10	–
imported	2 leaves	–	10	–
(Fancifoods)	2 leaves	–	5	–
(Krinos)	1 leaf	–	10	–
GRAPE SODA (*See* SOFT DRINK)				
GRAPEFRUIT				
canned/sections				
generic				
in juice	½ cup	–	46	–
in light syrup	½ cup	–	76	–

Food and Description	Amount	Fat Grams	Total Calories	% Fat Calories
in water	½ cup	–	44	–
(Kraft)	½ cup	–	50	–
(Nutradiet)	½ cup	–	40	–
(SW)				
in light syrup	½ cup	–	80	–
natural	⅔ cup	–	50	–
fresh/whole	½ medium	–	38	–
(Chiquita) ruby	½ medium	–	40	–
(Dole)	½ medium	–	50	–
(Ocean Spray)				
pink	½ medium	–	50	–
white	½ medium	–	45	–
GRAPEFRUIT JUICE/JUICE BLEND				
bottled, boxed, or canned				
(Dole) juice blend				
sunripe grapefruit/100%	8 fl oz	–	130	–
	10 fl oz	–	160	–
(Minute Maid)				
grapefruit	8 fl oz	–	97	–
pink grapefruit blend	8 fl oz	–	125	–
100% grapefruit	8 fl oz	–	100	–
(Mott's)	10 fl oz	–	120	–
(Ocean Spray)				
grapefruit juice	6 fl oz	–	60	–
pink grapefruit juice cocktail	6 fl oz	–	80	–
(Season's Best)	8 fl oz	–	90	–
	10 fl oz	–	110	–
	11.5 fl oz	–	120	–
(Seneca)	8 fl oz	–	90	–
(S&W)	6 fl oz	–	80	–
	8 fl oz	–	100	–
(TreeTop)	8 fl oz	–	100	–
	10 fl oz	–	130	–
	11.5 fl oz	–	140	–
(Tropicana)				
pure premium				
golden	6 fl oz	–	80	–
	8 fl oz	–	90	–
ruby red	6 fl oz	–	70	–
	8 fl oz	–	100	–
	10 fl oz	–	120	–
ruby red-orange	8 fl oz	–	120	–
Twister				
pink grapefruit	8 fl oz	–	120	–
	10 fl oz	–	140	–
	11.5 fl oz	–	160	–
ruby red-cranberry	8 fl oz	–	120	–
	10 fl oz	–	150	–

Food and Description	Amount	Fat Grams	Total Calories	% Fat Calories
(Welch's)	10 fl oz	–	130	–
	11.5 fl oz	–	150	–
GRAPEFRUIT JUICE DRINK (*See also* FRUIT PUNCH)				
bottled, boxed, or canned				
(Dole) Pacific pink grapefruit juice drink	8 fl oz	–	140	–
	16 fl oz	–	280	–
(Ocean Spray) ruby red grapefruit juice drink	6 fl oz	–	100	–
	8 fl oz	–	135	–
(Snapple) pink grapefruit cocktail	8 fl oz	–	120	–
(TreeTop) Desert Ice pink grapefruit juice cocktail	8 fl oz	–	120	–
frozen/prepared				
(Dole) Pacific pink grapefruit juice drink	8 fl oz	–	140	–
(Tropicana) Twister/light pink grapefruit juice drink	10 fl oz	–	40	–
GRAPEFRUIT PEEL/candied	1 oz	–	90	–
GRAVY (*See also* SAUCE; SEASONINGS)				
■ **CANNED OR JARRED**				
(Franco-American)				
au jus	¼ cup	–	10	–
beef	¼ cup	2.0	30	60%
chicken				
regular	¼ cup	4.0	40	90%
giblet	¼ cup	1.0	25	36%
cream	¼ cup	2.0	35	51%
mushroom	¼ cup	1.0	20	45%
pork	¼ cup	3.0	40	68%
turkey	¼ cup	1.0	25	36%
generic				
au jus	1 cup	0.5	38	12%
beef	1 cup	5.5	125	40%
brown	1 cup	4.0	100	36%
chicken	1 cup	14.0	190	66%
mushroom	1 cup	6.5	120	49%
turkey	1 cup	5.0	122	37%
(Heinz)				
au jus/bistro style	¼ cup	–	10	–
beef/homestyle				
regular	¼ cup	1.0	25	36%
w/onions	¼ cup	1.0	25	36%
brown/savory	¼ cup	1.0	25	36%
chicken				
classic	¼ cup	1.0	20	45%
fat-free	¼ cup	–	15	–
homestyle				
regular	¼ cup	2.0	35	51%

Food and Description	Amount	Fat Grams	Total Calories	% Fat Calories
w/mushrooms & onions	¼ cup	2.0	35	51%
country				
blue ribbon	¼ cup	1.0	25	36%
homestyle	¼ cup	1.0	25	36%
mushroom				
homestyle				
regular	¼ cup	1.0	25	36%
rich	¼ cup	0.5	20	23%
original/rich	¼ cup	0.5	20	23%
pork/homestyle	¼ cup	1.0	25	36%
turkey				
fat-free	¼ cup	–	15	–
homestyle	¼ cup	1.0	25	36%
(Libby's)				
chicken	¼ cup	4.0	60	60%
sausage/country	¼ cup	6.0	80	68%
(Pepperidge Farm) 98% fat-free				
chicken				
cream of	2 oz	1.0	30	30%
golden	2 oz	1.0	25	36%
rotisserie flavor	2 oz	1.0	25	36%
seasoned	2 oz	1.0	30	30%
mushroom/country	2 oz	0.5	30	15%
■ MIX (Note: Unless stated otherwise, 1 serving of mix = the amount in ¼ cup prepared)				
(Durkee) mix only				
au jus	1 serving	–	5	–
brown				
herb	1 serving	0.5	15	30%
mushroom	1 serving	–	15	–
onion	1 serving	–	15	–
original	1 serving	0.5	10	45%
chicken	1 serving	0.5	20	23%
country	1 serving	2.0	35	51%
homestyle	1 serving	0.5	15	30%
mushroom	1 serving	–	15	–
onion	1 serving	–	10	–
pork	1 serving	–	10	–
sausage	1 serving	2.0	35	51%
Swiss steak	1 serving	–	15	–
turkey	1 serving	–	20	–
(French's) mix only				
au jus	1 serving	–	5	–
brown				
herb	1 serving	0.5	15	30%
original	1 serving	0.5	10	45%
chicken	1 serving	0.5	25	18%
country	1 serving	2.0	35	51%
homestyle	1 serving	0.5	10	45%

Food and Description	Amount	Fat Grams	Total Calories	% Fat Calories
mushroom	1 serving	0.5	10	45%
onion	1 serving	–	15	–
pork	1 serving	–	10	–
sausage	1 serving	2.0	35	51%
Swiss steak	1 serving	–	15	–
turkey	1 serving	–	20	–
generic/prepared				
au jus	1 cup	1.0	32	28%
brown	1 cup	2.0	80	23%
chicken	1 cup	2.0	85	21%
mushroom	1 cup	1.0	70	13%
pork	1 cup	2.0	75	24%
turkey	1 cup	2.0	90	20%
(Jimmy Dean) country/mix only	1 Tbs	2.0	40	45%
(Knorr) mix only				
au jus	⅕ pkg	–	15	–
brown/classic	⅙ pkg	0.5	20	23%
brown & onion lyonnaise	⅕ pkg	0.5	20	23%
chicken	⅕ pkg	1.0	30	30%
hunter mushroom	⅕ pkg	1.0	25	36%
turkey	⅕ pkg	0.5	25	18%
(Lawry's) prepared				
beef	1 cup	1.5	80	17%
brown	1 cup	1.5	95	14%
chicken	1 cup	3.0	100	27%
turkey	1 cup	4.0	100	36%
(Loma Linda) Quik/mix only				
brown	1 Tbs	–	20	–
chicken	1 Tbs	–	20	–
country	1 Tbs	0.5	25	18%
mushroom	1 Tbs	–	15	–
onion	1 Tbs	–	20	–
(McCormick/Schilling) mix only				
au jus	½ tsp	–	5	–
brown				
herb	2 tsp	0.5	20	23%
regular	1 Tbs	0.5	20	23%
chicken	2 tsp	–	20	–
country				
regular	1⅓ Tbs	2.0	45	40%
sausage	4 tsp	1.5	40	34%
homestyle	1 Tbs	1.0	25	36%
mushroom	1 Tbs	0.5	20	23%
onion	2 tsp	0.5	20	23%
pork	1 Tbs	–	25	–
turkey	2 tsp	–	20	–
(Pillsbury) mix only				
au jus	2 tsp	–	10	–

Food and Description	Amount	Fat Grams	Total Calories	% Fat Calories
chicken	2 tsp	–	10	–
homestyle	2 tsp	–	10	–
(Weight Watchers) mix only				
brown				
regular	1 serving	–	5	–
w/mushroom	1 serving	–	10	–
w/onion	1 serving	–	10	–
chicken	1 serving	–	10	–
(Williams) mix only				
country				
regular	1 Tbs	2.0	40	45%
sausage flavored	1 Tbs	2.0	40	45%
GREAT NORTHERN BEAN				
canned				
(Bush's Best)	½ cup	–	70	–
(Eden)	½ cup	<1.0	110	4%
generic	½ cup	0.5	150	3%
(Green Giant)	½ cup	0.5	100	5%
(Joan of Arc)	½ cup	0.5	100	5%
(Luck's)				
mixed w/pinto beans	½ cup	0.5	130	3%
seasoned w/pork	½ cup	3.0	140	19%
(Seneca)	½ cup	0.5	150	3%
(Sun Vista)	½ cup	–	70	–
dry				
(Bean Cuisine)	½ cup	1.0	115	8%
generic/cooked	½ cup	0.5	105	4%
GREEK SOUP (*See* SOUP)				
GREEN BEAN/SNAP BEAN				
canned				
(Bush's Best)				
Blue Lake	½ cup	–	20	–
cut	½ cup	–	20	–
French style	½ cup	–	20	–
whole	½ cup	–	20	–
w/shelly beans	½ cup	–	35	–
(Del Monte)				
cut				
no salt added	½ cup	–	20	–
regular	½ cup	–	20	–
French style				
no salt added	½ cup	–	20	–
regular	½ cup	–	20	–
seasoned	½ cup	–	20	–
Italian cut	½ cup	–	30	–
whole	½ cup	–	20	–
(Festal)				
cut	½ cup	–	20	–

Food and Description	Amount	Fat Grams	Total Calories	% Fat Calories
French style	½ cup	–	20	–
(Freshlike)				
cut	½ cup	–	20	–
French style				
in water/no salt	½ cup	–	20	–
no salt added	½ cup	–	20	–
no salt or sugar added	½ cup	–	20	–
regular	½ cup	–	20	–
generic	½ cup	–	22	–
(Green Giant)				
cut				
50% less sodium	½ cup	–	20	–
regular	½ cup	–	20	–
French style	½ cup	–	20	–
kitchen sliced				
50% less sodium	½ cup	–	20	–
regular	½ cup	–	20	–
(Joan of Arc)				
cut				
50% less sodium	½ cup	–	20	–
regular	½ cup	–	20	–
French style	½ cup	–	20	–
(Libby)				
cut	½ cup	–	20	–
French style	½ cup	–	20	–
whole	½ cup	–	20	–
(S&W)				
cut	½ cup	–	20	–
cut green & wax	½ cup	–	20	–
dilled	1 oz	–	20	–
French style	½ cup	–	20	–
vertical pack	½ cup	–	20	–
whole	½ cup	–	20	–
(Seneca) all styles	½ cup	–	30	–
(Stokely)				
cut	½ cup	–	20	–
cut/no salt or sugar	½ cup	–	20	–
(Veg-All)				
cut	½ cup	–	20	–
French	½ cup	–	20	–
fresh/raw	½ cup	–	17	–
frozen				
(Birds Eye)				
cut	½ cup	–	25	–
French cut	½ cup	–	25	–
Italian	½ cup	–	30	–
whole				
deluxe	½ cup	–	45	–

Food and Description	Amount	Fat Grams	Total Calories	% Fat Calories
farm fresh	¾ cup	–	30	–
(C&W)				
French cut				
microwave	3 oz	–	25	–
regular	⅔ cup	–	30	–
haricots verts/tiny whole	¾ cup	–	25	–
Italian cut/microwave or regular	¾ cup	–	25	–
petite whole	¾ cup	–	25	–
(Freshlike)				
French style	3 oz	–	25	–
Italian style	3 oz	–	30	–
whole	3 oz	–	25	–
generic	½ cup	–	25	–
(Green Giant)				
cut	¾ cup	–	25	–
Harvest Fresh/cut	⅔ cup	–	25	–
(Seneca) all styles	¾ cup	–	30	–
(Veg-All)				
French	3 oz	–	30	–
Italian	3 oz	–	30	–
whole	3 oz	–	25	–
GREEN BEAN DISH (*See also* BEAN DISH; FROZEN ENTRÉE/DINNER; VEGETABLES, MIXED)				
(Birds Eye)				
Bavarian style	3.3 oz	5.0	100	45%
French cut w/toasted almonds	½ cup	3.5	70	45%
(Green Giant) Harvest Fresh w/almonds	⅔ cup	3.0	60	45%
GREEN ONION (*See* SCALLION)				
GRENADINE (*See* COCKTAIL MIXER)				
GRITS (*See* CORN GRITS; SOY GRITS)				
GROUND CHERRY				
raw	½ cup	0.5	37	12%
GROUPER				
cooked-dry heat	3 oz	1.0	100	9%
raw	3 oz	0.9	78	10%
GUACAMOLE (*See* DIP; SEASONINGS)				
GUAVA/fresh	1 medium	0.5	45	10%
GUAVA, STRAWBERRY				
raw	1 medium	<1.0	4	8%
	1 cup	1.5	169	8%
GUAVA BUTTER	1 Tbs	–	39	–
GUAVA JUICE/JUICE BLEND (*See also* FRUIT JUICE/JUICE DRINK, MIXED)				
(Kern's) nectar	6 fl oz	–	110	–
(Knudsen) guava-strawberry	8 fl oz	–	110	–
(Libby's) nectar	6 fl oz	–	110	–
(Welch's) frozen, prepared	8 fl oz	–	140	–

Food and Description	Amount	Fat Grams	Total Calories	% Fat Calories
GUAVA JUICE DRINK (*See also* FRUIT JUICE/JUICE DRINK, MIXED; FRUIT PUNCH; SOFT DRINK MIX)				
(Ocean Spray) Mauna Lai Hawaiian Guava Passion	6 fl oz	–	100	–
(Snapple) Gauva Mania	8 fl oz	–	110	–
GUAVA SAUCE/cooked	½ cup	–	43	–
GUINEA HEN/raw				
meat & skin	1 lb	23.0	568	36%
meat only	3.5 oz	2.5	110	20%
GUINEA PIG/raw	3 oz	1.7	82	19%
GUM				
(Bazooka)				
bubble	1 piece	–	15	–
soft				
regular	1 piece	–	30	–
sugarless	1 piece	–	20	–
(Beech-Nut)				
peppermint	1 piece	–	10	–
spearmint	1 piece	–	10	–
(Bubble Yum) bubble gum				
mega	1 piece	–	25	–
sugar-free	1 piece	–	15	–
variety	1 piece	–	25	–
(Bubblicious) assorted	1 piece	–	25	–
(Carefree) sugarless				
bubble gum	1 piece	–	10	–
cinnamon	1 piece	–	5	–
peppermint	1 piece	–	5	–
spearmint	1 piece	–	5	–
variety	1 piece	–	10	–
wintergreen	1 piece	–	10	–
(Chiclets) peppermint	1 piece	–	5	–
(Clorets)	1 piece	–	5	–
(Dentyne)				
Cinnaburst	1 piece	–	10	–
cinnamon	1 piece	–	10	–
regular	1 piece	–	10	–
sugar free	1 piece	–	5	–
(Dubble Bubble) bubble gum	1 piece	–	20	–
(Extra) sugar-free				
bubble gum				
classic	1 piece	–	5	–
original	1 piece	–	5	–
cinnamon	1 piece	–	5	–
peppermint	1 piece	–	5	–
spearmint	1 piece	–	5	–
winter fresh	1 piece	–	5	–

Food and Description	Amount	Fat Grams	Total Calories	% Fat Calories
(Freedent)				
peppermint	1 stick	–	10	–
spearmint	1 stick	–	10	–
winterfresh	1 stick	–	10	–
(Fruit Stripe)				
assorted	1 piece	–	10	–
bubble	1 piece	–	10	–
(Hubba Bubba)				
blueberry	1 piece	–	23	–
cola	1 piece	–	23	–
grape				
regular	1 piece	–	23	–
sugar-free	1 piece	–	13	–
original				
regular	1 piece	–	23	–
sugar-free	1 piece	–	14	–
raspberry	1 piece	–	23	–
strawberry	1 piece	–	23	–
generic/candy-coated pieces	12 pieces	–	63	–
(Trident)				
assorted	1 piece	–	5	–
cinnamon	1 piece	–	5	–
fresh mint	1 piece	–	5	–
original	1 piece	–	5	–
spearmint	1 piece	–	5	–
(Wrigley's)				
Big Red	1 stick	–	10	–
Doublemint	1 stick	–	10	–
Juicy Fruit	1 stick	–	10	–
spearmint	1 stick	–	10	–
winter fresh	1 stick	–	10	–

GUMBO (*See* SOUP; SEASONINGS)

H

Food and Description	Amount	Fat Grams	Total Calories	% Fat Calories
HADDOCK (*See also* SEAFOOD DINNER/ENTRÉE)				
breaded & fried	3 oz	9.7	194	45%
cooked-dry heat	3 oz	0.8	95	8%
raw	3 oz	0.6	74	7%

Food and Description	Amount	Fat Grams	Total Calories	% Fat Calories
smoked	3 oz	0.8	99	7%
HAKE (*See* WHITING)				
HALIBUT (*See also* SEAFOOD DINNER/ENTRÉE)				
Atlantic & Pacific				
batter-fried	3 oz	6.0	153	35%
broiled w/butter	3 oz	6.0	140	39%
cooked-dry heat	3 oz	2.5	119	19%
raw	3 oz	2.0	93	19%
smoked	3 oz	12.7	190	60%
Greenland				
raw	3 oz	12.0	160	68%
HAM (*See also* LUNCHEON MEAT; PORK; TURKEY)				
(Alpine Lace) cooked	2 oz	2.0	60	30%
(DAK)				
Danish/sliced	2 oz	2.0	60	30%
imported/sliced	2 oz	1.0	50	18%
Slender Slice	2 oz	1.0	60	15%
(Dubuque) canned patties	1 patty	11.0	140	71%
(Eckrich)				
Lean Supreme				
honey-smoked	1 slice	1.0	30	30%
Virginia baked	1 slice	0.5	30	15%
zip pack				
honey & clove	1 slice	1.0	30	30%
Virginia	1 slice	1.0	30	30%
(Fletcher's) Black Forest				
4% fat/fully cooked	3 oz	3.0	100	27%
generic				
cured				
boneless				
extra lean & regular				
cold	1 oz	2.0	45	40%
cold/chopped or diced	1 cup	10.5	230	41%
roasted	3 oz	6.5	140	42%
roasted/chopped or diced	1 cup	10.5	230	41%
extra lean/5% fat				
cold	1 oz	1.0	35	26%
cold/chopped or diced	1 cup	6.0	185	29%
roasted	3 oz	4 .0	125	32%
roasted/chopped or diced	1 cup	7.0	200	32%
regular/11% fat				
cold	1 oz	3.0	50	54%
cold/chopped or diced	1 cup	13.5	255	48%
roasted	3 oz	7.5	150	45%
roasted/chopped or diced	1 cup	12.5	250	45%
whole				
lean				
cold	1 oz	1.5	40	34%

Food and Description	Amount	Fat Grams	Total Calories	% Fat Calories
cold/chopped or diced	1 cup	7.0	210	30%
roasted	3 oz	4.0	135	27%
roasted/chopped or diced	1 cup	7.0	220	29%
lean & fat				
cold	1 oz	5.0	70	64%
cold/chopped or diced	1 cup	24.0	345	63%
roasted	3 oz	13.5	210	58%
roasted/chopped or diced	1 cup	22.0	340	58%
canned				
4% fat				
cold	1 oz	1.0	35	26%
cold/chopped or diced	1 cup	6.0	170	32%
roasted	3 oz	4.0	115	31%
roasted/chopped or diced	1 cup	6.5	190	31%
13% fat				
cold	1 oz	3.5	55	57%
cold/chopped or diced	1 cup	16.5	265	56%
roasted	3 oz	12.0	195	55%
roasted/chopped or diced	1 cup	19.5	320	55%
extra lean & regular				
cold	1 oz	2.0	40	45%
cold/chopped or diced	1 cup	9.5	200	43%
roasted	3 oz	6.5	145	40%
roasted/chopped or diced	1 cup	11.0	235	47%
country style center slice/lean & fat/cold	1 oz	3.5	60	53%
	4 oz	13.5	230	53%
patties, grilled	1 patty	17.5	205	77%
steak/extra lean/cold	2 oz	2.0	70	26%
(Healthy Choice) deli meats				
cooked	2 oz	1.5	60	23%
honey	2 oz	1.5	60	23%
smoked	2 oz	1.5	60	23%
Virginia	2 oz	1.5	60	23%
(Hillshire Farm)				
ham/10-oz pkg				
cooked	1 oz	<1.0	30	15%
lower salt	1 oz	1.0	30	30%
honey	1 oz	1.0	35	26%
luncheon meat				
brown sugar	1 oz	2.0	40	45%
genuine baked	1 oz	1.0	35	26%
honey	1 oz	2.0	40	45%
(Hormel)				
ham				
Black Label				
canned	3 oz	5.0	100	45%
chopped	1 oz	11.0	140	71%

Food and Description	Amount	Fat Grams	Total Calories	% Fat Calories
Cure 81/half ham	3 oz	5.0	100	45%
Curemaster	3 oz	3.0	80	34%
deli cooked	1 oz	1.0	29	31%
Light & Lean	3 oz	2.5	90	25%
Supreme Cut/canned				
1.5-lb ham	1 oz	1.0	31	29%
3-lb ham	1 oz	1.0	31	29%
chunk ham	2 oz	6.0	90	60%
patties				
ham	1 patty	17.0	180	85%
ham & cheese	1 patty	17.0	190	81%
(Louis Rich) baked cooked dinner slices	1 slice	1.5	80	17%
(Oscar Mayer)				
dinner slices	3 oz	3.0	80	34%
dinner steaks	1 steak	2.0	60	30%
Sweet Morsel smoked boneless pork shoulder butt	3 oz	15.0	180	75%
(Schwan's) Haugin's Farm/frozen	2 oz	2.0	60	30%
HAM & CHEESE LOAF (*See also* LUNCHEON MEAT)				
(Oscar Mayer)	1 slice	5.7	73	70%
HAM & CHEESE SPREAD	1 Tbs	2.8	37	68%
HAM SALAD (*See also* LUNCHEON MEAT)				
	1 Tbs	2.0	32	56%
	1 oz	4.0	61	59%
HAM SPREAD (*See* LUNCHEON MEAT SPREAD)				
HAMBURGER (*See also* BEEF; BEEF DISH/ENTRÉE; BUFFALO; FROZEN ENTRÉE/DINNER; TURKEY; VEGETARIAN FOODS; individual FAST FOOD listings)				
frozen or refrigerated				
(Hormel)				
bacon w/cheese	1 burger	22.0	440	45%
cheese	1 burger	20.0	400	45%
chili cheese	1 burger	23.0	450	46%
plain	1 burger	15.0	350	39%
(Jimmy Dean) mini beef w/cheese	2 burgers	14.0	270	47%
(Simplot) Micro Magic				
cheeseburger	1 burger	21.0	410	46%
plain	1 burger	15.0	340	40%
(White Castle)				
cheeseburger	2 burgers	17.0	310	49%
plain	2 burgers	14.0	270	47%
HAMBURGER HELPER (*See* BEEF DISH/ENTRÉE)				
HASH (*See* BEEF DISH/ENTRÉE; SAUSAGE DISH; TURKEY ENTRÉE/DINNER)				
HAZELNUT (*See* FILBERT)				
HAZELNUT SPREAD				
(Ferrero) Nutella chocolaty	1 Tbs	5.0	85	53%
(Roaster Fresh) hazelnut butter	2 Tbs	19.0	200	85%
HERBS (*See* SEASONINGS; individual listings)				

Food and Description	Amount	Fat Grams	Total Calories	% Fat Calories
HERRING (*See also* HERRING ROE)				
Atlantic				
breaded & fried	3 oz	18.0	279	58%
canned/in tomato sauce	2 oz	6.0	100	54%
cooked-dry heat	3 oz	9.9	172	52%
dried	1 oz	5.0	72	63%
kippered	~1.5 oz	5.0	87	51%
pickled	~½ oz	2.7	39	62%
	3 oz	15.0	220	61%
raw	3 oz	7.7	134	52%
(Lascco) chilled				
sour cream fillet	2 oz	7.0	120	53%
spice cut	2 oz	6.0	110	49%
wine snacks	2 oz	5.0	100	45%
(Nathan's) snacks in wine sauce	¼ cup	4.0	90	40%
Pacific				
cooked-dry heat	3 oz	15.0	215	63%
raw	3 oz	11.8	166	64%
HERRING ROE/raw	3 oz	1.7	111	14%
HICKORY NUT				
dried/shelled	1 oz	18.0	187	87%
HOKI/raw	3.5 oz	0.8	74	10%
HOLLANDAISE SAUCE (*See* SAUCE)				
HOMINY (*See also* CORN GRITS)				
canned				
generic	½ cup	<1.0	60	8%
(Allen's)				
golden	½ cup	<1.0	80	6%
Mexican	½ cup	<1.0	80	6%
white	½ cup	<1.0	70	6%
(Sun Vista)				
golden	½ cup	–	70	–
white	½ cup	0.5	65	7%
(Van Camp's)				
golden	½ cup	1.0	80	11%
white	½ cup	1.0	80	11%
HOMINY GRITS (*See* CORN GRITS)				
HONEY				
(Bee Maid)				
cinnamon	1 Tbs	–	70	–
natural/creamed	1 Tbs	–	60	–
regular	1 Tbs	–	60	–
(Burleson's)				
clover	1 Tbs	–	60	–
creamed	1 Tbs	–	60	–
natural	1 Tbs	–	60	–
raw	1 Tbs	–	60	–

Food and Description	Amount	Fat Grams	Total Calories	% Fat Calories
generic	1 Tbs	–	64	–
	½ cup	–	512	–
(Golden Blossom)	1 tsp	–	20	–
	1 Tbs	–	60	–
(Knott's Berry Farm)	1 Tbs	–	60	–
	1 oz	–	90	–
(Sioux)	1 Tbs	–	60	–
HONEY BUTTER				
(Downey's)				
cinnamon	1 Tbs	1.0	50	18%
original	1 Tbs	1.0	50	18%
HONEYDEW MELON/fresh				
cut up	1 cup	<1.0	50	9%
(Chiquita) cubed	1 cup	–	70	–
whole	⅒ melon	<1.0	47	10%
(Dole)	⅒ melon	–	50	–
HORSE/meat only				
roasted	4 oz	7.0	200	32%
roasted/chopped	1 cup	3.0	245	11%
HORSERADISH (See also SAUCE)				
fresh/raw	1 oz	–	18	–
jarred				
(Gold's) hot	1 tsp	–	4	–
(Hebrew National)				
red	1 Tbs	–	7	–
	½ cup	–	25	–
white	1 Tbs	–	7	–
	½ cup	–	25	–
(Kraft)				
cream style	1 tsp	–	5	–
prepared	1 tsp	–	5	–
(Rosoff's)				
red	1 Tbs	–	8	–
white	1 Tbs	–	7	–
(Silver Spring) cream style	1 tsp	–	–	–
HOT CROSS BUN (See PASTRY)				
HOT DOG (See FRANKFURTER; individual FAST FOOD listings)				
HUMMUS (See also DIP)				
homemade/USDA Standard Home Recipe	1 cup	21.0	420	45%
mix				
(Casbah) prepared	¼ cup	5.0	120	38%
HUNTER'S SOUP (See SOUP)				
HUSHPUPPY (See BREAD)				
HYACINTH BEAN				
mature				
boiled	½ cup	0.6	114	4%
raw	½ cup	2.0	350	5%
immature	½ cup	–	20	–

Food and Description	Amount	Fat Grams	Total Calories	% Fat Calories

ICE CREAM & ICE CREAM-LIKE FROZEN DESSERTS (*See also* FRUIT ICES, BARS, & POPS; ICE CREAM BARS, SANDWICHES, & FROZEN NOVELTIES; RICE FROZEN DESSERT; SHERBET; TOFU FROZEN DESSERT; YOGURT, FROZEN)
■ **(Baskin-Robbins)**
deluxe

Food and Description	Amount	Fat Grams	Total Calories	% Fat Calories
banana nut	½ cup	9.0	140	58%
banana strawberry	½ cup	6.0	130	42%
Baseball Nut	½ cup	8.0	150	48%
black walnut	½ cup	10.0	150	60%
blueberry cheesecake	⅓ cup	7.0	150	42%
Butterfinger	½ cup	8.0	160	45%
	reg scoop	15.0	300	45%
caramel chocolate crunch	½ cup	9.0	160	51%
cherry cheesecake	½ cup	7.0	150	40%
cherries jubilee	½ cup	6.0	130	42%
	reg scoop	11.0	240	41%
chewy Baby Ruth	½ cup	9.0	160	51%
chocolate	½ cup	8.0	150	48%
	reg scoop	14.0	270	47%
chocolate almond	½ cup	10.0	170	53%
	reg scoop	18.0	300	54%
chocolate chip	½ cup	9.0	150	48%
	reg scoop	15.0	260	52%
chocolate chip cookie dough	½ cup	10.0	170	53%
chocolate fudge	½ cup	9.0	160	45%
	reg scoop	15.0	290	47%
chocolate mousse royale	½ cup	9.0	170	48%
	reg scoop	16.0	320	45%
chocolate ribbon	½ cup	7.0	140	45%
chunks n chips	½ cup	9.0	160	51%
chunky Heath Bar	½ cup	9.0	170	48%
Cinnamon Tax Crunch	½ cup	8.0	160	45%
cookies 'n cream	½ cup	9.0	160	51%
	reg scoop	17.0	280	55%
French vanilla	½ cup	11.0	160	62%
	reg scoop	18.0	280	58%
fudge brownie	½ cup	10.0	170	53%
	reg scoop	18.0	320	51%

Food and Description	Amount	Fat Grams	Total Calories	% Fat Calories
German chocolate cake	½ cup	11.0	170	58%
	reg scoop	15.0	310	44%
Gold Medal Ribbon	½ cup	7.0	140	45%
Here Comes the Fudge	½ cup	7.0	150	42%
Jamoca	½ cup	13.0	240	49%
Jamoca almond fudge	½ cup	8.0	150	48%
	reg scoop	14.0	270	47%
lemon custard	½ cup	7.0	140	45%
mint chocolate chip	½ cup	9.0	150	54%
	reg scoop	15.0	260	52%
Naughty New Year's Resolution	½ cup	11.0	170	58%
New York cheesecake	½ cup	9.0	150	54%
nutty coconut	½ cup	11.0	170	58%
old fashioned butter pecan	½ cup	10.0	160	56%
	reg scoop	18.0	280	58%
Oregon blackberry	½ cup	6.9	130	48%
	reg scoop	12.0	231	47%
peach	½ cup	6.0	130	42%
	reg scoop	11.0	231	43%
peanut butter 'n chocolate	½ cup	11.0	180	55%
	reg scoop	20.0	330	55%
pink bubble gum	½ cup	7.0	150	42%
pistachio-almond	½ cup	11.0	160	62%
	reg scoop	18.0	290	56%
pralines 'n cream	½ cup	8.0	160	45%
	reg scoop	14.0	280	45%
Peter, Peter Pumpkin Cheezer	½ cup	8.0	150	48%
pumpkin pie	½ cup	6.0	130	42%
Quarterback Crunch	½ cup	9.0	160	51%
Reese's peanut butter	½ cup	10.0	170	53%
	reg scoop	18.0	302	54%
rocky road	½ cup	8.0	160	45%
	reg scoop	14.0	300	42%
rum raisin	½ cup	6.0	140	39%
s'mores	½ cup	7.5	170	40%
	reg scoop	13.0	302	39%
Snickidy Doo Dah	½ cup	8.0	170	42%
strawberry cheesecake	½ cup	7.0	150	42%
	reg scoop	13.0	260	45%
strawberry shortcake	½ cup	8.0	150	48%
Scunchous Crunch	½ cup	8.0	170	42%
Transylvania Twist	½ cup	8.0	160	45%
triple chocolate passion	½ cup	10.0	140	64%
vanilla	½ cup	8.0	140	51%
	reg scoop	14.0	240	53%
very berry strawberry	½ cup	6.0	120	45%
	reg scoop	10.0	220	41%
winter white chocolate	½ cup	8.0	150	48%

Food and Description	Amount	Fat Grams	Total Calories	% Fat Calories
world class chocolate	½ cup	8.0	150	48%
	reg scoop	14.0	280	45%
fat-free				
caramel banana surprise	½ cup	–	110	–
chocolate marshmallow	½ cup	–	110	–
chocolate vanilla twist	½ cup	–	100	–
chocolate wonder	½ cup	–	90	–
Jamoca swirl	½ cup	–	110	–
Just Peachy	½ cup	–	100	–
kookaberry kiwi	½ cup	–	100	–
peanut butter cream	½ cup	–	90	–
light				
almond buttercrunch	½ cup	4.0	120	30%
chocolate caramel nut	½ cup	4.0	130	28%
double raspberry	½ cup	2.0	90	20%
espresso 'n cream	½ cup	4.0	110	33%
pistachio creme chip	½ cup	4.0	120	30%
praline dream	½ cup	4.0	120	30%
rocky path	½ cup	4.0	130	28%
no sugar added				
berries 'n banana	½ cup	1.0	80	11%
Call Me Nuts	½ cup	2.0	100	18%
cherry cordial	½ cup	2.0	100	18%
chocolate chip	½ cup	2.5	100	23%
chocolate chocolate chip	½ cup	2.5	100	23%
chunky banana	½ cup	1.5	90	15%
coconut fudge	½ cup	1.5	110	12%
Jamoca Swiss almond	½ cup	2.5	100	23%
pineapple coconut	½ cup	1.5	90	15%
Raspberry Revelation	½ cup	1.0	100	9%
thin mint	½ cup	2.5	100	23%
vanilla Swiss almond	½ cup	2.0	110	16%
■ (Ben & Jerry's)				
original				
butter pecan	½ cup	26.0	310	75%
Cherry Garcia	½ cup	16.0	240	60%
chocolate chip cookie dough	½ cup	17.0	270	57%
chocolate fudge brownie	½ cup	14.0	250	50%
Chubby Hubby	½ cup	23.0	350	59%
Chunky Monkey	½ cup	19.0	280	61%
coconut almond fudge chip	½ cup	25.0	320	70%
coffee almond fudge	½ cup	20.0	290	62%
coffee toffee crunch	½ cup	19.0	280	61%
English toffee crunch	½ cup	21.0	310	61%
mint w/chocolate cookie	½ cup	17.0	260	59%
New York super fudge chunk	½ cup	20.0	290	62%
peanut butter cup	½ cup	26.0	370	63%
Rainforest Crunch	½ cup	23.0	300	69%

Food and Description	Amount	Fat Grams	Total Calories	% Fat Calories
vanilla	½ cup	17.0	230	67%
Wavy Gravy	½ cup	24.0	330	65%
smooth				
Aztec harvest coffee	½ cup	16.0	230	63%
deep dark chocolate	½ cup	15.0	260	52%
double chocolate fudge	½ cup	16.0	280	51%
mocha fudge	½ cup	16.0	270	53%
vanilla	½ cup	17.0	230	67%
vanilla bean	½ cup	17.0	230	67%
vanilla caramel fudge	½ cup	17.0	280	55%
white Russian	½ cup	16.0	250	58%
■ (Borden)				
Lady Borden				
butter pecan	½ cup	12.0	180	60%
olde fashioned recipe				
strawberry	½ cup	5.0	130	35%
vanilla	½ cup	7.0	130	48%
original				
strawberry	½ cup	6.0	130	42%
■ (Breyers)				
fat-free				
caramel praline crunch	½ cup	–	120	–
chocolate	½ cup	–	95	–
fudge twirl	½ cup	–	105	–
vanilla	½ cup	–	100	–
vanilla/strawberry	½ cup	–	90	–
light/reduced fat				
brownie marble fudge	½ cup	5.0	150	30%
chocolate chocolate chip	½ cup	5.0	150	30%
chocolate fudge twirl	½ cup	4.0	140	26%
fudge toffee parfait	½ cup	5.0	150	30%
heavenly hash	½ cup	5.0	150	30%
mint cookies in cream	½ cup	5.0	140	32%
mocha almond fudge	½ cup	6.0	160	34%
praline almond crunch	½ cup	5.0	140	32%
strawberry	½ cup	4.0	120	30%
Swiss almond fudge	½ cup	6.0	160	34%
vanilla	½ cup	4.5	130	31%
vanilla/chocolate/strawberry	½ cup	4.0	120	30%
no sugar added				
mint chocolate chip	½ cup	6.0	110	49%
vanilla	½ cup	5.0	90	50%
vanilla fudge twirl	½ cup	4.0	100	36%
vanilla/chocolate/strawberry	½ cup	5.0	100	45%
original				
banana strawberry	½ cup	3.0	140	19%
butter almond	½ cup	10.0	170	53%
butter pecan	½ cup	12.0	180	60%

Food and Description	Amount	Fat Grams	Total Calories	% Fat Calories
cherry vanilla	½ cup	7.0	140	45%
chocolate	½ cup	8.0	160	45%
chocolate chip	½ cup	10.0	170	53%
chocolate chip cookie dough	½ cup	9.0	170	42%
chocolate chocolate chip	½ cup	10.0	180	50%
coffee	½ cup	8.0	150	48%
cookies in cream	½ cup	9.0	170	48%
French vanilla	½ cup	10.0	170	53%
fudge twirl	½ cup	8.0	160	45%
mint chocolate chip	½ cup	10.0	170	53%
peach	½ cup	6.0	130	42%
praline almond	½ cup	8.0	170	42%
rocky road	½ cup	9.0	190	43%
rum raisin	½ cup	6.0	130	42%
strawberry	½ cup	6.0	130	42%
toffee bar crunch	½ cup	9.0	170	48%
vanilla	½ cup	8.0	150	48%
vanilla/black cherry	½ cup	8.0	160	45%
vanilla/chocolate	½ cup	8.0	160	45%
vanilla/chocolate/strawberry	½ cup	8.0	160	45%
vanilla fudge twirl	½ cup	8.0	160	45%
vanilla/orange sherbet	½ cup	5.0	140	32%
Romantica				
chocolate & vanilla	1 slice	10.0	180	50%
toffee & vanilla	1 slice	10.0	180	50%
Viennetta				
chocolate	1 slice	12.0	190	57%
mint	1 slice	11.0	190	52%
vanilla	1 slice	11.0	190	52%
■ (Dreyer's)				
fat-free				
black cherry vanilla swirl	½ cup	–	100	–
caramel praline crunch	½ cup	–	110	–
chocolate fudge				
no sugar added	½ cup	–	80	–
regular	½ cup	–	100	–
coffee fudge				
no sugar added	½ cup	–	80	–
regular	½ cup	–	100	–
cookie chunk	½ cup	–	110	–
marble fudge	½ cup	–	100	–
mint fudge	½ cup	–	100	–
raspberry vanilla swirl/no sugar added	½ cup	–	70	–
strawberry shortcake	½ cup	–	100	–
vanilla				
no sugar added	½ cup	–	80	–
regular	½ cup	–	90	–
vanilla chocolate swirl/no sugar added	½ cup	–	80	–

Food and Description	Amount	Fat Grams	Total Calories	% Fat Calories
vanilla 'n caramel/no sugar added	½ cup	–	80	–
Grand				
light				
brownies 'n fudge	½ cup	4.0	110	33%
butter pecan	½ cup	5.0	120	38%
cheesecake chunk	½ cup	5.0	120	38%
chocolate almond fudge	½ cup	5.0	120	38%
chocolate fudge mousse	½ cup	4.0	110	33%
cookie dough	½ cup	5.0	120	38%
cookies 'n cream	½ cup	4.0	110	33%
dreamy caramel cream	½ cup	4.0	110	33%
espresso fudge chip	½ cup	4.0	110	33%
French silk	½ cup	5.0	120	38%
malt ball 'n fudge	½ cup	5.0	110	41%
mint cookies 'n cream	½ cup	4.0	110	33%
mocha almond fudge	½ cup	4.0	110	33%
peanut butter cups	½ cup	5.0	120	38%
pralines 'n caramel	½ cup	4.0	120	30%
rocky road	½ cup	4.0	120	30%
vanilla	½ cup	4.0	100	36%
limited edition				
apple pie	½ cup	7.0	140	45%
championship sundae				
light	½ cup	4.0	120	30%
regular	½ cup	8.0	150	48%
egg nog	½ cup	7.0	140	45%
orange cream bar	½ cup	6.0	130	42%
peppermint				
light	½ cup	4.0	110	33%
regular	½ cup	8.0	140	51%
pumpkin	½ cup	7.0	140	45%
root beer float	½ cup	5.0	120	38%
turtle sundae	½ cup	9.0	160	51%
low-fat				
chocolate fudge chunk	½ cup	2.0	110	16%
cookies 'n cream	½ cup	2.0	110	16%
espresso chip	½ cup	2.0	100	18%
Heath toffee & caramel	½ cup	2.0	120	15%
rocky road	½ cup	2.0	110	16%
vanilla	½ cup	2.0	100	18%
no sugar added				
black cherry vanilla	½ cup	4.0	100	36%
chocolate	½ cup	4.0	100	36%
chocolate chip	½ cup	5.0	100	45%
marble fudge	½ cup	4.0	100	36%
mint fudge	½ cup	4.0	100	36%
mocha fudge	½ cup	4.0	100	36%
strawberry	½ cup	4.0	90	40%

Food and Description	Amount	Fat Grams	Total Calories	% Fat Calories
triple chocolate	½ cup	5.0	100	45%
vanilla	½ cup	4.0	100	36%
vanilla 'n caramel	½ cup	4.0	100	36%
regular				
almond praline	½ cup	8.0	160	45%
butter pecan	½ cup	9.0	160	51%
chocolate	½ cup	8.0	140	51%
Chocolate Chips!	½ cup	9.0	160	51%
coffee	½ cup	8.0	140	51%
cookie dough	½ cup	9.0	170	48%
cookies 'n cream	½ cup	8.0	150	51%
espresso chip	½ cup	8.0	150	48%
French vanilla	½ cup	10.0	160	56%
ice cream sandwich	½ cup	8.0	150	48%
marble fudge	½ cup	7.0	140	48%
Mint Chocolate Chips!	½ cup	9.0	160	51%
mocha almond fudge	½ cup	9.0	150	54%
mud pie	½ cup	8.0	150	48%
Neapolitan	½ cup	7.0	130	37%
real strawberry	½ cup	6.0	130	42%
rocky road	½ cup	10.0	170	53%
strawberry cheesecake chunk	½ cup	8.0	150	48%
super chocolate chunk	½ cup	11.0	180	55%
toasted almond	½ cup	9.0	150	54%
vanilla	½ cup	10.0	150	56%
vanilla bean	½ cup	9.0	150	54%
■ (Eagle Brand) all natural				
homestyle vanilla	½ cup	9.0	150	54%
■ (Edy's)				
fat-free				
black cherry vanilla swirl	½ cup	–	100	–
caramel praline crunch	½ cup	–	110	–
chocolate fudge				
no sugar added	½ cup	–	80	–
regular	½ cup	–	100	–
coffee fudge				
no sugar added	½ cup	–	80	–
regular	½ cup	–	100	–
cookie chunk	½ cup	–	110	–
marble fudge	½ cup	–	100	–
mint fudge	½ cup	–	100	–
raspberry vanilla swirl/no sugar added	½ cup	–	70	–
strawberry shortcake	½ cup	–	100	–
vanilla				
no sugar added	½ cup	–	80	–
regular	½ cup	–	90	–
vanilla chocolate swirl/no sugar added	½ cup	–	80	–
vanilla 'n caramel/no sugar added	½ cup	–	80	–

Food and Description	Amount	Fat Grams	Total Calories	% Fat Calories
Grand				
light				
brownies 'n fudge	½ cup	4.0	110	33%
butter pecan	½ cup	5.0	120	38%
cheesecake chunk	½ cup	5.0	120	38%
chocolate almond fudge	½ cup	5.0	120	38%
chocolate fudge mousse	½ cup	4.0	110	33%
cookie dough	½ cup	5.0	120	38%
cookies 'n cream	½ cup	4.0	110	33%
dreamy caramel cream	½ cup	4.0	110	33%
espresso fudge chip	½ cup	4.0	110	33%
French silk	½ cup	5.0	120	38%
mint cookies 'n cream	½ cup	4.0	110	33%
mocha almond fudge	½ cup	4.0	110	33%
peanut butter cups	½ cup	5.0	120	38%
pralines 'n caramel	½ cup	4.0	120	30%
rocky road	½ cup	4.0	120	30%
vanilla	½ cup	4.0	100	36%
limited edition				
apple pie	½ cup	7.0	140	45%
championship sundae				
light	½ cup	4.0	120	30%
regular	½ cup	8.0	150	48%
egg nog	½ cup	7.0	140	45%
orange cream bar	½ cup	6.0	130	42%
peppermint				
light	½ cup	4.0	110	33%
regular	½ cup	8.0	140	51%
pumpkin	½ cup	7.0	140	45%
root beer float	½ cup	5.0	120	38%
turtle sundae	½ cup	9.0	160	51%
low-fat				
chocolate fudge chunk	½ cup	2.0	110	16%
cookies 'n cream	½ cup	2.0	110	16%
espresso chip	½ cup	2.0	100	18%
Heath toffee & caramel	½ cup	2.0	120	15%
rocky road	½ cup	2.0	110	16%
vanilla	½ cup	2.0	100	18%
no sugar added				
black cherry vanilla	½ cup	4.0	100	36%
chocolate	½ cup	4.0	100	36%
chocolate chip	½ cup	5.0	100	45%
marble fudge	½ cup	4.0	100	36%
mint fudge	½ cup	4.0	100	36%
mocha fudge	½ cup	4.0	100	36%
strawberry	½ cup	4.0	90	40%
triple chocolate	½ cup	5.0	100	45%
vanilla	½ cup	4.0	100	36%

Food and Description	Amount	Fat Grams	Total Calories	% Fat Calories
vanilla 'n caramel	½ cup	4.0	100	36%
regular				
almond praline	½ cup	8.0	160	45%
banana split	½ cup	10.0	170	53%
brownie batter	½ cup	8.0	150	48%
butter pecan	½ cup	9.0	160	51%
cherry chocolate chip	½ cup	8.0	150	48%
chocolate	½ cup	9.0	140	58%
Chocolate Chips!	½ cup	8.0	160	45%
chocolate chocolate chip	½ cup	10.0	160	56%
chocolate fudge sundae	½ cup	10.0	170	53%
coffee	½ cup	8.0	140	51%
cookie dough	½ cup	9.0	170	48%
cookies 'n cream	½ cup	8.0	150	48%
double fudge brownie	½ cup	9.0	160	51%
espresso chip	½ cup	8.0	150	48%
French vanilla	½ cup	10.0	160	56%
ice cream sandwich	½ cup	8.0	150	48%
Mint Chocolate Chips!	½ cup	9.0	160	51%
real strawberry	½ cup	6.0	130	42%
rocky road	½ cup	10.0	170	53%
strawberry cheesecake chunk	½ cup	8.0	150	48%
vanilla	½ cup	10.0	150	50%
vanilla bean	½ cup	9.0	150	54%
vanilla chocolate strawberry	½ cup	7.0	130	48%
■ (Eskimo Pie)				
dairy dessert				
fudge ripple	½ cup	7.0	170	37%
vanilla	½ cup	7.0	140	45%
■ (Haagen-Dazs)				
Cordials				
Baileys Original Irish Cream	½ cup	18.0	280	58%
DiSaronno Amaretto	½ cup	15.0	260	52%
Extraas				
brownies à la mode	½ cup	18.0	280	58%
Cappuccino Commotion	½ cup	21.0	310	61%
Caramel Cone Explosion	½ cup	20.0	310	58%
Cookie Dough Dynamo	½ cup	19.0	300	57%
Peanut Butter Burst	½ cup	22.0	330	60%
Strawberry Cheesecake Craze	½ cup	18.0	290	56%
Triple Brownie Overload	½ cup	20.0	300	60%
regular				
butter pecan	½ cup	24.0	320	68%
chocolate	½ cup	18.0	270	60%
chocolate chip	½ cup	20.0	300	60%
coffee	½ cup	18.0	270	60%
cookies & cream	½ cup	17.0	270	57%
macadamia brittle	½ cup	20.0	300	60%

Food and Description	Amount	Fat Grams	Total Calories	% Fat Calories
rum raisin	½ cup	17.0	270	57%
strawberry	½ cup	16.0	250	58%
vanilla	½ cup	18.0	270	60%
vanilla fudge	½ cup	18.0	280	58%
vanilla Swiss almond	½ cup	21.0	310	61%
sorbet & cream				
orange	½ cup	9.0	200	41%
raspberry	½ cup	9.0	190	43%
■ (Healthy Choice)				
bananas Foster	½ cup	1.5	110	12%
Black Forest	½ cup	2.0	120	15%
butter pecan crunch	½ cup	2.0	120	15%
cappuccino chocolate chunk	½ cup	2.0	120	15%
cappuccino mocha fudge	½ cup	2.0	120	15%
cherry chocolate chunk	½ cup	2.0	110	16%
chocolate fudge mousse	½ cup	2.0	120	15%
cookies 'n cream	½ cup	2.0	120	15%
fudge brownie	½ cup	2.0	120	15%
fudge brownie à la mode	½ cup	2.0	120	15%
malt caramel cone	½ cup	2.0	120	15%
mint chocolate chip	½ cup	2.0	120	15%
orange sherbet & cream	½ cup	2.0	90	20%
peanut butter cookie dough	½ cup	2.0	120	15%
praline caramel cluster	½ cup	2.0	130	14%
rocky road	½ cup	2.0	140	13%
strawberry sorbet & cream	½ cup	2.0	90	20%
triple chocolate chunk	½ cup	2.0	110	16%
turtle fudge cake	½ cup	2.0	130	14%
vanilla	½ cup	2.0	100	18%
■ (Healthy Indulgence)				
low-fat				
butter pecan crunch	½ cup	2.0	120	15%
caramel praline	½ cup	2.0	130	14%
fudge brownie	½ cup	2.0	120	15%
heavenly hash	½ cup	2.0	120	15%
vanilla	½ cup	2.0	120	15%
■ (Kemp's)				
fat-free				
caramel praline	½ cup	–	120	–
fudge marble	½ cup	–	110	–
turtle fudge brownie	½ cup	–	120	–
vanilla	½ cup	–	100	–
premium				
almond praline	½ cup	8.0	160	45%
Bear Tracks	½ cup	9.0	170	48%
butter pecan	½ cup	11.0	170	58%
cookies 'n cream	½ cup	9.0	170	48%
chocolate chip	½ cup	10.0	170	53%

Food and Description	Amount	Fat Grams	Total Calories	% Fat Calories
Chocolate Monster	½ cup	8.0	170	42%
Mocha Madness	½ cup	8.0	160	45%
natural vanilla	½ cup	8.0	150	48%
premium fat-free				
caramel nutty crunch	½ cup	0.5	120	4%
fudge marble	½ cup	–	110	–
heavenly hash	½ cup	–	120	–
mint fudge brownie	½ cup	–	110	–
vanilla	½ cup	–	100	–
■ **(Knudsen)**				
3-gallon tub				
butter pecan	½ cup	8.0	150	48%
chocolate	½ cup	6.0	130	42%
chocolate chip	½ cup	7.0	140	45%
cookies in cream	½ cup	8.0	140	51%
French vanilla	½ cup	7.0	140	45%
rocky road	½ cup	7.0	140	45%
strawberry	½ cup	6.0	120	45%
vanilla	½ cup	7.0	130	48%
■ **(Lucerne)**				
light/dairy				
chocolate	½ cup	4.0	115	31%
cookie cream	½ cup	5.0	130	35%
mocha almond	½ cup	4.0	125	29%
rocky road	½ cup	4.0	130	28%
strawberry cream	½ cup	3.0	105	26%
regular				
chocolate chip	½ cup	8.0	150	48%
coffee	½ cup	7.0	140	45%
French vanilla	½ cup	8.0	150	48%
mint chocolate chip	½ cup	8.0	150	48%
Neapolitan	½ cup	7.0	140	45%
ranch pecan	½ cup	9.0	160	51%
rocky road	½ cup	8.0	150	48%
strawberry cheesecake	½ cup	6.0	140	39%
vanilla	½ cup	8.0	140	39%
■ **(Schwan's)**				
ice cream specialties				
grasshopper ice cream pie	⅛ pie	20.0	370	49%
holiday slice	1 slice	7.0	150	42%
ice cream nut roll	⅛ roll	16.0	250	58%
strawberry cheesecake ice cream pie	⅛ pie	14.0	330	38%
lite ice cream				
butter crunch	½ cup	3.5	120	26%
praline almondine sundae	½ cup	3.5	120	26%
vanilla	½ cup	3.0	100	27%
premium ice cream				
black raspberry	½ cup	7.0	140	45%

Food and Description	Amount	Fat Grams	Total Calories	% Fat Calories
butter crunch	½ cup	8.0	150	48%
butter pecan	½ cup	9.0	150	54%
butterscotch ripple	½ cup	7.0	140	45%
cherry nut	½ cup	7.0	140	45%
cherry vanilla	½ cup	7.0	140	45%
chip mint	½ cup	8.0	150	48%
chocolate	½ cup	7.0	140	45%
chocolate almond	½ cup	8.0	150	48%
chocolate chip	½ cup	8.0	150	48%
chocolate chip cookie dough	½ cup	8.0	150	48%
chocolate fudge ripple	½ cup	7.0	140	45%
chocolate marshmallow ripple	½ cup	5.0	140	32%
chunky chocolate supreme	½ cup	8.0	160	45%
cookies & cream	½ cup	8.0	160	45%
dark sweet cherry	½ cup	6.0	140	39%
French vanilla	½ cup	9.0	170	48%
holiday special	½ cup	6.0	150	36%
maple nut	½ cup	9.0	150	54%
Neapolitan	½ cup	7.0	140	45%
peach	½ cup	6.0	130	42%
peanut butter fudge ripple	½ cup	7.0	150	42%
pecan praline	½ cup	7.0	150	42%
peppermint stick	½ cup	7.0	150	42%
pink divinity	½ cup	7.0	150	42%
raspberry delight	½ cup	5.0	130	35%
raspberry ripple	½ cup	7.0	140	45%
rocky road	½ cup	6.0	150	36%
strawberry	½ cup	7.0	140	45%
Summer's Dream	½ cup	5.0	130	35%
vanilla	½ cup	7.0	140	45%
■ (Sealtest)				
fat-free				
chocolate	½ cup	–	100	–
vanilla	½ cup	–	100	–
vanilla fudge royale	½ cup	–	100	–
vanilla/chocolate/strawberry	½ cup	–	100	–
Gold				
cappuccino	½ cup	7.0	140	45%
caramel praline almond	½ cup	7.0	150	42%
cherry chocolate chunk	½ cup	7.0	140	45%
chocolate fudge brownie	½ cup	7.0	160	39%
Neapolitan	½ cup	6.0	110	49%
vanilla	½ cup	7.0	130	48%
regular				
butter pecan	½ cup	9.0	160	51%
chocolate	½ cup	7.0	140	45%
chocolate chip	½ cup	8.0	150	48%
chocolate chip cookie dough	½ cup	8.0	160	45%

Food and Description	Amount	Fat Grams	Total Calories	% Fat Calories
coffee	½ cup	7.0	140	45%
cookies n' cream	½ cup	7.0	140	45%
Cubic Scoops vanilla/orange	½ cup	8.0	140	51%
French vanilla	½ cup	8.0	140	51%
fudge royale	½ cup	7.0	150	42%
heavenly hash	½ cup	7.0	150	42%
maple walnut	½ cup	9.0	160	51%
mint chocolate chip	½ cup	8.0	150	48%
pistachio	½ cup	7.0	130	48%
spumoni	½ cup	7.0	140	45%
rainbow	½ cup	7.0	140	45%
strawberry	½ cup	6.0	130	42%
strawberry-chocolate-vanilla	½ cup	6.0	140	39%
vanilla	½ cup	7.0	140	45%
■ (Sweet 'N Low)				
butter pecan	½ cup	6.0	120	45%
chocolate	½ cup	2.0	90	20%
strawberry	½ cup	1.0	80	11%
vanilla	½ cup	2.0	80	23%
■ (Weight Watchers)				
Cookie Dough Craze	½ cup	3.5	140	23%
Oh! So Very Vanilla	½ cup	2.5	120	19%
Positively Praline Crunch	½ cup	3.0	140	19%
Triple Chocolate Tornado	½ cup	3.5	150	21%

ICE CREAM BARS, SANDWICHES, & FROZEN NOVELTIES (*See also* FRUIT ICES, BARS, & POPS; RICE FROZEN DESSERT; SHERBET; TOFU FROZEN DESSERT)

Food and Description	Amount	Fat Grams	Total Calories	% Fat Calories
■ (Baskin-Robbins)				
Chillyburger				
chocolate chip	1 piece	11.0	220	45%
mint chocolate chip	1 piece	11.0	220	45%
fountain ice-cream drink				
Cappy Blast w/whipped cream	1 drink	10.0	290	31%
Mocha Cappy Blast w/whipped cream	1 drink	11.0	330	30%
vanilla malt	1 drink	31.0	660	42%
sundae bar				
Jamoca almond fudge	1 bar	17.0	280	55%
peanut butter chocolate	1 bar	27.0	340	71%
pralines 'n cream	1 bar	17.0	280	55%
Tiny Toon bar				
chocolate chip	1 bar	17.0	240	64%
mint chocolate chip	1 bar	17.0	240	64%
vanilla	1 bar	16.0	210	69%
■ (Ben & Jerry's)				
novelties				
chocolate chip cookie dough	1 pop	28.0	450	56%
English toffee crunch	1 pop	23.0	340	61%
New York super fudge chunk	1 pop	31.0	390	72%
vanilla	1 pop	28.0	360	70%

Food and Description	Amount	Fat Grams	Total Calories	% Fat Calories
■ **(Breyers)**				
Breyers Cup	1 cup	10.0	90	10%
ice cream bar				
cookie dough	1 bar	17.0	280	55%
mint	1 bar	15.0	230	59%
vanilla				
plain	1 bar	15.0	230	59%
w/almonds	1 bar	17.0	250	61%
ice cream cone				
butter pecan	1 cone	17.0	300	51%
mint chocolate chip	1 cone	14.0	280	45%
ice cream sandwich	1 piece	11.0	250	40%
Viennetta/mini				
cappuccino/vanilla	1 piece	14.0	220	57%
vanilla	1 piece	14.0	220	57%
■ **CARNATION** (*See* (Nestle) in this section)				
■ **(Chiquita)**				
fruit & cream bar				
banana	1 bar	2.0	80	23%
blueberry	1 bar	1.0	80	11%
peach	1 bar	1.0	80	11%
raspberry	1 bar	1.0	80	11%
strawberry	1 bar	1.0	80	11%
strawberry-banana	1 bar	2.0	80	23%
■ **(Dove)**				
bar				
almond				
4 per pkg/3-oz bars	1 bar	19.0	280	61%
individual pkg/3.67-oz bar	1 bar	24.0	350	62%
caramel creme swirl/toffee chips/ 3-oz bar	1 bar	16.0	280	51%
chocolate w/dark chocolate coating				
4 per pkg/3-oz bars	1 bar	17.0	260	59%
individual pkg/3.67-oz bar	1 bar	21.0	330	57%
mocha cashew crunch/3-oz bar	1 bar	17.0	260	59%
vanilla				
w/dark chocolate coating				
4 per pkg/3-oz bars	1 bar	17.0	260	43%
individual pkg/3.67-oz bar	1 bar	21.0	330	57%
w/milk chocolate coating				
4 per pkg/3-oz bars	1 bar	17.0	260	43%
individual pkg/3.67-oz bar	1 bar	21.0	330	57%
w/white coating/3-oz bar	1 bar	17.0	270	57%
bite-size				
cherry royale	5 pieces	21.0	340	56%
double chocolate	5 pieces	21.0	330	57%
vanilla				
classic	5 pieces	21.0	330	57%

Food and Description	Amount	Fat Grams	Total Calories	% Fat Calories
French	5 pieces	21.0	330	57%
seasonal				
green mint & chocolate fudge truffle swirl bar w/dark chocolate coating/3-oz bar	1 bar	17.0	290	53%
Irish creme cordial/bite-size	5 pieces	22.0	340	58%
party peppermint/bite-size	5 pieces	22.0	360	55%
■ (Dreyer's)				
bar				
chocolate mocha crunch	1 bar	17.0	250	61%
cookies 'xn cream	1 bar	17.0	260	59%
rocky road	1 bar	19.0	270	63%
vanilla & almonds	1 bar	20.0	270	67%
cone				
caramel almond crunch	1 cone	20.0	350	51%
cookies 'n cream	1 cone	20.0	340	53%
double chocolate fudge	1 cone	26.0	390	60%
vanilla fudge sundae	1 cone	18.0	340	48%
■ (Edy's)				
bar				
chocolate mocha crunch	1 bar	17.0	250	61%
cookies 'n cream	1 bar	17.0	260	59%
rocky road	1 bar	19.0	270	63%
vanilla & almonds	1 bar	20.0	270	67%
cone				
caramel almond crunch	1 cone	20.0	350	51%
cookies 'n cream	1 cone	20.0	340	53%
double chocolate fudge	1 cone	26.0	390	60%
vanilla fudge sundae	1 cone	18.0	340	48%
■ (Eskimo Pie)				
butterscotch crunch	1 bar	11.0	170	58%
cherry	1 bar	10.0	150	60%
pecan w/milk chocolate coating	1 bar	15.0	190	71%
pudding	1 bar	1.5	80	17%
sandwich				
original	1 sandwich	6.0	180	30%
Sugar Freedom	1 sandwich	7.0	180	35%
sundae cone	1 cone	15.0	240	56%
vanilla				
original				
w/dark chocolate coating	1 bar	11.0	160	62%
w/milk chocolate coating	1 bar	12.0	180	60%
Sugar Freedom, w/crispy rice	1 bar	12.0	170	64%
w/dark chocolate coating	1 bar	12.0	180	60%
■ (Fudgetastics)				
sundae on a stick				
crunchy	1 bar	14.0	230	55%
plain	1 bar	15.0	220	61%

Food and Description	Amount	Fat Grams	Total Calories	% Fat Calories
■ **(Good Humor)**				
ice cream bar				
chocolate eclair	1 bar	10.0	220	41%
classic candy center crunch	1 bar	21.0	280	68%
classic strawberry shortcake	1 bar	11.0	210	47%
classic toasted almond	1 bar	11.0	230	43%
original	1 bar	13.0	230	51%
ice cream cone				
king cone/vanilla	5.5 oz	10.0	300	37%
ice cream cup				
chocolate milkshake	1 cup	5.0	230	20%
Reese's peanut butter cup	1 piece	16.0	220	65%
ice cream sandwich				
chocolate chip cookie	1 sandwich	15.0	320	42%
giant Neapolitan	1 sandwich	10.0	260	35%
giant vanilla	1 sandwich	10.0	240	38%
sidewalk sundae	1 sandwich	8.0	190	38%
■ **(Haagen-Dazs)**				
Extraas				
Caramel Cone Explosion				
multi-pack	1 cone	22.0	330	60%
single pack	1 cone	23.0	350	59%
Cookie Dough Dynamo/single pack	1 bar	25.0	380	59%
Iced Cappuccino				
multi-pack	1 bar	21.0	290	65%
single pack	1 bar	24.0	330	65%
Triple Brownie Overload				
multi-pack	1 bar	23.0	320	65%
single pack	1 bar	27.0	380	64%
regular				
chocolate w/dark chocolate coating				
multi-pack	1 bar	22.0	320	62%
single pack	1 bar	27.0	400	61%
coffee & almond crunch				
multi-pack	1 bar	21.0	290	65%
single pack	1 bar	26.0	360	65%
vanilla w/dark chocolate coating				
multi-pack	1 bar	22.0	320	62%
single pack	1 bar	27.0	400	61%
vanilla w/milk chocolate coating				
plain				
multi-pack	1 bar	20.0	280	64%
single pack	1 bar	27.0	370	66%
w/almonds				
multi-pack	1 bar	22.0	300	66%
single pack	1 bar	24.0	330	65%
■ **(Jackson's)**				
crunch bar	1 bar	11.0	170	58%

Food and Description	Amount	Fat Grams	Total Calories	% Fat Calories
fudge pop	1 pop	1.0	80	11%
sandwich	1 sandwich	7.0	180	35%
toffee bar	1 bar	14.0	200	63%
vanilla bar				
lite	1 bar	8.0	100	72%
regular	1 bar	13.0	190	62%
vanilla chocolate peanut cone	1 cone	18.0	330	49%
■ (Kemps)				
bar	1 bar	12.0	160	68%
sandwich				
cookies 'n cream	1 sandwich	7.0	120	53%
original	1 sandwich	6.0	160	34%
toffee bar	1 bar	8.0	110	65%
■ (Klondike)				
caramel crunch	1 bar	18.0	300	54%
Ice Cream Kone	1 cone	17.0	310	49%
krispy	1 bar	20.0	300	60%
Krunch Bar	1 bar	13.0	200	59%
vanilla w/milk chocolate coating	1 bar	20.0	290	62%
■ (M&M ★ Mars)				
Milky Way				
chocolate/milk chocolate/singles				
reduced fat/2-oz bar	1 bar	7.0	140	45%
stick/3-oz bar	1 bar	13.0	220	53%
vanilla/dark chocolate/singles				
reduced fat/2-oz bar	1 bar	7.0	140	45%
stick/3-oz bar	1 bar	13.0	220	53%
Snickers				
bar	1 bar	13.0	220	53%
ice cream cone	1 cone	15.0	290	47%
singles/2-oz bar	1 bar	13.0	200	59%
snack	4 bars	25.0	390	58%
3 Musketeers				
chocolate				
singles/2.75 oz-bar	1 bar	11.0	190	52%
6 per pkg, 2-oz bars	1 bar	9.0	150	54%
vanilla				
singles/2.75 oz bar	1 bar	11.0	190	52%
6 per pkg, 2-oz bars	1 bar	8.0	150	48%
■ MILKY WAY (See (M&M ★ Mars) in this section)				
■ (Natural Nectar)				
banana cream	1 bar	8.0	170	42%
coco fudge 'n cream	1 bar	8.0	170	42%
mocha	1 bar	14.0	300	42%
nectar	1 bar	15.0	300	45%
strawberries 'n cream	1 bar	5.0	120	38%
wildberry cream	1 bar	3.0	120	23%

Food and Description	Amount	Fat Grams	Total Calories	% Fat Calories
■ **(Nestle)**				
Bon Bons				
dark chocolate	5 pieces	13.0	190	62%
	8 pieces	21.0	310	61%
	9 pieces	24.0	350	62%
milk chocolate	5 pieces	14.0	200	63%
	8 pieces	23.0	330	63%
	9 pieces	26.0	370	63%
Butterfinger	1 bar	12.0	170	64%
Carnation strawberry sundae cup	6 oz	8.0	200	36%
Cool Creations				
cookies & cream	1 sandwich	11.0	240	41%
Lion King	1 cone	14.0	280	45%
Mickey Mouse bar	2.5 oz	7.0	110	57%
	4 oz	11.0	170	58%
mini sandwich	1 sandwich	5.0	110	41%
Crunch				
bar				
Crunch King	4 oz	19.0	270	63%
ice cream bar				
chocolate	3 oz	14.0	200	63%
vanilla	3 oz	14.0	200	63%
reduced fat	2.5 oz	7.0	130	48%
cone	1 cone	16.0	300	48%
nuggets	8 nuggets	20.0	300	60%
Drumstick				
chocolate	1 cone	19.0	340	50%
chocolate dipped	1 cone	17.0	340	45%
vanilla	1 cone	20.0	350	51%
vanilla caramel	1 cone	20.0	360	50%
vanilla fudge	1 cone	21.0	370	51%
Flintstones				
cool cream	2.75 oz	2.0	90	20%
push-up				
Pebbles treats	1 pop	6.0	120	45%
sherbet treats	1 pop	2.0	100	18%
Heath Bar	1 bar	12.0	160	68%
■ **(Polar Bar)**				
vanilla w/milk chocolate coating	1 bar	17.5	234	67%
■ **(Popsicle)**				
creamsicle	1 bar	3.0	110	25%
fudgsicle	1 bar	1.0	90	10%
pop-up				
orange	1 pop	1.0	80	11%
rainbow	1 pop	1.0	90	10%
supersicle double fudge bar	1 bar	2.0	150	12%
vanilla ice cream bar	1 bar	11.0	160	62%
vanilla sandwich	1 sandwich	8.0	190	38%

Food and Description	Amount	Fat Grams	Total Calories	% Fat Calories
■ (Schwan's)				
bar				
chocolate pudding	1 bar	9.0	160	51%
chocolate sundae crunch	1 bar	9.0	170	48%
English toffee	1 bar	14.0	200	57%
fudge stick	1 bar	1.5	110	12%
Gold'n Nugit	1 bar	16.0	260	55%
Krispie Krunch	1 bar	8.0	120	60%
peanut stick	1 bar	14.0	200	62%
rainbow stick	1 bar	1.0	90	10%
raspberry cordial	1 bar	13.0	210	56%
root beer float	1 bar	2.0	80	21%
Schwan bar	1 bar	14.0	200	57%
silver mint	1 bar	10.0	160	56%
strawberries & cream	1 bar	2.0	80	23%
strawberry fruit	1 bar	–	50	–
tin roof sundae	1 bar	16.0	250	58%
Trim Creations chocolate fudge stick	1 bar	–	50	–
cone				
pecan sundae	1 cone	12.0	270	40%
sundae cone	1 cone	10.0	210	47%
ice cream cup				
chocolate sundae	1 cup	5.0	120	38%
strawberry/nonfat	1 cup	–	80	–
strawberry sundae	1 cup	5.0	120	38%
vanilla				
nonfat	1 cup	–	80	–
regular	1 cup	6.0	110	49%
Push-Em				
chocolate malt	1 pop	2.5	90	25%
orange sherbet	1 pop	1.0	90	10%
strawberry shake	1 pop	2.5	90	25%
sandwich	1 sandwich	7.0	170	34%
■ (Sealtest)				
Colonel Crunch bar				
chocolate eclair	1 bar	7.0	160	39%
strawberry	1 bar	8.0	170	42%
cone				
olde nut sundae	1 cone	9.0	230	35%
ice cream cup				
chocolate	1 cup	7.0	140	45%
strawberry	1 cup	6.0	130	42%
vanilla				
fat-free	1 cup	–	100	–
no sugar added/reduced fat	1 cup	4.5	90	45%
regular	1 cup	7.0	140	45%
ice cream sandwich				
Chip Burrger	1 sandwich	15.0	320	42%

Food and Description	Amount	Fat Grams	Total Calories	% Fat Calories
Creamee Burrger	1 sandwich	17.0	310	49%
slice				
vanilla	1 slice	7.0	130	48%
specialty items				
Choco Taco	1 bar	17.0	320	48%
No. 1 Bar	1 bar	11.0	190	52%
Snoopy bar	1 bar	8.0	150	48%
sundae twist cup	1 cup	3.0	160	17%
WWF bar	1 bar	10.0	200	45%
X-Men	1 bar	5.0	140	32%
■ SNICKERS (See (M&M★Mars) in this section)				
■ 3 MUSKETEERS (See (M&M★Mars) in this section)				
■ (Weight Watchers)				
regular				
Arctic D'Lites	1 bar	7.0	130	48%
berries 'n creme mousse	2 bars	1.5	70	19%
caramel nut bar	1 bar	8.0	130	55%
chocolate dip	1 bar	6.0	100	54%
chocolate mousse bar	2 bars	1.0	70	13%
chocolate treat	1 bar	1.0	100	9%
crispy pralines 'n creme bar	1 bar	7.0	130	48%
English toffee crunch bar	1 bar	7.0	120	53%
orange vanilla treat	2 bars	1.0	70	13%
vanilla sandwich bar	1 bar	3.5	160	20%
Sweet Celebrations				
parfait				
double fudge brownie	5.3 oz	2.5	190	12%
praline toffee crunch	5.1 oz	3.0	190	14%
sundae				
chocolate chip cookie dough	5.43 oz	4.0	180	20%
ICE CREAM CONES & CUPS				
(Baskin-Robbins) cones				
sugar	1 cone	1.0	60	15%
waffle				
fresh-baked	1 cone	2.0	140	13%
large	1 cone	1.5	120	11%
(Colosso)				
bowl	1 bowl	1.0	73	12%
cone	1 cone	1.5	98	14%
(Comet)				
cones				
Oreo chocolate	1 cone	1.0	50	18%
sugar	1 cone	–	40	–
Teddy Grahams cinnamon	1 cone	0.5	60	8%
waffle	1 cone	0.5	70	6%
cups	1 cup	–	40	–
(Country Inn)	1 cone	–	18	–

Food and Description	Amount	Fat Grams	Total Calories	% Fat Calories
(Disney) cones				
cake	1 cone	–	17	–
sugar	1 cone	–	53	–
waffle	1 cone	<1.0	59	8%
(Joy)				
cones				
classic	1 cone	1	70	13%
sugar	1 cone	–	50	–
cups				
cake				
jumbo	1 cup	–	25	–
regular	1 cup	–	15	–
flavored color	1 cup	–	15	–
(Keebler) cups				
fudge-dipped	1 cup	1.5	35	39%
ice cream	1 cup	<1.0	15	30%
sugar	1 cone	–	45	–
(Little Debbie) ice cream cups	1 cup	–	15	–
ICE CREAM SANDWICH (*See* ICE CREAM BARS, SANDWICHES, & FROZEN NOVELTIES				
ICE CREAM TOPPING (*See also* CREAM; CUSTARD; WHIPPED TOPPING)				
bottled, canned, or jarred				
(Baskin-Robbins)				
butterscotch	2 oz	2.0	200	9%
hot fudge				
fat-free	1 oz	–	90	–
no sugar added	1 oz	–	90	–
regular	1 oz	3.0	100	27%
strawberry	1 oz	–	60	–
whipped cream	2 Tbs	2.5	30	75%
(Betty Crocker)				
confetti sprinkles	2 Tbs	2.0	110	16%
cookie 'n nut	2 Tbs	3.0	80	34%
ice cream critters	2 Tbs	1.5	90	15%
praline crunch	2 Tbs	5.0	100	45%
(Estee) chocolate syrup	2 Tbs	–	50	–
(Fisher) nut topping/peanut	1 oz	17.0	190	81%
(Hershey)				
Chocolate Shoppe toppings				
banana split fudge	1 Tbs	2.5	70	32%
butterscotch caramel	1 Tbs	1.0	70	13%
chocolate almond fudge	1 Tbs	2.0	70	26%
chocolate caramel fudge	1 Tbs	0.5	60	8%
chocolate marshmallow fudge	1 Tbs	2.0	70	26%
chocolate mint fudge	1 Tbs	2.0	80	23%
double chocolate fudge	1 Tbs	1.0	50	18%
hot fudge	1 Tbs	2.5	60	38%

Food and Description	Amount	Fat Grams	Total Calories	% Fat Calories
Chocolate Shoppe candy bar sprinkles				
candy coated milk chocolate	1 Tbs	2.5	70	32%
milk chocolate w/almonds	1 Tbs	4.0	80	45%
peanut butter	1 Tbs	4.0	80	45%
peppermint patty	1 Tbs	4.0	80	45%
sundae syrup				
chocolate mint	2 Tbs	–	110	–
double chocolate	2 Tbs	–	110	–
syrup				
chocolate				
lite	2 Tbs	–	50	–
malt	2 Tbs	–	100	–
original	2 Tbs	–	100	–
strawberry	1 Tbs	–	55	–
topping/canned				
chocolate fudge	1 Tbs	3.0	70	39%
(Kraft)				
butterscotch	2 Tbs	1.5	130	10%
caramel	2 Tbs	–	120	–
chocolate-flavored	2 Tbs	–	110	–
hot fudge	2 Tbs	4.0	140	26%
pineapple	2 Tbs	–	110	–
strawberry	2 Tbs	–	110	–
(Mrs. Richardson's) hot fudge/fat-free	2 Tbs	–	110	–
(Planter's) nut topping	2 Tbs	9.0	100	81%
(Smucker's)				
butterscotch & caramel syrup	2 Tbs	–	110	–
butterscotch & caramel topping				
regular	2 Tbs	–	130	–
special recipe	2 Tbs	1.0	130	7%
chocolate fudge	2 Tbs	1.5	130	10%
chocolate-flavored sundae syrup	2 Tbs	–	110	–
hot caramel	2 Tbs	3.0	120	23%
hot fudge				
light/fat-free	2 Tbs	–	90	–
original	2 Tbs	4.0	140	26%
special recipe	2 Tbs	4.0	140	26%
magic shell				
chocolate	2 Tbs	16.0	220	65%
chocolate fudge	2 Tbs	16.0	220	65%
chocolate nut	2 Tbs	16.0	220	65%
marshmallow topping	2 Tbs	–	120	–
peanut butter caramel	2 Tbs	4.5	150	27%
pecans in syrup	2 Tbs	11.0	190	52%
pineapple topping	2 Tbs	–	110	–
strawberry topping	2 Tbs	–	100	–
walnuts in syrup	2 Tbs	10.0	190	47%

Food and Description	Amount	Fat Grams	Total Calories	% Fat Calories
(Wax Orchards) fat-free				
amaretto fudge	2 Tbs	0.5	90	5%
classic fudge	2 Tbs	0.5	90	5%
orange passion fudge	2 Tbs	0.5	90	5%
peppermint stick fudge	2 Tbs	0.5	90	5%
homemade/USDA Standard Home Recipe				
chocolate sauce	1 Tbs	2.0	55	33%
hard sauce	1.2 oz	6.0	95	57%
lemon sauce	2 Tbs	1.5	60	8%

ICE MILK (*See* ICE CREAM & ICE CREAM-LIKE FROZEN DESSERTS)
ICE MILK BAR (*See* ICE CREAM BARS, SANDWICHES, & FROZEN NOVELTIES)
ICED TEA (*See* TEA)
ICES (*See* FRUIT ICES, BARS, & POPS)
ICING (*See* CAKE FROSTING/ICING)
INDIAN PUDDING (*See* PUDDING & MOUSSE)
INFANT FORMULA (*See* BABY/INFANT FORMULA)
ITALIAN SAUSAGE (*See* SAUSAGE)

J

Food and Description	Amount	Fat Grams	Total Calories	% Fat Calories
JACKFRUIT/raw	1 medium	–	107	–
JALAPEÑO (*See* MEXICAN FOOD; PEPPER)				
JAM/JELLY/PRESERVES				
(Bama)				
jam/red plum	2 tsp	–	30	–
jelly				
apple	2 tsp	–	30	–
grape	2 tsp	–	30	–
preserves				
peach	2 tsp	–	30	–
strawberry	2 tsp	–	30	–
(Cascadian Farm) organic				
conserve				
apricot	1 Tbs	–	40	–
blackberry	1 Tbs	–	40	–
blueberry	1 Tbs	–	40	–
red raspberry	1 Tbs	–	40	–
fancy fruit spread				
blackberry	1 Tbs	–	40	–

Food and Description	Amount	Fat Grams	Total Calories	% Fat Calories
blueberry	1 Tbs	–	40	–
dark cherry	1 Tbs	–	40	–
raspberry	1 Tbs	–	40	–
(Country Pure)				
jam				
apricot	2 tsp	–	35	–
blackberry	2 tsp	–	35	–
red cherry	2 tsp	–	35	–
red raspberry	2 tsp	–	35	–
strawberry	2 tsp	–	35	–
(Empress)				
jam				
Concord grape	2 tsp	–	35	–
grape	2 tsp	–	35	–
jelly				
apple	2 tsp	–	35	–
blackberry	2 tsp	–	35	–
mixed fruit	2 tsp	–	35	–
red currant	2 tsp	–	35	–
preserves				
apricot	2 tsp	–	35	–
apricot-pineapple	2 tsp	–	35	–
black cherry	2 tsp	–	35	–
black raspberry	2 tsp	–	35	–
blackberry/seedless	2 tsp	–	35	–
boysenberry	2 tsp	–	35	–
peach	2 tsp	–	35	–
peach-pineapple	2 tsp	–	35	–
plum	2 tsp	–	35	–
red cherry	2 tsp	–	35	–
red raspberry	2 tsp	–	35	–
strawberry	2 tsp	–	35	–
marmalade/California orange	2 tsp	–	35	–
(Estee)				
spreads				
apple spice	1 Tbs	–	10	–
apricot	1 Tbs	–	5	–
blackberry	1 Tbs	–	5	–
cherry	1 Tbs	–	5	–
grape	1 Tbs	–	10	–
orange	1 Tbs	–	10	–
peach	1 Tbs	–	5	–
red raspberry	1 Tbs	–	5	–
strawberry	1 Tbs	–	10	–
(Featherweight) fruit spreads/all flavors	1 Tbs	–	15	–
(Knott's Berry Farm)				
jelly				
jalapeño	1 tsp	–	18	–

Food and Description	Amount	Fat Grams	Total Calories	% Fat Calories
jelly/light				
apricot-pineapple	1 tsp	–	8	–
blackberry	1 tsp	–	8	–
raspberry	1 tsp	–	8	–
strawberry	1 tsp	–	8	–
preserves				
apricot	1 tsp	–	18	–
apricot-pineapple	1 tsp	–	18	–
bing cherry	1 tsp	–	18	–
blackberry/seedless	1 tsp	–	18	–
blueberry	1 tsp	–	18	–
boysenberry	1 tsp	–	18	–
Kadota fig	1 tsp	–	18	–
red cherry	1 tsp	–	18	–
red raspberry/seedless	1 tsp	–	18	–
strawberry	1 tsp	–	18	–
(Kraft)				
jam				
grape	1 Tbs	–	60	–
red plum	1 Tbs	–	60	–
strawberry	1 Tbs	–	50	–
jelly				
apple	1 Tbs	–	60	–
apple-strawberry	1 Tbs	–	50	–
blackberry	1 Tbs	–	50	–
grape	1 Tbs	–	50	–
guava	1 Tbs	–	50	–
red currant	1 Tbs	–	50	–
strawberry	1 Tbs	–	60	–
marmalade/orange	1 Tbs	–	50	–
preserves				
apricot	1 Tbs	–	50	–
blackberry	1 Tbs	–	50	–
peach	1 Tbs	–	50	–
pineapple	1 Tbs	–	50	–
red raspberry	1 Tbs	–	50	–
strawberry	1 Tbs	–	50	–
reduced-calorie fruit spread				
grape	1 Tbs	–	20	–
strawberry	1 Tbs	–	20	–
(Mary Ellen)				
jam				
apricot	1 Tbs	–	50	–
blackberry/seedless	1 Tbs	–	50	–
grape	1 Tbs	–	50	–
red raspberry	1 Tbs	–	50	–
strawberry	1 Tbs	–	50	–

Food and Description	Amount	Fat Grams	Total Calories	% Fat Calories
jelly				
grape	1 Tbs	–	50	–
strawberry	1 Tbs	–	50	–
(Poiret)				
100% pure fruit spreads				
apple	2 tsp	–	35	–
pear, apricot, apple	2 tsp	–	35	–
pear, black cherry	2 tsp	–	35	–
pear, strawberry	2 tsp	–	35	–
pear, strawberry, apple	2 tsp	–	35	–
(Polaner)				
jam				
grape	2 tsp	–	35	
jelly				
apple	2 tsp	–	35	–
currant	2 tsp	–	35	–
grape	2 tsp	–	35	–
mint	2 tsp	–	35	–
raspberry	2 tsp	–	35	–
strawberry	2 tsp	–	35	–
preserves				
apricot	2 tsp	–	35	–
black cherry	2 tsp	–	35	–
blackberry	2 tsp	–	35	–
blueberry	2 tsp	–	35	–
peach	2 tsp	–	35	–
red raspberry	2 tsp	–	35	–
strawberry	2 tsp	–	35	–
(Pritikin) fruit spread/all flavors	1 tsp	–	35	–
(R W Knudsen) all-fruit spread				
organic				
blackberry	1 Tbs	–	50	
blueberry	1 Tbs	–	50	–
red raspberry	1 Tbs	–	50	–
strawberry	1 Tbs	–	50	–
regular				
apricot	1 Tbs	–	50	–
black cherry	1 Tbs	–	50	–
blackberry	1 Tbs	–	50	–
blueberry	1 Tbs	–	50	–
boysenberry	1 Tbs	–	50	–
Concord grape	1 Tbs	–	50	–
orange	1 Tbs	–	50	–
peach	1 Tbs	–	50	–
red raspberry	1 Tbs	–	50	–
strawberry	1 Tbs	–	50	–
(Smucker's) fruit spreads				
homestyle/all flavors	1 Tbs	–	45	–

Food and Description	Amount	Fat Grams	Total Calories	% Fat Calories
jam/all flavors	1 Tbs	–	50	–
jelly/all flavors	1 Tbs	–	50	–
light fruit preserves/all flavors	1 Tbs	–	10	–
low-sugar/all flavors	1 Tbs	–	25	–
marmalade/orange	1 Tbs	–	50	–
preserves/all flavors	1 Tbs	–	50	–
Simply Fruit spread/all flavors	1 Tbs	–	40	–
(Sorrell Ridge)				
fruit spread				
apricot	1 Tbs	–	36	–
black cherry	1 Tbs	–	36	–
black raspberry	1 Tbs	–	36	–
blackberry	1 Tbs	–	36	–
boysenberry	1 Tbs	–	36	–
cherry	1 Tbs	–	36	–
concord grape	1 Tbs	–	36	–
orange marmalade	1 Tbs	–	36	–
peach	1 Tbs	–	36	–
plum good	1 Tbs	–	36	–
raspberry	1 Tbs	–	36	–
strawberry rhubarb	1 Tbs	–	36	–
wild blueberry	1 Tbs	–	36	–
(Welch's)				
jam/all flavors	1 Tbs	–	50	–
jelly/all flavors	1 Tbs	–	50	–
preserves/all flavors	1 Tbs	–	50	–
spread				
cherry	1 Tbs	–	50	–
strawberry	1 Tbs	–	50	–
Super Spreaders & Peanuts fruit spread/all flavors	1 Tbs	–	40	–
Totally Fruit				
apricot	1 Tbs	–	35	–
blackberry	1 Tbs	–	35	–
blueberry	1 Tbs	–	35	–
grape	1 Tbs	–	40	–
red raspberry	1 Tbs	–	35	–
strawberry	1 Tbs	–	35	–
JAPANESE FOOD (*See* ASIAN FOOD)				
JELL-O (*See* GELATIN)				
JELLY (*See* JAM/JELLY/PRESERVES)				
JERKY (*See* BEEF JERKY, STICKS, & STRIPS)				
JERUSALEM ARTICHOKE				
raw/sliced	½ cup	–	57	–
JEW'S EAR				
dried	½ cup	–	35	–
raw/sliced	½ cup	–	15	–

Food and Description	Amount	Fat Grams	Total Calories	% Fat Calories
JICAMA/YAM BEAN-TUBER				
cooked	½ cup	<1.0	46	10%
raw/sliced	1 cup	<1.0	50	9%
JUICE (*See* FRUIT JUICE/JUICE DRINK, MIXED; individual listings)				
JUJUBE				
dried	3 oz	0.9	246	3%
raw	3 oz	–	68	–

K

Food and Description	Amount	Fat Grams	Total Calories	% Fat Calories
KALE				
fresh/cooked	½ cup	–	21	–
frozen/cooked	½ cup	–	20	–
raw	½ cup	–	17	–
KANPYO/DRIED GOURD STRIP	3 strips	–	49	–
KASHA (*See* BUCKWHEAT GROATS)				
KELP (*See* SEAWEED)				
KETCHUP (*See* CATSUP)				
KIDNEY BEAN				
canned				
(Bush's Best)				
dark red	½ cup	–	70	–
light red	½ cup	–	70	–
(Eden)				
red/no salt added	½ cup	–	100	–
generic				
dark red	½ cup	<1.0	104	4%
red	½ cup	<1.0	108	4%
(Goya) habichuelas coloradas/red	½ cup	1.0	90	10%
(Green Giant)				
dark red	½ cup	–	110	–
light red	½ cup	–	110	–
(Hain) dark red	½ cup	–	110	–
(Hunt's)	½ cup	0.5	95	5%
(Joan of Arc)				
dark red	½ cup	–	110	–
light red	½ cup	–	110	–
(Progresso)				
cannellini/white	½ cup	0.5	130	3%

Food and Description	Amount	Fat Grams	Total Calories	% Fat Calories
red	½ cup	0.5	130	3%
(S&W) all types	½ cup	1.0	120	8%
(Seneca)	½ cup	0.5	120	4%
(Stokely)				
dark red	½ cup	1.0	110	8%
light red	½ cup	1.0	110	8%
(Trappey's)				
dark red	½ cup	–	90	–
jalapeño	½ cup	–	90	–
light red	½ cup	–	90	–
New Orleans style	½ cup	2.0	100	18%
(Van Camp's)				
dark red	½ cup	0.5	90	5%
light red	½ cup	0.5	90	5%
New Orleans style	½ cup	0.5	90	5%
dry				
(Arrowhead Mills)	¼ cup	0.5	160	3%
generic				
dark red				
boiled	½ cup	<1.0	112	4%
raw	½ cup	1.0	300	3%
red				
boiled	½ cup	<1.0	112	4%
raw	½ cup	1.0	310	3%
sprouted/raw				
mature seeds	1 oz	<1.0	8	15%
	½ cup	0.5	30	15%
KIELBASA (*See* SAUSAGE)				
KINGFISH				
cooked-dry heat	3 oz	11.0	219	45%
raw	3 oz	2.6	90	26%
KIWI JUICE/JUICE BLEND (*See also* FRUIT JUICE/JUICE DRINK, MIXED; FRUIT PUNCH; SOFT DRINK MIX; individual listings)				
(Snapple) kiwi-strawberry cocktail				
diet	8 fl oz	–	13	–
regular	8 fl oz	–	130	–
KIWIFRUIT				
fresh/raw	1 medium	<1.0	46	10%
	1 large	<1.0	55	8%
(Dole)	2 medium	1.0	90	10%
KNOCKWURST (*See* FRANKFURTER; SAUSAGE)				
KOHLRABI				
fresh/sliced				
cooked-drained	½ cup	–	24	–
raw	½ cup	–	19	–
KOOL-AID (*See* SOFT DRINK MIX)				
KRAUT (*See* SAUERKRAUT)				
KRAUT JUICE (*See* SAUERKRAUT JUICE)				

Food and Description	Amount	Fat Grams	Total Calories	% Fat Calories
KUMQUAT				
fresh/raw	1 medium	–	12	–

L

Food and Description	Amount	Fat Grams	Total Calories	% Fat Calories
LAMB				

(NOTE: All serving sizes are cooked portions, unless otherwise stated. "Lean" means lamb trimmed of all separable fat before cooking. "Lean & fat" means untrimmed and cooked or eaten as purchased. In most cases, 4 ounces of raw meat yields 3 ounces cooked.)

Food and Description	Amount	Fat Grams	Total Calories	% Fat Calories
domestic				
composite cuts/leg & shoulder				
lean				
braised/cubed	3 oz	7.5	190	36%
broiled				
cubed	3 oz	6.0	160	23%
ground	3 oz	17.0	240	64%
stewed/cubed	4 oz	10.0	255	35%
leg/foreshank				
lean				
braised	3 oz	5.0	160	28%
braised/diced	1 cup	8.5	260	29%
broiled/ground	3 oz	17.0	240	64%
stewed/diced	1 cup	8.5	265	29%
lean & fat				
braised	3 oz	11.5	210	49%
braised/diced	1 cup	19.0	340	50%
stewed	3 oz	11.5	210	49%
leg/shank				
lean				
roasted	3 oz	5.7	155	33%
roasted/diced	1 cup	9.0	250	32%
lean & fat				
roasted	3 oz	10.5	190	50%
roasted/diced	1 cup	17.5	315	50%
leg/sirloin				
lean				
roasted	3 oz	8.0	175	41%
roasted/diced	1 cup	13.0	290	40%

Food and Description	Amount	Fat Grams	Total Calories	% Fat Calories
lean & fat				
roasted	3 oz	17.5	250	63%
roasted/diced	1 cup	29.0	410	64%
leg/whole				
lean				
roasted	3 oz	6.5	165	35%
roasted/diced	1 cup	11.0	270	37%
lean & fat				
roasted	3 oz	14.0	220	57%
roasted/diced	1 cup	23.0	360	57%
loin				
lean				
broiled	3 oz	8.5	190	40%
roasted	3 oz	8.5	175	44%
lean & fat				
broiled	3 oz	19.5	270	65%
roasted	3 oz	20.0	265	68%
organs				
brain				
braised	3 oz	8.5	125	61%
pan-fried	3 oz	19.0	235	73%
heart				
braised	3 oz	7.0	160	39%
simmered	3 oz	7.0	160	39%
kidney				
braised	3 oz	3.0	120	23%
liver				
braised	3 oz	7.5	190	36%
pan-fried	3 oz	11.0	205	48%
lung/braised	3 oz	2.5	95	24%
pancreas/braised	3 oz	13.0	200	59%
spleen/braised	3 oz	4.0	135	27%
tongue/braised	3 oz	17.0	235	65%
rib				
lean				
broiled	3 oz	11.0	200	50%
roasted	3 oz	11.0	200	50%
lean & fat				
broiled	3 oz	25.0	305	74%
roasted	3 oz	25.5	305	75%
shoulder/arm				
lean				
braised	3 oz	12.0	235	46%
broiled	3 oz	7.5	170	40%
roasted	3 oz	8.0	165	44%
shoulder/blade				
lean				
braised	3 oz	14.0	245	51%

Food and Description	Amount	Fat Grams	Total Calories	% Fat Calories
broiled	3 oz	9.5	180	48%
roasted	3 oz	10.0	180	50%
lean & fat				
braised	3 oz	21.0	295	64%
broiled	3 oz	17.0	235	65%
roasted	3 oz	17.5	240	66%
shoulder/whole				
lean				
braised	3 oz	7.5	240	28%
braised/diced	1 cup	22.0	400	50%
broiled	3 oz	9.0	180	45%
roasted	3 oz	9.0	175	46%
roasted/diced	1 cup	10.0	320	28%
stewed	3 oz	7.5	240	28%
stewed/diced	1 cup	22.0	400	50%
lean & fat				
braised/diced	1 cup	34.0	485	63%
broiled	3 oz	22.0	315	63%
broiled/diced	1 cup	27.0	390	62%
roasted	3 oz	17.0	235	65%
roasted/diced	1 cup	28.0	385	65%
stewed	3 oz	21.0	295	64%
stewed/diced	1 cup	34.5	485	64%
New Zealand/frozen				
composite cuts				
lean/cooked	3 oz	7.5	175	39%
leg/foreshank				
lean				
braised	3 oz	5.0	160	28%
braised/diced	1 cup	8.5	260	29%
stewed	3 oz	5.0	160	28%
stewed/diced	1 cup	8.5	260	29%
lean & fat				
braised	3 oz	13.5	220	55%
braised/diced	1 cup	22.0	360	55%
stewed	3 oz	13.5	220	55%
stewed/diced	1 cup	22.0	360	55%
leg/whole				
lean				
roasted	3 oz	6.0	155	35%
roasted/diced	1 cup	10.0	255	35%
lean & fat				
roasted	3 oz	13.0	210	56%
roasted/diced	1 cup	22.0	345	57%
loin				
lean				
broiled	3 oz	7.0	170	37%
roasted	3 oz	7.0	170	37%

Food and Description	Amount	Fat Grams	Total Calories	% Fat Calories
lean & fat				
broiled	3 oz	20.5	270	68%
rib				
lean/roasted	3 oz	8.5	165	46%
lean & fat/roasted	3 oz	24.5	290	76%
shoulder/whole				
lean				
braised	3 oz	13.0	245	48%
braised/diced	1 cup	22.0	400	50%
stewed	3 oz	13.0	240	49%
stewed/diced	1 cup	22.0	400	50%
lean & fat				
braised	3 oz	22.0	305	65%
braised/diced	1 cup	35.5	490	65%
stewed	3 oz	21.5	300	65%
stewed/diced	1 cup	35.5	490	65%
LAMB DISH				
homemade/USDA Standard Home Recipe				
curry	1 cup	23.0	460	45%
stew	1 cup	7.0	165	38%
LAMB'S-QUARTERS				
fresh/cooked	1 cup	0.6	29	19%
LARD (See also FAT; OIL; PORK)	1 Tbs	12.8	115	100%
	1 cup	205.0	1850	100%
LASAGNA (See BEEF DISH/ENTRÉE; FROZEN ENTRÉE/DINNER; PASTA ENTRÉE/DINNER)				
LAVER (See SEAWEED)				
LECITHIN (See SOY LECITHIN)				
LEEK				
freeze-dried	¼ cup	–	3	–
fresh				
cooked	¼ cup	–	8	–
raw	¼ cup	–	16	–
	1 medium	–	17	–
LEMON/fresh	1 medium	–	17	–
	1 large	–	25	–
LEMON JUICE				
bottled				
generic	1 Tbs	–	5	–
	⅓ cup	–	17	–
(Realemon)	1 fl oz	–	6	–
(Seneca)	1 Tbs	–	5	–
fresh	1 Tbs	–	4	–
	⅓ cup	–	20	–
frozen				
generic	1 Tbs	–	3	–
(Sunkist)	1 oz	–	7	–

Food and Description	Amount	Fat Grams	Total Calories	% Fat Calories
LEMON PEEL				
candied				
generic	1 oz	–	90	–
(S&W)	58 pieces	–	80	–
grated	1 Tbs	–	–	–
LEMONADE/LEMONADE-FLAVORED DRINK (*See also* SOFT DRINK; SOFT DRINK MIX; TEA)				
bottled, boxed, or canned				
(Betty Crocker) Squeezit	6.76 fl oz	–	100	–
(Fruitopia)				
Cranberry Lemonade Vision	8 fl oz	–	117	–
Lemonade Love & Hope	8 fl oz	–	113	–
Pink Lemonade Euphoria	8 fl oz	–	117	–
Raspberry Psychic	8 fl oz	–	121	–
(Knudsen)				
cranberry	8 fl oz	–	120	–
natural	8 fl oz	–	120	–
organic	8 fl oz	–	120	–
(Snapple)				
cherry	8 fl oz	–	110	–
pink				
diet	8 fl oz	–	13	–
regular	8 fl oz	–	110	–
regular	8 fl oz	–	110	–
strawberry	8 fl oz	–	110	–
(Tropicana)	8 fl oz	–	120	–
	10 fl oz	–	140	–
	11.5 fl oz	–	160	–
(Welch's)	10 fl oz	–	160	–
	11.5 fl oz	–	190	–
frozen/prepared				
(Minute Maid)				
country style	8 fl oz	–	110	–
cranberry	8 fl oz	–	120	–
pink	8 fl oz	–	110	–
raspberry	8 fl oz	–	110	–
regular	8 fl oz	–	110	–
tropical	8 fl oz	–	120	–
(Mott's)	10 fl oz	–	160	–
(Seneca)	8 fl oz	–	110	–
mix/prepared				
(Country Time)				
pink				
sugar-free	8 fl oz	–	5	–
sweetened	8 fl oz	–	70	–
punch	8 fl oz	–	70	–
regular				
sugar-free	8 fl oz	–	5	–

Food and Description	Amount	Fat Grams	Total Calories	% Fat Calories
sweetened	8 fl oz	–	70	–
generic				
lemonade mix/powdered	4 fl oz	–	102	–
lemonade-flavored drink mix	8 fl oz			
LEMON-LIME DRINK (*See* SOFT DRINK; SOFT DRINK MIX; SPORTS DRINK)				
LENTIL (*See also* VEGETARIAN FOODS)				
canned				
cooked	½ cup	–	103	–
uncooked	½ cup	–	130	–
dry				
(Arrowhead Mills) green or red/raw	¼ cup	–	150	–
generic				
boiled	½ cup	–	115	–
raw	½ cup	1.0	374	2%
split	½ cup	1.0	379	2%
sprouted	½ cup	–	40	–
LENTIL SOUP (*See* SOUP)				
LETTUCE (*See also* SALAD GREENS, MIXED)				
Bibb	med head	–	21	–
butterhead	med head	–	21	–
cos/shredded	½ cup	–	2	–
iceberg	med head	–	70	13%
looseleaf or Simpson/shredded	½ cup	–	5	–
romaine/shredded	½ cup	–	4	–
LICHEE NUT/LYCHEE NUT/LITCHI NUT				
dried/shelled	1 oz	<1.0	80	4%
	3 oz	1.0	235	4%
raw	~6 nuts	0.5	40	10%
shelled & seeded	½ cup	0.5	65	7%
LIMA BEAN (*See also* BUTTER BEAN)				
canned				
(Bush's Best)				
green	½ cup	–	90	–
green & white	½ cup	–	80	–
(Del Monte) green	½ cup	–	80	–
(Dennison's) seasoned w/ham	½ cup	3.5	150	21%
(Freshlike)				
no salt	½ cup	–	80	–
regular	½ cup	–	80	–
(Green Giant) butter	½ cup	–	90	–
(Joan of Arc) butter	½ cup	–	90	–
(Luck's) seasoned w/pork				
giant	½ cup	3.0	150	18%
small	½ cup	2.0	140	13%
(Seneca)	½ cup	–	70	–
(Stokely)	½ cup	–	80	–
Fordhook	½ cup	–	80	–
no salt or sugar added	½ cup	–	80	–

Food and Description	Amount	Fat Grams	Total Calories	% Fat Calories
(Trappey's) baby				
green	½ cup	1.0	90	10%
white	½ cup	1.0	90	10%
(Van Camp's)	½ cup	–	80	–
(Veg-All)	½ cup	–	80	–
dried				
baby				
boiled	½ cup	–	115	–
uncooked	½ cup	1.0	330	3%
large				
boiled	½ cup	–	108	–
uncooked	½ cup	0.5	300	2%
frozen				
(Birds Eye)				
baby	½ cup	–	130	–
Fordhook	½ cup	–	100	–
(C&W) baby	½ cup	0.5	90	5%
(Green Giant) baby	½ cup	–	80	–
(Seneca)				
Fordhook	⅔ cup	–	90	–
regular	⅔ cup	–	110	–
(Veg-All)	½ cup	1.0	130	7%
LIMA BEAN DISH				
(Green Giant) frozen in butter sauce	½ cup	2.0	100	18%
LIME	1 medium	–	20	–
LIME JUICE				
bottled				
generic	1 Tbs	–	3	–
	⅓ cup	–	17	–
(Realime)	1 fl oz	–	6	–
fresh	⅓ cup	–	22	–
LIME JUICE DRINK (See also SOFT DRINK; SOFT DRINK MIX)				
(Knudsen) Key West lime	8 fl oz	–	100	–
LIMEADE/LIME DRINK				
bottled				
(Knudsen) Thirst Quencher/lime cactus	8 fl oz	–	120	–
frozen/prepared				
generic	8 fl oz	–	102	–
(Minute Maid)	8 fl oz	–	100	–
LING				
baked or broiled	3 oz	1.0	95	9%
raw	3 oz	0.5	75	6%
LINGCOD				
baked or boiled	3 oz	1.0	90	10%
raw	3 oz	1.0	75	12%

LINGUINE (See FROZEN ENTRÉE/DINNER; PASTA ENTRÉE/DINNER; VEGETARIAN FOODS)

Food and Description	Amount	Fat Grams	Total Calories	% Fat Calories
LIQUEUR (*See also* COCKTAIL)				
anisette	¾ fl oz	–	74	–
B & B	1 fl oz	–	94	–
Benedictine	¾ fl oz	–	69	–
brandy/fruit-flavored	1.5 fl oz	–	129	–
brandy/coffee	1.5 fl oz	–	132	–
Cherry Hering	1.5 fl oz	–	120	–
coffee	1.5 fl oz	–	174	–
coffee w/cream	1.5 fl oz	7.0	154	41%
creme de almonde	1.5 fl oz	–	151	–
creme de banana	1.5 fl oz	–	144	–
creme de cacao	1.5 fl oz	–	150	–
creme de cassis	1.5 fl oz	–	122	–
creme de menthe	1.5 fl oz	–	186	–
curaçao	¾ fl oz	–	54	–
Drambuie	1.5 fl oz	–	165	–
gin/citrus	1.5 fl oz	–	114	–
kirsch	1.5 fl oz	–	124	–
maraschino	1.5 fl oz	–	112	–
peppermint schnapps	1.5 fl oz	–	124	–
pernod	1.5 fl oz	–	117	–
rock & rye	1.5 fl oz	–	140	–
sloe gin	1.5 fl oz	–	124	–
Southern Comfort	1.5 fl oz	–	180	–
Tia Maria	1.5 fl oz	–	138	–
triple sec	1.5 fl oz	–	121	–
vodka/citrus	1.5 fl oz	–	150	–
LIQUOR, DISTILLED				
(NOTE: In all cases, the higher the proof [the % of alcohol], the higher the calories.)				
80 proof	1 fl oz	–	67	–
84 proof	1 fl oz	–	70	–
86 proof	1 fl oz	–	72	–
86.8 proof	1 fl oz	–	72	–
90 proof	1 fl oz	–	75	–
90.4 proof	1 fl oz	–	75	–
94 proof	1 fl oz	–	78	–
94.6 proof	1 fl oz	–	79	–
97 proof	1 fl oz	–	81	–
100 proof	1 fl oz	–	83	–
LIVER (*See* BEEF; CHICKEN; GOOSE; LAMB; PÂTÉ; PORK; TURKEY)				
LIVER LOAF (*See* LUNCHEON MEAT)				
LIVERWURST (*See* LUNCHEON MEAT)				
LOBSTER (*See also* SEAFOOD ENTRÉE/DINNER)				
fresh				
northern				
boiled	3 oz	0.5	83	5%
	1 cup	0.9	142	6%
raw/~5-oz lobster	1 lobster	1.0	140	6%

Food and Description	Amount	Fat Grams	Total Calories	% Fat Calories
spiny				
cooked-moist heat	3 oz	1.5	120	11%
raw	3 oz	1.0	95	10%
frozen				
(Langostino's) lobster tails/small/cooked	3 oz	1.0	105	9%
LOBSTER, IMITATION				
(Louis Kemp)				
chunk style	½ cup	–	80	–
flake style	½ cup	–	80	–
salad style	½ cup	–	80	–
LOBSTER BISQUE (*See* SOUP)				
LOBSTER PASTE	1 Tbs	2.0	39	46%
LOBSTER SALAD				
homemade/USDA Standard Home Recipe/made w/mayonnaise, tomato, celery, carrots, onion, & egg	3 oz	5.5	94	53%
LOGANBERRY				
canned				
in heavy syrup	½ cup	–	89	–
in water	½ cup	–	40	–
fresh	½ lb	1.5	140	10%
frozen	1 cup	0.5	80	5%
LOGANBERRY JUICE	8 oz	–	100	–
LOQUAT	1 medium	–	5	–
	½ lb	–	65	–
LOTUS ROOT				
cooked	½ cup	–	75	–
raw	10 slices	–	45	–
	1 root	–	60	–
LOTUS SEED				
dried	1 oz	0.5	94	5%
	1 cup	0.6	106	5%
raw	1 oz	–	25	–
LOX (*See* SALMON)				
LUNCHEON LOAF (*See* LUNCHEON MEAT)				
LUNCHEON MEAT (*See also* BEEF; CHICKEN; HAM; LUNCHEON MEAT SPREAD; TURKEY; VEGETARIAN FOODS)				
■ **(Armour/Armour Star)**				
beef				
chopped	2 oz	15.0	170	79%
dried/sliced	7 slices	1.5	450	20%
dried/sliced/"rinsed"	7 slices	1.0	45	20%
corned beef	2 oz	7.0	120	53%
ham				
chopped	2 oz	9.0	120	68%
deviled	3 oz	16.0	200	74%
potted meat	3 oz	8.0	120	68%
snack kit	1 kit	42.0	570	66%

Food and Description	Amount	Fat Grams	Total Calories	% Fat Calories
Treet				
50% less fat	2 oz	8.0	120	76%
original	2 oz	12.0	150	77%
turkey loaf	2 oz	8.0	110	65%
▦ (Ball Park)				
bologna				
beef	2 oz	16.0	180	80%
garlic	2 oz	16.0	170	85%
meat	2 oz	16.0	170	85%
regular	2 oz	16.0	180	80%
▦ (Bil Mar)				
beef				
Signature top round				
Cajun beef	2 oz	3.0	70	39%
deli	2 oz	2.0	70	26%
split	2 oz	3.0	70	39%
whole/cap off	2 oz	1.5	50	27%
West Virginia/smoked	6 slices	2.0	60	30%
ham/West Virginia				
honey pork	2 oz	1.5	60	27%
smoked	2 oz	2.0	60	30%
pastrami/West Virginia/smoked	6 slices	1.5	60	27%
turkey/Signature turkey breast				
cozzinni	2 oz	1.0	60	18%
deli	2 oz	0.5	50	9%
honey-smoked/fat-free	2 oz	–	60	–
natural	2 oz	1.5	60	23%
natural/smoked	2 oz	2.0	60	30%
peppered/fat-free	2 oz	–	50	–
reduced sodium	2 oz	–	50	–
skinless	2 oz	0.5	50	9%
smoked	2 oz	–	50	–
whole boneless/foil/raw	4 oz	4.5	140	29%
▦ (Bridgford)				
salami/hard	1 oz	12.0	130	83%
▦ (Butterball)				
chicken breast/skinless/browned	1 oz	–	25	–
turkey bologna	1 oz	5.0	60	75%
turkey breast				
skinless				
browned	1 oz	–	25	–
honey-roasted	1 oz	–	30	–
less sodium	1 oz	–	25	–
oven-roasted	1 oz	–	25	–
mesquite	1 oz	0.5	30	15%
smoked	1 oz	–	25	–
skin-on				
honey-roasted	1 oz	1.0	35	26%

Food and Description	Amount	Fat Grams	Total Calories	% Fat Calories
less sodium	1 oz	1.0	30	30%
oven-roasted	1 oz	1.0	30	30%
smoked	1 oz	1.0	30	30%
turkey ham				
10% water added	1 oz	1.0	35	26%
25% water added	1 oz	1.5	35	39%
turkey pastrami	1 oz	1.0	35	26%
turkey salami	1 oz	4.0	60	60%
■ (Carl Buddig)				
beef	1 pkg	5.0	100	45%
chicken	1 pkg	7.0	110	57%
corned beef	1 pkg	5.0	100	45%
ham				
lean/sliced				
brown sugar-baked	1 pkg	2.0	90	20%
roasted	1 pkg	2.0	90	20%
smoked	1 pkg	2.0	80	23%
original/sliced	1 pkg	7.0	120	53%
pastrami	1 pkg	5.0	100	45%
turkey				
lean/sliced				
honey-roasted	1 pkg	1.0	70	13%
roasted	1 pkg	1.0	70	13%
smoked	1 pkg	1.0	70	13%
original/sliced				
honey-roasted	1 pkg	5.0	110	41%
regular	1 pkg	7.0	110	57%
turkey ham	1 pkg	5.0	100	45%
■ (Deli Perfect)				
beef				
cooked	2 oz	1.0	50	18%
Italian-style	2 oz	1.0	50	18%
chicken breast				
browned	2 oz	1.0	60	15%
plain	2 oz	1.0	60	15%
corned beef	2 oz	1.0	50	18%
ham/Hygrade pixie	2 oz	1.0	45	20%
pastrami/beef	2 oz	1.0	50	18%
turkey breast/natural shape				
browned	2 oz	2.5	60	38%
regular	2 oz	2.5	60	38%
smoked	2 oz	1.5	60	23%
turkey ham	2 oz	2.5	60	38%
turkey roll/white	2 oz	5.0	80	56%
■ (Eckrich)				
bologna				
German	1 oz	7.0	80	90%
regular	1 oz	9.0	100	90%

Food and Description	Amount	Fat Grams	Total Calories	% Fat Calories
chicken breast/Lean Supreme				
oven-roasted oil-browned	1 slice	0.5	30	15%
ham/Lean Supreme				
honey & clove	1 slice	1.0	30	30%
honey-smoked	1 slice	1.0	30	30%
Virginia baked	1 slice	1.0	30	30%
turkey breast/Lean Supreme				
oven-roasted oil-browned	1 slice	1.0	30	30%
smoked	1 slice	1.0	30	30%
■ (Galileo)				
salami/Italian dry				
light	5 slices	4.0	60	60%
thin sliced	5 slices	8.0	110	65%
whole	1 oz	10.0	120	75%
■ GENERIC				
barbecue loaf/beef & pork	1 oz	3.0	49	55%
bologna				
beef	1 oz	8.0	89	81%
beef & pork	1 oz	8.0	89	81%
Lebanon/beef	1 oz	4.0	64	56%
pork	1 oz	5.6	70	72%
Braunschweiger/pork	1 oz	9.0	102	79%
corned beef loaf	1 oz	2.0	43	42%
Dutch loaf	1 oz	5.0	68	66%
headcheese/pork	1 oz	4.0	60	60%
liver cheese/pork	1 oz	7.0	86	73%
liverwurst/pork	1 oz	8.0	93	77%
luxury loaf	1 oz	1.0	40	23%
mother's loaf	1 oz	6.0	80	68%
olive loaf/pork	1 oz	4.7	67	63%
pastrami				
beef	1 oz	8.0	99	73%
turkey	2 oz	3.5	80	39%
peppered loaf/beef, pork	1 oz	1.8	42	39%
pickle & pimiento loaf/pork	1 oz	6.0	74	73%
picinic loaf/pork, beef	1 oz	4.7	66	64%
salami				
cooked				
beef	1 oz	5.9	74	72%
beef & pork	1 oz	5.7	71	72%
turkey	2 oz	7.8	111	63%
dry or hard/pork	1 oz	7.0	85	74%
salt pork/raw	1 oz	22.8	212	97%
souse loaf	1 oz	3.8	51	67%
turkey breast	~1.5 oz	0.7	47	13%
turkey ham	2 oz	2.9	73	36%
turkey roll				
light & dark meat	1 oz	2.0	42	42%

Food and Description	Amount	Fat Grams	Total Calories	% Fat Calories
light meat	1 oz	2.0	42	43%
■ (Healthy Choice)				
chicken breast	2 oz	–	45	–
corned beef	2 oz	1.5	60	23%
ham				
cooked	2 oz	1.5	60	23%
honey	2 oz	1.5	60	23%
smoked	2 oz	1.5	60	23%
Virginia	2 oz	1.5	60	23%
pastrami	2 oz	1.5	60	23%
roast beef				
medium	2 oz	1.5	60	23%
structured	2 oz	1.0	50	18%
turkey breast				
browned	2 oz	0.5	50	9%
honey-roasted/smoked	2 oz	–	60	–
skinless	2 oz	–	45	–
smoked	2 oz	–	50	–
■ (Hebrew National)				
bologna				
beef				
lite/reduced fat	1 oz	12.0	130	83%
regular	2 oz	16.0	180	80%
lean chub	2 oz	6.0	90	60%
midget/bullet stubbie	2 oz	16.0	180	80%
chicken/Deli Thin/oven-roasted	1.8 oz	0.5	45	10%
corned beef/Deli Express	2 oz	3.0	80	34%
pastrami/deli	2 oz	3.0	80	34%
salami/beef				
lite/reduced fat	2 oz	8.0	110	57%
midget/bullet stubbie	2 oz	14.0	170	74%
regular	2 oz	14.0	170	74%
tongue/Deli Express	2 oz	9.0	120	68%
turkey breast				
catering				
#1	2 oz	1.0	60	15%
#2	2 oz	0.5	50	8%
#3	2 oz	<1.0	45	10%
Deli Thin				
hickory-smoked	1.8 oz	0.5	55	8%
lemon-garlic	1.8 oz	0.5	45	10%
oven-roasted	1.8 oz	0.5	50	9%
■ (Hickory Farms)				
salami				
dry or hard	1 oz	10.0	120	75%
Genoa	1 oz	10.0	110	82%

Food and Description	Amount	Fat Grams	Total Calories	% Fat Calories
■ **(Hillshire Farm)**				
Lunch 'n Munch combinations				
light				
cooked ham	1 sandwich	2.0	35	51%
honey ham	1 sandwich	2.0	35	51%
smoked chicken	1 sandwich	2.0	35	51%
smoked turkey	1 sandwich	2.0	35	51%
original				
bologna/American	4.5 oz	37.0	480	60%
bologna/Amercian/Snickers	4.25 oz	34.0	490	62%
cooked ham/Swiss	4.5 oz	22.0	360	55%
cooked ham/Swiss/Oreo	4.25 oz	21.0	370	51%
cotto salami/Monterey jack	4.5 oz	32.0	440	65%
pepperoni/American	4.5 oz	46.0	570	73%
smoked chicken/Monterey jack	4.5 oz	20.0	350	51%
smoked chicken/Monterey jack/ Snickers	4.25 oz	23.0	400	52%
smoked turkey/cheddar	4.5 oz	21.0	350	54%
smoked turkey/cheddar/brownie	4.5 oz	22.0	400	50%
w/6 oz Hi-C				
bologna/American/Snickers	4.25 oz	34.0	590	52%
cooked ham/Swiss/Snickers	4.125 oz	21.0	470	40%
honey ham/cheddar/Snickers	4.25 oz	23.0	500	41%
smoked turkey/cheddar/brownie	4.5 oz	22.0	500	40%
luncheon meat				
beef/Deli Select				
oven-roasted/cured	1 slice	<1.0	10	27%
roast	1 slice	<1.0	10	27%
smoked	1 slice	<1.0	10	27%
bologna				
Deli Select/light	1 slice	1.0	12	75%
regular/light	1 slice	2.0	30	60%
chicken breast				
Deli Select				
oven-roasted	1 slice	<1.0	10	27%
smoked	1 slice	<1.0	10	27%
regular/smoked	1 slice	<1.0	20	23%
ham				
Deli Select				
baked	1 slice	<1.0	10	27%
brown sugar baked	1 slice	<1.0	10	27%
Cajun	1 slice	<1.0	10	27%
honey	1 slice	<1.0	10	27%
lower salt	1 slice	<1.0	10	27%
smoked	1 slice	<1.0	10	27%
luncheon meat				
brown sugar	1 oz	2.0	40	45%
genuine baked	1 oz	1.0	35	26%

Food and Description	Amount	Fat Grams	Total Calories	% Fat Calories
honey	1 oz	2.0	40	45%
regular				
brown sugar-baked	1 slice	<1.0	20	23%
cooked	1 oz	<1.0	30	15%
honey				
flavor pack	1 slice	<1.0	20	23%
10-oz pkg	1 oz	1.0	35	26%
lower salt	1 oz	1.0	30	30%
smoked	1 slice	<1.0	20	23%
pastrami				
Deli Select	1 slice	<1.0	10	27%
regular	1 slice	<1.0	18	25%
salami/hard	~1 oz	9.0	100	90%
turkey breast				
Deli Select				
honey-roasted	1 slice	<1.0	10	27%
oven-roasted	1 slice	<1.0	10	27%
smoked	1 slice	<1.0	10	27%
regular				
honey-cured	1 oz	2.0	35	51%
honey-roasted	1 slice	<1.0	20	23%
oven-roasted	1 slice	<1.0	20	23%
smoked				
flavor pack	1 slice	<1.0	20	23%
10-oz pkg	1 oz	1.0	35	26%
turkey ham/Deli Select	1 slice	<1.0	10	27%
■ (Hormel)				
beef				
chuck roast	2 oz	2.0	60	30%
dried/2.5-oz pkg	10 slices	1.5	50	27%
top round roast	2 oz	1.0	50	18%
chicken/chunk meat				
chicken	2 oz	3.0	70	39%
chicken breast				
no salt	2 oz	1.5	60	23%
regular	2 oz	1.5	60	23%
corned beef	2 oz	7.0	120	53%
ham				
chunk meat	2 oz	6.0	90	60%
Black Label				
canned	3 oz	5.0	84	54%
chopped	1 oz	11.0	140	71%
Cure 81/half	3 oz	5.0	100	45%
Curemaster	3 oz	3.0	80	34%
deli cooked	2 oz	2.5	60	38%
Light & Lean 97				
half ham	3 oz	2.5	90	25%
sliced	1 slice	1.0	25	36%

Food and Description	Amount	Fat Grams	Total Calories	% Fat Calories
patties				
plain	1 patty	17.0	180	85%
w/cheese	1 patty	17.0	190	80%
pork roast	2 oz	1.5	70	19%
salami				
Genoa				
Di Lusso	1 oz	9.0	120	68%
San Remo	1 oz	9.0	120	68%
Sandwich Maker	1 oz	11.0	120	83%
hard				
Homeland	1 oz	10.0	110	82%
Pillow Pack	4 slices	10.0	120	75%
Sandwich Maker	1 oz	10.0	110	82%
Spam				
less salt	2 oz	16.0	170	85%
lite	2 oz	8.0	110	65%
original	2 oz	16.0	170	85%
spread	4 Tbs	11.0	130	76%
turkey				
chunk meat				
turkey	2 oz	3.0	70	39%
white turkey	2 oz	1.0	60	15%
deli meat				
Light & Lean 97				
mesquite-smoked	1 slice	0.5	30	15%
sliced	1 slice	0.5	30	15%
smoked	3 oz	1.0	80	11%
mesquite-smoked	2 oz	1.0	60	15%
turkey ham/chunk meat	2 oz	4.0	70	51%
■ (Jimmy Dean)				
Tastefuls				
baked honey ham & cheese	1 pkg	33.0	490	61%
ham & turkey club w/cheddar cheese	1 pkg	29.0	490	53%
roast chicken & mozzarella	1 pkg	21.0	430	44%
roast turkey & Swiss	1 pkg	16.0	380	38%
■ (Johnsonville)				
bologna/country style				
beef ring	2 oz	15.0	170	79%
ring	2 oz	15.0	170	79%
■ (Kahn's)				
bologna				
beef				
8-oz pkg	1 slice	8.0	90	80%
family pack	1 slice	6.0	70	77%
giant/12-oz pkg	1 slice	8.0	90	80%
pounder	1 slice	8.0	90	80%
beef n' cheddar/8-oz pkg	1 slice	8.0	90	80%

Food and Description	Amount	Fat Grams	Total Calories	% Fat Calories
deluxe club				
8-oz pkg	1 slice	8.0	90	80%
family pack	1 slice	6.0	70	77%
giant/12-oz pkg	1 slice	8.0	90	80%
pounder	1 slice	8.0	90	80%
garlic/8-oz pkg	1 slice	8.0	90	80%
thick-sliced deluxe				
8-oz pkg	1 slice	13.0	140	84%
giant/12-oz pkg	1 slice	10.0	110	82%
thin-sliced deluxe/8-oz pkg	1 slice	5.0	60	75%
Dutch loaf/8-oz pkg	1 slice	7.0	80	79%
ham				
chopped/8-oz pkg	1 slice	3.0	50	54%
cooked/5-oz pkg	1 slice	1.0	30	30%
low salt/5-oz pkg	1 slice	1.0	30	30%
ham & cheese loaf	1 slice	6.0	70	77%
ham bologna/12-oz pkg	1 slice	8.0	90	80%
honey loaf/8-oz pkg	1 slice	2.0	40	45%
jalapeño loaf/8-oz pkg	1 slice	6.0	70	77%
liver loaf	1 slice	15.0	170	79%
P&B loaf/8-oz pkg	1 slice	2.0	40	45%
pepper loaf/8-oz pkg	1 slice	2.0	40	45%
pickle loaf				
beef/family pack	1 slice	5.0	60	75%
regular				
8-oz pkg	1 slice	7.0	80	79%
family pack	1 slice	6.0	70	77%
salami				
beef				
8-oz pkg	1 slice	6.0	70	77%
family pack	1 slice	5.0	60	75%
cooked/8-oz pkg	1 slice	4.0	60	60%
cotto/family pack	1 slice	3.0	45	60%
souse loaf/8-oz pkg	1 slice	7.0	90	70%
spice loaf				
beef/family pack	1 slice	5.0	60	75%
regular				
8-oz pkg	1 slice	7.0	80	79%
family pack	1 slice	6.0	70	77%
■ (Libby's)				
canned				
deviled meat	3 oz	13.0	160	73%
potted meat	3 oz	13.0	160	73%
■ (Louis Rich)				
chicken				
breast, oven roasted deluxe	1 slice	0.5	30	15%
Carving Board				
classic baked	2 slices	0.5	40	11%

Food and Description	Amount	Fat Grams	Total Calories	% Fat Calories
grilled	2 slices	0.5	40	11%
honey-glazed	2 slices	0.5	45	10%
Deli-Thin				
breast, oven roasted	4 slices	1.5	60	23%
white meat, oven roasted	1 slice	2.5	40	56%
ham/Carving Board				
baked	2 slices	1.5	50	27%
honey-glazed				
thin-carved	6 slices	1.5	70	19%
traditional	2 slices	1.5	50	27%
smoked	2 slices	1.5	45	30%
turkey				
breast/fully cooked/skinless				
fat-free				
barbecued	2 oz	–	60	–
hickory-roasted	2 oz	–	60	–
hickory-smoked	2 oz	–	50	–
oven-roasted	2 oz	–	50	–
breast/sliced				
Carving Board				
hickory-smoked	2 slices	0.5	40	11%
oven-roasted				
thin-carved	6 slices	0.5	60	8%
traditional carved	2 slices	0.5	40	11%
fat-free				
hickory-smoked	1 slice	–	25	–
oven-roasted	1 slice	–	25	–
Deli-Thin	4 slices	–	40	–
regular				
hickory-smoked	1 slice	–	50	–
honey-roasted	1 slice	–	60	–
oven-roasted	1 slice	–	50	–
breast & white meat/sliced				
Deli-Thin				
hickory-smoked	4 slices	1.0	50	18%
oven-roasted	4 slices	1.0	50	18%
regular				
hickory-smoked	1 slice	0.5	30	15%
honey-roasted	1 slice	0.5	30	15%
oven-roasted	1 slice	0.5	30	15%
smoked	1 slice	1.0	30	30%
chunk specialty/breast & white meat	2 oz	1.0	60	15%
turkey bologna	1 slice	3.5	50	63%
turkey ham				
chopped/sliced	1 slice	2.5	45	50%
chunk specialty	2 oz	3.0	70	39%
Deli-Thin/sliced	4 slices	1.5	60	23%
honey-cured/sliced	1 slice	1.0	30	30%

Food and Description	Amount	Fat Grams	Total Calories	% Fat Calories
regular/sliced	1 slice	1.0	35	26%
turkey pastrami				
chunk specialty	2 oz	2.0	70	26%
sliced	1 slice	1.0	30	30%
turkey salami				
chunk specialty/cooked	2 oz	9.0	120	68%
cooked/sliced	1 slice	2.5	40	56%
cotto/sliced	1 slice	2.5	40	56%
▩ (Mr. Turkey)				
chicken/smoked	6 slices	–	50	–
turkey				
breast				
honey-cured/variety pack	1 slice	–	25	–
oven-roasted				
regular	6 slices	–	50	–
variety pack	1 slice	–	25	–
smoked				
regular	6 slices	–	60	–
variety pack	1 slice	–	25	–
sliced/smoked	2 oz	1.0	60	15%
white meat/variety pack	1 slice	0.5	30	15%
turkey bologna				
regular	2 oz	11.0	130	76%
variety pack	1 slice	5.0	70	64%
turkey ham				
regular	2 oz	2.5	60	38%
smoked/variety pack	1 slice	1.5	35	39%
turkey pastrami				
chub	2 oz	3.0	70	39%
dark	2 oz	3.0	70	39%
turkey salami				
regular	2 oz	7.0	100	63%
variety pack	1 slice	3.0	50	54%
▩ (Oscar Mayer)				
Lunchables lunch combinations				
deluxe				
chicken/turkey	1 pkg	23.0	390	53%
turkey/ham	1 pkg	21.0	370	51%
Fun Pack				
bologna/wild cherry	1 pkg	28.0	530	48%
ham/fruit punch	1 pkg	20.0	440	41%
pizza				
mozzarella/fruit punch	1 pkg	15.0	450	30%
pepperoni/orange	1 pkg	17.0	480	32%
turkey/Pacific cooler	1 pkg	20.0	450	40%
turkey/surfer cooler	1 pkg	15.0	430	31%
low-fat w/drink				
ham/fruit punch	1 pkg	10.0	360	25%

Food and Description	Amount	Fat Grams	Total Calories	% Fat Calories
ham/Surfer Cooler	1 pkg	11.0	390	25%
turkey/Pacific Cooler	1 pkg	9.0	360	23%
regular				
bologna/American	1 pkg	35.0	470	67%
ham/cheddar	1 pkg	22.0	360	55%
ham/Swiss	1 pkg	20.0	340	53%
pizza				
pepperoni/mozzarella	1 pkg	15.0	330	41%
2 cheese	1 pkg	13.0	330	35%
salami/American	1 pkg	30.0	430	63%
turkey/cheddar	1 pkg	20.0	350	52%
turkey/Monterey jack	1 pkg	21.0	350	54%
luncheon meat				
beef roast/Deli-Thin	4 slices	1.5	60	23%
bologna				
Free/fat-free	1 slice	–	20	–
light				
beef	1 slice	4.0	60	60%
pork, chicken, & beef	1 slice	4.0	60	60%
regular				
beef	1 slice	8.0	90	80%
garlic	1 slice	12.0	130	83%
pork, chicken, & beef	1 slice	8.0	90	80%
Wisconsin-made ring	2 oz	16.0	180	80%
Braunschweiger liver sausage	2 slices	16.0	170	85%
chicken breast				
Free/fat-free	4 slices	–	45	–
honey glazed/Deli-Thin	4 slices	1.0	60	15%
ham				
Deli-Thin				
boiled	4 slices	2.0	50	36%
honey	4 slices	2.0	60	30%
smoked, cooked	4 slices	2.0	50	36%
Free/fat-free				
baked	3 slices	–	40	–
honey	3 slices	–	45	–
smoked	3 slices	–	35	–
Healthy Favorites				
baked	4 slices	1.5	50	27%
honey	4 slices	1.5	60	23%
smoked, cooked	4 slices	1.5	50	27%
regular				
baked	3 slices	1.0	60	15%
boiled	3 slices	2.5	60	38%
chopped	1 slice	3.0	50	54%
honey	3 slices	2.5	70	32%
lower sodium	3 slices	2.5	70	32%
smoked/cooked	3 slices	2.5	60	38%

Food and Description	Amount	Fat Grams	Total Calories	% Fat Calories
ham & cheese loaf	1 slice	5.0	70	64%
headcheese	1 slice	4.0	50	72%
honey loaf	1 slice	1.0	35	26%
liver cheese/pork fat-wrapped	1 slice	10.0	120	75%
old-fashioned loaf	1 slice	5.0	60	75%
olive loaf	1 slice	6.0	70	77%
pickle & pimiento loaf	1 slice	6.0	80	68%
salami				
cotto				
beef	2 slices	7.0	90	70%
pork, chicken, & beef	2 slices	9.0	110	74%
for beer	3 slices	9.0	110	74%
Genoa	3 slices	9.0	100	81%
hard				
Deli-Thin	4 slices	11.0	130	76%
regular	3 slices	9.0	100	81%
Machiaeh/beef	2 slices	10.0	120	75%
spiced luncheon loaf	1 slice	5.0	70	64%
turkey				
breast				
oven roasted				
Free/fat-free	4 slices	–	40	–
regular	1 slice	0.5	25	18%
smoked/free/fat-free	4 slices	–	40	–
breast & white meat/Deli-Thin				
roasted	4 slices	1.0	50	18%
smoked/honey-roasted	4 slices	1.0	50	18%
white meat/oven-roasted	1 slice	1.0	30	30%
■ (Perdue)				
chicken bologna	2 slices	9.0	130	62%
■ (Reser's)				
salami/cooked	2 oz	11.0	140	71%
■ (Sara Lee)				
deli				
beef				
Angus/sliced/peppered	2 oz	2.0	70	26%
top round/sliced				
cap	2 oz	2.0	70	26%
choice cap	2 oz	2.0	70	26%
chicken breast/plain	2 oz	1.0	60	15%
corned beef/sliced				
regular	2 oz	4.5	90	45%
top round	2 oz	2.0	70	26%
ham				
Bavarian baked	2 oz	4.0	80	45%
Bavarian baked/honey	2 oz	4.0	80	45%
brown sugar	2 oz	1.5	60	23%
honey/spiral-sliced	2 oz	2.5	80	28%

Food and Description	Amount	Fat Grams	Total Calories	% Fat Calories
honey-cured	2 oz	1.5	60	23%
natural smoked	2 oz	2.0	70	26%
pastrami				
eye of round beef	2 oz	6.0	100	54%
pork roast				
sliced	2 oz	3.0	70	39%
sliced bellas	2 oz	3.5	80	39%
turkey breast				
honey cured	2 oz	–	60	–
natural smoked	2 oz	2.0	60	30%
oven-roasted	2 oz	1.5	60	23%
peppered	2 oz	–	50	–
plain	2 oz	1.5	60	23%
smoked/skinless	2 oz	1.0	60	15%
turkey ham				
Black Forest	2 oz	3.0	70	39%
honey-cured	2 oz	3.0	70	39%
turkey pastrami	2 oz	0.5	60	8%
■ SPAM (See (Hormel) in this section)				
LUNCHEON MEAT SPREAD (See also PÂTÉ)				
generic				
beef	1 tbs	2.5	34	67%
	1 oz	5.0	67	67%
chicken	1 oz	3.0	55	49%
deviled ham	¼ cup	18.0	198	82%
ham & cheese	1 tbs	2.8	37	68%
ham salad	1 oz	4.0	61	59%
pork	1 tbs	2.5	34	67%
	1 oz	5.0	67	67%
turkey	~2 oz	6.0	100	54%
(Hormel)				
deviled ham	4 Tbs	12.0	150	72%
liverwurst	4 Tbs	10.0	130	69%
potted meat	4 Tbs	7.0	100	63%
(Libby's) Spredables				
chicken	⅓ cup	9.0	140	58%
ham	⅓ cup	4.5	110	37%
tuna	⅓ cup	8.0	130	55%
turkey	⅓ cup	10.0	150	60%
(Oscar Mayer)				
Braunschweiger liver sausage	2 oz	17.0	190	80%
sandwich spread	2 oz	10.0	130	69%
(Swanson)				
chicken/chunky	¼ cup	8.0	120	60%
(Underwood)				
chicken/chunky	¼ cup	8.0	120	60%
ham				
deviled	¼ cup	14.0	160	79%

Food and Description	Amount	Fat Grams	Total Calories	% Fat Calories
honey	¼ cup	16.0	180	80%
liverwurst	¼ cup	14.0	160	79%
roast beef	¼ cup	11.0	130	76%
LUPIN				
boiled	½ cup	2.0	98	18%
raw	½ cup	8.0	330	22%

M

Food and Description	Amount	Fat Grams	Total Calories	% Fat Calories
MACADAMIA NUT				
generic				
dried	1 oz	21.0	200	95%
dry-roasted	1 oz	21.0	193	98%
oil-roasted	1 oz	21.7	204	96%
	¼ cup	24.0	250	86%
(Mauna Loa)				
brittle	1 oz	8.0	150	48%
chocolate-covered	1 oz	13.0	170	69%
honey-roasted	1 oz	17.0	200	77%
roasted/salted/shelled	1 oz	21.0	210	90%
MACARONI (See PASTA)				
MACARONI & CHEESE (See FROZEN ENTRÉE/DINNER; PASTA ENTRÉE/DINNER; VEGETARIAN FOODS)				
MACAROON (See COOKIE)				
MACE/ground	1 tsp	0.6	8	68%
MACKEREL (See also SEAFOOD ENTRÉE/DINNER)				
Atlantic				
cooked-dry heat	3 oz	15.0	223	61%
raw	3 oz	11.8	174	61%
jack/canned/drained				
(Empress)	4 oz	8.0	140	51%
generic	1 cup	12.0	296	36%
king				
cooked-dry heat	3 oz	5.5	135	37%
raw	3 oz	1.7	89	17%
Pacific/mixed species				
cooked-dry heat	3 oz	8.5	170	45%
raw	3 oz	6.5	135	43%

Food and Description	Amount	Fat Grams	Total Calories	% Fat Calories
Spanish				
cooked-dry heat	3 oz	5.0	134	34%
raw	3 oz	5.0	118	38%
MAHI MAHI				
cooked-dry heat	3 oz	1.0	95	9%
Hawaiian style/frozen/skinless-boneless	4 oz	1.0	100	9%
raw	3 oz	0.6	72	8%
MALT (See BARLEY MALT; MILK MIX)				
MALT LIQUOR (See BEER, ALE, & MALT LIQUOR)				
MAMEY APPLE/MAMMEY APPLE/MAMMEE APPLE				
raw				
peeled/no seeds	3 oz	<1.0	42	6%
whole	1 medium	4.4	445	9%
MANDARIN ORANGE (See also TANGERINE)				
canned				
(Del Monte)	5.5 oz	<1.0	100	5%
(Dole) in light syrup	½ cup	<1.0	76	6%
(Empress)	½ cup	–	80	–
generic				
in juice	1 cup	–	92	–
in light syrup	1 cup	0.5	125	4%
(S&W)				
natural style	½ cup	–	60	–
sections in heavy syrup	½ cup	<1.0	76	6%
fresh/raw				
sections	½ cup	–	45	–
whole	1 medium	–	35	–
MANDARIN ORANGE JUICE/JUICE BLEND				
bottled, boxed, or canned				
(Dole) 100% juice blend/Mandarin	8 fl oz	–	160	–
tangerine	10 fl oz	–	200	–
frozen or refrigerated				
(Dole) Mandarin tangerine				
frozen/prepared	8 fl oz	–	140	–
refrigerated	4 fl oz	–	70	–
	8 fl oz	–	140	–
MANGO/fresh				
diced or sliced	1 cup	0.5	110	4%
whole	1 medium	0.5	135	3%
MANGO JUICE/JUICE BLEND/JUICE DRINK (See also FRUIT PUNCH)				
bottled				
(Kern's) nectar	6 fl oz	–	110	–
	11.5 fl oz	–	210	–
(Knudsen)				
Mango Montage	8 fl oz	–	110	–
mango-peach	8 fl oz	–	120	–
(Libby's) nectar	6 fl oz	–	110	–

Food and Description	Amount	Fat Grams	Total Calories	% Fat Calories
(Snapple) cocktail				
Mango Mad				
regular	8 fl oz	–	110	–
diet	8 fl oz	–	13	–
(TreeTop) More Mango	8 fl oz	–	120	–
mix				
(Tang) drink mix/mango flavored	¼ cup	–	100	–
MANICOTTI (*See* FROZEN ENTRÉE/DINNER; PASTA ENTRÉE/DINNER)				
MAPLE SYRUP (*See also* PANCAKE/WAFFLE SYRUP)				
	1 Tbs	–	50	–
MARGARINE, MARGARINE SPREAD, & SPRAY				
(Autumn) spread	1 Tbs	8.0	80	100%
(Blue Bonnet)				
lower fat				
stick	1 Tbs	6.0	50	100%
tub	1 Tbs	4.5	45	100%
regular/soft or stick	1 Tbs	11.0	100	100%
spread				
Better Blend				
stick	1 Tbs	11.0	90	100%
tub	1 Tbs	11.0	90	100%
48% vegetable oil	1 Tbs	6.0	60	100%
75% vegetable oil	1 Tbs	11.0	90	100%
whipped				
soft	1 Tbs	7.0	70	100%
stick	1 Tbs	7.0	70	100%
(Brummel & Brown) w/yogurt				
tub	1 Tbs	5.0	50	100%
stick	1 Tbs	5.0	50	100%
(Canola Harvest) soft	1 Tbs	11.0	100	100%
(Chiffon)				
soft stick	1 Tbs	11.0	100	100%
soft tub	1 Tbs	11.0	100	100%
whipped	1 Tbs	7.0	70	100%
(Fleischmann's)				
corn oil spread				
extra light	1 Tbs	6.0	50	100%
fat-free/squeeze	1 Tbs	–	5	–
light				
soft or stick	1 Tbs	8.0	80	100%
squeeze	1 Tbs	10.0	90	100%
diet	1 Tbs	6.0	50	100%
soft or stick	1 Tbs	11.0	100	100%
whipped	1 Tbs	7.0	70	100%
generic				
hard	1 pat	4.0	35	100%
	1 Tbs	11.0	100	100%
	4 oz	91.0	810	100%

Food and Description	Amount	Fat Grams	Total Calories	% Fat Calories
soft	1 Tbs	11.0	100	100%
	4 oz	92.0	813	100%
spread				
40% fat/soft	1 Tbs	5.7	50	100%
	4 oz	44.0	393	100%
60% fat				
hard	1 pat	3.0	25	100%
	1 Tbs	9.0	75	100%
	4 oz	69.0	610	100%
soft	1 Tbs	9.0	75	100%
	4 oz	69.0	613	100%
squeeze	1 tsp	4.0	35	100%
whipped/hard or soft	1 Tbs	7.0	70	100%
(Gold-N-Sweet) canola	1 Tbs	11.0	100	100%
(Gregg's) Gold-n-Soft-Lite spread	1 Tbs	7.0	70	100%
(Hain) safflower				
regular	1 Tbs	11.0	100	100%
unsalted	1 Tbs	11.0	100	100%
(Heartlight) canola	1 Tbs	11.0	100	100%
(Hollywood) safflower				
regular	1 Tbs	11.0	100	100%
unsalted sweet	1 Tbs	11.0	100	100%
(I Can't Believe It's Not Butter)				
light spread				
stick	1 Tbs	7.0	60	100%
tub	1 Tbs	7.0	60	100%
regular	1 Tbs	10.0	90	100%
spray	4 sprays	0.4	4	100%
	10 sprays	1.0	10	100%
	1 Tbs	5.5	55	100%
squeeze	1 Tbs	9.0	80	100%
(Imperial)				
A La Mode	1 Tbs	7.5	70	100%
A La Mode stick	1 Tbs	11.0	100	100%
light	1 Tbs	6.0	60	100%
quarters	1 Tbs	11.0	100	100%
Savory Squeeze				
buttery	1 Tbs	10.0	90	100%
garlic & herb	1 Tbs	10.0	90	100%
soft	1 Tbs	11.0	100	100%
soft diet	1 Tbs	6.0	50	100%
whipped	1 Tbs	5.6	50	100%
(Kraft) Touch of Butter				
47% fat/tub	1 Tbs	7.0	60	100%
70% fat/stick	1 Tbs	7.0	60	100%
(Land O'Lakes)				
Country Morning Blend				
stick	1 Tbs	11.0	100	100%

Food and Description	Amount	Fat Grams	Total Calories	% Fat Calories
light	1 Tbs	6.0	50	100%
unsalted	1 Tbs	11.0	100	100%
tub				
light	1 Tbs	6.0	50	100%
regular	1 Tbs	11.0	100	100%
premium corn oil				
stick	1 Tbs	11.0	100	100%
tub	1 Tbs	11.0	100	100%
soy oil				
stick	1 Tbs	11.0	100	100%
tub	1 Tbs	11.0	100	100%
spread w/sweet cream				
stick				
salted	1 Tbs	10.0	90	100%
unsalted	1 Tbs	10.0	90	100%
tub	1 Tbs	8.0	80	100%
(Mazola)				
reduced calorie				
extra light	1 Tbs	6.0	50	100%
light corn oil	1 Tbs	6.0	50	100%
regular	1 Tbs	11.0	100	100%
(Miracle Brand) whipped				
soft	1 Tbs	7.0	60	100%
stick	1 Tbs	7.0	70	100%
(Mrs. Filberts)				
corn oil family spread	1 Tbs	7.0	60	100%
golden quarters	1 Tbs	11.0	100	100%
soft corn	1 Tbs	11.0	100	100%
soft gold	1 Tbs	11.0	100	100%
vegetable oil	1 Tbs	7.0	65	100%
(Nabisco) Move Over Butter				
stick	1 Tbs	10.0	90	100%
tub	1 Tbs	10.0	90	100%
whipped	1 Tbs	7.0	60	100%
(Nucanola)	1 Tbs	10.0	90	100%
(Nucoa)				
Heart Beat/corn oil	1 Tbs	3.0	25	100%
Smartbeat				
regular	1 Tbs	2.0	20	100%
unsalted	1 Tbs	2.0	20	100%
soft	1 Tbs	10.0	90	100%
stick	1 Tbs	11.0	100	100%
(Parkay)				
diet	1 Tbs	6.0	50	100%
liquid				
regular	1 Tbs	9.0	80	100%
spread	1 Tbs	9.0	80	100%
soft or stick	1 Tbs	11.0	100	100%

Food and Description	Amount	Fat Grams	Total Calories	% Fat Calories
vegetable oil spread				
40%/light	1 Tbs	7.0	60	100%
50%	1 Tbs	7.0	60	100%
53%	1 Tbs	7.0	70	100%
70%	1 Tbs	10.0	90	100%
whipped/soft or stick	1 Tbs	7.0	70	100%
(Promise)				
extra light	1 Tbs	6.0	50	100%
fat-free	1 Tbs	–	5	–
regular	1 Tbs	10.0	90	100%
sunflower oil	1 Tbs	10.0	90	100%
ultra/tub	1 Tbs	4.0	35	100%
(Saffola)	1 Tbs	11.0	100	100%
(Shedd's Spread)				
churn style	1 Tbs	7.0	60	100%
classic 64% spread/stick	1 Tbs	7.0	60	100%
corn oil spread	1 Tbs	7.0	60	100%
Country Crock	1 Tbs	7.0	70	100%
original	1 Tbs	9.0	80	100%
quarters spread	1 Tbs	9.0	80	100%
squeeze	1 Tbs	9.0	80	100%
whipped honey spread	1 Tbs	9.0	90	90%
(Weight Watchers)				
Country Cottage spread/tub	1 Tbs	4.0	45	100%
light spread/tub				
regular	1 Tbs	4.0	45	100%
sodium-free	1 Tbs	4.0	45	100%
reduced fat	1 Tbs	7.0	60	100%
(Willow Run Print) sticks	1 Tbs	11.0	100	100%
MARINADE (*See also* SEASONINGS)				
bottled or jarred				
(Andre Prost) hot adobo	1 Tbs	–	10	–
(Girard's) lemon dill	2 Tbs	14.0	130	97%
(Golden Dipt)				
Cajun style	1 Tbs	4.5	60	68%
ginger teriyaki	1 Tbs	3.0	60	45%
honey mustard/fat-free	1 Tbs	–	25	–
honey soy/fat-free	1 Tbs	–	30	–
lemon herb	1 Tbs	9.0	80	100%
white wine Dijon/fat-free	1 Tbs	–	10	–
(Lawry's)				
citrus grill	1 Tbs	–	15	–
Hawaiian	1 Tbs	–	20	–
herb garlic	1 Tbs	–	10	–
lemon pepper	1 Tbs	0.5	10	45%
mesquite	1 Tbs	–	5	–
red wine	1 Tbs	–	5	–
teriyaki	1 Tbs	–	25	–

Food and Description	Amount	Fat Grams	Total Calories	% Fat Calories
(Mr. Marinade)				
Cajun	1 Tbs	–	10	–
honey mustard	1 Tbs	–	20	–
Italian	1 Tbs	–	10	–
red wine	1 Tbs	–	15	–
teriyaki	1 Tbs	–	10	–
white wine	1 Tbs	0.5	15	30%
(S&W)				
mesquite	1 Tbs	–	10	–
teriyaki				
lite	1 Tbs	–	25	–
regular	1 Tbs	–	25	–
mix/mix only				
(Durkee) beef	⅒ pkg	–	–	–
(French's) meat	⅒ pkg	–	–	–
(Kikkoman)	1 oz	–	60	–
(Lawry's)				
chicken sauté				
country Dijon	2 Tbs	1.0	40	23%
garlic Italian	2 Tbs	2.0	30	60%
seasoned	1 Tbs	–	10	–
teriyaki	1 Tbs	–	25	–
(Marinade-Magic)				
fajitas	½ tsp	–	5	–
grilled chicken	¾ tsp	–	10	–
lemon beef	½ tsp	–	10	–
(McCormick/Schilling)				
chicken				
Italian	2 tsp	–	20	–
mesquite	2 tsp	–	20	–
fajita	¼ tsp	–	1	–
Grill Mates				
mesquite	2 tsp	–	15	–
Oriental	2 tsp	–	15	–
Southwest	2 tsp	–	15	–
zesty herb	2 tsp	–	10	–
meat/original	1 tsp	–	15	–
MARINARA SAUCE (See SAUCE)				
MARIONBERRY				
(Schwan's) frozen/no sugar	3.5 oz	–	60	–
MARJORAM/dried	1 tsp	–	2	–
MARMALADE (See JAM/JELLY/PRESERVES)				
MARSHMALLOW				
(Campfire)				
large	2 pieces	–	40	–
miniature	10 pieces	–	17	–
	24 pieces	–	40	–
generic/large or small	1 oz	–	95	–

Food and Description	Amount	Fat Grams	Total Calories	% Fat Calories
(Kraft)				
Funmallows				
large	4 pieces	–	110	–
miniature	10 pieces	–	18	–
	½ cup	–	100	–
Jet Puffed	5 pieces	–	110	–
Miniatures	½ cup	–	100	–
Teddy Bear/cocoa flavored	½ cup	–	100	–
MARSHMALLOW CREME				
(Kraft)	2 Tbs	–	40	–
MATZO (*See also* CRACKER; MATZO MEAL & MIX)				
generic				
egg	1 matzo	<1.0	111	4%
egg & onion	1 matzo	0.5	111	4%
plain	1 matzo	<1.0	112	4%
whole wheat	1 matzo	<1.0	100	5%
(Goodman's) Passover				
egg	1 matzo	1.0	130	7%
plain	1 matzo	–	130	–
(Manischewitz)				
American	1 matzo	2.0	115	16%
apple cinnamon	1 matzo	–	110	–
egg 'n onion	1 matzo	1.0	110	8%
everything onion	1 matzo	0.5	110	4%
honey spice	12 crackers	1.0	110	8%
	1 matzo	1.0	110	8%
miniatures	13 crackers	0.5	110	4%
Passover				
egg	10 crackers	2.0	110	16%
plain	1 matzo	–	130	–
savory garlic	1 matzo	–	100	–
thin salted	1 matzo	–	10	–
thin tea/daily	1 matzo	–	100	–
thins/dietetic	1 matzo	1.0	100	9%
unsalted/daily	1 matzo	–	110	–
wheat	10 crackers	1.0	90	10%
whole wheat	1 matzo	1.0	110	8%
MATZO MEAL & MIX (*See also* SOUP)				
meal				
(Goodman's) Passover	1 cup	1.0	514	2%
(Manischewitz)	1 cup	1.0	510	2%
mix				
(Manischewitz) matzo ball/mix only	2 Tbs	–	50	–
MAYONNAISE/MAYONNAISE-TYPE DRESSING (*See also* SALAD DRESSING)				
(Bama) regular	1 Tbs	11.0	100	100%
(Bennett's) real	1 Tbs	12.0	110	98%
(Best Foods)				
Dijonnaise blend	1 tsp	1.0	10	90%

Food and Description	Amount	Fat Grams	Total Calories	% Fat Calories
light	1 Tbs	5.0	50	90%
real	1 Tbs	11.0	100	99%
reduced fat	1 Tbs	3.0	40	68%
(Estee)	1 Tbs	5.0	50	90%
(Featherweight) soyamaise mayo dressing	1 Tbs	11.0	100	99%
(Hain)				
canola				
light/reduced calorie	1 Tbs	5.0	60	75%
regular	1 Tbs	11.0	100	100%
cold-processed	1 Tbs	12.0	110	98%
eggless	1 Tbs	12.0	110	98%
light	1 Tbs	6.0	60	90%
real	1 Tbs	12.0	110	98%
safflower	1 Tbs	12.0	110	98%
(Hellman's)				
Dijonnaise blend	1 tsp	1.0	10	90%
light	1 Tbs	5.0	50	90%
real	1 Tbs	11.0	100	100%
reduced fat	1 Tbs	3.0	40	68%
(Hollywood)				
canola	1 Tbs	11.0	100	100%
safflower	1 Tbs	11.0	100	98%
(Kraft)				
mayonnaise				
Kraft Free/nonfat	1 Tbs	–	10	–
light	1 Tbs	5.0	50	90%
real	1 Tbs	11.0	100	99%
Miracle Whip				
light	1 Tbs	3.0	40	68%
nonfat	1 Tbs	–	15	–
original	1 Tbs	7.0	70	90%
(Life All Natural) egg-free	1 Tbs	8.0	70	100%
(Nasoya) tofu Nayonaise	1 Tbs	4.0	40	90%
(Nucoa) Heart Beat corn oil	1 Tbs	4.0	40	90%
(Smart Beat)				
canola oil	1 Tbs	4.0	40	90%
corn oil	1 Tbs	4.0	40	90%
(Spectrum) canola				
eggless lite	1 Tbs	3.0	30	90%
real	1 Tbs	12.0	100	100%
(Weight Watchers)				
fat free	1 Tbs	–	10	–
light				
low-sodium	1 Tbs	2.0	25	72%
regular	1 Tbs	2.0	25	72%
whipped	1 Tbs	–	15	–
(Westbrae) canola	1 Tbs	11.0	100	99%

MEAL REPLACEMENT (*See* NUTRITIONAL SUPPLEMENT)

Food and Description	Amount	Fat Grams	Total Calories	% Fat Calories
MEAT LOAF (*See* FROZEN ENTRÉE/DINNER)				
MEAT SEASONING (*See* MARINADE; SEASONINGS)				
MEAT SPREAD (*See* LUNCHEON MEAT SPREAD)				
MEAT SUBSTITUTE (*See* VEGETARIAN FOODS; individual listings)				
MEAT TENDERIZER (*See also* MARINADE; SEASONINGS)				
generic/seasoned	1 tsp	–	2	–
(Tone's)				
seasoned	1 tsp	–	7	–
unseasoned	1 tsp	–	7	–
MEATBALL (*See* BEEF; BEEF DISH/ENTRÉE; FROZEN ENTRÉE/DINNER; PASTA ENTRÉE/DINNER)				
MELBA TOAST (*See* CRACKER)				
MELON (*See also* individual listings)				
balls/frozen				
(C&W) mixed/no sugar added	⅔ cup	–	40	–
generic				
cantaloupe & honeydew	1 lb	1.0	145	6%
sweetened	1 cup	0.5	245	2%
unsweetened	½ cup	0.5	60	8%
MELON DRINK/JUICE DRINK (*See also* FRUIT PUNCH; SOFT DRINK; SOFT DRINK MIX)				
(Snapple) Melonberry Cocktail	8 fl oz	–	120	–
(TreeTop) Wonder Melon juice drink	8 fl oz	–	120	–
MEXICAN FOOD (*See also* BEEF DISH/ENTRÉE; BREAKFAST SANDWICH; DIP; FROZEN ENTRÉE/DINNER; PASTA ENTRÉE/DINNER; RICE DISH; SAUCE; SEASONINGS; TOMATO; TOMATO SAUCE; TORTILLA CHIPS; VEGETARIAN FOODS)				
■ **BEANS** (*See* Chili Beans; Ranchero Beans; Refried Beans in this section)				
■ **BURRITO**				
frozen				
(BR Brand)				
bean & cheese	5 oz	6.0	290	19%
beef & bean	5 oz	15.0	400	34%
green chili	5 oz	9.0	340	24%
red chili	5 oz	5.0	290	16%
(Don Miguel)				
breakfast				
bacon & egg	1 burrito	27.0	520	47%
sausage	1 burrito	27.0	510	48%
smoked ham	1 burrito	17.0	420	36%
Lean Olé!				
bean & cheese	1 burrito	4.0	380	9%
chicken, beans, & rice	1 burrito	5.0	380	12%
steak, beans, & rice	1 burrito	4.0	380	9%
regular				
beef steak & bean w/jalapeño peppers	1 burrito	8.0	350	21%
chicken & cheese	1 burrito	14.0	410	31%

Food and Description	Amount	Fat Grams	Total Calories	% Fat Calories
shredded beef & cheese	1 burrito	11.0	390	25%
shredded beef, cheddar cheese sauce, & green chilies				
hot & spicy	1 burrito	7.0	270	23%
regular	1 burrito	6.0	230	23%
skinless chicken	4.5 oz	5.0	240	19%
	7 oz	8.0	360	20%
steak strips/beef steak & bean	1 burrito	8.0	370	19%
3 cheeses/bean & cheese	4.5 oz	8.0	280	26%
	7 oz	13.0	420	28%
(El Charrito)				
bean & cheese				
grande	6 oz	8.0	380	19%
regular	5 oz	8.0	320	23%
beef & bean				
grande	6 oz	16.0	430	33%
regular	5 oz	12.0	350	31%
grande	6 oz	14.0	410	31%
green chili beef & bean	5 oz	16.0	370	39%
green chili grande	6 oz	15.0	410	33%
jalapeño grande	6 oz	15.0	410	33%
red chili beef & bean	5 oz	18.0	380	43%
red chili grande	6 oz	15.0	410	45%
red hot beef	5 oz	17.0	340	45%
red hot beef & bean	5 oz	18.0	540	30%
(El Monterey) reduced fat				
bean & cheese	1 burrito	4.0	220	16%
beef & bean	1 burrito	6.0	240	23%
(Healthy Choice)				
beef & bean ranch				
medium	1 burrito	7.0	290	22%
mild	1 burrito	7.0	300	21%
chicken con queso	1 burrito	6.0	280	19%
(Hormel) Quick Meal				
beef	1 burrito	13.0	300	39%
cheese	1 burrito	6.0	350	15%
red chili	1 burrito	11.0	280	35%
(Old El Paso)				
bean & cheese	1 burrito	9.0	290	28%
beef & bean				
hot	1 burrito	10.0	320	28%
medium	1 burrito	10.0	320	28%
mild	1 burrito	9.0	330	25%
pizza				
cheese	1 burrito	9.0	320	25%
pepperoni	1 burrito	10.0	260	35%
sausage	1 burrito	9.0	260	31%

Food and Description	Amount	Fat Grams	Total Calories	% Fat Calories
(Patio)				
britos				
beef & bean	6 oz	19.0	420	41%
nacho beef	6 oz	18.0	410	40%
nacho cheese	6 oz	13.0	360	33%
spicy chicken & cheese	6 oz	16.0	400	36%
burritos				
bean & cheese	5 oz	5.0	270	17%
chicken	5 oz	4.0	260	14%
hot beef & bean red chili	5 oz	5.0	260	34%
mild beef & bean green chili	5 oz	5.0	260	33%
red chili	5 oz	6.0	270	20%
red hot beef & bean	5 oz	7.0	280	38%
(Ruiz)				
beef steak	1 burrito	6.0	270	20%
chicken	1 burrito	7.0	290	22%
Monterey shredded beef & cheese	1 burrito	10.0	310	29%
(Schwan's) beef & bean	4.3 oz	13.0	260	45%
mix				
(Del Monte) burrito filling mix	½ cup	1.0	110	8%
(Old El Paso)				
kit				
mix & 1 tortilla	1 piece	3.5	190	16%
prepared	1 piece	7.0	280	23%
seasoning/mix only	2 tsp	–	20	–
■ BURRO				
frozen				
(Chi-Chi's)				
beef	1 burro	19.0	570	30%
chix	1 burro	16.0	530	27%
■ CHILI (*See also* BEEF DISH/ENTRÉE; SEASONINGS)				
canned				
(Armour Star) beef				
w/beans				
hot	1 cup	28.0	440	57%
regular	1 cup	28.0	440	57%
Western style	1 cup	32.0	460	63%
w/o beans	1 cup	38.0	470	73%
(Chili Man)				
beef w/beans				
hot	1 cup	27.0	430	57%
regular	1 cup	27.0	430	57%
turkey w/beans	1 cup	8.0	300	24%
(Dennison's) beef				
con carne/chunky w/beans	1 cup	16.0	340	42%
hot				
w/beans	1 cup	18.0	370	44%
w/o beans	1 cup	22.0	350	57%

Food and Description	Amount	Fat Grams	Total Calories	% Fat Calories
hot & chunky w/beans	1 cup	15.0	330	41%
jalapeño w/beans	1 cup	18.0	370	44%
lite w/beans	1 cup	4.0	200	18%
original	1 cup	17.0	360	43%
reduced fat	1 cup	7.0	290	22%
Select w/beans				
caliente hot & spicy	1 cup	6.0	240	15%
homestyle mild	1 cup	7.0	250	25%
w/beans	7 oz	16.0	300	48%
	1 cup	17.0	360	43%
w/o beans	1 cup	22.0	360	55%
(Don Miguel) XLNT chili con carne	1/3 cup	20.0	250	72%
w/o beans				
(Gebhardt) beef w/beans	1 cup	15.0	320	42%
(Health Valley) fat-free				
burrito flavor	½ cup	–	80	–
enchilada flavor	½ cup	–	80	–
fajita flavor	½ cup	–	80	–
mild w/black beans	½ cup	–	80	–
mild w/3 beans	½ cup	–	80	–
spicy w/black beans	½ cup	–	80	–
(Hormel)				
beef				
w/beans				
chunky	1 cup	16.0	330	44%
hot	1 cup	17.0	340	45%
regular	1 cup	17.0	340	45%
w/o beans				
hot	1 cup	30.0	410	66%
regular	1 cup	30.0	410	66%
turkey				
w/beans	1 cup	3.0	220	12%
w/o beans	1 cup	3.0	190	14%
vegetarian	1 cup	–	200	–
(Just Rite) beef w/beans	1 cup	27.0	380	64%
(Libby's) beef				
w/beans	1 cup	27.0	420	58%
w/o beans	1 cup	37.0	480	69%
(Nile Spice) vegetarian/chili 'n beans				
mild	7 oz	1.0	160	6%
spicy	7 oz	2.0	170	11%
(Old El Paso) beef w/beans	1 cup	7.0	200	32%
(Stagg)				
beef				
Chunkero w/beans	1 cup	15.0	330	41%
classic w/beans	1 cup	16.0	330	44%
country w/beans	1 cup	16.0	330	44%
dynamite hot w/beans	1 cup	15.0	330	41%

Food and Description	Amount	Fat Grams	Total Calories	% Fat Calories
Laredo w/beans	1 cup	12.0	300	36%
steakhouse straight	1 cup	22.0	360	55%
chicken/ranch house w/beans	1 cup	6.0	270	20%
(Worthington) vegetarian	1 cup	15.0	290	47%
homemade/USDA Standard Home Recipe				
beef	1 cup	15.0	400	34%
kit/mix/seasoning				
(Durkee)				
mild/mix only	1 cup	0.5	30	15%
pot-o-chili/mix only	1 cup	–	30	–
regular/mix only	1 cup	–	30	–
Texas red/mix only	1 cup	1.0	45	20%
(Fantastic Foods) vegetarian				
mix only	⅛ cup	–	50	–
prepared	½ cup	–	50	–
(French's) Chili-O/mix only				
mild	1 cup	0.5	30	15%
onion	1 cup	–	40	–
original	1 cup	–	30	–
Texas style	1 cup	1.0	45	20%
(Gebhardt) quick/mix only	1 pkg	1.0	80	11%
(Hunt's) Chili Fixings	½ cup	1.0	84	11%
(Knorr) 4 bean chili/mix only	1 serving	1.5	230	6%
(McCormick/Schilling) mix only				
Cincinnati	⅙ pkg	1.0	80	11%
Texas	⅕ pkg	1.5	50	27%
(Old El Paso) mix only	1 Tbs	0.5	25	18%
(Spice Islands) Quick Meal				
regular/prepared	1 pkg	1.5	110	12%
spicy three bean/prepared	1 pkg	1.5	180	8%
(Tabasco) 7 spice chili recipe	½ cup	0.5	50	9%
microwave container				
(Hormel) micro cup meal				
hot w/beans	1 cup	11.0	250	40%
regular				
10.5 oz w/beans	1 cup	17.0	410	37%
w/beans	1 cup	11.0	250	40%
w/o beans	1 cup	17.0	290	53%
(Libby's) Diner w/beans	1 container	22.0	320	62%
(Lunch Bucket)	7.5 oz	12.0	260	42%
■ CHILI BEANS (See also individual bean listings)				
(Bush's Best) hot	½ cup	–	70	–
(Dennison's) in chili gravy	½ cup	–	110	–
(Gebhardt)	½ cup	1.0	135	7%
(Green Giant)				
caliente style/dry	½ cup	1.0	100	9%
extra spicy	½ cup	1.0	110	8%
Mexican	½ cup	1.5	120	11%

Food and Description	Amount	Fat Grams	Total Calories	% Fat Calories
(Hunt's)	½ cup	1.0	90	10%
(Joan of Arc)				
caliente style/dry	½ cup	1.0	100	9%
extra spicy	½ cup	1.0	110	8%
Mexican	½ cup	1.5	120	11%
(Luck's) pintos in chili gravy	½ cup	1.0	120	8%
(S&W)	½ cup	1.0	130	7%
(Sun Vista)	½ cup	1.0	110	8%
(Van Camp's) Mexican	1 cup	2.5	210	11%
■ CHILI MAC (*See* PASTA ENTRÉE/DINNER)				
■ CHILIES (*See* Peppers in this section)				
■ CHIMICHANGA				
frozen				
(Chi-Chi's)				
beef	1 piece	27.0	630	39%
chix	1 piece	23.0	600	35%
(Don Miguel)				
beef steak & bean				
hot	1 piece	12.0	380	28%
mucho bistec	1 piece	12.0	400	27%
chicken	1 piece	12.0	390	28%
(Old El Paso)				
beef	1 piece	20.0	370	49%
chicken	1 piece	16.0	350	41%
(Posada) sliced beef	1 piece	17.0	380	40%
(Schwan's)				
beef	1 piece	10.0	230	39%
chicken	1 piece	10.0	230	39%
homemade w/beef & cheese	4 oz	15.6	282	50%
■ CHURRO				
frozen				
(Tio Pepe's) cinnamon/6-oz pkg	1 piece	5.0	110	41%
■ DIP (*See* DIP)				
■ ENCHILADA				
frozen				
(Chi-Chi's)				
baja	1 piece	17.0	580	26%
chix suprema	1 piece	23.0	580	36%
(El Charrito)				
beef				
grande/4 per pkg	16.5 oz	47.0	890	48%
6 per pkg	16.25 oz	49.0	880	50%
3 per pkg	11 oz	31.0	560	50%
beef & cheese/6 per pkg	16.25 oz	42.0	880	43%
cheese				
6 per pkg	16.25 oz	30.0	780	35%
3 per pkg	11 oz	20.0	470	38%
chicken(3)	11 oz	13.0	440	27%

Food and Description	Amount	Fat Grams	Total Calories	% Fat Calories
(Weight Watchers)				
chicken enchiladas suiza	9 oz	8.0	250	29%
nacho grande chicken	9 oz	8.0	290	25%
■ FLAUTA				
frozen				
(Schwan's) apple	2 oz	7.0	170	26%
■ GAZPACHO (See SOUP)				
■ GUACAMOLE (See DIP)				
■ MENUDO				
(Gebhardt) mix/mix only	1 tsp	–	5	–
(Juanita's) hot & spicy	1 cup	7.0	170	37%
(Pico Pica)	1 cup	9.0	200	41%
■ MEXICAN CRISP				
(Old El Paso)	5 crisps	9.0	150	54%
■ NACHOS				
frozen/microwaveable				
(Real Fresh) muy fresco	3.5 oz	9.0	140	51%
■ PEPPERS				
(Chi-Chi's)				
diced tomatoes & green chilies	¼ cup	–	20	–
green chili				
diced	2 Tbs	–	10	–
whole	¾ pepper	–	10	–
jalapeño				
wheels	19 pieces	–	10	–
whole	2½ medium	–	10	–
(Del Monte)				
chipotle/in spice sauce	2 Tbs	–	20	–
hot yellow chili	4 peppers	–	10	–
jalapeño				
nachos	2 Tbs	–	5	–
pickled				
sliced	2 Tbs	–	5	–
whole	2 Tbs	–	5	–
whole	1 medium	–	3	–
(La Victoria) jalapeño				
marinated	1 Tbs	–	4	–
nacho	1 Tbs	–	2	–
(Old El Paso)				
green chili				
chopped	2 Tbs	–	5	–
whole	1 medium	–	10	–
jalapeño				
sliced	2 Tbs	–	15	–
whole				
peeled	3 medium	–	10	–
pickled	2 medium	–	5	–

Food and Description	Amount	Fat Grams	Total Calories	% Fat Calories
(Ortega)				
green chili				
diced	1 oz	–	8	–
sliced	1 oz	–	8	–
strips	1 oz	–	8	–
whole	1 oz	–	8	–
hot chili				
diced	1 oz	–	8	–
whole	1 oz	–	8	–
(Pancho Villa)				
green chili/diced	2 Tbs	–	5	–
(Rosarita)				
green chili				
diced	2 Tbs	–	6	–
whole	2 Tbs	–	5	–
jalapeño				
diced	2 Tbs	–	5	–
nacho sliced	2 Tbs	–	4	–
whole	2 Tbs	–	8	–
(Vlasic) jalapeño/Mexican hot	1 medium	–	8	–
■ RANCHERO BEANS				
(Chi-Chi's)	½ cup	0.5	100	5%
■ REFRIED BEANS				
(Chi-Chi's)				
fat-free	½ cup	–	80	–
original	½ cup	6.0	100	54%
vegetarian	½ cup	–	80	–
(Del Monte) plain	½ cup	2.0	130	14%
(Fantastic Foods) instant dry				
mix only	⅓ cup	1.0	160	6%
prepared	½ cup	1.0	160	6%
(Gebhardt)				
jalapeño	½ cup	3.0	105	26%
no-fat	½ cup	<1.0	90	5%
traditional	½ cup	3.0	110	25%
vegetarian	½ cup	2.0	115	16%
(Hain) vegetarian/black bean	½ cup	0.5	110	4%
(Old El Paso)				
beans & cheese	½ cup	3.5	130	17%
beans & green chillies	½ cup	0.5	110	4%
beans & sausage	½ cup	13.0	200	59%
black beans	½ cup	2.0	120	15%
fat-free	½ cup	–	110	–
regular	½ cup	2.0	110	16%
spicy	½ cup	3.0	140	19%
vegetarian	½ cup	1.0	100	9%
(Rosarita)				
bacon	½ cup	3.0	116	23%

Food and Description	Amount	Fat Grams	Total Calories	% Fat Calories
green chile	½ cup	3.0	110	25%
green chiles & lime/no-fat	½ cup	–	100	–
low-fat black beans	½ cup	<1.0	105	4%
nacho cheese	½ cup	3.0	137	20%
onion	½ cup	3.0	114	23%
original	½ cup	2.5	130	17%
spicy	½ cup	2.5	120	19%
traditional				
no-fat	½ cup	–	120	–
regular	½ cup	3.0	125	22%
vegetarian	½ cup	2.0	120	18%
zesty salsa/no-fat	½ cup	–	120	–
(Taco Bell)	⅓ cup	2.5	100	23%
■ SALSA (*See* SAUCE)				
■ SANCHO				
frozen				
(Schwan's) beef & bean	5.5 oz	14.0	320	39%
■ SAUCE				
(Chi-Chi's)				
enchilada	¼ cup	1.5	30	45%
picante				
hot	2 Tbs	–	10	–
medium	2 Tbs	–	10	–
mild	2 Tbs	–	10	–
salsa				
hot	2 Tbs	–	10	–
medium	2 Tbs	–	10	–
mild	2 Tbs	–	10	–
pico de gallo	2 Tbs	–	10	–
salsa verde medium	2 Tbs	–	15	–
salsa verde mild	2 Tbs	–	15	–
taco/thick & chunky	1 Tbs	–	15	–
(Contadina) Italian salsa				
crushed red pepper	2 Tbs	0.5	20	23%
sweet bell pepper	2 Tbs	0.5	20	23%
(Del Monte)				
picante				
hot	2 Tbs	–	10	–
medium	2 Tbs	–	10	–
salsa				
fire roasted/medium	2 Tbs	–	10	–
garlic	2 Tbs	–	10	–
Mexicana	2 Tbs	–	5	–
taquera	2 Tbs	–	5	–
thick & chunky				
hot	2 Tbs	–	10	–
medium	2 Tbs	–	10	–
mild	2 Tbs	–	10	–

Food and Description	Amount	Fat Grams	Total Calories	% Fat Calories
verde	2 Tbs	–	10	–
(Doritos) salsa				
medium	2 Tbs	–	15	–
mild	2 Tbs	–	15	–
(Eagle) salsa				
medium	2 Tbs	–	10	–
mild	2 Tbs	–	10	–
(El Molino)				
enchilada/hot	2 Tbs	1.0	16	56%
taco/red mild	1 Tbs	–	10	–
(Enrico's) salsa/chunky style				
hot				
no salt added	2 Tbs	–	8	–
regular	2 Tbs	–	8	–
mild				
no salt added	2 Tbs	–	8	–
regular	2 Tbs	–	8	–
(Gebhardt)				
chili hot dog	¼ cup	3.0	60	45%
enchilada	¼ cup	2.0	35	51%
hot	1 tsp	–	5	–
(Guiltless Gourmet) salsa/medium	2 Tbs	–	10	–
(Hain) salsa/green chili				
hot	¼ cup	–	20	–
mild	¼ cup	–	20	–
(Heinz) chili	1 Tbs	–	17	–
(Heluva Good Cheese) salsa				
cheese	2 Tbs	6.0	80	68%
thick & chunky				
hot	2 Tbs	–	10	–
mild	2 Tbs	–	10	–
(Hunt's)				
burrito/Manwich	¼ cup	–	25	–
Mexican/Manwich	¼ cup	–	26	–
pepper				
hot	1 tsp	–	1	–
original	1 tsp	–	1	–
picante				
medium	2 Tbs	–	11	–
mild	2 Tbs	–	11	–
salsa				
alfresco				
medium	2 Tbs	–	10	–
mild	2 Tbs	–	10	–
regular				
hot	2 Tbs	–	27	–
medium	2 Tbs	–	27	–
mild	2 Tbs	–	27	–

Food and Description	Amount	Fat Grams	Total Calories	% Fat Calories
taco/Manwich	¼ cup	–	30	–
(Kaukauna)				
nacho cheese	1 oz	6.0	80	68%
salsa/Mexican	1 oz	<1.0	14	32%
(La Victoria)				
salsa				
brava	1 Tbs	–	6	–
casera	1 Tbs	–	4	–
green chili	1 Tbs	–	5	–
green jalapeño	1 Tbs	–	4	–
omelet	1 Tbs	–	6	–
picante	1 Tbs	–	5	–
ranchera	1 Tbs	–	6	–
red jalapeño	1 Tbs	–	6	–
suprema	1 Tbs	–	5	–
Victoria	1 Tbs	–	4	–
taco				
green	1 Tbs	–	4	–
red	1 Tbs	–	6	–
(Louise's) salsa/fat-free				
BBQ black bean	1 oz	–	10	–
black bean	1 oz	–	10	–
medium	1 oz	–	10	–
mild	1 oz	–	10	–
nacho queso	1 oz	–	15	–
(Newman's Own) salsa				
hot	1 Tbs	–	6	–
medium	1 Tbs	–	6	–
mild	1 Tbs	–	6	–
(Old El Paso)				
enchilada				
green chili	¼ cup	1.5	30	45%
hot	¼ cup	1.0	25	36%
mild	¼ cup	1.5	30	45%
picante				
regular				
hot	2 Tbs	–	10	–
medium	2 Tbs	–	10	–
mild	2 Tbs	–	10	–
thick & chunky				
hot	2 Tbs	–	10	–
medium	2 Tbs	–	10	–
mild	2 Tbs	–	10	–
salsa				
green chili	2 Tbs	–	10	–
homestyle				
medium	2 Tbs	–	5	–
mild	2 Tbs	–	5	–

Food and Description	Amount	Fat Grams	Total Calories	% Fat Calories
pico de gallo				
hot	2 Tbs	–	5	–
medium	2 Tbs	–	5	–
salsa verde/medium	2 Tbs	–	10	–
thick & chunky				
hot	2 Tbs	–	10	–
medium	2 Tbs	–	10	–
mild	2 Tbs	–	10	–
taco				
extra chunky				
medium	1 Tbs	–	5	–
mild	1 Tbs	–	5	–
regular				
hot	1 Tbs	–	5	–
medium	1 Tbs	–	5	–
mild	1 Tbs	–	5	–
tomatoes & green chilies	¼ cup	–	10	–
tomatoes & jalapeños	¼ cup	–	15	–
(Ortega) salsa/green chili				
mild	2 Tbs	–	10	–
medium	2 Tbs	–	8	–
hot	2 Tbs	–	10	–
(Pace)				
picante/Velveeta/con queso				
medium	2 Tbs	8.0	100	72%
mild	2 Tbs	8.0	100	72%
salsa/thick & chunky	2 Tbs	–	12	–
(Pancho Villa)				
taco	2 Tbs	–	15	–
(Progresso)				
salsa/Italian				
hot	2 Tbs	–	10	–
medium	2 Tbs	–	10	–
mild	2 Tbs	–	10	–
(Rosarita)				
enchilada/mild	¼ cup	1.0	23	39%
picante/zesty jalapeno				
hot	2 Tbs	–	8	–
medium	2 Tbs	–	8	–
mild	2 Tbs	–	8	–
salsa				
extra chunky/medium	2 Tbs	–	7	–
green tomatillo/medium	2 Tbs	–	8	–
roasted/mild	2 Tbs	–	10	–
traditional				
medium	2 Tbs	–	7	–
mild	2 Tbs	–	7	–

Food and Description	Amount	Fat Grams	Total Calories	% Fat Calories
(Ro*Tel) salsa/diced tomatoes & green chilies				
extra hot	½ cup	–	20	–
regular	½ cup	–	20	–
(S&W) salsa				
mild	¼ cup	–	16	–
ready-cut tomatoes				
medium	¼ cup	–	20	–
mild	¼ cup	–	20	–
w/chipotle	¼ cup	–	20	–
w/cilantro	¼ cup	–	20	–
(Sonora Valley) salsa				
hot	1 oz	–	10	–
mild	1 oz	–	10	–
(Sun Vista)				
picante				
hot	2 Tbs	–	10	–
mild	2 Tbs	–	5	–
salsa				
hot	2 Tbs	–	5	–
mild	2 Tbs	–	5	–
(Taco Bell)				
picante				
hot	2 Tbs	–	20	–
medium	2 Tbs	–	20	–
mild	2 Tbs	–	15	–
salsa				
hot	2 Tbs	–	20	–
medium	2 Tbs	–	20	–
mild	2 Tbs	–	15	–
taco	⅙ pkg	–	5	–
(Tostitos)				
picante				
hot	2 Tbs	–	15	–
medium	2 Tbs	–	15	–
mild	2 Tbs	–	15	–
salsa				
con queso/restaurant style	2 Tbs	2.0	40	45%
hot	2 Tbs	–	15	–
medium	2 Tbs	–	15	–
mild	2 Tbs	–	15	–
(Wise)				
picante	2 Tbs	–	12	–
(Wolf)				
chili hot dog	⅙ cup	2.0	40	45%
■ SOMBRERO				
frozen				
(Sabatasso's)	1 piece	24.0	420	51%

Food and Description	Amount	Fat Grams	Total Calories	% Fat Calories
■ **SPANISH RICE** (*See* RICE DISH)				
■ **TACO** (*See also* BREAKFAST SANDWICH; Taco Seasoning in this section; Taco Shell in this section)				
boxed kit				
(Old El Paso)				
w/taco shell				
mix & 2 shells only	2 pieces	7.0	140	45%
prepared	2 tacos	13.0	270	43%
w/tortilla				
mix & 2 tortillas only	2 pieces	3.5	210	15%
prepared	2 tacos	10.0	380	24%
(Pancho Villa)				
mix & 2 shells only	2 pieces	8.0	150	48%
prepared	2 tacos	13.0	270	43%
frozen				
(Owens) Border Breakfasts				
ham	2 tacos	6.0	90	60%
sausage	2 tacos	12.0	190	57%
(Schwan's) taco barquito	~5 oz	18.0	350	46%
homemade/USDA Standard Home Recipe				
beef	~3 oz	7.0	153	41%
beef w/cheese	~3 oz	9.0	182	45%
■ **TACO SEASONING** (*See also* SEASONINGS)				
(Durkee) mix only				
family	1 serving	–	10	–
mild	1 serving	–	15	–
regular	1 serving	–	15	–
salad	1 serving	–	20	–
(French's) mix only				
mild	1 serving	–	15	–
onion	1 serving	–	20	–
regular	1 serving	–	15	–
(Old El Paso) mix only				
40% less sodium	2 tsp	–	20	–
regular	2 tsp	–	20	–
(Ortega)				
mix only	1 oz	1.0	90	10%
prepared	1 oz	4.0	60	60%
(Taco Bell) mix only	2 Tbs	–	20	–
■ **TACO SHELL**				
(Azteca) super	1 shell	12.0	200	54%
(Chi-Chi's)	2 shells	8.0	170	40%
(Gebhardt)	3 shells	8.5	155	32%
(Old El Paso)				
mini	7 shells	10.0	160	56%
regular	3 shells	10.0	170	53%
super	2 shells	12.0	190	57%
white corn	3 shells	10.0	170	53%

Food and Description	Amount	Fat Grams	Total Calories	% Fat Calories
(Pancho Villa)	3 shells	11.0	190	52%
(Rosarita)	3 shells	8.5	155	32%
(Taco Bell)	2 shells	4.0	100	36%
■ TAMALE				
canned				
(Derby)	3 tamales	17.0	253	60%
(Gebhardt)				
jumbo	2 tamales	25.0	330	68%
original	2 tamales	20.0	270	67%
(Hormel)				
beef	3 tamales	21.0	280	68%
	7.5 oz	21.0	290	65%
chicken	3 tamales	10.0	210	43%
hot/spicy	3 tamales	21.0	280	68%
jumbo	2 tamales	20.0	270	67%
(Old El Paso)	3 tamales	19.0	330	52%
(Van Camp's)	8 oz	16.0	290	50%
(Wolf)	1 cup	24.0	350	62%
frozen				
(Delimex)	1 tamale	11.0	240	41%
(Schwan's)	4 tamales	15.0	320	42%
homemade/USDA Standard Home Recipe				
beef	~2.5 oz	9.5	183	48%
■ TAQUITO				
frozen				
(Delimex)				
beef	5 pieces	15.0	370	36%
chicken	5 pieces	20.0	410	44%
generic/beef/shredded	8 oz	25.0	490	46%
(Schwan's)				
beef	5 pieces	15.0	360	38%
white chicken	5 pieces	16.0	370	39%
■ TOMATILLO				
canned or jarred				
(La Costena)	4 medium	2.5	40	56%
(La Victoria) entero	1 Tbs	–	6	–
■ TORTILLA				
(Azteca)				
corn	1 small	–	45	–
flour				
8" dia	1 tortilla	3.0	130	21%
salad bake & fill	1 tortilla	12.0	200	54%
small	1 tortilla	2.0	80	23%
taco salad shell	1 tortilla	12.0	200	54%
(El Charito)				
corn	2 tortillas	1.0	95	9%
flour	2 tortillas	4.0	170	21%

Food and Description	Amount	Fat Grams	Total Calories	% Fat Calories
(Mission)				
corn				
regular size	2 tortillas	1.5	100	14%
super size	1 tortilla	1.0	80	11%
flour/burrito-size/99% fat-free	1 tortilla	0.5	160	3%
original	1 tortilla	5.0	200	23%
(Old El Paso)				
flour	1 tortilla	3.0	150	18%
soft taco	2 tortillas	3.5	180	45%
(Tyson)				
corn/enchilada style	1 tortilla	<1.0	50	8%
flour				
burrito style	1 tortilla	4.0	170	21%
fajita style	1 tortilla	2.0	90	20%
large	1 tortilla	4.0	180	20%
small	1 tortilla	2.0	105	17%
soft taco	1 tortilla	3.0	120	23%
whole wheat	1 tortilla	3.0	120	23%
◨ **TORTILLA CHIPS** (See TORTILLA CHIPS)				
◨ **TORTILLA MIX**				
(Quaker) corn				
harina preparada para tortillas	⅓ cup	4.0	160	23%
masa harina	¼ cup	1.0	110	8%
◨ **TOSTACO SHELL**				
corn				
(Old El Paso)	1 shell	5.0	100	45%
◨ **TOSTADA**				
frozen				
(Van de Kamp's) beef supreme	8.5 oz	30.0	530	51%
homemade/USDA Standard Home recipe				
beef	~3 oz	7.0	153	41%
beef w/cheese	~3 oz	9.0	182	45%
◨ **TOSTADA SHELL**				
corn				
(Old El Paso)	1 shell	3.0	55	49%
(Ortega)	1 shell	2.0	50	36%
(Pancho Villa)	1 shell	3.0	55	49%
(Rosarita)	1 shell	3.0	60	45%
MEXICAN POTATO (See JICAMA)				
MILK (See also MILK SUBSTITUTE; RICE DRINK; SOYMILK)				
buffalo	1 cup	17.0	236	65%
carob	1 cup	3.0	160	17%
cow				
buttermilk				
(A&P)	1 cup	1.0	90	10%
(Borden) Golden Churn/1.5% fat	1 cup	4.0	120	30%
(Crowley)	1 cup	4.0	110	33%
(Friendship) 1.5% fat	1 cup	4.0	120	30%

Food and Description	Amount	Fat Grams	Total Calories	% Fat Calories
generic/cultured	1 cup	2.0	100	18%
	1 quart	9.0	396	20%
(Knudsen) 2% fat/reduced fat	1 cup	5.0	120	38%
(Land O'Lakes)	1 cup	2.0	100	18%
(Saco) dry	4 Tbs	<1.0	80	5%
chocolate-flavored				
(Anderson & Erickson) skim	1 cup	1.0	130	7%
(Borden) Dutch 2% fat/reduced fat	1 cup	5.0	180	25%
generic				
1% fat/light	1 cup	2.5	160	14%
2% fat/reduced fat	1 cup	5.0	180	25%
whole	1 cup	8.5	210	36%
(Hershey)				
2% fat/reduced fat	1 cup	5.0	190	23%
whole milk	1 cup	9.0	210	39%
(Kemp's) Swiss style 1% fat/light	1 cup	3.0	170	16%
(Land O'Lakes)				
1% fat/light	1 cup	3.0	160	17%
skim/fat-free	1 cup	–	140	–
whole	1 cup	8.0	210	34%
(Lucerne) 2% fat/reduced fat	1 cup	5.0	200	23%
(Meadow Gold) whole	1 cup	8.0	210	34%
(Nestle) whole	1 cup	9.0	210	39%
(Pevely)	1 cup	8.0	210	34%
condensed/sweetened				
(Borden) Eagle	⅓ cup	9.0	320	25%
(Carnation)	1 oz	3.0	123	22%
	3.5 fl oz	8.7	321	24%
	⅓ cup	9.0	318	26%
(Dairy Sweet)	⅓ cup	9.0	320	25%
generic	¼ cup	6.6	244	24%
evaporated				
(Carnation)				
low-fat	3.5 oz	1.9	85	20%
	½ cup	3.0	110	25%
skim	3.5 fl oz	–	80	–
	½ cup	–	100	–
whole	3.5 fl oz	7.6	134	51%
	½ cup	10.0	170	53%
generic				
low-fat	¼ cup	1.5	55	25%
skim	¼ cup	–	50	–
whole	¼ cup	4.8	84	51%
(Milnot)				
skim	2 Tbs	–	25	–
	½ cup	–	100	–
whole	2 Tbs	2.0	40	45%
	½ cup	8.0	150	48%

Food and Description	Amount	Fat Grams	Total Calories	% Fat Calories
(Pet)				
regular	½ cup	10.0	170	53%
skim	½ cup	–	100	–
fresh				
(A&P)				
1% fat/light	1 cup	3.0	100	27%
2% fat/reduced fat	1 cup	5.0	120	38%
(Borden)				
skim/fat-free/protein-fortified	1 cup	1.0	100	9%
1% fat/light w/*L. acidophilus*	1 cup	2.0	100	18%
hi-protein 2% fat/reduced fat	1 cup	5.0	140	32%
whole	1 cup	8.0	150	48%
(Crowley)				
1% fat/light	1 cup	2.0	100	18%
2% fat/reduced fat	1 cup	5.0	120	38%
(Darigold)				
1% fat/light	1 cup	2.0	100	18%
2% fat/reduced fat	1 cup	5.0	120	38%
generic				
skim/fat-free				
regular	1 cup	0.6	90	6%
w/nonfat milk solids added	1 cup	0.6	90	6%
1% fat/light/w/nonfat milk solids added	1 cup	2.4	104	21%
2% fat/reduced fat/w/nonfat milk solids added	1 cup	4.7	125	34%
whole				
vitamin D	1 cup	8.0	150	48%
w/added calcium	1 cup	8.0	150	48%
(Knudsen)				
Nice 'n Light/1% fat/light	1 cup	3.0	130	21%
2% fat/reduced fat	1 cup	5.0	140	32%
(Land O'Lakes)				
1% fat/light	1 cup	3.0	100	27%
2% fat/reduced fat	1 cup	5.0	120	38%
(Pevely) ½% fat	1 cup	1.0	90	10%
(Real) whole w/vitamins A & D	1 cup	8.0	150	48%
(Viva) 2% fat/reduced fat/ w/extra calcium	1 cup	5.0	120	38%
(Weight Watchers) skim/fat-free	1 cup	–	90	–
lactose-reduced (*See* MILK SUBSTITUTE)				
powdered dry				
(Alba) nonfat, prepared	1 cup	–	80	–
(Carnation) skim/mix only	⅓ cup	–	80	–
generic				
nonfat/skim				
mix only	¼ cup	–	100	–
prepared	1 cup	–	80	–

Food and Description	Amount	Fat Grams	Total Calories	% Fat Calories
whole				
mix only	¼ cup	8.5	159	48%
prepared	1 cup	8.5	150	48%
(Lucerne) skim/prepared	1 cup	–	80	–
(Milkman) low-fat/prepared	1 cup	1.0	90	9%
	1 quart	5.0	380	12%
(Saco) nonfat				
mix only	⅓ cup	–	80	–
prepared	1 cup	–	80	–
(Sanalac) nonfat/prepared	1 cup	–	80	–
goat				
canned evaporated				
(Meyenberg)	4 oz	8.0	150	48%
carton				
powder mixed w/water	1 cup	8.0	150	48%
refrigerated	1 cup	8.0	150	48%
fresh	1 cup	10.0	168	54%
human	1 cup	11.0	170	58%
reindeer	8 fl oz	48.6	580	75%
sheep	8 fl oz	17.0	264	58%
MILK MIX (*See also* BREAKFAST DRINK; COCOA; MILK SHAKE)				
(Alba)				
chocolate marshmallow	1 pkt	–	60	–
milk chocolate	1 pkt	–	60	–
mocha	1 pkt	–	60	–
(Alpine)				
Bavarian chocolate cream				
light	1 pouch	1.5	60	23%
original	1 pouch	6.0	160	34%
Irish cream				
light	1 pouch	1.5	60	23%
original	1 pouch	6.0	160	34%
Swiss mocha				
light	1 pouch	1.5	60	23%
original	1 pouch	6.0	160	34%
(Baker's) chocolate	1 oz	2.0	120	15%
(Caracoa) carob/instant/prepared	8 fl oz	1.0	145	6%
(Carnation) mix only				
banana	2 Tbs	–	90	–
chocolate malted	3 heaping Tbs	0.8	79	9%
	3.5 oz	3.8	375	9%
malted/original	3 heaping Tbs	2.0	90	20%
	3.5 oz	8.5	411	19%
milk chocolate				
fat-free	1 envelope	–	25	–
low-calorie	1 envelope	–	70	–

Food and Description	Amount	Fat Grams	Total Calories	% Fat Calories
no sugar added	3 Tbs	–	50	–
regular	3 Tbs	1.0	110	8%
rich chocolate				
original	3 Tbs	1.0	110	8%
w/chocolate marshmallows	3 Tbs	1.0	110	8%
w/marshmallows	3 Tbs	1.0	110	8%
(Choco Milk) chocolate				
mix only	1 oz	1.0	110	8%
prepared w/whole milk	8 fl oz	10.0	264	34%
(El Molino) carob				
mix only	1 Tbs	<1.0	40	11%
prepared w/whole milk	8 fl oz	9.0	190	43%
(Featherweight) chocolate	1 pouch	1.0	40	23%
generic				
carob				
mix only	1 Tbs	<1.0	45	10%
prepared w/whole milk	8 fl oz	9.0	195	42%
chocolate malted				
mix only	1 heaping Tbs	1.0	85	11%
prepared w/whole milk	8 fl oz	9.0	235	35%
chocolate syrup				
prepared w/whole milk	8 fl oz	8.5	232	33%
syrup only	2 Tbs	0.5	82	6%
(Ghirardelli)				
chocolate hazelnut	2.5 Tbs	1.5	80	17%
double chocolate	2.5 Tbs	1.5	80	17%
mocha	2.5 Tbs	1.5	80	17%
(Hershey)				
Hot Cocoa Collection				
chocolate almond	1 envelope	3.0	150	18%
chocolate amaretto	1 envelope	3.0	150	18%
chocolate mint	1 envelope	3.0	150	18%
chocolate raspberry	1 envelope	3.0	150	18%
Dutch chocolate	1 envelope	3.0	150	18%
French vanilla	1 envelope	2.5	140	16%
Irish cream	1 envelope	3.0	150	18%
Swiss mocha	1 envelope	2.0	140	13%
syrup/chocolate malted	2 Tbs	–	100	–
(Kraft) malted				
chocolate/instant				
mix only	3 Tbs	1.0	80	11%
prepared w/2% milk	1 cup	6.0	200	27%
natural				
mix only	3 Tbs	2.0	90	20%
prepared w/2% milk	1 cup	7.0	210	30%
(Land O'Lakes) Chocolate Supreme Cocoa Classic				
amaretto	1 pkt	5.0	160	28%

Food and Description	Amount	Fat Grams	Total Calories	% Fat Calories
black cherry	1 pkt	5.0	160	28%
cinnamon	1 pkt	5.0	160	28%
French vanilla	1 pkt	5.0	160	28%
hazelnut	1 pkt	5.0	160	28%
Irish cream	1 pkt	5.0	160	28%
lite	1 pkt	2.0	80	23%
mint	1 pkt	5.0	160	28%
mocha	1 pkt	5.0	160	28%
raspberry	1 pkt	5.0	160	28%
(Nestle) mix only				
Milo chocolate-flavored hot or cold drink mix	3 Tbs	2.0	80	23%
Quik				
chocolate				
no sugar added	2 Tbs	1.0	40	23%
regular	2 Tbs	0.5	90	5%
strawberry	2 Tbs	–	90	–
(Ovaltine) chocolate malted				
classic/traditional				
mix only	4 Tbs	–	80	–
prepared w/2% milk	8 fl oz	5.0	210	21%
lite				
mix only	2 Tbs	–	50	–
prepared w/skim milk	8 fl oz	0.6	170	32%
original				
mix only	4 Tbs	–	80	–
prepared w/2% milk	8 fl oz	5.0	210	21%
rich chocolate				
mix only	4 Tbs	–	80	–
prepared w/2% milk	8 fl oz	5.0	210	21%
(PDQ) malted/prepared w/whole milk	8 fl oz	5.0	180	25%
(Swiss Miss) mix only				
almond mocha	1 pkt	3.0	145	19%
chocolate raspberry	1 pkt	3.0	145	19%
Chocolate Sensations	1 pkt	4.0	150	24%
chocolate truffle	1 pkt	2.5	140	16%
cocoa				
diet	1 pkt	–	25	–
fat-free	1 pkt	–	50	–
lite	1 pkt	<1.0	70	6%
regular	1 pkt	3.0	140	19%
sugar-free	¼ cup	1.0	70	13%
cocoa & cream	1 pkt	5.0	150	30%
English toffee	1 pkt	2.0	140	13%
milk chocolate				
regular	1 pkt	1.0	110	8%
sugar-free	1 pkt	–	50	–

Food and Description	Amount	Fat Grams	Total Calories	% Fat Calories
mini marshmallows				
regular	1 pkt	1.0	110	8%
sugar-free	1 pkt	1.0	50	18%
rich chocolate				
regular	1 pkt	1.0	110	8%
sugar-free	1 pkt	–	50	–
white chocolate	1 pkt	1.0	110	8%
(Ultra Slim Fast) creamy hot cocoa/ mix only	1 pkg	<1.0	190	2%
(Weight Watchers) chocolate & marshmallow/mix only	1 pkt	–	70	–
MILK SHAKE (*See also* individual FAST FOOD listings)				
canned				
(Frostee)				
chocolate-flavored drink	1 cup	8.0	200	36%
strawberry-flavored drink	1 cup	7.0	180	35%
(Real) Sport Shake				
chocolate	10 fl oz	10.0	310	29%
strawberry	10 fl oz	10.0	270	33%
fountain drink/made w/whole milk				
(Baskin Robbins) vanilla	1 shake	31.0	660	42%
generic				
chocolate	10 fl oz	10.0	360	25%
strawberry	10 fl oz	9.0	350	23%
vanilla	10 fl oz	9.0	340	27%
frozen				
(M&M★Mars) low-fat chocolate-malt	1 cup	3.0	220	12%
(Micro Magic)				
chocolate	11.5 fl oz	8.0	340	21%
strawberry	11.5 fl oz	9.0	340	24%
vanilla	11.5 fl oz	13.0	380	31%
mix				
(Alba 77) Dairy Shake/mix only				
chocolate	1 pkt	–	70	–
double fudge	1 pkt	0.5	70	6%
strawberry	1 pkt	–	70	–
vanilla	1 pkt	–	70	–
(Weight Watchers) chocolate fudge	1 pkt	1.0	80	11%
refrigerated				
(Hershey) box/chocolate shake	7 fl oz	4.5	220	18%
(Killer) shake				
Choco Loco	8 fl oz	6.0	240	23%
Radically Vanilla	8 fl oz	5.0	220	20%
Totally Chocolate	8 fl oz	5.0	230	20%
MILK SUBSTITUTE (*See also* RICE DRINK; SOYMILK; YOGURT DRINK)				
(Better Than Milk)				
carob	1 cup	5.0	130	35%
chocolate	1 cup	5.0	125	36%

Food and Description	Amount	Fat Grams	Total Calories	% Fat Calories
light	1 cup	–	80	–
natural	1 cup	5.0	90	50%
(Dairy Ease) lactose-reduced milk				
skim/fat-free	1 cup	–	90	–
1% fat/light	1 cup	2.0	100	18%
2% fat/reduced fat	1 cup	5.0	120	38%
(Lactaid)				
chocolate/1% fat	1 cup	3.0	160	17%
regular				
calcium-fortified	1 cup	<1.0	90	5%
skim/fat-free	1 cup	–	90	–
1% fat/light	1 cup	2.5	100	23%
2% fat/reduced fat	1 cup	5.0	120	38%
(Meadow Farms)	1 cup	5.0	120	38%
(Nutritious Foods) First Alternative	1 cup	2.0	90	20%
(Vance's) Darifree nondairy beverage	1 cup	–	90	–
MILKFISH/raw	3 oz	6.0	125	43%
MILLET (See also CEREAL; FLOUR)				
(Arrowhead Mills)	¼ cup	1.5	150	9%
generic/pearl				
cooked	4 oz	1.0	135	7%
	1 cup	2.0	287	6%
dry/raw	1 oz	1.0	107	8%
	1 cup	8.0	756	10%
MINCEMEAT (See PIE FILLING & GLAZE)				
MINERAL WATER (See WATER)				
MINESTRONE (See SOUP)				
MISO				
(Eden)				
barley/mugi	1 Tbs	<1.0	25	18%
brown rice/genmai	1 Tbs	1.0	25	72%
rice/shiro	1 Tbs	1.0	35	51%
soybean/hacho	1 Tbs	2.0	35	51%
soybean & rice/kome	1 Tbs	1.0	25	72%
generic	½ cup	8.5	285	27%
w/barley malt/mugi-koji	1 oz	1.0	55	16%
w/rice malt/kome-koji				
dark yellow	1 oz	1.5	53	25%
sweet	1 oz	1.0	62	15%
w/soybean malt/mame-koji	1 oz	4.0	65	55%
(Westbrae) pasteurized				
barley	1 tsp	–	10	–
brown rice	1 tsp	–	10	–
red	1 tsp	–	10	–
soybean	1 tsp	–	12	–
MOLASSES				
(Brer Rabbit)				
dark	1 Tbs	–	60	–

Food and Description	Amount	Fat Grams	Total Calories	% Fat Calories
light	1 Tbs	–	60	–
generic				
Barbados	1 Tbs	–	54	–
	1 oz	–	111	–
	1 cup	–	889	–
light/lst extraction	1 Tbs	–	50	–
	1 oz	–	103	–
	1 cup	–	827	–
medium/2nd extraction	1 Tbs	–	46	–
	1 oz	–	95	–
	1 cup	–	761	–
treacle/black	1 Tbs	–	53	–
(Mott's) Grandma's				
gold label	1 Tbs	–	70	–
green label	1 Tbs	–	70	–
(Plantation) blackstrap/3rd extraction	1 Tbs	–	43	–
	1 oz	–	87	–
	1 cup	–	699	–
MONKFISH				
cooked-dry heat	3 oz	2.0	85	21%
raw	3 oz	1.0	64	14%
MOOSE/boneless				
raw	3 oz	4.8	152	28%
roasted	3 oz	1.0	115	8%
roasted/diced	1 cup	1.5	190	7%
MORTADELLA (See SAUSAGE)				
MOTH BEAN				
boiled	½ cup	0.5	105	4%
raw	½ cup	1.5	335	4%
MOUNTAIN YAM				
Hawaiian/cooked	1 cup	–	119	–
MOUSSE (See PUDDING & MOUSSE)				
MUFFIN (See also BREAKFAST SANDWICH; PASTRY, TOASTER)				
■ **FROZEN**				
(Pepperidge Farm) Wholesome Choice				
apple oatmeal	1 muffin	3.5	160	20%
blueberry	1 muffin	2.5	140	16%
bran w/raisins	1 muffin	2.5	150	15%
corn	1 muffin	3.0	150	18%
(Sara Lee)				
food service				
almond paradise/4¼-oz muffin	1 muffin	18.0	410	37%
apple cranberry nut				
large muffin/4¼ oz	1 muffin	23.0	440	47%
small muffin/2⅛ oz	1 muffin	12.0	220	49%
banana nut				
individually wrapped	1 muffin	19.0	380	45%
large muffin/4¼ oz	1 muffin	24.0	430	50%

Food and Description	Amount	Fat Grams	Total Calories	% Fat Calories
mini-muffin	2 muffins	8.0	180	40%
reduced fat	1 muffin	10.0	280	32%
small muffin/2⅛ oz	1 muffin	9.0	220	37%
blueberry				
individually wrapped	1 muffin	17.0	380	40%
large muffin/4¼ oz	1 muffin	18.0	400	41%
mini-muffin	2 muffins	9.0	190	43%
reduced fat	1 muffin	9.0	310	26%
small muffin/2⅛ oz	1 muffin	10.0	220	41%
blueberries & cheese streusel/ large muffin/4¼ oz	1 muffin	18.0	430	38%
bran/individually wrapped	1 muffin	20.0	430	42%
carrot nut				
individually wrapped	1 muffin	23.0	450	46%
large muffin/4¼ oz	1 muffin	21.0	470	40%
cheese streusel				
individually wrapped	1 muffin	19.0	410	42%
large muffin/4¼ oz	1 muffin	22.0	440	45%
small muffin/2⅛ oz	1 muffin	11.0	220	45%
chocolate chunk				
individually wrapped	1 muffin	17.0	410	37%
mini-muffin	2 muffins	9.0	200	41%
small muffin/2⅛ oz	1 muffin	11.0	230	43%
corn				
individually wrapped	1 muffin	25.0	480	47%
large muffin/4¼ oz	1 muffin	26.0	490	48%
mini-muffin	2 muffins	11.0	210	47%
small muffin/2⅛ oz	1 muffin	13.0	240	49%
cranberry nut/mini-muffin	2 muffins	9.0	200	41%
double chocolate chunk/ large muffin/4¼ oz	1 muffin	18.0	440	37%
lemon poppy seed/large muffin/ 4¼ oz	1 muffin	22.0	460	43%
oat bran raisin/small muffin/2⅛ oz	1 muffin	6.0	190	28%
orange streusel/large muffin/4¼ oz	1 muffin	19.0	450	39%
peaches & cheese streusel/ large muffin/4¼ oz	1 muffin	13.0	380	31%
sweet harvest/large muffin/4¼ oz	1 muffin	24.0	460	47%
retail				
blueberry	1 muffin	11.0	220	45%
corn	1 muffin	14.0	260	48%
(Schwan's) frozen batter/blueberry	1 muffin	8.0	180	40%
(Weight Watchers) Breakfast On-The-Go!				
banana nut	1 muffin	5.0	190	24%
blueberry	1 muffin	5.0	250	18%
chocolate chcocolate chip	1 muffin	4.0	200	18%
harvest honey bran	1 muffin	4.0	220	16%

Food and Description	Amount	Fat Grams	Total Calories	% Fat Calories
■ HOMEMADE				
USDA Standard Home Recipe (Note: Unless otherwise noted, homemade muffins were prepared with whole milk)				
apple	2 oz	6.0	165	33%
blueberry	2 oz	6.0	165	33%
bran	2 oz	6.5	160	36%
corn				
prepared w/2% milk	2 oz	6.5	180	33%
prepared w/whole milk	2 oz	7.0	185	34%
orange	2 oz	7.0	180	33%
plain	2 oz	5.0	155	28%
■ MIX				
(Arrowhead Mills) mix only				
wheat bran	⅓ cup	2.0	150	12%
wheat-free oat bran	⅓ cup	4.0	160	23%
(Betty Crocker)				
fat-free				
apple cinnamon				
mix only	¼ cup	–	120	–
prepared	1 muffin	–	120	–
blueberry				
mix only	3 Tbs	–	120	–
prepared	1 muffin	–	120	–
original				
banana nut				
mix only	3 Tbs	2.5	130	17%
prepared	1 muffin	5.0	150	30%
cinnamon streusel				
mix only	¼ cup	7.0	160	39%
prepared	1 muffin	7.0	170	37%
lemon poppy seed				
mix only	¼ cup	2.0	140	13%
prepared	1 muffin	7.0	190	33%
twice the blueberry				
mix only	¼ cup	1.5	120	11%
prepared	1 muffin	4.0	140	26%
(Dromedary) corn/prepared	1 muffin	5.0	130	35%
(Duncan Hines)				
bakery style				
blueberry				
mix only	1/12 pkg	5.0	170	26%
prepared	1 muffin	6.0	190	28%
cinnamon swirl				
mix only	1/12 pkg	6.0	190	28%
prepared	1 muffin	7.0	200	32%
honey nut				
mix only	1/12 pkg	7.0	200	32%
prepared	1 muffin	7.0	200	32%

Food and Description	Amount	Fat Grams	Total Calories	% Fat Calories
original				
blueberry				
mix only	1/12 pkg	4.5	150	27%
prepared	1 muffin	5.0	160	28%
chocolate chip				
mix only	1/12 pkg	7.0	180	35%
prepared	1 muffin	8.0	190	38%
raspberry				
mix only	1/12 pkg	4.5	150	27%
prepared	1 muffin	4.5	160	25%
(Flako) corn/prepared	1 muffin	4.0	120	30%
generic/corn/prepared	1 muffin	6.0	145	37%
(Gold Medal)				
banana nut				
mix only	1/6 pkg	5.0	140	32%
prepared	1 muffin	8.0	170	42%
caramel nut				
mix only	1/6 pkg	3.5	130	24%
prepared	1 muffin	7.0	170	37%
corn				
mix only	1/6 pkg	1.0	110	8%
prepared	1 muffin	6.0	160	38%
(Krusteaz)				
fat-free				
apple cinnamon				
mix & fruit	1/4 cup	–	130	–
prepared	1 muffin	–	140	–
blueberry				
mix & fruit	1/4 cup	–	120	–
prepared	1 muffin	–	130	–
corn honey cornbread & muffin				
mix only	1/4 cup	–	120	–
prepared	1 muffin	–	120	–
original				
almond poppy seed				
mix only	1/3 cup	4.5	170	24%
prepared	1 muffin	5.0	180	25%
apple cinnamon				
mix & fruit	1/3 cup	4.0	160	23%
blueberry				
mix & fruit	1/3 cup	5.0	170	26%
prepared	1 muffin	6.0	180	30%
blueberry bran				
mix & fruit	1/3 cup	6.0	180	30%
prepared	1 muffin	6.0	190	28%
honey bran				
mix only	1/4 cup	4.0	150	24%
prepared	1 muffin	4.5	160	25%

Food and Description	Amount	Fat Grams	Total Calories	% Fat Calories
lemon poppy seed				
mix only	⅓ cup	4.5	170	24%
prepared	1 muffin	5.0	180	25%
oat bran/mix only	⅓ cup	5.0	190	24%
(Martha White)				
apple cinnamon				
mix only	⅓ cup	3.0	150	18%
prepared	1 muffin	3.0	160	17%
banana nut				
mix only	⅓ cup	7.0	170	37%
prepared	1 muffin	7.0	190	33%
blueberry/mix only	1 muffin	3.0	160	17%
lemon poppy seed/mix only	¼ cup	4.0	150	24%
strawberry				
mix only	⅓ cup	4.0	160	23%
prepared	1 muffin	4.0	170	21%
(Robin Hood)				
apple cinnamon				
mix only	⅙ pkg	4.0	130	28%
prepared	1 muffin	8.0	170	42%
banana nut				
mix only	⅙ pkg	5.0	140	32%
prepared	1 muffin	8.0	170	42%
blueberry				
mix only	⅙ pkg	3.0	120	23%
prepared	1 muffin	6.0	160	34%
caramel nut				
mix only	⅙ pkg	3.5	130	24%
prepared	1 muffin	7.0	170	37%
■ READY TO SERVE				
(Arnold) English				
Bran'nola	1 muffin	1.5	130	10%
extra crisp	1 muffin	1.0	120	8%
raisin	1 muffin	1.0	150	6%
sourdough	1 muffin	1.0	120	8%
(Awrey's)				
apple				
1.5-oz muffin	1 muffin	6.0	130	42%
2.5-oz muffin	1 muffin	10.0	220	41%
apple streusel/4.2-oz muffin	1 muffin	13.0	340	34%
apple w/banana nut/4.2-oz muffin	1 muffin	16.0	260	55%
blueberry				
4.2-oz muffin	1 muffin	14.0	360	35%
1.5-oz muffin	1 muffin	5.0	130	35%
2.5-oz muffin	1 muffin	8.0	210	34%
corn				
1.5-oz muffin	1 muffin	5.0	130	42%
2.5-oz muffin	1 muffin	8.0	220	33%

Food and Description	Amount	Fat Grams	Total Calories	% Fat Calories
cranberry/1.5-oz muffin	1 muffin	4.0	120	30%
oat bran/2.75-oz muffin	1 muffin	7.0	180	35%
pineapple raisin oat bran/ 2.75-oz muffin	1 muffin	6.0	180	30%
raisin bran				
4.2-oz muffin	1 muffin	12.0	320	34%
1.5-oz muffin	1 muffin	4.0	110	33%
2.5-oz muffin	1 muffin	7.0	190	33%
(Dunkin' Donuts)				
English	1 muffin	1.0	130	7%
low-fat				
banana	1 muffin	1.5	240	6%
blueberry	1 muffin	1.5	220	6%
cranberry orange	1 muffin	1.5	230	6%
regular				
apple n' spice	1 muffin	8.0	300	24%
banana nut	1 muffin	10.0	310	29%
blueberry	1 muffin	8.0	280	26%
chocolate chip	1 muffin	16.0	400	36%
corn	1 muffin	12.0	340	32%
cranberry orange nut	1 muffin	9.0	290	25%
honey raisin bran	1 muffin	10.0	330	27%
oat-bran				
apple	1 muffin	9.0	270	30%
blueberry	1 muffin	9.0	350	23%
plain	1 muffin	11.0	290	34%
raisin-nut	1 muffin	12.0	310	35%
(Earth Grains)				
English				
plain	1 muffin	1.0	150	6%
raisin	1 muffin	1.0	150	6%
wheatberry	1 muffin	1.0	150	6%
whole wheat	1 muffin	2.0	170	11%
(Entenmann's)				
blueberry				
fat-free	1 muffin	–	120	–
original	1 muffin	7.0	160	39%
generic				
blueberry	1 muffin	4.0	160	23%
English				
cracked wheat	1 muffin	1.0	158	6%
plain	1 muffin	1.0	140	6%
sourdough	1 muffin	1.0	130	7%
w/raisins	1 muffin	1.0	146	6%
whole wheat	1 muffin	1.6	130	11%
oat bran	1 muffin	4.0	155	23%
(Home Pride) muffin loaf				
apple cinnamon	1 piece	6.0	110	49%

Food and Description	Amount	Fat Grams	Total Calories	% Fat Calories
blueberry	1 piece	5.0	110	41%
raspberry	1 piece	5.0	110	41%
(Hostess)				
mini muffin				
apple cinnamon	5 muffins	16.0	260	55%
blueberry	5 muffins	13.0	240	49%
raisin walnut	5 muffins	16.0	280	51%
muffin loaf				
blueberry	1 muffin	19.0	440	39%
raspberry	1 muffin	19.0	440	39%
regular muffin				
oat bran	1 muffin	8.0	160	45%
oat bran banana nut	1 muffin	6.0	150	36%
(Oroweat) Master's Best English				
blueberry	1 muffin	1.0	170	5%
cinnamon raisin	1 muffin	1.0	170	5%
extra crisp	1 muffin	0.5	130	3%
health nut raisin	1 muffin	3.0	170	16%
oat bran	1 muffin	1.0	150	6%
oat nut raisin	1 muffin	2.0	160	11%
raisins, dates, pecans	1 muffin	3.0	200	14%
sourdough	1 muffin	1.0	140	6%
winter wheat	1 muffin	8.0	220	33%
(Pepperidge Farm) English				
cinnamon raisin	1 muffin	2.0	140	6%
plain	1 muffin	1.0	130	7%
seven-grain	1 muffin	1.0	130	7%
sourdough	1 muffin	1.0	130	7%
(Roman Meal) English	1 muffin	1.0	130	7%
(Sara Lee) English				
blueberry	1 muffin	1.0	140	6%
cinnamon raisin	1 muffin	1.0	140	6%
classic	1 muffin	1.5	130	10%
sourdough	1 muffin	1.0	135	7%
(SunMaid) English/raisin	1 muffin	1.0	60	15%
(Thomas')				
English				
original				
blueberry	1 muffin	1.0	140	6%
cinnamon raisin	1 muffin	1.0	160	6%
cranberry	1 mufin	1.0	140	6%
honey wheat	1 muffin	1.0	110	8%
oat bran	1 muffin	1.0	120	8%
plain	1 muffin	1.0	120	8%
raisin	1 muffin	1.0	140	6%
sourdough	1 muffin	1.0	120	8%
sandwich size				
Onion Em's	1 muffin	1.5	180	8%

Food and Description	Amount	Fat Grams	Total Calories	% Fat Calories
plain	1 muffin	2.0	190	9%
Sourdough Em's	1 muffin	2.0	200	9%
Wheat Em's	1 muffin	1.5	180	8%
Toast-R-Cakes				
banana	1 muffin	5.0	110	41%
blueberry	1 muffin	3.0	100	27%
cinnamon apple	1 muffin	3.0	100	27%
corn	1 muffin	4.0	110	33%
raisin bran	1 muffin	3.0	90	30%
strawberry	1 muffin	4.0	110	33%
(Wolferman's) English/deluxe				
apple strudel	1 muffin	5.0	250	18%
blueberry				
mini	1 muffin	–	80	–
regular	1 muffin	1.0	220	4%
cinnamon & raisin				
mini	1 muffin	0.5	80	6%
regular	1 muffin	2.0	240	8%
cranberry				
mini	1 muffin	0.5	80	6%
regular	1 muffin	1.0	240	4%
golden raisin	1 muffin	1.5	250	5%
heartland harvest	1 muffin	1.0	230	4%
honey nut	1 muffin	2.5	240	9%
jalapeño cheese	1 muffin	3.0	250	11%
low-sodium	1 muffin	1.0	220	4%
mixed berry				
mini	1 muffin	–	80	–
regular	1 muffin	1.0	230	4%
natural cheese	1 muffin	2.5	230	10%
oatmeal cinnamon	1 muffin	3.5	250	13%
original				
mini	1 muffin	–	70	–
regular	1 muffin	1.0	220	4%
sourdough				
mini	1 muffin	–	70	–
regular	1 muffin	1.0	220	4%
sun-dried tomato & herb	1 muffin	4.0	250	14%
MULBERRY/fresh	1 cup	0.6	61	8%
MULLET/striped				
cooked-dry heat	3 oz	4.0	127	28%
raw	3 oz	3.0	99	27%
MUNG BEAN				
dried				
(Arrowhead Mills)	¼ cup	0.5	160	3%
generic				
boiled	6 oz	–	107	–
raw	½ cup	1.0	361	3%

Food and Description	Amount	Fat Grams	Total Calories	% Fat Calories
sprouted				
canned	½ cup	–	8	–
cooked	½ cup	–	13	–
raw	½ cup	–	16	–
stir-fried	½ cup	–	31	–
MUNGO BEAN				
boiled	½ cup	–	95	–
raw	½ cup	2.0	365	5%
MUSHROOM				
canned or jarred				
(BinB) broiled in butter				
pieces & stems	1 can	–	30	–
sliced	1 can	–	30	–
sliced w/garlic	1 can	0.5	35	13%
whole	1 can	–	30	–
(Cara Mia)				
marinated	1 oz	1.0	13	69%
seasoned/whole	1 oz	–	7	–
(Empress)				
button				
pieces & stems	2 oz	–	14	–
sliced	2 oz	–	14	–
whole	2 oz	–	14	–
straw/broken	2 oz	–	10	–
generic				
Oriental straw	2 oz	–	12	–
shiitake	4 oz	–	45	–
white/canned in butter sauce	2 oz	1.0	30	30%
(Green Giant) white				
pieces & stems	½ cup	–	30	–
sliced	½ cup	–	30	–
whole	½ cup	–	30	–
(Libby's)	1 oz	–	70	–
(Seneca)				
shiitake	½ cup	–	25	–
white				
brine pack	½ cup	–	25	–
marinated				
food service	1 oz	0.5	15	30%
retail	1 oz	9.0	90	90%
pickled	1 oz	–	5	–
teriyaki-sliced	½ cup	–	80	–
water pack	½ cup	–	25	–
dried				
shiitake	1 piece	<1.0	11	3%
	1 oz	<1.0	84	3%
	1 lb	4.5	1343	3%

Food and Description	Amount	Fat Grams	Total Calories	% Fat Calories
fresh				
enoki/raw	1 large	–	2	–
oyster/raw	2 oz	–	14	–
shitake/cooked	4 oz	–	40	
white				
boiled	½ cup	–	21	–
fried or sautéed in butter	10 small	10.0	100	90%
raw				
pieces	½ cup	–	10	–
whole	1 medium	–	5	–
frozen				
(Freshlike)	3.5 oz	–	30	–
(Seneca)	½ cup	–	20	–
(Veg-All)	3.5 oz	–	30	–
MUSHROOM DISH (*See also* FROZEN ENTRÉE/DINNER; VEGETABLES, MIXED; individual FAST FOOD listings)				
(Pasta Pasta Pasta) frozen stuffed Italian mushrooms	2 mushrooms	5.0	90	50%
MUSHROOM SOUP (*See* SOUP)				
MUSKELLUNGE/NORTH AMERICAN PIKE				
raw	3 oz	2.0	93	19%
MUSKMELON (*See* CANTALOUPE)				
MUSKRAT				
roasted	3 oz	10.0	200	45%
roasted/diced	1 cup	13.0	260	45%
MUSSEL				
fresh/blue				
cooked-moist heat	3 oz	3.8	147	23%
raw	3 oz	1.9	73	23%
	1 cup	3.0	129	21%
frozen				
(Sanford) New Zealand Greenshell on half	3 oz	2.5	100	23%
MUSTARD				
dry	1 tsp	<1.0	12	38%
prepared				
(Best Foods) Dijonnaise	1 tsp	1.0	10	90%
(Featherweight)	1 Tbs	–	–	–
(French's)				
bold 'n spicy	1 Tbs	–	5	–
Dijon	1 tsp	0.5	10	45%
(Grey Poupon)				
country Dijon	1 tsp	–	6	–
Dijon	1 tsp	–	6	–
Parisian	1 tsp	–	6	–
(Gulden's)				
creamy mild	1 Tbs	–	6	–
Diablo	1 Tbs	–	8	–

Food and Description	Amount	Fat Grams	Total Calories	% Fat Calories
spicy brown	1 Tbs	–	8	–
(Hain) stone ground				
no salt added	1 Tbs	1.0	14	64%
regular	1 Tbs	1.0	14	64%
(Hebrew National) deli mustard				
original	1 Tbs	–	4	–
w/horseradish	1 Tbs	–	4	–
(Heinz)				
mild yellow	1 Tbs	–	8	–
spicy brown	1 Tbs	1.0	14	64%
(Hellmann's) Dijonnaise	1 tsp	1.0	10	90%
(Jack Daniel's)				
Dijon	1 tsp	–	5	–
honey Dijon	1 tsp	–	10	–
horseradish	1 tsp	–	5	–
Old No. 7	1 tsp	–	5	–
peppercorn	1 tsp	–	5	–
spicy brown	1 tsp	–	5	–
Tennessee Dijon	1 tsp	–	5	–
(Kraft)				
horseradish	1 tsp	–	5	–
prepared	1 tsp	–	–	–
(Luizianne) Creole	1 Tbs	–	10	–
(Plochman's)				
Dijon	1 Tbs	1.0	11	82%
spicy brown	1 Tbs	1.0	11	82%
stone ground	1 Tbs	1.0	11	82%
yellow	1 Tbs	1.0	11	82%
(Reckitt & Colman)				
classic yellow	1 tsp	<1.0	4	68%
dry	1 Tbs	2.0	29	62%
French				
bold 'n spicy	1 Tbs	–	5	–
Dijon	1 tsp	0.5	10	45%
(Savoir Faire)				
country style	1 tsp	–	5	–
Dijon	1 tsp	–	5	–
(Silver Spring) Beer 'n Brat horseradish	1 tsp	–	–	–
(Westbrae)				
Mt. Fuji	1 tsp	–	–	–
natural stone-ground	1 tsp	–	–	–
yellow	1 tsp	–	–	–
MUSTARD GREENS				
canned				
(Glory Foods)	½ cup	0.5	50	9%
fresh				
boiled	½ cup	–	11	–
raw	½ cup	–	7	–

Food and Description	Amount	Fat Grams	Total Calories	% Fat Calories
frozen				
generic				
boiled/drained	½ cup	–	14	–
chopped	½ cup	–	15	–
	10 oz	–	60	–
(Pictsweet)	3.3 oz	–	20	–
MUSTARD SAUCE (See SAUCE)				
MUSTARD SEED				
yellow/whole	1 tsp	1.0	15	60%
MUSTARD SPINACH/fresh				
boiled-drained	½ cup	–	14	–
raw/chopped	½ cup	–	17	–

N

Food and Description	Amount	Fat Grams	Total Calories	% Fat Calories
NACHOS (See MEXICAN FOOD)				
NAPOLEON (See PASTRY)				
NATAL PLUM (See CARISSA)				
NATTO	½ cup	9.7	187	47%
NAVY BEAN				
canned				
(Bush's Best)	½ cup	–	60	–
(Eden Foods) organic	½ cup	0.5	110	4%
(Luck's) seasoned w/pork	½ cup	4.0	140	26%
(Trappey's) seasoned w/bacon	½ cup	1.5	110	12%
dried				
boiled	½ cup	0.5	130	3%
raw	½ cup	1.5	345	4%
sprouted/raw	½ cup	–	35	–
NAVY BEAN SOUP (See SOUP)				
NECTARINE/fresh				
sliced	1 cup	1.0	70	13%
whole	1 medium	1.0	70	13%
NEUFCHATEL CHEESE (See CHEESE; CHEESE SPREAD)				
NEWBURG SAUCE (See SAUCE)				

NONDAIRY FROZEN DESSERT (See ICE CREAM & ICE CREAM-LIKE FROZEN DESSERTS; ICE CREAM BARS, SANDWICHES, & FROZEN NOVELTIES; RICE FROZEN DESSERT; SHERBET; TOFU FROZEN DESSERT)
NOODLE (See ASIAN FOOD; PASTA)

Food and Description	Amount	Fat Grams	Total Calories	% Fat Calories
NOODLE SOUP (*See* SOUP)				
NORI (*See* SEAWEED)				
NUTMEG/ground	1 tsp	0.8	11	66%
NUTRITION BAR (*See* GRANOLA/GRANOLA-TYPE BAR)				
NUTRITIONAL SUPPLEMENT (*See also* BREAKFAST BAR, BREAKFAST DRINK;				
GRANOLA/GRANOLA-TYPE BAR)				
(Boost) canned				
chocolate	8 fl oz	4.0	240	15%
chocolate mocha	8 fl oz	4.0	240	15%
strawberry	8 fl oz	4.0	240	15%
vanilla	8 fl oz	4.0	240	15%
(California Slim) mix only				
chocolate shake	1 serving	<1.0	100	5%
citrus juice	1 serving	<1.0	90	5%
fruit juice	1 serving	<1.0	90	5%
mocha shake	1 serving	<1.0	100	5%
vanilla shake	1 serving	<1.0	100	5%
(Dynatrim)				
Dutch chocolate				
mix only	1 serving	1.0	100	9%
prepared w/1% milk	8 fl oz	4.0	220	16%
strawberry royale				
mix only	1 serving	1.0	100	9%
prepared w/1% milk	8 fl oz	4.0	220	16%
vanilla royale				
mix only	1 serving	1.0	100	9%
prepared w/1% milk	8 fl oz	4.0	220	16%
Ensure (*See* (Ross) in this section)				
(Nestle) Sweet Succes				
canned				
cool mint chocolate	10 fl oz	3.0	200	14%
chocolate raspberry truffle	10 fl oz	3.0	200	14%
creamy milk chocolate	10 fl oz	3.0	200	14%
creamy vanilla delight	10 fl oz	3.0	200	14%
dark fudge chocolate	10 fl oz	3.0	200	14%
mocha supreme	10 fl oz	3.0	200	14%
rich chocolate almond	10 fl oz	3.0	200	14%
strawberries 'n' cream	10 fl oz	3.0	200	14%
instant				
chocolate raspberry truffle				
mix only	1 scoop	1.5	90	15%
prepared w/skim milk	9 fl oz	1.5	180	8%
classic chocolate chip				
mix only	1 scoop	2.0	90	20%
prepared w/skim milk	9 fl oz	2.0	180	10%
creamy milk chocolate				
mix only	1 scoop	1.5	90	15%
prepared w/skim milk	9 fl oz	1.5	180	8%

Food and Description	Amount	Fat Grams	Total Calories	% Fat Calories
creamy vanilla delight				
mix only	1 scoop	1.5	90	5%
prepared w/skim milk	9 fl oz	1.5	180	8%
dark chocolate fudge				
mix only	1 scoop	1.5	90	15%
prepared w/skim milk	9 fl oz	1.5	180	8%
mocha supreme				
mix only	1 scoop	1.5	90	15%
prepared w/skim milk	9 fl oz	1.5	180	8%
rich chocolate almond				
mix only	1 scoop	1.5	90	15%
prepared w/skim milk	9 fl oz	1.5	180	8%
(Nutrament) energy food				
chocolate	12 fl oz	10.0	360	25%
vanilla	12 fl oz	10.0	360	25%
(Pedia-Sure) liquid nutrition w/fiber				
for children 1-10 years				
chocolate	8 fl oz	11.8	237	45%
vanilla	8 fl oz	11.8	237	45%
(Resource) fruit nutritional drink				
plus/Swiss chocolate	8 fl oz	13.0	360	33%
regular				
French vanilla	8 fl oz	9.0	250	32%
strawberry	8 fl oz	9.0	250	32%
Swiss chocolate	8 fl oz	9.0	250	32%
(Ross) Ensure				
high-protein				
banana	8 fl oz	6.0	225	24%
chocolate royale	8 fl oz	6.0	225	24%
vanilla supreme	8 fl oz	6.0	225	24%
wild berry	8 fl oz	6.0	225	24%
light				
strawberry	8 fl oz	3.0	200	14%
plus				
chocolate	8 fl oz	13.0	355	32%
coffee	8 fl oz	13.0	355	32%
eggnog	8 fl oz	13.0	355	32%
strawberry	8 fl oz	13.0	355	32%
vanilla	8 fl oz	13.0	355	32%
regular				
black walnut	8 fl oz	9.0	250	32%
chocolate	8 fl oz	9.0	250	32%
coffee	8 fl oz	9.0	250	32%
eggnog	8 fl oz	9.0	250	32%
strawberry	8 fl oz	9.0	250	32%
vanilla	8 fl oz	9.0	250	32%
w/fiber				
butter pecan	8 fl oz	9.0	260	31%

Food and Description	Amount	Fat Grams	Total Calories	% Fat Calories
chocolate	8 fl oz	9.0	260	31%
vanilla	8 fl oz	9.0	260	31%
(Sego) liquid diet food				
lite				
chocolate				
Dutch	1 can	3.0	150	18%
regular	1 can	3.0	150	18%
strawberry	1 can	4.0	150	24%
vanilla				
French	1 can	4.0	150	24%
regular	1 can	4.0	150	24%
very				
chocolate	1 can	1.5	240	6%
chocolate malt	1 can	1.5	240	6%
strawberry	1 can	5.0	240	19%
vanilla	1 can	5.0	240	19%
(Sustacal)				
original				
chocolate	8 fl oz	6.0	240	23%
vanilla	8 fl oz	6.0	240	23%
plus				
chocolate	8 fl oz	14.0	360	35%
vanilla	8 fl oz	14.0	360	35%
(Ultra Slim*Fast)				
instant/mix only				
chocolate royale	1 scoop	1.0	110	8%
French vanilla	1 scoop	0.5	110	4%
strawberry supreme	1 scoop	0.5	120	4%
ready-to-drink meal				
apple-cranberry-raspberry	11.5 fl oz	1.5	220	6%
chocolate fudge	11 fl oz	3.0	220	12%
chocolate royale	11 fl oz	3.0	220	12%
coffee	11 fl oz	3.0	220	12%
French vanilla	11 fl oz	3.0	220	12%
golden apple	11.5 fl oz	1.5	220	6%
milk chocolate	11 fl oz	3.0	230	12%
orange-strawberry-banana	11.5 fl oz	1.5	220	6%
pineapple	11.5 fl oz	1.5	220	6%
strawberry supreme	11 fl oz	3.0	230	12%
NUTS (See NUTS, FORMULATED; NUTS, MIXED; individual listings)				
NUTS, FORMULATED/wheat based				
macadamia-flavored	1 oz	16.0	176	82%
other flavors	1 oz	18.0	184	88%
unflavored	1 oz	16.0	177	81%
NUTS, MIXED (See also ICE CREAM TOPPINGS; individual nut listings)				
(Eagle)				
honey-roasted/cashew & peanut mix	¼ cup	14.0	180	90%

Food and Description	Amount	Fat Grams	Total Calories	% Fat Calories
oil-roasted				
deluxe w/o peanuts	¼ cup	17.0	200	77%
lightly salted	¼ cup	17.0	200	77%
original	¼ cup	17.0	200	77%
(Fisher)				
honey-roasted/peanut-cashew mix	1 oz	13.0	170	69%
oil-roasted				
deluxe	1 oz	16.0	180	80%
25% more cashews	1 oz	16.0	180	80%
generic				
dry-roasted/w/peanuts	1 oz	15.0	170	79%
oil-roasted				
w/peanuts	1 oz	16.0	175	82%
w/o peanuts	1 oz	16.0	175	82%
(Guy's)	1 oz	16.0	180	80%
(Planters)				
dry-roasted	1 oz	14.0	170	74%
honey-roasted	1 oz	13.0	140	84%
oil-roasted				
deluxe	1 oz	16.0	170	85%
lightly salted	1 oz	15.0	170	79%
mixed	1 oz	15.0	170	79%
no Brazil nuts				
regular	1 oz	15.0	170	79%
unsalted	1 oz	15.0	170	79%
Select				
cashews w/almonds & macadamias	1 oz	16.0	170	85%
cashews w/almonds & pecans	1 oz	15.0	170	79%
sesame nut mix	1 oz	12.0	150	72%
unsalted	1 oz	15.0	170	79%

Food and Description	Amount	Fat Grams	Total Calories	% Fat Calories
OAT BRAN (*See* BRAN; CEREAL)				
OATS (*See also* CEREAL)				
(Arrowhead Mills)				
groats	¼ cup	3.0	160	17%
rolled flakes	⅓ cup	2.5	130	17%
steel-cut	¼ cup	3.0	170	16%

Food and Description	Amount	Fat Grams	Total Calories	% Fat Calories
generic/whole-grain	1 oz	2.0	110	16%
	1 cup	10.8	607	16%
OCEAN PERCH (*See also* FROZEN ENTRÉE/DINNER; SEAFOOD ENTRÉE/DINNER)				
Atlantic				
breaded & fried	3 oz	11.0	185	54%
cooked-dry heat	3 oz	1.8	103	16%
raw	3 oz	1.0	80	11%
OCTOBER BEAN/canned				
(Luck's) seasoned w/pork	½ cup	3.0	140	19%
OCTOPUS (*See also* SQUID; SEAFOOD ENTRÉE/DINNER)				
cooked-moist heat	3 oz	2.0	140	13%
raw	3 oz	0.9	70	11%
OIL (*See also* ASIAN FOOD/SAUCES & SEASONINGS; COOKING SPRAY)				
all vegetable & fish oils	1 Tbs	14.0	120	100%
	1 cup	218.0	1927	100%

(NOTE: We all need to watch even our use of "healthier" (less saturated) oils in order to keep our total fat intake within acceptable boundaries. Because it is so important to select the least saturated oil that fits your needs, I have listed the most commonly used oils and fats below, showing the percentages of saturated fat, polyunsaturated fat, and monounsaturated fat in each. Those that contain less saturated fat are listed first. Data are based on information from *USDA Nutritive Value of American Foods in Common Units, 1988.* REMEMBER—NO VEGETABLE OIL CONTAINS CHOLESTEROL!)

Vegetable Oils	% Saturated	% Unsaturated	
		% Poly	% Mono
Canola	7%	35%	58%
Almond	8%	19%	73%
Safflower	9%	78%	13%
Sunflower	11%	69%	20%
Corn	13%	62%	25%
Olive	14%	12%	74%
Walnut	14%	67%	19%
Sesame	15%	43%	42%
Soybean	15%	43%	42%
Margarine			
liquid/tub	17%	37%	46%
stick	20%	33%	47%
whipped	20%	30%	50%
Peanut	18%	33%	49%
Soybean/cottonseed blend	19%	50%	31%
Wheat germ	20%	50%	31%
Shortening (vegetable)	27%	26%	47%
Cottonseed	27%	55%	18%
Palm	52%	10%	38%
Cocoa butter	62%	3%	35%
Palm kernel	87%	2%	11%
Coconut	92%	2%	6%

Animal Fats	% Saturated	% Unsaturated
Goose	27%	73%
Chicken	30%	70%
Turkey	30%	70%
Duck	34%	66%
Salt pork	36%	64%
Lard	41%	59%
Beef tallow	52%	48%
Butter		
stick	66%	34%
whipped	69%	31%

OKRA (*See also* VEGETABLES, MIXED)

	Portion			
canned	½ cup	–	25	–
fresh				
boiled	½ cup	–	25	–
raw	½ cup	–	19	–
frozen				
(Freshlike)				
cut	3.3 oz	–	25	–
whole	3.3 oz	–	30	–
generic/cooked	½ cup	–	34	
(Pictsweet)				
cut	3.3 oz	–	25	–
microwave	2.5 oz	–	20	–
(Stilwell) breaded	21 pieces	1.0	70	13%
(Veg-All)				
cut	3.3 oz	–	25	–
whole	3.3 oz	–	30	–
OLIVE				
(Alma) black/Greek	2 large	3.0	30	90%
(Early California) pitted/all sizes	~1 oz	3.0	30	90%
(Fancifoods)				
green/stuffed or plain	3 olives	2.0	25	72%
queen/plain	2 colossal	2.0	25	72%
generic				
green/pickled	10 small	3.6	33	98%
	10 large	4.9	45	98%
	10 giant	8.0	76	95%
ripe				
Ascolano				
sliced	1 cup	18.6	174	94%
whole	10 extra large	6.5	61	96%
	10 mammoth	7.7	72	96%
	10 giant	9.5	89	96%
	10 jumbo	11.0	105	94%

Food and Description	Amount	Fat Grams	Total Calories	% Fat Calories
Manzanillo				
sliced	1 cup	18.6	174	96%
whole	10 small	4.0	38	95%
	10 medium	4.7	44	96%
	10 large	5.5	51	97%
	10 extra large	6.5	61	96%
Mission				
sliced	1 cup	27.0	248	98%
whole	10 small	5.9	54	98%
	10 medium	6.9	63	99%
	10 large	8.0	73	99%
	10 extra large	9.5	87	98%
Sevillano				
sliced	1 cup	12.8	126	91%
whole	10 giant	6.5	64	91%
	10 jumbo	7.8	76	92%
	10 colossal	9.7	95	92%
	10 super colossal	11.6	114	92%
salt-cured/Greek style/whole	10 medium	6.9	65	96%
	10 extra large	9.5	89	96%
(Janet Lee)	8 small	3.0	30	90%
	10 medium	3.0	30	90%
	10 large	3.0	30	90%
(Krinos) Calamata	4 olives	4.0	45	80%
(Lindsay) pickled/pitted				
Ascolano	10 jumbo	6.0	70	77%
	10 colossal	8.0	90	80%
	10 super colossal	10.0	120	75%
Manzanilla	10 small	3.5	40	79%
	10 medium	4.0	45	80%
	10 large	5.0	50	90%
	10 extra large	6.0	65	83%
Mission	10 small	3.5	40	79%
	10 medium	4.0	45	80%
	10 large	5.0	50	90%
	10 extra large	6.0	65	83%
mixed				
chopped	1 oz	3.0	30	90%
sliced	1 oz	3.0	30	90%
	½ cup	6.5	70	84%
Sevillano	10 jumbo	6.0	70	77%
	10 colossal	8.0	90	80%
	10 super colossal	10.0	120	75%
(Progresso) oil-cured	6 olives	6.0	80	68%

Food and Description	Amount	Fat Grams	Total Calories	% Fat Calories
(S&W) ripe				
black/pitted	3 extra large	2.5	25	90%
	3 jumbo	2.0	25	72%
	3 super colossal	4.5	45	90%
green				
Manzanilla/stuffed	3 olives	2.0	25	72%
queen	2 olives	2.0	20	90%
stuffed	1 olive	1.0	10	90%
	2 olives	1.5	15	90%
(Santa Barbara Olive Co.)				
Cajun	0.5 oz	1.5	15	90%
California black	0.5 oz	1.5	15	90%
country	0.5 oz	2.0	25	72%
garlic	0.5 oz	1.5	15	90%
pitted	0.5 oz	2.0	25	72%
stuffed	0.5 oz	1.5	15	90%
Italian/pitted	0.5 oz	1.5	15	90%
jalapeño	0.5 oz	1.5	15	90%
pimento-stuffed martini	0.5 oz	1.5	15	90%
OLIVE LOAF (See LUNCHEON MEAT.)				
OLIVE OIL (See OIL)				
OLIVE SALAD				
(Progresso) drained	2 Tbs	2.5	25	90%
OMELET (See EGG DISH/MEAL)				
ONION (See also SCALLION; VEGETABLES, MIXED)				
canned or jarred				
(Durkee) French-fried	1 oz	15.0	175	77%
generic/chopped	½ cup	–	20	–
(Green Giant) whole	½ cup	–	35	–
(Heinz) sweet	1 oz	–	40	–
(S&W)				
cocktail	12 pieces	–	5	–
small/whole	½ cup	–	40	–
tiny/whole	½ cup	–	40	–
(Vlasic) cocktail				
lightly spiced	1 oz	–	4	–
plain	1 oz	–	4	–
dried				
flakes	1 Tbs	–	16	–
	¼ cup	–	45	–
powder/ground	1 tsp	–	7	–
	1 Tbs	–	23	–
fresh/all types/mature				
cooked	1 cup	–	60	–
raw				
chopped	1 Tbs	–	4	–
	½ cup	–	20	–

Food and Description	Amount	Fat Grams	Total Calories	% Fat Calories
whole				
(Dole)	1 medium	–	60	–
frozen				
(Birds Eye) small/whole	½ cup	–	30	–
(C&W) petite/whole	⅔ cup	–	30	–
(Freshlike) whole	3.3 oz	–	35	–
generic	10 oz	–	100	–
ONION, GREEN OR SPRING (See SCALLION)				
ONION DISH (See also FROZEN ENTRÉE/DINNER; VEGETABLES, MIXED; VEGETARIAN FOODS)				
frozen				
(Birds Eye) small onions w/cream sauce	½ cup	3.0	100	27%
(Bland Farms) Vidalia O's	6 rings	7.0	180	35%
(Farm Rich) onion rings				
batter dipt	4 oz	13.0	260	45%
Onion O's	5 pieces	9.0	190	43%
generic/onion rings/pan-fried in oven	7 rings	19.0	285	60%
(Mrs. Paul's) crispy onion rings	2.5 oz	12.0	190	57%
(Ore-Ida)				
chopped onions	¾ cup	–	25	–
onion rings				
classic	4 pieces	12.0	220	49%
gourmet	4 pieces	11.0	220	45%
Onion Ringers	6 rings	13.0	230	51%
ONION POWDER	1 tsp	–	7	–
ONION RINGS (See ONION DISH; individual FAST FOOD listings)				
ONION SOUP (See SOUP)				
OPOSSUM				
braised or roasted	3 oz	8	190	38%
roasted/diced	1 cup	14.5	310	42%
ORANGE (See also MANDARIN ORANGE)				
fresh				
California				
navel				
peeled sections	1 cup	–	75	–
whole	1 medium	–	65	–
Valencia				
peeled sections	1 cup	0.5	90	5%
whole	1 medium	–	60	–
(Dole)	1 medium	–	50	–
Florida				
peeled sections	1 cup	0.5	85	5%
whole	1 medium	<1.0	70	4%
ORANGE DRINK/JUICE DRINK BLEND (See also SOFT DRINK; SOFT DRINK MIX; TEA)				
bottled, boxed, or canned				
(Bama)	8.45 fl oz	–	120	–

Food and Description	Amount	Fat Grams	Total Calories	% Fat Calories
(Betty Crocker) Squeezit Smarty Arty	6.75 fl oz	–	110	–
(Capri Sun)	6.75 fl oz	–	100	–
(Hi-C)	7.7 fl oz	–	110	–
	8 fl oz	–	120	–
Bright & Early beverage	8 fl oz	–	120	–
drink box	8.45 fl oz	–	120	–
(Knudsen) orange juice float	8 fl oz	–	140	–
(Ocean Spray) Refreshers/ orange-cranberry	6 fl oz	–	100	–
(Powerade) orange	8 fl oz	–	72	–
(Snapple) orangeade	8 fl oz	–	120	–
(Tropicana) Twister orange-cranberry				
light	8 fl oz	–	30	–
	10 fl oz	–	35	–
regular	8 fl oz	–	130	–
	10 fl oz	–	160	–
	11.5 fl oz	–	160	–
orange-peach	8 fl oz	–	120	–
	10 fl oz	–	150	–
orange-raspberry				
light	8 fl oz	–	35	–
	10 fl oz	–	45	–
regular	8 fl oz	–	120	–
	10 fl oz	–	150	–
orange-strawberry-banana	8 fl oz	–	120	–
	10 fl oz	–	140	–
	11.5 fl oz	–	160	–
orange-strawberry-guava	8 fl oz	–	120	–
	10 fl oz	–	140	–
(Welch's) orange-pineapple	11.5 fl oz	–	180	–
frozen				
(Tropicana) Twister/concentrate/undiluted				
orange-cranberry	2 fl oz	–	130	–
orange-peach	2 fl oz	–	120	–
orange-raspberry	2 fl oz	–	120	–
orange-strawberry-banana	2 fl oz	–	120	–
(Welch's) Welchade/orange	8 fl oz	–	140	–
mix				
(Tang) breakfast drink/mix only				
regular	2 Tbs	–	100	–
sugar-free	⅛ tub	–	5	–
ORANGE JUICE/JUICE BLEND (*See also* FRUIT PUNCH)				
bottled, boxed, or canned				
(Chiquita)				
Citrus Adventure/orange-tangerine	8 fl oz	–	120	–
tropical orange/light	8 fl oz	–	30	–

Food and Description	Amount	Fat Grams	Total Calories	% Fat Calories
(Citrus Hill)				
plus calcium	6 fl oz	–	90	–
select	6 fl oz	–	90	–
(Dole)				
orange juice	10 fl oz	–	140	–
orange juice cooler	8.45 fl oz	–	130	–
generic				
sweetened	8 fl oz	–	119	–
unsweetened	8 fl oz	–	104	–
(Knudsen) orange-mango	8 fl oz	–	110	–
(Minute Maid)				
orange juice				
juice box	8.45 fl oz	–	120	–
refrigerated				
calcium rich	8 fl oz	–	120	–
country style	8 fl oz	–	110	–
premium choice	8 fl oz	–	110	–
country style	8 fl oz	–	110	–
pulp-free	8 fl oz	–	110	–
orange juice blend	8 fl oz	–	125	–
(Mott's) blend	10 fl oz	–	130	–
(Ocean Spray)				
100% orange juice	6 fl oz	–	80	–
orange juice cocktail	6 fl oz	–	100	–
(S&W)				
regular	6 fl oz	–	90	–
unsweetened	6 fl oz	–	83	–
(Season's Best)				
calcium	8 fl oz	–	110	–
homestyle	8 fl oz	–	110	–
regular	8 fl oz	–	110	–
	10 fl oz	–	130	–
	11.5 fl oz	–	140	–
vitamin	8 fl oz	–	110	–
(Seneca)				
orange	8 fl oz	–	120	–
orange-grapefruit	8 fl oz	–	110	–
orange-pineapple	8 fl oz	–	110	–
(Sunkist)				
fresh-squeezed	6 fl oz	–	80	–
regular	6 fl oz	–	85	–
(TreeTop)	5.5 fl oz	–	80	–
	8 fl oz	–	120	–
	10 fl oz	–	150	–
	11.5 fl oz	–	170	–
(Tropicana)				
orange-pineapple	8 fl oz	–	130	–
	10 fl oz	–	130	–

Food and Description	Amount	Fat Grams	Total Calories	% Fat Calories
Pure Premium				
+ calcium	8 fl oz	–	110	–
+ calcium & vitamin c	8 fl oz	–	110	–
+ fiber	8 fl oz	–	120	–
+ vitamins	8 fl oz	–	110	–
regular	8 fl oz	–	110	–
	10 fl oz	–	130	–
Tropics				
orange-kiwi passion	8 fl oz	–	100	–
orange-peach-mango	8 fl oz	–	110	–
orange-pineapple	8 fl oz	–	110	–
orange-strawberry-banana	8 fl oz	–	110	–
(Welch's)				
juice	10 fl oz	–	130	–
	11.5 fl oz	–	170	–
juice blend	11.5 fl oz	–	170	–
juice cocktail	8 fl oz	–	120	–
frozen				
generic/concentrate/undiluted	6 oz	<1.0	340	1%
(Gold-N-Rich) concentrate/prepared	8 fl oz	–	110	–
(Minute Maid) concentrate/prepared				
calcium-rich	8 fl oz	–	120	–
country style	8 fl oz	–	110	–
original	8 fl oz	–	110	–
pulp free	8 fl oz	–	110	–
reduced acid	8 fl oz	–	110	–
(Seneca) concentrate/undiluted				
Awake	2 oz	–	120	–
orange	2 oz	–	110	–
orange plus	2 oz	–	130	–
Valencia	2 oz	–	110	–
(Tropicana) concentrate/undiluted				
all types	2 oz	–	110	–
homemade/USDA Standard Home Recipe	8 fl oz	0.5	110	4%
ORANGE PEEL				
candied				
generic	1 oz	–	90	–
(S&W)	58 pieces	–	80	–
fresh	1 Tbs	–	–	–
ORANGE ROUGHY (See also SEAFOOD ENTRÉE/DINNER)				
cooked-dry heat	3 oz	1.0	80	11%
raw	3 oz	6.0	110	50%
OREGANO/ground	1 tsp	–	5	–
ORIENTAL FOOD (See ASIAN FOOD; FROZEN ENTRÉE/DINNER; PASTA ENTRÉE/DINNER; RICE DISH; VEGETARIAN FOODS; individual listings)				
OYSTER (See also SEAFOOD ENTRÉE/DINNER)				
canned				
(Bumble Bee) whole	½ cup	4.0	100	36%

Food and Description	Amount	Fat Grams	Total Calories	% Fat Calories
(Empress) whole	½ cup	4.0	100	36%
(Geisha) whole	⅓ cup	2.5	60	38%
generic				
Eastern	3 oz	2.0	58	31%
	1 cup	6.0	170	32%
Pacific	1 cup	5.0	220	20%
	12 oz	7.5	310	22%
(Reese) smoked	2 oz	1.0	45	50%
(S&W)				
smoked	2 oz	6.0	100	54%
whole	2 oz	3.0	70	39%
fresh				
eastern				
battered & fried	3 oz	10.0	180	50%
	6 medium	11.0	175	57%
breaded & fried	3 oz	11.0	170	58%
	6 medium	11.0	175	57%
meat only	1 cup	4.0	160	23%
raw	6 medium	2.0	50	30%
steamed	3 oz	4.5	120	34%
	6 medium/ ~1.5 oz	2.0	60	30%
Pacific/western				
raw	3 oz	2.0	70	26%
steamed	1 medium	1.0	40	23%
	3 oz	4.0	140	26%

OYSTER DISH (*See also* FROZEN ENTRÉE/DINNER; SEAFOOD ENTRÉE/DINNER; SOUP)

homemade/USDA Standard Home Recipe

oyster stew/6 oysters per cup	1 cup	15.5	235	59%
oysters Rockefeller	4 oysters	2.5	85	26%

P

Food and Description	Amount	Fat Grams	Total Calories	% Fat Calories
PANCAKE (*See also* PANCAKE & WAFFLE MIX)				
frozen				
(Aunt Jemima)				
blueberry	3 pancakes	3.5	210	15%

Food and Description	Amount	Fat Grams	Total Calories	% Fat Calories
buttermilk	3 pancakes	3.0	180	15%
low-fat	3 pancakes	1.5	130	10%
original	3 pancakes	3.0	200	10%
(Downyflake) regular	3 pancakes	7.0	270	23%
(Krusteaz)				
blueberry	3 pancakes	5.0	260	17%
buttermilk	3 pancakes	5.0	270	17%
mini	6 pancakes	2.5	120	19%
(Pillsbury) Hungry Jack				
blueberry	3 pancakes	3.5	230	14%
buttermilk	3 pancakes	4.0	240	15%
original				
mini	11 pancakes	4.0	230	14%
regular	3 pancakes	4.0	240	15%
(Schwan's) buttermilk	3 pancakes	5.0	260	17%
(Swanson)				
Budget Breakfast				
eggs & silver dollar pancakes	1 meal	14.0	250	50%
silver dollar pancakes & sausage	1 meal	18.0	340	41%
Kids' Breakfast Blast				
6 mini pancakes w/syrup	1 meal	8.0	320	23%
Great Starts				
pancakes & sausages	1 meal	25.0	490	46%
pancakes w/bacon	1 meal	20.0	400	45%
(Van's) multigrain/nondairy	2 pancakes	1.5	180	8%
homemade/USDA Standard Home Recipe				
buckwheat/6" dia	3 pancakes	9.0	410	20%
buttermilk/6" dia	3 pancakes	15.0	490	28%
plain				
4" dia	1 pancake	2.0	62	29%
6" dia	1 pancake	5.0	169	27%
mix (Note: Unless otherwise stated, data are for dry mix only.)				
(Arrowhead Mills)				
blue corn	⅓ cup	2.0	150	12%
buckwheat	⅓ cup	1.5	140	10%
buttermilk	¼ cup	0.5	120	4%
gluten-free	¼ cup	2.0	130	14%
griddle lite	½ cup	3.0	260	10%
kamut	¼ cup	1.0	130	7%
multigrain	¼ cup	0.5	120	4%
oat bran	⅓ cup	1.5	140	10%
whole grain	¼ cup	0.5	120	4%
wild rice	¼ cup	1.0	140	6%
(Betty Crocker)				
complete				
buttermilk				
mix only	⅓ cup	3.0	200	14%

Food and Description	Amount	Fat Grams	Total Calories	% Fat Calories
prepared	3 pancakes	3.0	200	14%
original				
mix only	⅓ cup	3.0	210	13%
prepared	3 pancakes	3.0	210	13%
(Estee) pancake mix	⅓ cup	–	180	–
(Featherweight) complete	5 Tbs	2.0	160	11%
generic/prepared/4" dia				
buckwheat	1 pancake	2.0	60	30%
buttermilk	1 pancake	1.0	75	12%
plain	1 pancake	1.0	75	12%
whole wheat	1 pancake	3.0	90	30%
(Hungry Jack)				
buttermilk				
mix only	⅓ cup	1.5	160	8%
prepared				
made w/2% milk, oil, & egg	1 serving	13.0	290	40%
made w/skim milk, oil, & egg whites	1 serving	6.0	230	42%
buttermilk complete				
mix only	⅓ cup	1.5	160	8%
prepared	1 serving	1.5	160	8%
Extra Lights				
mix only	⅓ cup	1.5	160	8%
prepared				
made w/2% milk, oil, & egg	1 serving	8.0	240	30%
made w/skim milk, oil, & egg whites	1 serving	6.0	230	23%
Extra Lights complete				
mix only	⅓ cup	2.0	150	12%
prepared	1 serving	2.0	150	12%
original				
mix only	⅓ cup	1.5	150	9%
prepared				
made w/2% milk, oil, & egg whites	1 serving	13.0	290	40%
made w/skim milk, oil, & egg whites	1 serving	6.0	220	25%
premeasured packet	½ pkt	3.5	200	16%
(Krusteaz)				
blueberry				
mix only	½ cup	3.0	210	13%
prepared	3 pancakes	3.0	210	13%
buckwheat				
mix only	½ cup	4.0	280	13%
prepared	3 pancakes	4.0	280	13%
buttermilk				
fat-free				
mix only	½ cup	–	190	–
prepared	½ cup	–	190	–
original				
mix only	½ cup	3.0	200	14%
prepared	3 pancakes	3.0	200	14%

Food and Description	Amount	Fat Grams	Total Calories	% Fat Calories
harvest apple spice				
mix only	½ cup	3.0	210	13%
prepared	3 pancakes	3.0	210	13%
oat bran/lite				
mix only	½ cup	1.0	140	6%
prepared	3 pancakes	1.0	140	6%
old fashioned				
mix only	¼ cup	0.5	120	4%
prepared	3 pancakes	9.0	230	35%
whole wheat & honey				
mix only	½ cup	1.5	230	6%
prepared	3 pancakes	1.5	230	6%
(Martha White)				
Flapstax				
batter	¼ cup	1.0	80	11%
prepared	1 pancake	1.0	80	11%
light crust/mix only	2 oz	3.0	120	23%
(Pepperidge Farm) old-fashioned				
buttermilk	¼ cup	1.0	140	6%
corn	¼ cup	1.0	130	7%
home style	¼ cup	1.0	140	6%
whole wheat	¼ cup	1.0	130	7%
(Robin Hood) buttermilk				
mix only	⅓ cup	4.0	170	21%
prepared	3 pancakes	6.0	220	25%
PANCAKE & WAFFLE MIX (See also PANCAKE)				
(Aunt Jemima)				
buckwheat	¼ cup	1.0	120	8%
complete				
buttermilk				
reduced calorie	⅓ cup	1.5	140	10%
regular	⅓ cup	2.0	190	9%
original	⅓ cup	0.5	150	3%
whole wheat	¼ cup	0.5	130	3%
(Bisquick) Shake 'N Pour				
blueberry				
mix only	½ cup	4.0	220	16%
prepared	3 pancakes	4.0	220	16%
buttermilk				
mix only	½ cup	3.0	200	14%
prepared	3 pancakes	3.0	200	14%
original				
mix only	½ cup	3.0	210	13%
prepared	3 pancakes	3.0	210	13%
(Feam) mix only				
buckwheat	½ cup	3.0	235	12%
Rich Earth	½ cup	2.0	190	10%
7-grain buttermilk	½ cup	2.0	200	9%

Food and Description	Amount	Fat Grams	Total Calories	% Fat Calories
stone ground whole wheat	½ cup	2.0	220	8%
unbleached wheat & soya	½ cup	2.0	235	8%
generic/blue corn	⅓ cup	2.0	200	9%
(Manischewitz) potato/mix only	3 Tbs	1.0	80	11%
PANCAKE & WAFFLE SYRUP (*See also* MAPLE SYRUP)				
(Aunt Jemima)				
butter lite	¼ cup	–	100	–
butter rich	¼ cup	–	210	–
lite	¼ cup	–	100	–
original	¼ cup	–	210	–
(Brer Rabbit)				
dark	2 Tbs	–	120	–
light	2 Tbs	–	120	–
(Cary's)				
pure maple	2 Tbs	–	100	–
sugar-free	¼ cup		35	
(Estee)				
blueberry	¼ cup	–	80	–
maple	¼ cup	–	80	–
(Featherweight) lite				
blueberry syrup	¼ cup	–	80	–
maple	¼ cup	–	80	–
(Golden Griddle)	4 Tbs	–	220	–
(Hungry Jack)				
butter maple				
lite	¼ cup	–	100	–
regular	¼ cup	–	210	–
original				
lite	¼ cup	–	100	–
regular	¼ cup	–	210	–
(Karo) pancake	1 Tbs	–	60	–
	4 Tbs	–	240	–
(Knott's Berry Farm)				
blackberry	2 Tbs	–	110	–
blueberry	2 Tbs	–	120	–
blueberry				
light	2 Tbs	–	50	–
regular	2 Tbs	–	120	–
boysenberry				
light	2 Tbs	–	50	–
regular	2 Tbs	–	120	–
country	2 Tbs	–	110	–
microwavable				
light	2 Tbs	–	45	–
w/30% real maple syrup	2 Tbs	–	110	–
strawberry	2 Tbs	–	120	–
(Log Cabin)				
Country Kitchen				
butter	¼ cup	–	200	–

Food and Description	Amount	Fat Grams	Total Calories	% Fat Calories
lite	¼ cup	–	100	–
regular	¼ cup	–	200	–
original				
lite	¼ cup	–	100	–
regular	¼ cup	–	200	–
(Mrs. Butterworth's)				
lite	¼ cup	–	100	–
regular	¼ cup	–	200	–
(Mrs. Richardson's)				
lite	¼ cup	–	100	–
original recipe	¼ cup	–	210	–
(Nabisco) Vermont Maid	1 Tbs		50	–
(Polaner)				
blueberry	¼ cup	–	200	–
raspberry	¼ cup	–	200	–
strawberry	¼ cup	–	200	–
(S&W) reduced calorie				
blueberry	¼ cup	–	60	–
butter flavor	¼ cup	–	60	–
maple	¼ cup	–	60	–
strawberry	¼ cup	–	60	–
(Smucker's) fruit				
light	¼ cup	–	130	–
natural	¼ cup	–	210	–
PAPAW/fresh	½ lb	2.0	194	9%
PAPAYA/fresh				
cubed-peeled	1 cup	–	60	–
whole	½ medium	–	80	–
PAPAYA JUICE/NECTAR (*See also* FRUIT PUNCH)				
bottled, boxed, or canned				
generic	1 cup	–	145	–
(Goya)	6 fl oz	–	110	–
(Kern's)	6 fl oz	–	110	–
(Knudsen)				
papaya juice				
papaya-lime juice	8 fl oz	–	115	–
nectar	11.5 fl oz	–	210	–
Thirst Quencher	8 fl oz	–	130	–
(Libby's)	6 fl oz	–	110	–
PAPRIKA/ground	1 tsp	–	6	–
PARFAIT (*See* CANDY; ICE CREAM BARS, SANDWICHES, & FROZEN NOVELTIES; PUDDING & MOUSSE)				
PARSLEY				
dried	1 tsp	–	1	–
freeze-dried	any amount	–	–	–
fresh	10 sprigs	–	3	–
	½ cup	–	10	–

Food and Description	Amount	Fat Grams	Total Calories	% Fat Calories
PARSNIP/fresh				
cooked	½ cup	–	66	–
raw/sliced	½ cup	–	50	–
PASSION FRUIT/GRANADILLA				
fresh	1 medium	–	18	–
	½ lb	–	106	–
PASSION FRUIT JUICE/JUICE BLEND (See also FRUIT PUNCH)				
bottled, boxed, or canned				
(Snapple) Passion Supreme	10 fl oz	–	160	–
fresh				
purple	1 cup	–	126	–
yellow	1 cup	–	149	–
frozen				
(Welch's) passion fruit	8 fl oz	–	140	–
PASTA				
(American Beauty) dry/uncooked				
angel hair	2 oz	1.0	210	4%
capellini	2 oz	1.0	210	4%
curly roni	2 oz	1.0	210	4%
egg noodles				
extra wide	2 oz	3.0	220	12%
fine	2 oz	3.0	220	12%
krinkly	2 oz	3.0	220	12%
wide	2 oz	3.0	220	12%
elbow roni	2 oz	1.0	210	4%
fettuccine	2 oz	3.0	220	12%
lasagna	2 oz	1.0	210	4%
mostaccioli	2 oz	1.0	210	4%
rainbow shells	2 oz	1.0	210	4%
rainbow twirls	2 oz	1.0	210	4%
roni mac	2 oz	1.0	210	4%
rotelle	2 oz	1.0	210	4%
rotini	2 oz	1.0	210	4%
salad mac	2 oz	1.0	210	4%
seashell	2 oz	1.0	210	4%
shell roni				
large	2 oz	1.0	210	4%
regular	2 oz	1.0	210	4%
shells/medium	2 oz	1.0	210	4%
spaghetti				
regular	2 oz	1.0	210	4%
thin	2 oz	1.0	210	4%
vermicelli	2 oz	1.0	210	4%
(Antoine's) dry/uncooked				
farfelle	1 cup	1.0	210	4%
fettuccini w/herbs	1 cup	3.0	220	12%
fusilli tricolore	¾ cup	1.0	210	4%
gernelli	½ cup	1.0	210	4%

Food and Description	Amount	Fat Grams	Total Calories	% Fat Calories
radiatore tricolore	⅔ cup	1.0	210	4%
spicy spirals	¾ cup	1.0	210	4%
tagliatelle	1 cup	3.0	220	12%
(Contadina) fresh/refrigerated				
angel's hair	1¼ cups	3.0	240	11%
fettuccine				
cholesterol-free	1 cup	2.5	240	9%
regular	1 cup	3.5	250	13%
linguine/egg	1¼ cups	4.0	260	14%
ravioli				
beef	1¼ cups	21.0	350	54%
cheese				
light	1 cup	7.0	240	26%
regular	1¼ cups	18.0	280	58%
chicken & rosemary	1¼ cups	19.0	330	52%
4-cheese	1¼ cups	12.0	280	39%
garden vegetable/lite	1 cup	5.0	240	19%
gorgonzola cheese & walnut	1¼ cups	15.0	380	36%
vegetable	1¼ cups	9.0	290	28%
tagliatelle/spinach	1¼ cups	6.0	270	21%
tortellini				
cheese	¾ cup	9.0	260	31%
cheese (spinach)	¾ cup	9.0	260	31%
cheese & basil	1 cup	16.0	360	40%
chicken & prosciutto	1 cup	20.0	360	50%
chicken & vegetable	¾ cup	10.0	270	33%
4-cheese	¾ cp	6.0	260	21%
mushroom	1 cup	8.0	310	23%
sausage	1 cup	15.0	330	41%
(Creamette) dry/uncooked				
egg noodles				
enriched/wide	2 oz	3.0	220	12%
no egg yolk	2 oz	2.5	210	11%
stroganoff	2 oz	2.5	210	11%
wide & broad	2 oz	2.5	210	11%
regular				
dumpling	2 oz	2.5	210	11%
extra wide	2 oz	2.5	210	11%
fine	2 oz	2.5	210	11%
kluski	2 oz	3.0	220	12%
enriched pasta				
elbow macaroni	2 oz	1.0	210	4%
fettuccine	2 oz	1.0	210	4%
lasagna	2 oz	1.0	210	4%
linguini	2 oz	1.0	210	4%
manicotti/8-oz pkg	3 pieces	1.0	180	5%
mostaccioli	2 oz	1.0	210	4%
rainbow rotini	2 oz	1.0	210	4%

Food and Description	Amount	Fat Grams	Total Calories	% Fat Calories
ribbons/no egg yolk	2 oz	1.0	210	4%
rigatoni	2 oz	1.0	210	4%
rotini	2 oz	1.0	210	4%
shells/jumbo	6 pieces	1.0	210	4%
spaghetti				
regular	2 oz	1.0	210	4%
thin	2 oz	1.0	210	4%
spinach				
egg	2 oz	3.0	220	12%
no egg	2 oz	1.0	210	4%
tri-color	2 oz	1.0	210	4%
vermicelli	2 oz	1.0	210	4%
(De Boles) dry/uncooked				
angel hair/Jerusalem artichoke				
garlic & parsley	2 oz	1.0	210	4%
tomato & basil	2 oz	1.0	210	4%
whole wheat	2 oz	2.0	210	4%
fettuccine/Jerusalem artichoke				
regular	2 oz	1.0	210	4%
spinach	2 oz	1.0	210	4%
lasagna				
Jerusalem artichoke	2 oz	1.0	210	4%
whole wheat	2 oz	2.0	210	9%
linguine/Jerusalem artichoke	2 oz	1.0	210	4%
ribbon/whole wheat	2 oz	2.0	210	9%
rigatoni/Jerusalem artichoke	2 oz	1.0	210	4%
rotini				
Jerusalem artichoke	2 oz	1.0	210	4%
vegetable				
primavera	2 oz	1.0	210	4%
tomato & basil	2 oz	1.0	210	4%
wheat				
garlic & parsley	2 oz	1.0	210	4%
tricolor primavera	2 oz	1.0	210	4%
shells				
wheat-free corn	2 oz	1.0	210	4%
whole wheat	2 oz	2.0	210	9%
spaghetti				
Jerusalem artichoke	2 oz	1.0	210	4%
whole wheat	2 oz	2.0	210	9%
ziti				
Jerusalem artichoke	2 oz	1.0	210	4%
(De Cecco) dry/cooked				
capellini	4 oz	1.0	210	4%
egg noodle	4 oz	3.0	210	13%
fusilli	4 oz	1.0	210	4%
lasagna	4 oz	1.0	210	4%
linguini	4 oz	1.0	210	4%

Food and Description	Amount	Fat Grams	Total Calories	% Fat Calories
penne rigati	4 oz	1.0	210	4%
pennete	4 oz	1.0	210	4%
rigatoni	4 oz	1.0	210	4%
rotelle	2 oz	1.0	210	4%
spaghetti	4 oz	1.0	210	4%
spaghettini	4 oz	1.0	210	4%
spinach wheat	4 oz	1.0	210	4%
(Dell'Alpe) homemade style/dry/uncooked				
angel hair	1¼ cups	3.0	220	12%
fettuccine				
hot	1¼ cups	3.0	220	12%
parsley & Parmesan	1¼ cups	3.0	220	12%
spinach	1¼ cups	3.0	220	12%
spinach & egg	1¼ cups	3.0	220	12%
tri-color	1¼ cups	3.0	220	12%
(Di Giorno) refrigerated				
angel's hair	2 oz	1.0	160	6%
fettuccine				
regular	2.5 oz	1.5	190	7%
spinach	2.5	1.5	190	7%
linguine				
herb	2.5 oz	1.5	190	7%
regular	2.5	1.5	190	7%
ravioli				
Italian herb-cheese	1 cup	13.0	350	33%
Italian sausage	¾ cup	12.0	340	32%
stuffed pasta/light varieties				
cheese & garlic	1 cup	2.0	270	7%
tomato & cheese	1 cup	3.0	280	10%
tortellini				
cheese	¾ cup	6.0	260	21%
meat	¾ cup	9.0	290	28%
tortelloni				
chicken & herbs	1 cup	5.0	260	17%
hot red pepper-cheese	1 cup	9.0	310	26%
mozzarella-garlic	1 cup	9.0	300	27%
mushroom	1 cup	7.0	290	22%
(Eden) organic/dry				
extra fine pasta/wheat/cooked	4 oz	–	228	–
noodles/Japanese buckwheat/uncooked				
regular	2 oz	1.0	190	10%
w/mugwort leaf	2 oz	0.5	190	2%
ribbons/cooked				
wheat				
paella ribbons w/saffron	4 oz	–	228	–
Provençal	4 oz	–	228	–
whole wheat/spinach	4 oz	–	212	–
shells/wheat vegetable/cooked	4 oz	1.0	228	4%

Food and Description	Amount	Fat Grams	Total Calories	% Fat Calories
spirals				
wheat vegetable	4 oz	1.0	228	4%
whole wheat				
sesame rice	4 oz	1.0	212	4%
vegetable	4 oz	1.0	212	4%
(Fantastic Foods)				
couscous				
wheat				
cooked	⅝ cup	–	210	–
uncooked	¼ cup	–	210	–
whole wheat				
cooked	¾ cup	0.5	180	3%
uncooked	¼ cup	0.5	180	3%
(Foulds) No Yolks/dry/uncooked				
egg noodle				
broad	2 oz	0.5	210	2%
substitute	2 oz	2.0	210	9%
generic				
chow mein noodles	1 cup	11.0	220	45%
egg noodles				
cooked	1 cup	2.0	200	9%
flakes	2 oz	3.0	220	12%
uncooked	8 oz	10.0	881	10%
macaroni				
cooked				
firm	1 cup	1.0	190	5%
tender				
cold	1 cup	<1.0	115	4%
hot	1 cup	1.0	155	6%
uncooked	8 oz	2.7	838	3%
pastini/dry				
carrot	4 oz	2.0	420	4%
egg	1 cup	7.0	651	10%
spinach	4 oz	2.0	415	4%
spaghetti/cooked				
firm	1 cup	1.0	190	5%
tender	1 cup	1.0	155	6%
(Golden Grain) dry				
egg noodles	2 oz	2.0	210	9%
pasta	2 oz	1.0	200	5%
(Grandma's) frozen/cooked				
egg noodles/wide country style	4 oz	2	175	10%
(Health Valley) dry/uncooked				
elbows				
whole wheat	2 oz	1.0	202	5%
whole wheat w/4 vegetables	2 oz	1.0	202	5%
lasagna				
spinach	2 oz	1.0	170	5%

Food and Description	Amount	Fat Grams	Total Calories	% Fat Calories
whole wheat w/wheat germ spaghetti	2 oz	1.0	170	5%
amaranth	2 oz	1.0	170	5%
oat bran	2 oz	1.0	120	7%
whole wheat	2 oz	1.0	170	5%
whole wheat amaranth	2 oz	1.0	200	5%
whole wheat w/spinach	2 oz	1.0	170	5%
(Hodgson Mill) dry/cooked				
bows/semolina veggie	4 oz	1.0	200	4%
egg noodles				
semolina veggie	4 oz	3.0	220	12%
whole wheat	4 oz	3.0	220	12%
whole wheat-spinach	4 oz	3.0	220	12%
elbows/whole wheat	4 oz	1.0	190	5%
fettuccine/whole wheat	4 oz	1.0	190	5%
lasagna/whole wheat	4 oz	1.0	190	5%
rotini/semolina veggie	4 oz	1.0	200	4%
shells/medium/whole wheat	4 oz	1.0	190	5%
spaghetti				
whole wheat	4 oz	1.0	190	5%
whole wheat-spinach	4 oz	2.0	190	9%
spirals/whole wheat	4 oz	1.0	190	5%
wagon wheels/semolina veggie	4 oz	1.0	200	4%
(Mallard's) refrigerated				
ravioli/spinach & ricotta cheese	1 cup	8.0	265	27%
(Manischewitz) dry/cooked				
egg noodles				
fine	1½ cups	3.0	220	12%
flakes	⅓ cup	3.0	220	12%
medium	1¼ cups	3.0	220	12%
wide	1¾ cups	3.0	220	12%
large egg bows	⅓ cup	3.0	220	12%
matzo farfel	1 cup	1.0	180	5%
wide cut/yolk-free	1¾ cups	1.0	210	4%
(Martha Gooch) dry/cooked				
egg noodles				
dumplings	4 oz	3.0	220	12%
extra wide	4 oz	3.0	220	12%
wide	4 oz	3.0	220	12%
elbow macaroni/big	4 oz	1.0	210	4%
rotini	4 oz	1.0	210	4%
shell macaroni	4 oz	1.0	210	4%
spaghetti				
long	4 oz	1.0	210	4%
thin	4 oz	1.0	210	4%
(Mendocino Pasta Co.) dry/uncooked				
fettuccine				
garlic-basil	1 cup	1.5	180	8%

Food and Description	Amount	Fat Grams	Total Calories	% Fat Calories
lemon-pepper	1 cup	1.5	180	8%
spinach & chive	1 cup	1.5	180	8%
tomato-basil	1 cup	1.5	180	8%
rotelle/garden rainbow	¾ cup	1.5	180	8%
(Monterey Pasta Co.) refrigerated				
ravioli/snow crab	3 oz	3.0	205	13%
(Mueller's) dry/uncooked				
egg noodles				
golden rich	2 oz	3.0	220	12%
regular	2 oz	3.0	220	12%
elbows	2 oz	1.0	210	4%
lasagna	2 oz	1.0	210	4%
macaroni	2 oz	1.0	210	4%
ready-cut	2 oz	1.0	210	4%
ruffles	2 oz	1.0	210	4%
sea shells	2 oz	1.0	210	4%
spaghetti				
regular	2 oz	1.0	210	4%
thin	2 oz	1.0	210	4%
tri-color twist trio	2 oz	1.0	210	4%
twists	2 oz	1.0	210	4%
vermicelli	2 oz	1.0	210	4%
wide/yolk-free	2 oz	1.0	210	4%
(Nature's Cuisine) dry/uncooked				
long spaghetti				
artichoke	2 oz	2.0	210	9%
sesame	2 oz	2.0	190	9%
spinach	2 oz	2.0	190	9%
wheat & soya	2 oz	1.0	220	4%
(Pasta La Bella) dry/uncooked				
penne rigate	¾ cup	1.0	210	4%
pepi rigate	¾ cup	1.0	210	4%
radiatore	¾ cup	1.0	210	4%
rotelle	1¼ cups	1.0	210	4%
rotini/garden	¾ cup	1.0	210	4%
shells/medium	¾ cup	1.0	210	4%
spaghetti	2 oz	1.0	210	4%
ziti	2 oz	1.0	210	4%
(Pennsylvania Dutch) dry/uncooked				
alphabets/egg	2 oz	2.5	210	11%
bott boi/egg/no yolks	2 oz	2.5	210	11%
bows/egg	2 oz	2.5	210	11%
egg noodles				
broad	2 oz	2.5	210	11%
fine	2 oz	2.5	210	11%
homestyle	2 oz	2.5	210	11%
kluski	2 oz	3	220	12%
medium	2 oz	2.5	210	11%

Food and Description	Amount	Fat Grams	Total Calories	% Fat Calories
stroganoff	2 oz	2.5	210	11%
wide & broad	2 oz	2.5	210	11%
(Pritikin) dry, cooked				
spaghetti/whole wheat/thin	⅛ box	1.0	190	5%
spirals/3-component	⅔ cup	1.0	190	5%
(Quinoa) wheat-free				
elbows	2 oz	2.0	180	10%
garden pagodas	2 oz	2.0	180	10%
pasta	2 oz	2.0	180	10%
rotini	2 oz	1.0	210	4%
shells	2 oz	2.0	180	10%
spaghetti	2 oz	1.0	210	4%
(Reames) frozen egg noodles	½ cup	2.0	170	11%
(Ronzoni) dry/uncooked				
egg noodles				
regular	2 oz	2.0	210	9%
spinach	2 oz	3.0	220	12%
fettuccini	2 oz	1.0	210	4%
fusilli	2 oz	1.0	210	4%
lasagne	2 oz	1.0	210	4%
macaroni				
regular	2 oz	1.0	210	4%
spinach	2 oz	1.0	210	4%
mostaccioli	2 oz	1.0	210	4%
rigatoni	2 oz	1.0	210	4%
rotelle	2 oz	1.0	210	4%
rotini/tri-color	2 oz	1.0	210	4%
shells				
jumbo	2 oz	1.0	210	4%
medium	2 oz	1.0	210	4%
tubettini	2 oz	1.0	210	4%
(San Giorgio) dry				
light & fluffy				
dumplings	1 oz	1.0	210	4%
egg noodles				
extra wide	1 oz	2.5	210	11%
medium	1 oz	2.5	210	11%
spinach	1 oz	2.5	210	11%
wide	1 oz	2.5	210	11%
regular				
acine di pepe	1 oz	1.0	210	4%
alphabets	2 oz	1.0	210	4%
bows/pot pie	2 oz	3.0	220	12%
capellini	1 oz	1.0	210	4%
fusilli/cut	1 oz	1.0	210	4%
ditalini	2 oz	1.0	210	4%
elbow macaroni	1 oz	1.0	210	4%
flakes	2 oz	1.0	210	4%

Food and Description	Amount	Fat Grams	Total Calories	% Fat Calories
kluske	2 oz	3.0	220	12%
lasagne/rippled	2 oz	1.0	210	4%
linguine	1 oz	1.0	210	4%
mafalda	1 oz	1.0	210	4%
manicotti	1 oz	1.0	210	4%
mixed types				
Italian trio	2 oz	1.0	210	4%
rainbow medley	1 oz	1.0	210	4%
mostaccioli/ridged	1 oz	1.0	210	4%
mustaccioli rigati	2 oz	1.0	210	4%
orzo	1 oz	1.0	210	4%
pastina/baby	2 oz	1.0	210	4%
shells/rainbow	1 oz	1.0	210	4%
racing wheels/pot pie	2 oz	3.0	220	12%
rigatoni	1 oz	1.0	210	4%
rotelle	2 oz	1.0	210	4%
rotini	1 oz	1.0	210	4%
shells				
jumbo	1 oz	1.0	210	4%
large	1 oz	1.0	210	4%
small	1 oz	1.0	210	4%
spaghetti	1 oz	1.0	210	4%
spaghettini	1 oz	1.0	210	4%
squares/pot pie	2 oz	3.0	220	12%
tubettini	2 oz	1.0	210	4%
twirls/rainbow	1 oz	1.0	210	4%
ziti/cut	1 oz	1.0	210	4%
vermicelli	2 oz	1.0	210	4%
(Sinatra's)				
angel hair	½ cup	1.5	170	19%
fettuccine				
spinach	½ cup	1.0	150	6%
white	½ cup	1.5	170	19%
(Trio's) refrigerated				
ravioli				
cheese/low-fat	1 cup	3.0	300	9%
garlic-cheese-cracked pepper	1 cup	10.0	340	26%
tortellini				
garlic & herbs cheese	1 cup	8.0	320	23%
tri-color	1 cup	8.0	320	23%
(Westbrae Natural) dry/uncooked				
angel hair/corn	2 oz	2.0	210	9%
elbows/corn	2 oz	2.0	210	9%
lasagna/whole wheat/no egg				
plain	2 oz	2.0	210	9%
spinach	2 oz	2.0	210	9%
shells/corn	2 oz	2.0	210	9%

Food and Description	Amount	Fat Grams	Total Calories	% Fat Calories
spaghetti				
corn	2 oz	2.0	210	9%
whole wheat/no egg				
plain	2 oz	2.0	210	9%
spinach	2 oz	2.0	210	9%

PASTA ENTRÉE/DINNER (*See also* ASIAN FOOD; FROZEN ENTRÉE/DINNER; VEGETARIAN FOODS; individual listings)

■ **CANNED**

(Chef Boyardee)

ABC's & 123's				
plain	1 cup	–	200	–
w/meatballs	1 cup	9.0	280	29%
beef ravioli	1 cup	5.0	230	20%
Beefaroni	1 cup	7.0	260	24%
Beefogetti w/meatballs	1 cup	7.0	250	25%
cheese ravioli in tomato sauce				
plain	1 cup	–	210	–
w/beef	1 cup	3.0	220	12%
cheese tortellini	1 cup	1.0	230	4%
Chili Mac	1 cup	11.0	260	38%
dinosaurs				
plain	1 cup	–	210	–
w/meatballs	1 cup	9.0	270	30%
fettuccine	1 cup	6.0	230	23%
lasagna	1 cup	11.0	270	37%
macaroni & cheese	1 cup	1.5	180	8%
mini-bites cheese ravioli & meatballs	1 cup	11.0	270	37%
mini-cannelloni	1 cup	9.0	260	31%
mini-beef ravioli	1 cup	5.0	230	20%
rigatoni	1 cup	7.0	250	25%
roller coasters	1 cup	7.0	250	25%
Sir Chomps-A-Lot/bite-size				
beef ravioli	1 cup	4.0	210	17%
lasagna	1 cup	3.0	210	13%
O-rings	1 cup	10.0	260	35%
ravioli	1 cup	–	210	–
spaghetti & meatballs	1 cup	10.0	250	36%
Spider Man				
plain	1 cup	–	190	–
w/meatballs	1 cup	8.0	250	29%
Street Sharks				
plain	1 cup	–	210	–
w/meatballs	1 cup	8.0	250	29%
Teenage Mutant Ninja Turtles Versus Shredder				
plain	1 cup	–	170	–
w/meatballs	1 cup	9.0	260	31%

Food and Description	Amount	Fat Grams	Total Calories	% Fat Calories
Tic Tac Toes				
plain	1 cup	–	190	–
w/meatballs	1 cup	10.0	260	35%
X-Men				
plain	1 cup	–	210	–
w/meatballs	1 cup	8.0	270	27%
generic/macaroni & cheese	1 cup	9.6	228	38%
(Hormel)				
chili mac	7.5 oz	9.0	200	41%
lasagna	7.5 oz	14.0	250	50%
spaghetti & meatballs	7.5 oz	7.0	210	30%
(Hunt's) homestyle separates				
beef ravioli	1 cup	8.0	221	33%
beef stew	1 cup	4.0	155	23%
noodles & beef	1 cup	4.0	151	24%
noodles & chicken				
cacciatore	1 cup	6.0	176	30%
regular	1 cup	6.0	176	31%
w/mushrooms	1 cup	4.0	199	18%
rigatoni w/Italian garden style sauce	1 cup	5.0	165	27%
(Libby's) Diner				
beef ravioli	7.75 oz	9.0	230	35%
lasagna	7.75 oz	7.0	200	32%
macaroni & beef	7.75 oz	9.0	220	37%
macaroni & cheese	7.75 oz	20.0	320	56%
pasta spirals & chicken	7.75 oz	4.0	130	28%
spaghetti & meatballs	7.75 oz	5.0	190	24%
(Progresso)				
beef ravioli	1 cup	5.0	260	17%
cheese ravioli	1 cup	2.0	220	8%
(Read) Italian pasta salad	½ cup	2.5	90	25%
(Van Camp's)				
Chili-Mac	1 cup	20.0	320	56%
Noodle Weenee	1 cup	8.0	240	30%
Spaghettee Weenee	1 cup	7.0	240	26%
(Wolf) Chili-Mac	1 cup	20.0	320	56%
■ FROZEN				
(Birds Eye)				
Easy Recipe/prepared				
Alfredo vegetables	2¼ cups	25.0	370	61%
Pasta Secrets/prepared				
creamy peppercorn	1 cup	15.0	300	45%
primavera	1 cup	10.0	230	39%
white cheddar	1 cup	10.0	240	38%
zesty garlic	1 cup	10.0	240	38%
(Campbell's) Specialty Kitchens				
fettuccine w/chicken Florentine	1 cup	15.0	330	14%

Food and Description	Amount	Fat Grams	Total Calories	% Fat Calories
(Chicago Brother's) gourmet				
lasagna w/meat sauce	1 cup	15.0	310	44%
vegetable lasagna	1 cup	8.0	210	34%
(Fazzio's)				
breaded meat ravioli	6 pieces	6.0	250	22%
cannelloni	10 oz	20.0	410	44%
meat ravioli/toasted	6 pieces	16.0	340	42%
pizza rav's/toasted/pepperoni & sausage	6 pieces	19.0	350	49%
(Green Giant) Pasta Accents				
Alfredo	2 cups	8.0	210	34%
creamy cheddar	2⅓ cups	8.0	250	29%
Florentine	2 cups	9.0	310	26%
garden herb seasoning	2 cups	7.0	230	27%
garlic seasoning	2 cups	10.0	260	35%
primavera	2¼ cups	12.0	320	34%
white cheddar sauce	1¾ cups	12.0	300	36%
(Hanover) pasta salad				
Italian	½ cup	–	60	–
Milano	½ cup	–	60	–
Oriental	½ cup	–	80	–
primavera	½ cup	–	50	–
(Michael Angelo's)				
cheese ravioli	4 oz	7.5	218	31%
eggplant Parmesan	1 cup	21.0	300	63%
lasagna				
regular	1 cup	22.0	410	48%
sausage	1 cup	20.0	410	44%
stuffed pasta shells	4 oz	9.0	210	39%
(Pasta Pasta Pasta) lasagna bowl	1 bowl	15.0	330	41%
(Renaissance) Cafe Pasta				
jumbo stuffed shells	2 pieces	15.0	290	47%
lasagna				
meat	8 oz	18.0	370	44%
vegetable				
plain	8 oz	7.0	260	24%
w/italian sausage	8 oz	12.0	320	34%
ravioli				
beef	10 pieces	14.0	330	38%
cheese	10 pieces	10.0	280	32%
tortellini				
beef	1 cup	7.0	260	24%
cheese	1 cup	6.0	240	23%
chicken	1 cup	3.0	210	13%
(Wolfgang Puck's)				
lasagna				
4-cheese	5 oz	13.0	200	59%
spicy chicken	1 cup	15.0	260	52%

Food and Description	Amount	Fat Grams	Total Calories	% Fat Calories
ravioli				
mushroom & spinach	13 oz	18.0	260	62%
spicy chicken	2 cups	24.0	360	60%
■ HOMEMADE				
USDA Standard Home Recipe				
lasagna/~2½" x 4" piece				
w/meat/~7 oz	1 piece	12.0	325	33%
w/o meat/~8 oz	1 piece	9.5	317	27%
macaroni & cheese	1 cup	22.0	430	46%
manicotti				
w/meat sauce	~5 oz	11.0	235	42%
w/tomato sauce	5 oz	10.0	223	45%
ravioli				
cheese				
w/meat sauce	~9 oz	17.0	360	43%
w/tomato sauce	~9 oz	15.0	340	40%
w/o sauce	~8.5 oz	17.0	430	36%
meat				
w/tomato sauce	~9 oz	17.0	385	40%
w/o sauce	~8.5 oz	23.0	550	38%
rigatoni w/meat sauce	1 cup	16.0	347	41%
spaghetti dinner				
w/meatballs & tomato sauce	1 cup	11.7	332	32%
w/red clam sauce	1 cup	7.0	226	28%
w/tomato sauce & cheese	1 cup	8.8	280	28%
w/white clam sauce	1 cup	19.0	345	50%
■ MICROWAVE CONTAINER				
(Chef Boyardee)				
microwave bowl				
ABC's & 123's w/meatballs	1 bowl	9.0	230	35%
beef ravioli	1 bowl	3.0	180	15%
Beefaroni	1 bowl	3.0	190	14%
cheese ravioli	1 bowl	3.0	190	14%
chicken & pasta	1 bowl	1.0	150	6%
dinosaurs w/meatballs	1 bowl	8.0	230	31%
lasagna	1 bowl	8.0	230	31%
macaroni & cheese	1 bowl	1.0	160	6%
meat tortellini	1 bowl	2.5	220	10%
Sir Chomps-A-Lot bite-size ravioli				
beef	1 bowl	2.0	180	10%
cheese	1 bowl	–	170	–
spaghetti & meatballs	1 bowl	6.0	200	27%
spaghetti rings & meatballs	1 bowl	8.0	240	30%
Teenage Mutant Ninja Turtles Versus Shredder w/meatballs	1 bowl	7.0	220	29%
Tic Tac Toe's w/meatballs	1 bowl	8.0	220	33%
microwave bowl main meals				
fettuccine in meat sauce	1 bowl	9.0	320	25%

Food and Description	Amount	Fat Grams	Total Calories	% Fat Calories
hearty lasagna	1 bowl	11.0	300	33%
meat tortellini	1 bowl	4.0	300	12%
noodles & chicken	1 bowl	1.0	170	5%
ravioli suprema				
beef	1 bowl	5.0	270	17%
cheese	1 bowl	5.0	280	16%
spaghetti	1 bowl	6.0	230	23%
ziti	1 bowl	–	250	–
(Franco American)				
Garfield w/tomato & cheese	1 cup	2.0	190	9%
Gargoyles w/meatballs	1 cup	11.0	260	38%
Shnookums & meat	1 cup	11.0	260	38%
Sonic the hedgehog w/meatballs	1 cup	11.0	280	35%
spaghetti w/tomato & cheese	1 cup	2.0	210	9%
SpaghettiOs w/meatballs	1 cup	11.0	260	38%
Teddy Os w/tomato & cheese	1 cup	2.0	190	9%
Where's Waldo w/meatballs	1 cup	11.0	260	38%
(Hormel)				
Kid's Kitchen				
beefy macaroni	1 cup	6.0	190	28%
mini ravioli	1 cup	7.0	240	26%
noodle rings & chicken	1 cup	5.0	150	30%
spaghetti & mini meatballs	1 cup	8.0	220	33%
spaghetti rings	1 cup	2.0	190	9%
spaghetti rings & franks	1 cup	6.0	230	23%
spaghetti rings & meatballs	1 cup	7.0	250	25%
micro cup meals				
chili mac	1 cup	9.0	200	41%
lasagna	1 cup	14.0	250	50%
lasagna & beef in tomato sauce	1 cup	19.0	359	48%
macaroni & cheese	1 cup	11.0	260	38%
noodles & chicken				
regular size	1 cup	9.0	200	41%
10.5 oz container	1 cup	11.0	270	37%
ravioli w/tomato sauce	1 cup	11.0	270	37%
spaghetti & meatballs	1 cup	7.0	210	30%
Top Shelf two-minute entrées				
beef ravioli	1 bowl	9.0	300	27%
Italian lasagna	1 bowl	16.0	340	42%
spaghetti w/meatballs	1 bowl	11.0	300	33%
(Lunch Bucket)				
beef ravioli	1 container	3.5	180	18%
elbows 'n tomato sauce	1 container	2.0	160	11%
Italian style pasta	1 container	1.0	130	7%
lasagna	1 container	3.0	160	17%
macaroni 'n beef	1 container	4.5	180	23%
macaroni 'n cheese	1 container	7.0	190	33%
pasta 'n chicken	1 container	5.0	150	30%

Food and Description	Amount	Fat Grams	Total Calories	% Fat Calories
spaghetti 'n meat sauce	1 container	3.0	160	17%
(Knorr) microwavable pasta in a cup				
fettuccine	1 cup	4.0	220	16%
Oriental noodles	1 cup	3.0	210	13%
pasta twists	1 cup	4.5	210	19%
three cheese macaroni	1 cup	4.0	220	16%
vegetable stew	1 cup	2.0	160	11%
(Mayacamas) Just Enough cup				
Alfredo	1 cup	0.5	70	6%
mushroom & pea	1 cup	0.5	80	6%
tomato & basil	1 cup	–	100	–
■ MIX				
(Annie's)				
Alfredo w/garlic & garden basil				
mix only	½ cup	3.5	200	16%
prepared	¾ cup	9.0	250	32%
mild Mexican shells & cheddar				
mix only	½ cup	3.0	200	14%
prepared	¾ cup	9.0	250	32%
petite pasta shells & cheddar				
mix only	½ cup	3.0	200	14%
prepared	¾ cup	9.0	250	32%
whole wheat shells & cheddar				
mix only	½ cup	4.5	200	20%
prepared	¾ cup	10.0	250	36%
(Bean Cuisine)				
country French beans w/gemelli				
mix only	1 serving	1.0	217	4%
prepared	1 cup	10.5	316	30%
Florentine beans w/bow ties				
mix only	1 serving	2.0	162	11%
prepared	1 cup	5.5	216	23%
pasta & beans w/radiatore				
mix only	1 serving	0.5	162	3%
prepared	1 cup	4.5	215	19%
(Betty Crocker) Suddenly Salad				
Caesar				
mix only	⅔ cup	1.0	170	5%
prepared				
low-fat recipe	¾ cup	3.0	190	14%
regular recipe	¾ cup	10.0	250	36%
classic				
mix only	¾ cup	1.0	170	5%
prepared				
low-fat recipe	¾ cup	3.0	18	15%
regular recipe	¾ cup	7.0	220	29%
creamy macaroni				
mix only	⅓ cup	1.0	140	6%

Food and Description	Amount	Fat Grams	Total Calories	% Fat Calories
prepared				
low-fat recipe	¾ cup	1.5	210	6%
regular recipe	¾ cup	20.0	320	56%
garden Italian/98% fat-free				
mix only	½ cup	1.0	130	7%
prepared	¾ cup	1.0	130	7%
ranch & bacon				
mix only	¾ cup	1.0	150	6%
prepared				
low-fat recipe	¾ cup	2.0	180	10%
regular recipe	¾ cup	9.0	320	53%
(Casbah) couscous pilaf/prepared	1 cup	<1.0	200	2%
(Creamette)				
macaroni & cheese				
mix only	2.5 oz	2.0	250	7%
prepared	1 cup	18.0	390	39%
Master-a-Meal lasagna dinner				
mix only	1.5 oz	1.0	150	6%
prepared	1 cup	11.0	310	32%
noodle & cheese fettuccine dinner				
mix only	1.5 oz	4.0	210	17%
prepared	1 cup	12.0	280	39%
(De Boles)				
artichoke elbow macaroni & cheese				
mix only	2 oz	2.0	210	9%
prepared	¾ cup	7.0	220	29%
artichoke shells & cheddar				
mix only	2 oz	2.0	210	9%
prepared	¾ cup	7.0	220	29%
wheat elbow mac & cheese				
mix	2 oz	3.0	210	13%
prepared	¾ cup	8.0	200	36%
(Fantastic Foods)				
couscous cup/prepared				
black bean salsa	1 pkg	1.5	240	6%
Creole vegetable	1 pkg	1.5	220	6%
nacho cheddar	1 pkg	3.0	200	14%
sweet corn	1 pkg	1.0	180	5%
Italian herb pasta salad				
mix only	⅔ cup	1.5	170	8%
prepared	1 cup	1.5	170	8%
macaroni & cheese				
cheddar				
mix only	⅜ cup	1.5	200	7%
prepared	1 cup	1.5	200	7%
Parmesan				
mix only	⅜ cup	1.5	200	7%
prepared	1 cup	1.5	200	7%

Food and Description	Amount	Fat Grams	Total Calories	% Fat Calories
savory couscous pilaf				
mix only	⅓ cup	1.0	240	4%
prepared	1 cup	1.0	240	4%
spicy Oriental				
mix only	⅔ cup	3.0	200	14%
prepared	1 cup	3.0	200	14%
(Farmhouse) Noodles & Sauce/prepared				
chicken	½ box	2.0	235	8%
creamy garlic	½ box	3.0	260	10%
fettuccine Alfredo	½ box	4.0	250	14%
herb & butter	½ box	2.0	250	7%
Parmesan	½ box	3.0	245	11%
stroganoff	½ box	3.0	250	11%
(Formagg) alternative/mix only				
macaroni & cheese sauce	⅔ cup	2.0	190	9%
pasta primavera	⅔ cup	2.0	190	9%
penne pasta Alfredo	⅔ cup	2.0	190	9%
vegetable pasta & Caesar Italian garden	⅔ cup	2.0	190	9%
(Golden Grain) Pasta Roni/prepared				
angel hair				
w/herbs	1 cup	14.0	320	39%
w/Parmesan cheese	1 cup	14.5	320	41%
corkscrew pasta				
w/creamy garlic sauce	1 cup	24.5	420	53%
w/four cheese sauce	1 cup	18.0	410	40%
fettuccine				
w/Alfredo sauce	1 cup	25.0	470	48%
w/broccoli au gratin	1 cup	10.0	290	31%
w/chicken sauce	1 cup	13.5	320	38%
w/mild cheddar sauce	1 cup	10.5	300	32%
w/Romanoff sauce	1 cup	19.0	410	42%
w/stroganoff sauce	1 cup	14.0	370	34%
linguine				
w/chicken & broccoli	1 cup	16.0	370	39%
w/creamy chicken Parmesan	1 cup	18.5	410	41%
Oriental style pasta w/stir-fry sauce	1 cup	12.0	290	37%
penne w/herb & butter sauce	1 cup	24.5	430	51%
rigatoni				
w/tomato basil	1 cup	9.0	240	34%
w/white cheddar & broccoli sauce	1 cup	19.0	400	43%
shells w/white cheddar sauce	1 cup	16.0	390	37%
tenderthin pasta				
w/broccoli & mushroom	1 cup	24.0	460	47%
w/Parmesan sauce	1 cup	17.0	400	38%
vermicelli w/garlic & olive oil sauce	1 cup	15.5	360	39%
(Hain) Pasta & Sauce/mix only				
creamy Parmesan	¼ pkg	3.0	150	18%

Food and Description	Amount	Fat Grams	Total Calories	% Fat Calories
creamy Swiss	¼ pkg	4.0	170	21%
fettuccine Alfredo	¼ pkg	4.0	180	20%
Italian herb	¼ pkg	2.0	110	16%
primavera	¼ pkg	4.0	140	26%
tangy cheddar	¼ pkg	6.0	180	30%
(Knorr) spicy couscous/mix only	¼ pkg	1.0	150	6%
(Kraft)				
cheddar cheese-egg noodle dinner				
mix only	2.5 oz	4.5	270	15%
prepared	1 cup	21.0	430	44%
chicken-egg noodle dinner				
mix only	2.5 oz	5.0	270	17%
prepared	1 cup	12.0	330	33%
macaroni & cheese				
dinosaurs				
mix only	2.5 oz	3.0	260	10%
prepared	1 cup	17.0	390	39%
mild white cheddar				
mix only	2.5 oz	3.0	260	10%
prepared	1 cup	17.0	390	39%
original				
deluxe				
mix only	3.5 oz	10.0	320	28%
prepared	1 cup	10.0	320	28%
regular				
mix only	2.5 oz	2.5	260	9%
prepared	1 cup	17.0	390	39%
Santa mac				
mix only	2.5 oz	3.0	260	10%
prepared	1 cup	17.0	390	39%
spirals				
mix only	2.5 oz	3.0	260	10%
prepared	1 cup	17.0	390	39%
Super Mario Bros.				
mix only	2.5 oz	3.0	260	10%
prepared	1 cup	17.0	390	39%
teddy bears				
mix only	2.5 oz	3.0	260	10%
prepared	1 cup	17.0	390	39%
The Flintstones				
mix only	2.5 oz	3.0	260	10%
prepared	1 cup	17.0	390	39%
thick 'n creamy				
mix only	2.5 oz	2.5	260	9%
prepared	1 cup	10.0	320	28%
pasta salad				
classic ranch w/bacon				
mix only	2.5 oz	23.0	360	58%

Food and Description	Amount	Fat Grams	Total Calories	% Fat Calories
prepared	¾ cup	23.0	360	58%
creamy Caesar				
mix only	2.5 oz	22.0	360	57%
prepared	¾ cup	22.0	350	57%
golden primavera				
mix only	2.6 oz	12.0	280	39%
prepared	¾ cup	12.0	280	39%
Italian/light				
mix only	2.5 oz	2.0	190	9%
prepared	¾ cup	2.0	190	9%
Parmesan peppercorn				
mix only	2/5 oz	25.0	360	63%
prepared	¾ cup	25.0	360	63%
spaghetti dinner				
mild American				
mix only	2.5 oz	1.5	200	7%
prepared	1 cup	4.5	270	15%
tangy Italian				
mix only	2 oz	2.0	200	9%
prepared	1 cup	4.5	270	15%
w/meat sauce				
mix only	5.5 oz	11.0	330	30%
prepared	1 cup	11.0	330	30%
Velveeta rotini & cheese				
broccoli				
mix only	4.5 oz	16.0	400	36%
prepared	1 cup	16.0	400	36%
Velveeta shells & cheese				
bacon				
mix only	4 oz	14.0	360	35%
prepared	1 cup	14.0	360	35%
original				
mix only	4 oz	13.0	360	33%
prepared	1 cup	13.0	360	33%
salsa				
mix only	4.5 oz	14.0	380	33%
prepared	1 cup	14.0	380	33%
(Lipton) mix only				
Golden Sauté pasta				
angel hair chicken broccoli	⅓ cup	1.5	210	6%
angel hair Parmesan	⅓ cup	5.0	240	19%
chicken herb Parmesan	½ cup	3.0	230	12%
chicken stir-fry	½ cup	2.0	220	8%
garlic butter	½ cup	3.0	230	12%
herb & garlic penne	⅓ cup	3.0	230	12%
Noodles & Sauce				
Alfredo	⅔ cup	7.0	250	25%
Alfredo broccoli	⅔ cup	7.0	260	24%

Food and Description	Amount	Fat Grams	Total Calories	% Fat Calories
Alfredo carbonara	⅔ cup	7.0	260	24%
beef	⅔ cup	3.5	220	14%
butter	⅔ cup	8.0	260	19%
butter & herb	⅔ cup	7.0	250	25%
cheddar bacon	⅔ cup	4.5	230	18%
cheese	⅔ cup	4.5	250	16%
chicken	⅔ cup	4.5	235	18%
chicken broccoli	⅔ cup	4.0	225	26%
chicken tetrazzini	⅔ cup	5.0	220	20%
creamy chicken	⅔ cup	6.0	235	23%
Parmesan	⅔ cup	8.0	250	29%
Romanoff	⅔ cup	7.0	265	24%
sour cream & chive	⅔ cup	8.0	260	28%
stroganoff	⅔ cup	4.0	210	17%
Pasta & Sauce				
cheddar broccoli	½ cup	3.5	260	12%
chicken primavera	¾ cup	3.0	220	12%
creamy garlic	⅔ cup	6.0	260	21%
herb tomato	⅔ cup	2.0	240	8%
Italian cheese bow ties	¾ cup	5.0	230	20%
rotini primavera	½ cup	5.0	240	19%
three cheese	½ cup	5.0	240	19%
(Near East) couscous				
herbed chicken				
mix only	1 serving	0.5	190	2%
prepared	1 serving	3.5	220	14%
Mediterranean curry				
mix only	1 serving	0.5	190	2%
prepared	1 serving	3.5	220	14%
Moroccan pasta				
prepared	1¼ cups	6.0	260	21%
Parmesan				
mix only	1 serving	1.5	200	7%
prepared	1 serving	2.5	220	10%
roasted garlic & olive oil				
mix only	1 serving	1.5	200	7%
prepared	1 serving	4.5	230	18%
tomato lentil				
mix only	1 serving	0.5	190	2%
prepared	1 serving	3.5	220	14%
(Ragu) Pasta Toss				
herbs & olive oil/tomato & garlic	½ cup	8.0	120	60%
(Ramen) noodles (See SOUP)				
(Spice Islands) Quick Meal/prepared				
creamy tomato basil	1 pkg	2.0	200	9%
garlic & herb	1 pkg	1.0	160	6%
pasta prima	1 pkg	2.0	170	11%
spinach & mushroom	1 pkg	1.5	180	8%

Food and Description	Amount	Fat Grams	Total Calories	% Fat Calories
(Uncle Ben's) Country Inn pasta & sauce mix/mix only				
angel hair Parmesan	2.2 oz	5.0	245	18%
broccoli & white cheddar	2.2 oz	5.0	240	19%
butter & herb	2 oz	5.8	230	23%
creamy garlic	2.4 oz	4.8	261	16%
fettuccine Alfredo	2.25 oz	6.0	310	17%
herb linguine	2.2 oz	3.5	240	13%
mushroom fettuccine	2.25 oz	5.6	250	20%
vegetable Alfredo	2.2 oz	4.5	240	17%
Velveeta (See (Kraft) in this section)				
(Villa Lorenzo) Pasta for One/mix only				
Alfredo	2.3 oz	8.0	270	27%
butter & herbs	2.3 oz	7.0	270	23%
cream sauce & mushrooms	2.3 oz	6.0	260	21%
pesto & herbs	2.3 oz	6.0	260	21%
3 cheese & broccoli	2.3 oz	6.0	260	21%
zesty tomato	2.3 oz	3.0	250	11%

PASTA SAUCE (See SAUCE)
PASTRAMI (See LUNCHEON MEAT)
PASTRY (See also CAKE; DONUT; PASTRY, TOASTER; PASTRY DOUGH; PIE CRUST)
■ **FROZEN OR REFRIGERATED**

Food and Description	Amount	Fat Grams	Total Calories	% Fat Calories
(Chef Pierre) food service				
apple dumpling w/cinnamon sauce	1 dumpling	23.0	540	38%
(Dutch) mini cream puffs	2 pieces	10.0	110	82%
(Pepperidge Farm)				
cinnamon roll	1 roll	12.0	250	43%
cloud				
dark chocolate	2 pastries	38.0	580	60%
milk chocolate	2 pastries	38.0	580	60%
Danish/individually wrapped/pocket				
apple	1 Danish	9.0	210	39%
cheese	1 Danish	10.0	200	45%
cinnamon raisin	1 Danish	12.0	250	43%
raspberry	1 Danish	9.0	210	39%
dumpling				
apple	1 dumpling	11.0	290	34%
cherry	1 dumpling	9.0	280	29%
peach	1 dumpling	11.0	300	33%
fruit square/apple	1 square	10.0	210	43%
turnover				
apple				
mini	1 turnover	8.0	140	51%
regular	1 turnover	14.0	330	38%
w/vanilla icing	1 turnover	14.0	360	35%
blueberry	1 turnover	16.0	340	42%
cherry				
mini	1 turnover	8.0	140	51%
regular	1 turnover	13.0	320	37%

Food and Description	Amount	Fat Grams	Total Calories	% Fat Calories
w/vanilla icing	1 turnover	13.0	340	34%
peach				
mini	1 turnover	8.0	160	45%
regular	1 turnover	15.0	340	40%
raspberry				
regular	1 turnover	14.0	330	38%
w/vanilla icing	1 turnover	14.0	360	35%
strawberry/mini	1 turnover	7.0	140	45%
(Pillsbury)				
sweet roll				
apple cinnamon roll w/icing	1 roll	5.0	140	32%
caramel roll	1 roll	7.0	170	37%
cinnamon raisin roll w/icing	1 roll	7.0	180	35%
cinnamon roll w/icing	1 roll	5.0	140	32%
orange sweet roll w/icing	1 roll	7.0	170	37%
turnover				
apple	2 turnovers	17.0	350	44%
cherry	2 turnovers	17.0	360	43%
(Rhodes) cinnamon roll/prepared	1 roll	10.0	240	38%
(Rich's) iced chocolate eclair	1 eclair	9.0	190	43%
(Sara Lee)				
food service				
apple twist	1 pastry	21.0	420	45%
cheese butterfly	1 pastry	25.0	450	50%
cherry cheese	1 pastry	20.0	380	47%
cinnamon almond bear claw	1 pastry	21.0	410	46%
cinnamon roll/indvidually wrapped	1 roll	20.0	470	38%
cinnamon supreme				
2⅛-oz roll	1 roll	10.0	240	38%
4¼-oz roll	1 roll	20.0	470	38%
Danish				
demi-Danish				
apple	1 Danish	6.0	120	45%
cheese	1 Danish	8.0	130	55%
cinnamon raisin	1 Danish	8.0	140	51%
pecan	1 Danish	9.0	150	54%
raspberry	1 Danish	6.0	130	42%
individually wrapped				
apple	1 Danish	13.0	300	39%
cheese	1 Danish	14.0	240	53%
cinnamon raisin	1 Danish	16.0	350	41%
iced cheese	1 Danish	19.0	340	50%
nut caramel	1 Danish	15.0	300	45%
raspberry	1 Danish	12.0	320	34%
tray pack				
apple	1 Danish	14.0	310	41%
cheese	1 Danish	14.0	310	41%
cinnamon raisin	1 Danish	15.0	350	39%

Food and Description	Amount	Fat Grams	Total Calories	% Fat Calories
retail				
butter cinnamon roll				
plain	1 roll	14.0	300	42%
w/1 pkt icing	1 roll	14.0	350	36%
eclair	1 eclair	9.0	190	43%
(Schwan's) cinnamon w/icing	1 roll	4.5	240	17%
(Weight Watchers)				
eclair				
chocolate	1 eclair	4.0	150	24%
triple chocolate	1 eclair	5.0	160	28%
glazed cinnamon roll	1 roll	5.0	200	23%
■ HOMEMADE				
USDA Standard Home Recipe				
apple dumpling	1 average	16.0	275	52%
baklava	2 oz	18.0	250	65%
eclair	3.5 oz	14.5	260	50%
strudel	~4 oz	8.0	265	27%
■ READY TO SERVE				
(Dolly Madison) snack				
apple sweet roll	1 roll	6.0	230	23%
bear claw	1 pastry	11.0	310	32%
cherry bun	1 bun	7.0	230	27%
cherry sweet roll	1 roll	6.0	210	26%
cinnamon roll	1 roll	7.0	220	29%
cream cheese Danish	1 Danish	15.0	380	39%
English cruller	1 cruller	14.0	260	48%
honey bun				
3-oz bun	1 bun	20.0	360	50%
3.75-oz bun	1 bun	25.0	450	50%
honey wheat cinnamon roll	1 roll	8.0	240	30%
honey wheat cinnamon twirl	1 pastry	14.0	450	28%
lemon sweet roll	1 roll	7.0	230	27%
pecan roller	1 roll	7.0	210	30%
raspberry sweet roll	1 roll	7.0	230	27%
(Dunkin' Donuts)				
apple fritter	1 fritter	13.0	300	39%
Bismark	1 pastry	14.0	310	41%
bow tie	1 pastry	10.0	250	36%
coffee roll				
chocolate frosted	1 roll	14.0	290	43%
cinnamon raisin	1 roll	13.0	330	35%
maple frosted	1 roll	13.0	300	39%
plain	1 roll	13.0	280	42%
vanilla frosted	1 roll	13.0	300	39%
eclair	1 eclair	12.0	290	62%
glazed fritter	1 fritter	13.0	290	40%
tart				
apple	1 tart	10.0	290	31%

Food and Description	Amount	Fat Grams	Total Calories	% Fat Calories
blueberry	1 tart	10.0	300	30%
lemon	1 tart	11.0	280	35%
raspberry	1 tart	10.0	310	29%
strawberry	1 tart	10.0	310	29%
turnover				
apple	1 turnover	15.0	350	39%
blueberry	1 turnover	15.0	370	36%
lemon	1 turnover	15.0	350	39%
raspberry	1 turnover	15.0	380	36%
strawberry	1 turnover	15.0	380	36%
(Entenmann's)				
fat-free				
apple bun	1 bun	–	150	–
apricot Danish twist	⅛ pastry	–	150	–
Black Forest pastry	⅑ pastry	–	130	–
blueberry cheese bun	1 bun	–	140	–
cinnamon apple twist	⅛ pastry	–	150	–
cinnamon raisin bun	1 bun	–	160	–
lemon twist	⅛ pastry	–	130	–
pineapple cheese bun	1 bun	–	140	–
raspberry cheese bun	1 bun	–	160	–
raspberry cheese pastry	⅑ pastry	–	140	–
raspberry twist	⅛ pastry	–	140	–
original				
apple puff	1 puff	12.0	260	42%
apple strudel	¼ strudel	14.0	310	41%
chocolate eclair	1 eclair	9.0	250	32%
cinnamon bun	1 bun	10.0	220	41%
cinnamon filbert ring	⅙ pastry	17.0	270	57%
pecan Danish ring	⅛ pastry	15.0	230	59%
raspberry twist	⅛ pastry	11.0	220	45%
walnut Danish ring	⅛ pastry	14.0	230	55%
generic				
cinnamon bun/~2 oz				
frosted	1 bun	5.0	185	24%
plain	1 bun	5.0	174	26%
cream puff/2" high/3⅓" dia				
shell only	2 oz	10.0	135	66%
w/custard filling	1 puff	18.0	303	54%
Danish/4½" dia/~2 oz				
plain	1 Danish	12.0	220	49%
w/fruit	1 Danish	13.0	235	50%
eclair w/custard filling & chocolate icing	1 eclair	13.6	239	51%
hot cross bun/2 oz	1 bun	8.0	190	38%
Napoleon	1 medium	15.0	285	47%
(Health Valley) fat-free tart				
baked apple cinnamon	1 tart	–	150	–
California strawberry	1 tart	–	150	–

Food and Description	Amount	Fat Grams	Total Calories	% Fat Calories
chocolate fudge	1 tart	–	150	–
cranberry apple	1 tart	–	150	–
mountain blueberry	1 tart	–	150	–
red raspberry	1 tart	–	150	–
sweet red cherry	1 tart	–	150	–
(Hostess) snack				
honey bun				
glazed	1 bun	19.0	320	53%
iced/frosted	1 bun	20.0	390	46%
(Lance) snack				
honey bun	1 bun	3.0	85	32%
pecan twirl	2 pieces	9.0	220	37%
Swiss roll	1 roll	9.0	170	48%
(Little Debbie) snack				
boxed				
honey bun	1 pkg	13.0	210	56%
pecan spinwheel	1 pkg	4.0	110	33%
individual packages				
honey bun				
3-oz bun	1 bun	23.0	380	54%
3.98-oz bun	1 bun	28.0	460	55%
pecan spinwheel	1 pkg	9.0	220	37%
(Sara Lee) fresh				
Danish				
apple cinnamon	⅛ Danish	6.0	220	25%
cinnamon crumb	⅛ Danish	7.0	200	32%
pecan twist	⅛ Danish	11.0	230	43%
raspberry	⅛ Danish	7.0	230	27%
(TastyKake) snack				
honey bun				
glazed	1 bun	17.0	350	44%
iced	1 bun	17.0	350	44%
pastry pocket				
apple	1 pastry	23.0	380	54%
cheese	1 pastry	27.0	410	59%
cherry	1 pastry	20.0	370	49%
pecan twirl	1 pkg	9.0	220	37%
whirly twirl	1 pkg	14.0	260	48%
PASTRY, TOASTER				
(Kellogg's) Pop Tarts				
bite-size minis/frosted				
chocolate	1 pouch	4.0	170	21%
grape	1 pouch	4.0	170	21%
strawberry	1 pouch	4.0	170	21%
regular				
frosted				
blueberry	1 pastry	5.0	200	23%

Food and Description	Amount	Fat Grams	Total Calories	% Fat Calories
brown sugar/cinnamon	1 pastry	7.0	210	30%
cherry	1 pastry	5.0	200	23%
chocolate fudge	1 pastry	5.0	200	23%
grape	1 pastry	5.0	200	23%
raspberry	1 pastry	6.0	210	26%
s'mores	1 pastry	5.0	200	23%
strawberry	1 pastry	5.0	200	23%
vanilla cream	1 pastry	5.0	200	23%
unfrosted				
apple cinnamon	1 pastry	5.0	210	21%
blueberry	1 pastry	7.0	210	30%
brown sugar cinnamon	1 pastry	9.0	220	37%
cherry	1 pastry	5.0	200	23%
milk chocolate graham	1 pastry	6.0	210	26%
raspberry	1 pastry	6.0	210	26%
strawberry	1 pastry	5.0	200	23%
(Nabisco)				
SnackWell's/iced				
apple cinnamon	1 pastry	1.0	170	5%
blueberry	1 pastry	1.0	170	5%
fudge	1 pastry	1.0	160	6%
Toastettes tarts				
frosted				
apple	1 pastry	5.0	190	24%
blueberry	1 pastry	5.0	190	24%
brown sugar cinnamon	1 pastry	5.0	190	24%
cherry	1 pastry	5.0	190	24%
fudge	1 pastry	5.0	200	23%
strawberry	1 pastry	5.0	190	24%
unfrosted/strawberry	1 pastry	5.0	190	24%
(Pillsbury) Toaster Strudel				
apple	1 pastry	7.0	180	35%
blueberry	1 pastry	7.0	180	35%
cherry	1 pastry	7.0	180	35%
cinnamon	1 pastry	8.0	190	38%
cream cheese	1 pastry	10.0	190	47%
cream cheese & blueberry	1 pastry	9.0	190	43%
cream cheese & strawberry	1 pastry	9.0	190	43%
French toast style	1 pastry	7.0	190	33%
raspberry	1 pastry	7.0	180	35%
strawberry	1 pastry	7.0	180	35%
PASTRY DOUGH (*See also* PIE CRUST)				
(Athens Foods) mini fillo dough shell	2 shells	2.0	45	40%
(Fillo) pastry dough sheet	1⅓ leaves	–	80	–
(Pepperidge Farm)				
patty shell	1 shell	14.0	230	55%
puff pastry dough sheet	⅙ sheet	11.0	200	50%

Food and Description	Amount	Fat Grams	Total Calories	% Fat Calories
PÂTÉ				
(Bonavita) Swiss/vegetarian	1 oz	4.0	60	60%
generic/canned				
chicken liver	1 tbs	1.7	26	59%
	1 oz	3.7	57	58%
goose liver/foie gras				
regular	1 tbs	5.7	60	86%
	1 oz	12.0	131	82%
smoked	1 Tbs	5.5	60	82%
	1 oz	12.0	131	82%
(Sell's) liver	¼ cup	14.0	160	79%
PEA (*See also* BLACK-EYED PEA; PEA DISH; PIGEON PEA; PURPLE HULL PEA; SNOW PEA; VEGETABLES, MIXED)				
canned				
(Del Monte) sweet				
no salt added	½ cup	–	60	–
regular	½ cup	–	60	–
very young small	½ cup	–	60	–
(Freshlike)				
garden sweet	½ cup	–	50	–
small	½ cup	–	50	–
generic				
Alaska/early or June				
drained	½ cup	–	75	–
undrained	½ cup	–	67	–
green	½ cup	–	59	–
sweet				
drained	½ cup	–	68	–
undrained	½ cup	–	71	–
(Green Giant) sweet				
50% less sodium	½ cup	–	60	–
regular	½ cup	–	60	–
(LeSueur)				
early	½ cup	–	60	–
sweet				
50% less sodium	½ cup	–	60	–
regular	½ cup	–	60	–
(Libby) sweet/drained	½ cup	–	60	–
(Luck's) seasoned w/pork				
crowder	½ cup	3.0	120	23%
field peas w/snaps	½ cup	3.0	130	21%
(S&W)				
petit pois/early June	½ cup	–	70	–
sweet	½ cup	–	70	–
(Seneca)	½ cup	–	70	–
(Stokely)				
early/June	½ cup	–	60	–
sweet	½ cup	–	60	–

Food and Description	Amount	Fat Grams	Total Calories	% Fat Calories
(Tendersweet)	½ cup	–	70	–
(Val Vista) early June	½ cup	–	80	–
dried				
(Arrowhead Mills) green split	¼ cup	0.5	170	3%
generic				
split	1 cup	<1.0	280	2%
whole	1 cup	<1.0	280	2%
fresh				
green				
cooked	½ cup	–	67	–
raw	½ cup	–	63	–
split/field				
boiled	½ cup	–	115	–
raw	½ cup	1.0	348	3%
sugar snap				
(Dole)	½ cup	–	30	–
frozen				
(Birds Eye)				
green	½ cup	–	70	–
portion pack	3 oz	–	70	–
sugar snap deluxe	½ cup	–	45	–
tender deluxe	½ cup	–	60	–
(C&W)				
petite				
microwave box	⅔ cup	0.5	70	6%
no salt added	⅔ cup	0.5	70	6%
regular	⅔ cup	0.5	70	6%
sugar snap	⅔ cup	–	35	–
(Chun King) Chinese	1.5 oz	–	20	–
generic/edible-podded/boiled	½ cup	–	54	–
(Green Giant)				
sugar snap				
Harvest Fresh	⅔ cup	–	50	–
regular	¾ cup	–	35	–
sweet				
Harvest Fresh	⅔ cup	–	60	–
regular	⅔ cup	–	70	–
(La Choy)				
(LeSueur)				
baby early/Harvest Fresh	⅔ cup	–	70	–
baby sweet	⅔ cup	–	60	–
early June				
plain	⅔ cup	–	60	–
w/mushrooms	¾ cup	–	60	–
(Seneca)	⅔ cup	–	80	–
(Veg-All)	3.3 oz	–	60	–

PEA, BLACK-EYED (See BLACK-EYED PEA)

Food and Description	Amount	Fat Grams	Total Calories	% Fat Calories
PEA, PIGEON (*See* PIGEON PEA)				
PEA, PURPLE HULL (*See* PURPLE HULL PEA)				
PEA, SNOW (*See* SNOW PEA)				
PEA DISH (*See also* PEA; VEGETABLES, MIXED)				
(Green Giant) frozen sweet peas in butter sauce	¾ cup	2.0	100	18%
(LeSueur) frozen baby early peas in butter sauce	¾ cup	2.0	100	18%
PEACH				
can or cup				
(Del Monte)				
cling				
halves				
in extra light syrup/lite	½ cup	–	60	–
in heavy syrup	½ cup	–	100	–
melba/in heavy syrup	½ cup	–	100	–
sliced				
in extra light syrup/lite	½ cup	–	60	–
in heavy syrup	½ cup	–	100	–
in pear & peach juices/Fruit Naturals	½ cup	–	60	–
whole/spiced/in heavy syrup	½ cup	–	100	–
freestone				
halves/in heavy syrup	½ cup	–	100	–
sliced				
in extra light syrup/lite	½ cup	–	60	–
in heavy syrup	½ cup	–	100	–
fruit cups				
diced				
in extra light syrup/lite	4.25 oz	–	60	–
in heavy syrup	4.25 oz	–	90	–
in light syrup	3.50 oz	–	70	–
in pear & peach juices/ Fruit Naturals	4.25 oz	–	60	–
generic				
sliced				
in heavy syrup	1 cup	–	190	–
in juice	1 cup	–	109	–
in water	1 cup	–	58	–
spiced/in syrup	1 cup	–	180	–
whole/in heavy syrup	½ cup	–	90	–
(Hunt's)				
halves	½ cup	–	100	–
sliced	½ cup	–	100	–
(Libby's) lite/in juice				
halves	½ cup	–	50	–
sliced	½ cup	–	50	–

Food and Description	Amount	Fat Grams	Total Calories	% Fat Calories
(S&W)				
ready-cut				
California Sun	½ cup	–	80	–
clingstone				
halves/in heavy syrup	½ cup	–	100	–
sliced				
in heavy syrup	½ cup	–	100	–
in peach juice/natural style	½ cup	–	90	–
freestone				
halves/in heavy syrup	½ cup	–	100	–
sliced/in heavy syrup	½ cup	–	100	–
Sweet Memory w/cinnamon	½ cup	–	70	–
Tropical Sun	½ cup	–	80	–
whole/spiced/in heavy syrup	1 peach	–	100	–
dried				
(Del Monte) sun-dried	⅓ cup	–	90	–
generic/halves				
cooked				
w/sugar	½ cup	<1.0	165	3%
w/o sugar	½ cup	<1.0	100	5%
uncooked	½ cup	0.6	191	2%
	10 medium	0.9	341	2%
(Mariani)	¼ cup	–	140	–
(Sun Maid)	¼ cup	–	100	–
(SunSweet)	¼ cup	–	140	–
fresh				
peeled/sliced	½ cup	–	37	–
whole	1 medium	–	37	–
(Dole)	2 medium	–	70	–
frozen				
(Big Valley) freestone	⅔ cup	–	50	–
(C&W) sliced	⅔ cup	–	50	–
generic/sliced				
sweetened	1 cup	<1.0	235	2%
unsweetened	3.5 oz	<1.0	45	10%
	1 cup	<1.0	132	3%
PEACH BUTTER				
(Smucker's)	1 tsp	–	15	–
PEACH JUICE/JUICE BLEND/JUICE DRINK (See also FRUIT PUNCH; SOFT DRINK; SOFT DRINK MIX)				
bottled, boxed, or canned				
(Dole) orchard peach 100% juice blend	8 fl oz	–	140	–
	10 fl oz	–	170	–
(Goya) nectar	6 fl oz	–	110	–
(Kern's) nectar	11.5 fl oz	–	210	–
(Knudsen)				
After the Fall/Georgia peach	8 fl oz	–	100	–
Thirst Quencher/nectar	8 fl oz	–	120	–

Food and Description	Amount	Fat Grams	Total Calories	% Fat Calories
(Libby's) nectar	8 fl oz	–	130	–
(Smucker's)	8 fl oz	–	120	–
(TreeTop) Peach Quake	8 fl oz	–	120	–
frozen/prepared				
(Dole) Orchard Peach 100% juice blend	8 fl oz	–	140	–
(Mott's) Fruit Basket				
orchard peach juice cocktail	8 fl oz	–	130	–
PEANUT				
(Ballpark)	1 oz	15.0	180	75%
(Eagle)				
lightly salted	1 oz	15.0	180	75%
oil honey-roasted	1 oz	13.0	170	69%
roasted	1 oz	15.0	180	75%
(Fisher)				
dry/honey-roasted	1 oz	13.0	150	78%
golden roasted	1 oz	14.0	170	74%
honey-roasted	1 oz	14.0	160	79%
oil-roasted	1 oz	15.0	170	79%
salted in shell/shelled	1 oz	14.0	170	74%
Spanish/roasted	1 oz	16.0	180	80%
(Frito Lay)				
hot	¼ cup	21.0	280	68%
salted	1 oz	15.0	180	75%
generic				
all types				
boiled	½ cup	7.0	102	62%
dried	1 oz	14.0	161	78%
dry-roasted				
lite	1 oz	9.0	135	60%
regular	1 oz	13.9	164	76%
honey-roasted	1 oz	13.0	170	69%
oil-roasted	1 oz	13.8	163	76%
	½ cup	35.5	418	76%
Spanish				
oil-roasted	1 oz	14.0	160	78%
	½ cup	36.0	425	76%
raw	1 oz	13.7	162	76%
	½ cup	36.0	415	78%
Valencia				
oil-roasted	1 oz	14.0	165	76%
	½ cup	37.0	424	78%
raw	1 oz	13.0	160	73%
	½ cup	35.0	420	75%
Virginia				
oil-roasted	1 oz	13.7	160	77%
	½ cup	35.0	415	76%
raw	1 oz	13.5	160	76%
	½ cup	35.5	410	78%

Food and Description	Amount	Fat Grams	Total Calories	% Fat Calories
(Guy's)				
dry-roasted	1 oz	14.0	170	74%
Spanish/salted	1 oz	14.0	170	74%
(Lance)				
honey-toasted	¼ cup	14.0	200	63%
	1⅜ oz	15.0	220	61%
roasted	1¾ oz	14.0	190	66%
salted				
long tube	¼ cup	14.0	180	70%
	2⅛ oz	15.0	190	74%
regular	⅞ oz	12.0	150	72%
	1⅛ oz	15.0	200	68%
(Laura Scudder's)				
Spanish	1 oz	15.0	180	75%
Virgina	1 oz	15.0	180	75%
(Planters)				
all types				
dry-roasted	1 oz	14.0	170	74%
lightly salted	1 oz	14.0	160	79%
	1.75 oz	25.0	290	78%
unsalted	1 oz	14.0	160	79%
honey dry-roasted	1.7 oz	19.0	260	69%
honey-roasted	1 oz	13.0	160	73%
oil-roasted	2 oz	24.0	340	77%
cocktail	1 oz	14.0	170	74%
lightly salted	1 oz	15.0	170	79%
unsalted	1 oz	14.0	160	79%
fun size	2 bags	14.0	170	74%
heat hot spicy	1 oz	14.0	160	79%
	1.7 oz	25.0	290	78%
	2 oz	29.0	330	79%
lightly salted	1.75 oz	27.0	300	81%
Munch 'N Go singles	2.5 oz	36.0	410	79%
Munch 'N Go	3 Tbs	15.0	170	79%
Pennant	1 oz	14.0	170	74%
salted	1.7 oz	25.0	290	78%
sweet n crunchy	1 oz	7.0	140	45%
Spanish				
raw	1 oz	13.0	150	78%
oil-roasted	1 oz	14.0	170	74%
(Weight Watchers) honey-roasted	0.7 oz	5.0	100	45%
PEANUT BUTTER				
(Arrowhead Mills) 100% Valencia/sodium-free				
creamy	2 Tbs	15.0	200	68%
crunchy	2 Tbs	15.0	200	68%
(Bama)				
creamy	2 Tbs	17.0	200	77%
crunchy	2 Tbs	17.0	200	77%

Food and Description	Amount	Fat Grams	Total Calories	% Fat Calories
(Country Pure)				
chunky	2 Tbs	16.0	190	76%
creamy	2 Tbs	16.0	190	76%
(Erewhon)				
chunky				
regular	2 Tbs	14.0	190	66%
unsalted	2 Tbs	14.0	190	66%
creamy				
regular	2 Tbs	14.0	190	66%
unsalted	2 Tbs	14.0	190	66%
(Estee)				
creamy	2 Tbs	15.0	190	71%
crunchy	2 Tbs	15.0	190	71%
(Featherweight)				
chunky	2 Tbs	15.0	190	71%
creamy	2 Tbs	15.0	190	71%
generic				
chunky	2 Tbs	16.0	188	77%
	½ cup	64.0	760	76%
	1 cup	132.0	1526	78%
creamy	2 Tbs	16.0	188	77%
	½ cup	64.0	760	76%
	1 cup	131.0	1526	78%
(Health Valley)				
chunky				
no salt	2 Tbs	14.0	170	74%
regular	2 Tbs	14.0	170	74%
creamy				
no salt	2 Tbs	14.0	170	74%
regular	2 Tbs	14.0	170	74%
(Jif)				
original				
creamy	2 Tbs	16.0	190	76%
extra crunchy	2 Tbs	16.0	190	76%
reduced fat				
creamy	2 Tbs	12.0	190	57%
crunchy	2 Tbs	12.0	190	57%
Simply Jif				
creamy	2 Tbs	16.0	190	76%
crunchy	2 Tbs	16.0	190	76%
(Knott's Berry Farm)				
creamy	2 Tbs	16.0	190	76%
crunchy	2 Tbs	16.0	190	76%
(Laura Scudder's)				
old fashioned				
creamy				
regular	2 Tbs	16.0	200	72%
unsalted	2 Tbs	16.0	200	72%

Food and Description	Amount	Fat Grams	Total Calories	% Fat Calories
nutty				
regular	2 Tbs	16.0	200	72%
unsalted	2 Tbs	16.0	200	72%
reduced fat/creamy	2 Tbs	12.0	200	54%
(Nu Made)				
chunky	2 Tbs	16.0	190	76%
creamy	2 Tbs	16.0	190	76%
(Peter Pan)				
creamy				
regular	2 Tbs	16.0	190	75%
very low sodium	2 Tbs	17.0	200	77%
crunchy				
regular	2 Tbs	16.0	190	75%
very low sodium	2 Tbs	17.0	200	77%
Smart Choice spread				
creamy	2 Tbs	11.0	180	55%
crunchy	2 Tbs	12.0	190	57%
whipped				
creamy	2 Tbs	13.0	150	78%
crunchy	2 Tbs	13.0	150	78%
(President's Choice) Too Good to Be True				
creamy	2 Tbs	18.0	210	77%
crunchy	2 Tbs	18.0	210	77%
(Real)				
creamy	2 Tbs	16.0	190	75%
crunchy	2 Tbs	16.0	190	75%
(Reese's)				
creamy	2 Tbs	16.0	200	72%
crunchy	2 Tbs	16.0	200	72%
(Roaster Fresh) gourmet/unsalted	2 Tbs	14.0	170	74%
(Skippy)				
reduced fat				
creamy	2 Tbs	12.0	190	57%
super chunk	2 Tbs	12.0	180	60%
roasted honey nut/creamy	2 Tbs	17.0	190	81%
super chunk	2 Tbs	17.0	190	81%
	1 cup	138.0	1560	80%
(Smucker's)				
Goober peanut butter & jelly	3 Tbs	13.0	230	51%
old fashioned natural				
chunky	2 Tbs	16.0	200	72%
creamy	2 Tbs	16.0	200	72%
original				
chunky	2 Tbs	16.0	200	72%
creamy	2 Tbs	16.0	200	72%
stabilized				
chunky	2 Tbs	15.0	190	71%
creamy	2 Tbs	15.0	190	71%

Food and Description	Amount	Fat Grams	Total Calories	% Fat Calories
(Westbrae) natural				
chunky				
regular	2 Tbs	16.0	190	76%
no salt	2 Tbs	16.0	190	76%
creamy/no salt	2 Tbs	16.0	190	76%
PEANUT BUTTER FLAVORED BAKING CHIPS (See BAKING BITS, CHIPS, CHUNKS, & PIECES)				
PEANUT FLOUR (See FLOUR)				
PEAR				
candied	1 oz	–	86	–
canned				
(Del Monte)				
halves				
in extra light syrup/lite	½ cup	–	60	–
in pear juice/Fruit Naturals	½ cup	–	60	–
in heavy syrup	½ cup	–	100	–
sliced				
in extra light syrup/lite	½ cup	–	60	–
in heavy syrup	½ cup	–	100	–
generic/solids & liquid				
in extra heavy syrup	1 cup	<1.0	250	1%
in extra light syrup	1 cup	<1.0	115	2%
in heavy syrup	1 cup	<1.0	190	2%
in juice	1 cup	<1.0	125	1%
in light syrup	1 cup	<1.0	140	2%
in water	1 cup	<1.0	70	2%
(Libby's) lite				
halves	½ cup	–	60	–
sliced	½ cup	–	60	–
(S&W)				
Bartlett halves/in heavy syrup	½ cup	–	90	–
quartered/in heavy syrup	½ cup	–	90	–
sliced/in pear juice	½ cup	–	80	–
dried				
generic				
cooked				
sweetened	½ cup	0.5	200	2%
unsweetened	½ cup	0.5	165	3%
uncooked	½ cup	0.5	240	2%
(Mariani) dried	¼ cup	–	150	–
fresh				
Bartlett	1 medium	1.0	100	9%
California Sun/ready-cut	½ cup	–	80	–
D'Anjou				
sliced	1 cup	0.7	97	6%
whole	1 medium	1.0	120	8%
(Dole)	1 medium	1.0	100	9%

Food and Description	Amount	Fat Grams	Total Calories	% Fat Calories
PEAR JUICE/NECTAR				
canned				
(Goya) nectar	6 fl oz	–	120	–
(Kern's) nectar	6 fl oz	–	120	–
(Knudsen) Rogue River pear juice	8 fl oz	–	120	–
(Libby's) nectar	6 fl oz	–	110	–
PECAN				
(Azar)				
chips	1 oz	21.0	210	90%
halves	1 oz	21.0	210	90%
pieces	1 oz	21.0	210	90%
(Fisher)				
chopped	1 oz	19.0	190	90%
ground	1 oz	19.0	190	90%
raw	1 oz	19.0	190	90%
generic				
dried	1 oz	19.0	190	90%
halves	1 cup	73.0	721	91%
dry-roasted	1 oz	18.0	187	87%
	10 extra large	28.7	277	93%
fresh				
in shell	10 large	24.5	236	93%
shelled	2 oz	40.0	390	92%
chopped	1 Tbs	5.0	52	87%
	1 cup	84.0	811	93%
ground	1 cup	67.6	653	93%
halves	10 large	6.0	62	87%
	10 jumbo	10.0	96	94%
	10 mammoth	12.8	124	93%
	1 cup	76.9	742	93%
oil-roasted	1 oz	20.0	195	92%
(Planters)				
chips	2 oz	40.0	390	92%
halves				
Gold Measure	2 oz	40.0	390	92%
regular	1 oz	20.0	190	95%
honey-roasted	1 oz	16.0	180	80%
pieces	1 oz	20.0	190	95%
PECAN FLOUR (See FLOUR)				
PECTIN (See FRUIT PECTIN)				
PEPPER (See also MEXICAN FOOD; PEPPER, GROUND; SEASONINGS)				
canned or jarred				
(Hebrew National)				
filet peppers	1 oz	–	9	–
hot cherry	1 oz	–	11	–
red filet peppers	1 oz	–	9	–

Food and Description	Amount	Fat Grams	Total Calories	% Fat Calories
(Heinz)				
banana/hot	1 pepper	–	6	–
hot rings/slices	1 pepper	–	4	–
mild sweet	1 pepper	–	8	–
sweet pepper momentos	1 pepper	–	6	–
(Progresso)				
cherry/drained	2 Tbs	2.0	30	60%
fried-drained	2 Tbs	5.0	60	75%
hot cherry	1 pepper	–	15	–
pepper salad/drained	2 Tbs	2.0	25	72%
roasted	½ piece	–	10	–
Tuscan/drained	3 peppers	–	10	–
(Rosoff's) sweet	1 oz	–	9	–
(Schorr's) filet	1 oz	–	9	–
(Trappey's)				
hot/in vinegar	15 peppers	–	9	–
jalapeño/hot				
sliced	21 slices	–	4	–
whole	1 pepper	–	11	–
Serrano/hot	3 peppers	–	7	–
tempero/Greek peperoncini/mild	1 pepper	–	7	–
torrido/Santa Fe grande/hot	1 pepper	–	10	–
(Vlasic)				
banana/hot	1 oz	–	4	–
cherry				
hot	1 oz	–	10	–
mild	1 oz	–	8	–
Greek pepperoncini salad				
hot	1 oz	–	10	–
mild	1 oz	–	4	–
Mexican hot	1 oz	–	8	–
Mexican tiny hot	1 oz	–	6	–
dried				
green	1 Tbs	–	1	–
red	1 Tbs	–	1	–
freeze-dried/sweet red or green	1 Tbs	–	1	–
	½ cup	–	10	–
fresh				
green chili/hot				
chopped	½ cup	–	16	–
whole	1 medium	–	15	–
jalapeño				
chopped	½ cup	–	20	–
whole	2 medium	–	14	–
red chili/hot				
chopped	½ cup	–	17	–
whole	1 medium	–	18	–

Food and Description	Amount	Fat Grams	Total Calories	% Fat Calories
red or green/sweet				
chopped	½ cup	–	12	–
whole	1 medium	–	18	–
yellow/sweet				
chopped	10 strips	–	14	–
whole	1 medium	–	50	–
frozen				
(Birds Eye) green & red, stir-fry	3 oz	–	25	–
(C&W) green & red/strips	3 oz	–	25	–
(Southland) sweet				
green, diced	2 oz	–	10	–
green & red/cut	2 oz	–	15	–
PEPPER, GROUND (See also PEPPER; SEASONINGS)				
(Durkee)				
black	1 tsp	–	8	–
red/cayenne	1 tsp	–	8	–
white	1 tsp	–	9	–
generic				
black	1 tsp	–	5	–
	1 Tbs	–	15	–
chili	1 tsp	–	9	–
red/cayenne	1 tsp	–	5	–
	1 Tbs	–	15	–
white	1 tsp	–	7	–
	1 Tbs	–	20	–
(Lawry's) lemon	1 tsp	–	6	–
PEPPER DISH (See also FROZEN ENTRÉE/DINNER; VEGETARIAN FOODS)				
homemade/USDA Standard Home Recipe				
stuffed pepper				
w/beef & bread crumbs	1 medium	10.5	325	29%
w/beef & rice	½ medium	13.0	219	53%
w/rice only	~5 oz	11.9	198	54%
PEPPER POT SOUP (See SOUP)				
PEPPERONI (See SAUSAGE)				
PERCH (See OCEAN PERCH; WHITE PERCH)				
PERSIMMON				
Japanese/kaki				
dried	1 medium	<1.0	93	5%
fresh	1 medium	<1.0	118	4%
native/fresh	1 medium	–	32	–
PESTO SAUCE (See SAUCE)				
PHEASANT/raw				
breast meat	~6 oz	5.9	243	22%
giblets	3 oz	4.0	119	30%
leg meat	~4 oz	4.6	143	29%
meat & skin	~1 lb	42.0	825	46%
meat only	~¾ lb	12.8	470	25%
PHYLLO DOUGH (See PASTRY DOUGH)				

Food and Description	Amount	Fat Grams	Total Calories	% Fat Calories
PICANTE SAUCE (*See* MEXICAN FOOD; SAUCE)				
PICCALILLI (*See* PICKLE RELISH)				
PICKLE				
(Arnold's)				
dill				
German	1 oz	–	–	–
hot	1 oz	–	–	–
kosher	1 oz	–	–	–
kosher/spears	1 oz	–	–	–
regular	1 oz	–	–	–
hamburger slices	1 oz	–	–	–
(Claussen)				
bread 'n butter				
chips	4 slices	–	20	–
sandwich slices	2 slices	–	20	–
half sours/New York deli style	½ pickle	–	5	–
hamburger dills slices/chips	10 slices	–	5	–
kosher dills				
halves	½ pickle	–	5	–
mini	1 pickle	–	5	–
sandwich slices	2 slices	–	5	–
slices	4 slices	–	5	–
spears	1 spear	–	5	–
whole	½ pickle	–	5	–
(Del Monte)				
dill				
halves	¼ pickle	–	5	–
hamburger chips	5½ chips	–	5	–
tiny kosher	1½ pickles	–	5	–
sweet				
chips	5 chips	–	40	–
gherkins	2 pickles	–	40	–
midget	3 pickles	–	40	–
whole				
8- or 22-oz jar	2 pickles	–	40	–
12-oz jar	1 pickle	–	40	–
(Featherweight) dill/whole	1 medium	–	5	–
generic				
bread & butter	3 slices	–	16	–
dill				
deli style halves	1 oz	–	4	–
genuine	1 oz	–	2	–
hamburger	1 oz	–	2	–
whole	1 medium	–	15	–
gherkins	1 small	–	22	–
hamburger chips	1 oz	–	2	–
(Hebrew National)				
half-sour	1 oz	–	4	–

Food and Description	Amount	Fat Grams	Total Calories	% Fat Calories
kosher				
barrel cured dill				
hot	1 pouch	–	23	–
regular	1 pouch	–	23	–
chips	1 oz	–	4	–
halves	1 oz	–	4	–
large	1 oz	–	4	–
spears	1 oz	–	4	–
whole	1 oz	–	4	–
kraut sour garlic	1 oz	–	3	–
(Heinz)				
hot garlic	1 oz	–	6	–
kosher				
dill				
baby	1 oz	–	4	–
chips	1 oz	–	4	–
spears	1 oz	–	4	–
whole	1 oz	–	4	–
halves	1 piece	–	9	–
old fashioned				
chips	1 oz	–	4	–
deli halves	1 oz	–	4	–
whole	1 oz	–	4	–
slices	1 oz	–	3	–
whole	1 oz	–	2	–
pickled cucumbers	2 spears	–	13	–
Polish syle				
dill	1 oz	–	4	–
dill/spears	1 oz	–	4	–
Polskie ogorki	1 oz	–	6	–
processed dill	1 oz	–	2	–
sour	1 oz	–	3	–
sweet				
gherkins/midget or regular	1 oz	–	35	–
mixed	1 oz	–	40	–
pickles	1 oz	–	35	–
salad cubes	1 oz	–	30	–
slices	1 oz	–	35	–
sweet cucumber				
slices	1 oz	–	20	–
stix	1 oz	–	25	–
(Mrs. Klein's) fancy imported				
pepperoncini	1 oz	–	5	–
Southern hot mix	1 oz	–	–	–
(Mt. Olive)				
bread & butter	1 oz	–	25	–
dill	1 oz	–	–	–

Food and Description	Amount	Fat Grams	Total Calories	% Fat Calories
kosher dill	1 oz	–	–	–
baby	1 oz	–	–	–
chips	1 oz	–	–	–
strips	1 oz	–	–	–
sweet	1 oz	–	35	–
cucumber strips	1 oz	–	20	–
midgets	1 oz	–	35	–
(Rosoff's)				
kosher				
halves	1 oz	–	4	–
whole	1 oz	–	4	–
sour				
half spears	1 oz	–	4	–
halves	1 oz	–	4	–
(Schorr's)				
bread & butter	1 oz	–	12	–
kosher				
deli	1 oz	–	4	–
halves	1 oz	–	4	–
spears	1 oz	–	4	–
whole	1 oz	–	4	–
sour				
garlic whole	1 oz	–	3	–
half spears	1 oz	–	4	–
halves	1 oz	–	4	–
(Steinfeld's)				
garlic dills	1 oz	–	5	–
Greek pepperoncini	1 oz	–	5	–
homestyle dills	1 oz	–	5	–
kosher				
dills	1 oz	–	5	–
spears	1 oz	–	5	–
Polish dills	1 oz	–	5	–
sandwich builders				
bread & butter	1 oz	–	–	–
kosher dill	1 oz	–	5	–
baby	1 oz	–	5	–
tiny	1 oz	–	5	–
Polish dill	1 oz	–	–	–
zesty dill	1 oz	–	–	–
sweet	1 oz	–	30	–
cucumber chips	1 oz	–	30	–
(Vlasic)				
Half-The-Salt				
hamburger dill chips	1 oz	–	2	–
kosher crunchy dills	1 oz	–	4	–
kosher dill spears	1 oz	–	4	–
sweet butter chips	1 oz	–	30	–

Food and Description	Amount	Fat Grams	Total Calories	% Fat Calories
kosher				
baby dills	1 oz	–	4	–
crunchy dills	1 oz	–	4	–
dill gherkins	1 oz	–	4	–
dill spears	1 oz	–	4	–
snack chunks	1 oz	–	4	–
no garlic				
crunchy dills	1 oz	–	4	–
dill spears	1 oz	–	4	–
refrigerated				
deli bread & butter	1 oz	–	25	–
deli dill halves	1 oz	–	4	–
regular				
bread & butter chunks	1 oz	–	25	–
original dills				
original dills	1 oz	–	2	–
Polish snack chunks	1 oz	–	4	–
zesty crunchy dills	1 oz	–	4	–
zesty dill snack chunks	1 oz	–	4	–
zesty dill spears	1 oz	–	4	–
sweet butter chips	1 oz	–	30	–
sweet butter stix	1 oz	–	18	–
PICKLE RELISH				
(Arnold's) sweet	1 Tbs	–	15	–
(Claussen) sweet	1 Tbs	–	15	–
(Del Monte)				
hamburger	1 Tbs	–	20	–
hot dog	1 Tbs	–	15	–
sweet	1 Tbs	–	20	–
(Hebrew National) sweet/green	1 Tbs	–	18	–
(Heinz)				
piccalilli	1 oz	–	30	–
relish				
dill	1 Tbs	–	–	–
hamburger	1 Tbs	–	15	–
hot dog	1 Tbs	–	15	–
sweet	1 Tbs	–	30	–
(Mt. Olive) sweet	1 Tbs	–	20	–
(Vlasic)				
piccalilli				
green tomato	1 oz	–	35	–
hot	1 oz	–	35	–
relish				
dill	1 oz	–	2	–
hamburger	1 oz	–	40	–
hot dog	1 oz	<1.0	40	11%
India	1 oz	–	30	–
sweet	1 oz	–	30	–

Food and Description	Amount	Fat Grams	Total Calories	% Fat Calories
PIE & COBBLER (*See also* PIE CRUST; PIE FILLING & GLAZE)				
■ **FROZEN OR REFRIGERATED**				
(Amy's) apple pie	1 pie	12.0	280	39%
(Banquet) pie				
apple	4 oz	13.0	300	39%
banana	⅓ pie	21.0	350	54%
cherry	4 oz	14.0	290	43%
chocolate	⅓ pie	20.0	360	50%
coconut cream	⅓ pie	20.0	350	51%
lemon	⅓ pie	20.0	360	50%
mincemeat	4 oz	13.0	310	38%
peach	4 oz	12.0	260	42%
pumpkin	⅙ pie	8.0	250	29%
(Chef Pierre) food service				
condensed/10" pie				
ice box				
chocolate	1/9 pie	11.0	310	32%
coconut	1/9 pie	12.0	330	33%
lemon	⅛ pie	10.0	380	24%
lime	⅛ pie	9.0	360	20%
tropical				
Key West lime	⅛ pie	16.0	460	31%
country fruit cobbler				
apple	1/18 cobbler	9.0	230	35%
blackberry	1/18 cobbler	10.0	260	35%
cherry	1/18 cobbler	9.0	260	31%
peach	1/18 cobbler	9.0	240	34%
creme de la cream pie				
banana	1/10 pie	17.0	300	51%
cappuccino	⅛ pie	29.0	430	61%
chocolate	1/9 pie	28.0	400	63%
coconut	1/10 pie	20.0	350	51%
cookies & cream	1/9 pie	28.0	410	61%
double chocolate	1/10 pie	19.0	360	48%
lemon	1/9 pie	24.0	360	60%
toffee crunch	1/9 pie	29.0	430	61%
gourmet silk pie				
chocolate peanut butter	⅛ pie	35.0	500	63%
French silk	⅛ pie	35.0	490	64%
meringue pie				
gourmet				
chocolate	1/10 pie	12.0	320	34%
coconut	1/10 pie	14.0	340	37%
lemon	1/10 pie	8.0	290	25%
regular				
chocolate	1/10 pie	12.0	320	34%
coconut	⅛ pie	14.0	340	37%
lemon	⅛ pie	9.0	290	28%

Food and Description	Amount	Fat Grams	Total Calories	% Fat Calories
lime	⅛ pie	15.0	440	31%
prebaked individually wrapped slices				
apple				
24 pack	1 slice	11.0	300	33%
48 pack	1 slice	9.0	270	30%
cherry				
24 pack	1 slice	11.0	290	34%
48 pack	1 slice	11.0	280	35%
ice box lemon	1 slice	9.0	260	30%
Southern pecan	1 slice	23.0	470	44%
prebaked 10" pie				
full crust				
apple	1/10 pie	15.0	350	39%
cherry	1/10 pie	17.0	380	40%
Hi-Pie				
apple	1/10 pie	19.0	350	49%
blueberry	1/9 pie	19.0	380	45%
cherry	1/9 pie	17.0	360	43%
peach	1/9 pie	19.0	370	46%
lattice top				
apple	1/9 pie	12.0	320	34%
blueberry	1/9 pie	12.0	330	32%
cherry	1/9 pie	12.0	310	35%
peach	1/9 pie	12.0	300	36%
specialty pie				
Boston cream	1/10 pie	7.0	220	29%
chocolate chip pecan	⅛ pie	34.0	560	55%
French coconut	⅛ pie	22.0	490	40%
pumpkin	1/9 pie	11.0	330	30%
Southern pecan	⅛ pie	27.0	570	43%
sweet potato	⅛ pie	19.0	410	42%
traditional cream/10" pie				
banana	⅙ pie	22.0	400	50%
chocolate	⅙ pie	23.0	410	50%
coconut	⅙ pie	25.0	430	52%
lemon	⅙ pie	23.0	420	49%
lime	⅙ pie	23.0	420	49%
unbaked pie				
gourmet Hi-Pie				
apple				
9" pie	⅛ pie	21.0	370	51%
10" pie	1/10 pie	27.0	440	55%
Apple Razz/10" pie	1/10 pie	23.0	380	54%
apple w/butter10" pie	1/10 pie	23.0	410	50%
apple-cranberry w/icing/10" pie	1/10 pie	22.0	440	45%
blackberry/10" pie	1/10 pie	20.0	410	44%
blueberry				
9" pie	⅛ pie	18.0	390	42%

Food and Description	Amount	Fat Grams	Total Calories	% Fat Calories
10" pie	1/10 pie	20.0	410	44%
cherry				
9" pie	1/8 pie	19.0	370	46%
10" pie	1/10 pie	20.0	400	45%
Dutch apple/9" pie	1/8 pie	18.0	390	42%
Fruits of the Forest/10" pie	1/10 pie	19.0	350	49%
peach				
9" pie	1/8 pie	19.0	340	50%
10" pie	1/10 pie	18.0	360	45%
peach & apricot/10" pie	1/10 pie	21.0	380	50%
rhubarb/10" pie	1/10 pie	18.0	360	45%
regular/10" pie				
apple				
original	1/10 pie	16.0	340	42%
reduced fat	1/8 pie	5.0	270	17%
blackberry	1/10 pie	16.0	360	40%
blueberry	1/10 pie	16.0	350	41%
boysenberry	1/10 pie	16.0	360	40%
cherry	1/10 pie	15.0	330	41%
coconut custard	1/8 pie	16.0	320	45%
Dutch apple	1/10 pie	14.0	360	35%
egg custard	1/8 pie	9.0	240	34%
lemon krunch	1/8 pie	17.0	430	36%
mince	1/10 pie	18.0	370	44%
peach	1/10 pie	16.0	340	42%
pumpkin	1/8 pie	11.0	280	35%
raisin	1/10 pie	16.0	350	40%
red raspberry	1/10 pie	18.0	360	45%
strawberry-rhubarb	1/10 pie	18.0	360	45%
(Marie Callender's) cobbler				
apple	1/4 cobbler	18.0	350	46%
berry				
10-oz cobbler	4 oz	19.0	350	49%
17-oz cobbler	1/4 cobbler	19.0	390	44%
blueberry	1/4 cobbler	18.0	340	48%
cherry	1/4 cobbler	19.0	390	44%
peach				
10-oz cobbler	4 oz	16.0	340	42%
17-oz cobbler	1/4 cobbler	18.0	370	44%
(Mrs. Smith's) pie				
apple				
lattice/ready to serve/8" pie	1/5 pie	13.0	310	38%
regular				
8" pie	1/6 pie	11.0	270	37%
9" pie	1/8 pie	14.0	310	41%
10" pie	1/10 pie	12.0	280	39%
old fashioned/special recipe/9" pie	1/8 pie	16.0	350	41%
apple-cranberry/8" pie	1/6 pie	11.0	280	35%

Food and Description	Amount	Fat Grams	Total Calories	% Fat Calories
banana cream/8" pie	¼ pie	14.0	280	45%
berry/8" pie	⅙ pie	11.0	280	35%
blackberry/8" pie	⅙ pie	11.0	280	35%
blueberry/8" pie	⅙ pie	11.0	260	38%
Boston cream/8" pie	⅛ pie	5.0	170	26%
cherry				
lattice top/ready to serve/8" pie	⅕ pie	13.0	320	37%
old fashioned/special recipe/9" pie	⅛ pie	13.0	320	37%
regular				
8" pie	⅙ pie	11.0	270	37%
9" pie	⅛ pie	14.0	350	36%
10" pie	⅒ pie	11.0	280	35%
chocolate cream/8" pie	¼ pie	17.0	330	46%
coconut cream/8" pie	¼ pie	19.0	340	50%
coconut custard/8" pie	⅕ pie	12.0	280	39%
Dutch apple				
old fashioned/special recipe/9" pie	⅑ pie	12.0	310	35%
regular				
8" pie	⅙ pie	13.0	320	37%
9" pie	⅛ pie	14.0	350	36%
10" pie	⅒ pie	12.0	320	34%
French silk/8" pie	⅕ pie	21.0	410	46%
lemon cream/8" pie	¼ pie	15.0	300	45%
lemon meringue/8" pie	⅕ pie	8.0	300	24%
mince/8" pie	⅙ pie	11.0	300	33%
peach				
regular/8" pie	⅙ pie	11.0	260	38%
old fashioned/special recipe/9" pie	⅛ pie	13.0	310	38%
pecan				
8" pie	⅕ pie	23.0	520	40%
10" pie	⅛ pie	23.0	500	41%
pumpkin, hearty				
8" pie	⅕ pie	8.0	250	29%
9" pie	⅛ pie	7.0	240	26%
pumpkin custard				
8" pie	⅕ pie	8.0	270	27%
9" pie	⅛ pie	8.0	230	31%
10" pie	⅑ pie	8.0	250	29%
red raspberry/8" pie	⅙ pie	11.0	280	35%
strawberry/8" pie	⅕ pie	11.0	290	34%
strawberry rhubarb/8" pie	⅙ pie	11.0	280	35%
(Pet-Ritz)				
cobbler				
apple	⅙ cobbler	12.0	280	39%
apple crumb	⅙ cobbler	9.0	280	29%
blackberry	⅙ cobbler	11.0	260	38%
blackberry crumb	⅙ cobbler	9.0	280	29%
blueberry	⅙ cobbler	11.0	280	35%

Food and Description	Amount	Fat Grams	Total Calories	% Fat Calories
cherry	⅙ cobbler	11.0	300	33%
cherry crumb	⅙ cobbler	8.0	260	28%
peach	⅙ cobbler	9.0	230	35%
peach crumb	⅙ cobbler	7.0	230	27%
strawberry	⅙ cobbler	9.0	260	31%
cream pie				
banana	¼ pie	13.0	270	43%
chocolate	¼ pie	13.0	290	40%
coconut	¼ pie	13.0	270	43%
fudge vanilla	¼ pie	15.0	300	45%
key lime	¼ pie	13.0	270	43%
lemon	¼ pie	13.0	270	43%
peanut butter chocolate	¼ pie	15.0	300	45%
pumpkin	¼ pie	13.0	270	43%
(Sara Lee's) homestyle/9" pie				
apple	⅛ pie	17.0	330	46%
blueberry	⅛ pie	15.0	350	39%
cherry	⅛ pie	16.0	320	45%
chocolate cream	⅕ pie	32.0	500	58%
coconut cream	⅕ pie	31.0	480	58%
Dutch apple	⅛ pie	15.0	350	39%
lemon meringue	⅙ pie	11.0	350	28%
peach	⅛ pie	14.0	320	39%
pecan	⅛ pie	24.0	520	42%
pumpkin	⅛ pie	11.0	260	38%
(Schwan's) old fashioned				
apple	1/12 pie	13.0	270	43%
cherry	1/10 pie	15.0	320	42%
pumpkin	1/10 pie	10.0	250	36%
(Weight Watchers)				
chocolate mocha	2.75 oz	4.0	170	21%
chocolate mousse	2.75 oz	4.0	190	19%
Mississippi mud	5.04 oz	5.0	180	25%
praline pecan mousse	2.71 oz	3.5	170	19%
triple chocolate caramel mousse	2.75 oz	4.0	200	18%

■ HOMEMADE

USDA Standard Home Recipe (Note: Pie crust was made with enriched flour & vegetable shortening.)

Food and Description	Amount	Fat Grams	Total Calories	% Fat Calories
fried pie				
apple	4.5 oz	20.0	400	45%
blueberry	4.5 oz	20.0	400	45%
cherry	4.5 oz	20.0	400	45%
lemon	4.5 oz	20.0	400	45%
peach	4.5 oz	20.0	400	45%
strawberry	4.5 oz	20.0	400	45%
regular 9" pie				
apple	⅙ pie	18.0	405	40%
banana cream	⅙ pie	13.0	300	39%

Food and Description	Amount	Fat Grams	Total Calories	% Fat Calories
banana custard	⅙ pie	14.0	336	38%
blackberry	⅙ pie	17.0	384	40%
blueberry	⅙ pie	17.0	380	40%
butterscotch	⅛ pie	12.5	304	37%
cherry	⅙ pie	18.0	410	40%
chess	⅙ pie	24.0	485	45%
chocolate	⅙ pie	22.0	433	46%
chocolate meringue	⅙ pie	18.0	383	42%
coconut cream	⅙ pie	23.0	455	45%
coconut custard	⅙ pie	19.0	357	48%
custard	⅙ pie	17.0	330	46%
grasshopper	⅙ pie	23.0	460	45%
key lime	⅙ pie	19.0	460	37%
lemon chiffon	⅙ pie	13.6	338	36%
lemon meringue	⅙ pie	14.0	355	36%
mincemeat	⅙ pie	18.0	428	38%
peach	⅙ pie	17.0	405	38%
pecan	⅙ pie	32.0	575	50%
pineapple	⅙ pie	17.0	400	38%
pineapple chiffon	⅙ pie	13.0	311	38%
pineapple custard	⅙ pie	13.0	334	35%
pumpkin	⅙ pie	17.0	320	48%
raisin	⅙ pie	17.0	427	36%
rhubarb	⅙ pie	17.0	400	38%
shoo-fly	⅛ pie	13.0	395	30%
squash	⅙ pie	20.0	360	50%
strawberry	⅙ pie	10.0	246	37%
strawberry-rhubarb	⅛ pie	23.0	430	48%
sweet potato	⅙ pie	17.0	324	47%
vanilla cream	⅛ pie	17.0	350	44%
■ **MIX**				
(Betty Crocker) dessert mix/refrigerated				
banana cream				
mix only	⅑ pkg	4.0	160	23%
prepared	⅑ dessert	11.0	250	40%
chocolate French silk				
mix only	⅛ pkg	4.0	180	20%
prepared	⅛ dessert	11.0	270	37%
coconut cream				
mix only	⅑ pkg	7.0	200	32%
prepared	⅛ dessert	13.0	290	40%
cookies & cream				
mix only	⅙ pkg	7.0	280	23%
prepared	⅙ dessert	16.0	380	38%
Sunkist Lemon Supreme				
mix only	⅑ pkg	7.0	270	23%
prepared	⅑ dessert	13.0	320	37%

Food and Description	Amount	Fat Grams	Total Calories	% Fat Calories
(Jell-O) No-Bake Dessert				
chocolate silk				
mix only	⅛ pkg	4.5	190	21%
prepared w/2% milk & margarine	⅛ pie	16.0	310	46%
coconut cream				
mix only	⅛ pkg	4.5	190	21%
prepared w/2% milk & margarine	⅛ pie	19.0	330	52%
(Linsey's Kitchen) Dessert Solutions				
banana cream pie kit				
mix only	⅛ pie	11.0	230	43%
prepared	⅛ pie	12.0	330	33%
(Royal) No-Bake Pie Mix				
Mississippi mud				
mix only	⅛ pkg	6.0	250	22%
prepared	⅛ pie	14.5	370	35%
■ READY TO SERVE				
(Aunt Fanny's) individual pie				
apple	1 pie	23.0	460	45%
berry	1 pie	22.0	430	46%
cherry	1 pie	22.0	400	50%
peach	1 pie	22.0	430	46%
(Break Cake) snack/fried pie				
apple	1 pie	14.0	255	49%
cherry	1 pie	14.0	250	50%
(Dolly Madison) snack/packaged				
apple	1 pie	23.0	510	41%
blueberry	1 pie	24.0	520	42%
cherry	1 pie	24.0	530	41%
chocolate	1 pie	27.0	570	43%
lemon	1 pie	25.0	530	42%
peach	1 pie	23.0	500	41%
pecan	1 pie	22.0	540	37%
pineapple	1 pie	22.0	490	40%
(Drake's) snack/packaged				
apple	2 pies	16.0	400	36%
blueberry	2 pies	18.0	420	39%
cherry	2 pies	18.0	420	39%
(Entenmann's) pie				
fat-free				
apple beehive	⅕ pie	–	270	–
cherry beehive	⅕ pie	–	270	–
original				
apple/homestyle	⅙ pie	14.0	300	42%
coconut custard	⅕ pie	19.0	340	50%
lemon	⅙ pie	17.0	340	45%
(Hostess) snack/packaged				
apple	1 pie	21.0	440	43%
blueberry	1 pie	21.0	440	43%

Food and Description	Amount	Fat Grams	Total Calories	% Fat Calories
cherry	1 pie	21.0	450	42%
lemon	1 pie	21.0	440	42%
peach	1 pie	21.0	440	42%
(Lance) snack/packaged				
pecan	3 oz	17.0	350	44%
(McMillin's) snack/individually packaged				
apple	1 pie	23.0	430	48%
berry	1 pie	23.0	430	48%
cherry	1 pie	24.0	430	50%
lemon	1 pie	25.0	450	50%
peach	1 pie	24.0	430	50%
strawberry	1 pie	20.0	400	45%
(Tastykake) snack				
apple	1 pie	12.0	290	37%
blueberry	1 pie	11.0	320	31%
cherry	1 pie	12.0	320	34%
coconut creme	1 pie	20.0	390	46%
French apple	1 pie	12.0	360	30%
lemon	1 pie	12.0	320	34%
peach	1 pie	11.0	300	33%
pineapple	1 pie	12.0	290	37%
pineapple cheese	1 pie	12.0	320	34%
pumpkin	1 pie	14.0	330	38%
strawberry	1 pie	12.0	310	35%
Tastyklair	1 pie	20.0	410	44%
PIE CRUST (*See also* PASTRY)				
■ **FROZEN**				
(Chef Pierre) food service/unbaked				
deep dish/9" crust	⅛ crust	8.0	130	55%
regular/10" crust	⅑ crust	7.0	110	57%
vegetable shortening				
9" crust	⅑ crust	8.0	130	55%
10" crust	⅑ crust	8.0	120	60%
generic/9" crust	⅛ crust	4.8	80	53%
	1 crust	38.0	650	53%
(Mrs. Smith's)				
8" crust	⅛ crust	5.0	80	56%
9" crust	⅛ crust	5.0	90	50%
9⅝" crust	⅛ crust	7.0	120	53%
(Oronoque)				
deep dish/9" dia	⅙ crust	9.0	130	62%
regular/9" dia	⅙ crust	8.0	120	60%
(Pepperidge Farm) patty shells	1 shell	14.0	230	55%
(Pet-Ritz)				
deep dish				
all vegetable shortening	⅛ crust	7.0	100	58%
9" crust	⅛ crust	6.0	100	62%
graham cracker	⅙ crust	6.0	110	49%

Food and Description	Amount	Fat Grams	Total Calories	% Fat Calories
regular				
all vegetable shortening	⅛ crust	6.0	90	60%
9" crust	⅛ crust	5.0	80	60%
tart shell				
3" dia	1 shell	10.0	150	60%
6" dia	¼ shell	7.0	110	57%
■ HOMEMADE				
USDA Standard Home Recipe/9" crust				
cookie-type				
chocolate wafer				
baked	⅛ crust	8.0	140	51%
chilled	⅛ crust	8.0	140	51%
graham cracker				
baked	⅛ crust	7.0	150	42%
chilled	⅛ crust	7.0	150	42%
vanilla wafer				
baked	⅛ crust	7.5	120	56%
chilled	⅛ crust	7.5	120	56%
regular				
baked	⅛ crust	7.0	120	53%
	1 crust	63.0	960	59%
unbaked	⅛ crust	7.0	115	55%
	1 crust	63.0	920	62%
■ MIX				
(Betty Crocker) 9" crust/prepared	⅛ crust	8.0	110	65%
generic				
mix only	1 oz	8.5	150	51%
9" crust/prepared	⅛ crust	6.0	100	54%
(Krusteaz)				
mix only	2 Tbs	5.0	90	50%
9" crust/baked	⅛ crust	5.0	90	50%
(Nabisco)				
Honey Maid/graham				
9" crust/prepared	⅙ crust	7.0	140	45%
Nilla/cookie crumb				
crumbs only	2 Tbs	2.5	70	32%
9" crust/prepared	⅙ crust	8.0	140	51%
Oreo/cookie crumb				
crumbs only	2 Tbs	3.0	80	34%
9" crust/prepared	⅙ crust	7.0	140	45%
(Pillsbury) mix only	2 Tbs	6.0	100	54%
■ READY TO USE				
(Flako) 9" crust	⅙ crust	15.0	250	54%
(Keebler) Ready Crust				
butter-flavored	⅛ crust	5.0	110	41%
chocolate	⅛ crust	5.0	120	38%
graham cracker	⅛ crust	6.0	120	45%
single serve	1 tart	5.0	100	45%

Food and Description	Amount	Fat Grams	Total Calories	% Fat Calories
(Pillsbury) refrigerated/all ready	¼ crust	15.0	240	56%
(Wonderslim) fat-free				
chocolate	⅛ crust	–	70	–
original	⅛ crust	–	70	–
PIE FILLING & GLAZE (*See also* PUDDING & MOUSSE)				
■ CANNED OR JARRED				
(Borden) None Such mincemeat				
condensed	¼ pkg	2.0	220	8%
ready to use				
original	⅓ cup	1.0	200	5%
w/brandy & rum	⅓ cup	2.0	220	8%
(Comstock)				
apple				
cinnamon n' spice	⅓ cup	–	100	–
French	⅓ cup	–	100	–
original	⅓ cup	–	90	–
reduced calorie	⅓ cup	–	50	–
apricot	⅓ cup	–	100	–
banana cream	⅓ cup	1.5	100	14%
blackberry	⅓ cup	–	110	–
blueberry	⅓ cup	–	100	–
cherry				
dark sweet	⅓ cup	–	100	–
lite	⅓ cup	–	60	–
original	⅓ cup	–	90	–
chocolate cream	⅓ cup	1.5	120	11%
coconut cream	⅓ cup	3.0	110	25%
lemon	⅓ cup	1.0	150	6%
peach	⅓ cup	–	100	–
pineapple	⅓ cup	–	110	–
pumpkin	⅓ cup	–	90	–
raisin	⅓ cup	–	120	–
raspberry	⅓ cup	–	100	–
strawberry	⅓ cup	–	100	–
(Libby's) pumpkin pie mix	½ cup	–	100	–
(Musselman's)				
apple				
deluxe	⅓ cup	–	120	–
plus	⅓ cup	–	120	–
turnover/diced	⅓ cup	–	120	–
apricot	⅓ cup	–	150	–
blackberry				
plus	⅓ cup	–	120	–
regular	⅓ cup	–	120	–
blueberry				
plus	⅓ cup	–	145	–
regular	⅓ cup	–	120	–
boysenberry	⅓ cup	–	120	–

Food and Description	Amount	Fat Grams	Total Calories	% Fat Calories
cherry				
plus	⅓ cup	–	110	–
regular	⅓ cup	–	120	–
gooseberry	⅓ cup	–	180	–
lemon				
French	⅓ cup	1.0	180	5%
regular	⅓ cup	2.0	200	9%
mincemeat	⅓ cup	1.0	190	5%
peach				
plus	⅓ cup	–	115	–
regular	⅓ cup	–	150	–
pineapple	⅓ cup	–	110	–
pumpkin	⅓ cup	–	170	–
raisin	½ cup	–	130	–
raspberry				
black	⅓ cup	–	190	–
red	⅓ cup	–	190	–
strawberry				
plus	⅓ cup	–	140	–
regular	⅓ cup	–	120	–
strawberry-rhubarb	⅓ cup	–	120	–
(S&W) mincemeat	¼ cup	2.5	180	13%
(Thank You)				
apple				
cinnamon n' spice	⅓ cup	–	100	–
French	⅓ cup	–	100	–
original	⅓ cup	–	90	–
reduced calorie	⅓ cup	–	50	–
apricot	⅓ cup	–	100	–
banana cream	⅓ cup	1.5	100	14%
blackberry	⅓ cup	–	110	–
blueberry	⅓ cup	–	100	–
cherry				
dark sweet	⅓ cup	–	100	–
lite	⅓ cup	–	60	–
original	⅓ cup	–	90	–
chocolate cream	⅓ cup	1.5	120	11%
coconut cream	⅓ cup	3.0	110	25%
lemon	⅓ cup	1.0	150	6%
peach	⅓ cup	–	100	–
pineapple	⅓ cup	–	110	–
pumpkin	⅓ cup	–	90	–
raisin	⅓ cup	–	120	–
raspberry	⅓ cup	–	100	–
strawberry	⅓ cup	–	100	–
(Wilderness)				
banana cream	⅓ cup	1.5	100	14%
chocolate cream	⅓ cup	1.5	120	11%

Food and Description	Amount	Fat Grams	Total Calories	% Fat Calories
coconut cream	⅓ cup	3.0	110	25%
pumpkin	⅓ cup	–	90	–

■ **MIX** (Note: Unless stated otherwise, 1 serving of mix = the amount in ½ cup prepared.)

Food and Description	Amount	Fat Grams	Total Calories	% Fat Calories
(Calhoun Bend Mill)				
apple-cinnamon crisp/mix only	¼ cup	–	140	–
cherry-oatmeal crunch/mix only	¼ cup	0.5	140	3%
chocolate-fudge/mix only	3 Tbs	5.0	140	32%
peach cobbler/mix only	¼ cup	–	150	–
pecan/mix only	⅛ cup	–	110	–
strawberry				
mix only	1 oz	<1.0	110	4%
prepared	1 serving	7.0	256	25%
(Durkee) lemon/mix only	1 Tbs	–	50	–
(Jell-O) pudding & pie filling				
Americana pudding & custard				
custard				
mix only	1 serving	–	80	–
prepared w/2% milk	½ cup	2.5	140	16%
rice pudding				
mix only	1 serving	–	100	–
prepared w/2% milk	½ cup	2.5	160	14%
tapioca pudding				
mix only	1 serving	–	80	–
prepared w/2% milk	½ cup	2.5	140	16%
cook & serve				
original				
banana cream				
mix only	1 serving	–	80	–
prepared w/2% milk	½ cup	2.5	140	16%
butterscotch				
mix only	1 serving	–	90	–
prepared w/2% milk	½ cup	2.5	160	14%
chocolate				
mix only	1 serving	–	90	–
prepared w/2% milk	½ cup	2.5	150	15%
chocolate fudge				
mix only	1 serving	–	90	–
prepared w/2% milk	½ cup	2.5	150	15%
coconut cream				
mix only	1 serving	2.5	90	25%
prepared w/2% milk	½ cup	5.0	150	30%
flan				
mix only	1 serving	–	80	–
prepared w/2% milk	½ cup	2.5	140	16%
lemon				
mix only	1 serving	–	50	–
prepared w/sugar, egg yolks, & water	½ cup	2.0	140	13%

Food and Description	Amount	Fat Grams	Total Calories	% Fat Calories
milk chocolate				
mix only	1 serving	–	90	–
prepared w/2% milk	½ cup	2.5	150	15%
vanilla				
mix only	1 serving	–	80	–
prepared w/2% milk	½ cup	2.5	140	16%
sugar-free/reduced calorie				
chocolate				
mix only	1 serving	–	30	–
prepared w/2% milk	½ cup	2.5	90	25%
vanilla				
mix only	1 serving	–	20	–
prepared w/2% milk	½ cup	2.5	80	28%
instant				
fat-free/sugar-free/reduced calorie				
banana				
mix only	1 serving	–	25	–
prepared w/skim milk	½ cup	–	70	–
butterscotch				
mix only	1 serving	–	25	–
prepared w/skim milk	½ cup	–	70	–
chocolate				
mix only	1 serving	–	35	–
prepared w/skim milk	½ cup	–	80	–
chocolate fudge				
mix only	1 serving	–	35	–
prepared w/skim milk	½ cup	–	80	–
pistachio				
mix only	1 serving	–	30	–
prepared w/skim milk	½ cup	–	70	–
vanilla				
mix only	1 serving	–	25	–
prepared w/skim milk	½ cup	–	70	–
original				
banana cream				
mix only	1 serving	–	90	–
prepared w/2% milk	½ cup	2.5	150	15%
butter pecan				
mix only	1 serving	0.5	100	5%
prepared w/2% milk	½ cup	3.0	160	17%
butterscotch				
mix only	1 serving	–	90	–
prepared w/2% milk	½ cup	2.5	150	15%
chocolate				
mix only	1 serving	–	100	–
prepared w/2% milk	½ cup	2.5	160	14%
chocolate fudge				
mix only	1 serving	–	100	–

Food and Description	Amount	Fat Grams	Total Calories	% Fat Calories
prepared w/2% milk	½ cup	3.0	160	17%
coconut cream				
mix only	1 serving	2.0	100	18%
prepared w/2% milk	½ cup	4.5	160	25%
French vanilla				
mix only	1 serving	–	90	–
prepared w/2% milk	½ cup	2.5	150	15%
lemon				
mix only	1 serving	–	90	–
prepared w/2% milk	½ cup	2.5	150	15%
milk chocolate				
mix only	1 serving	0.5	100	5%
prepared w/2% milk	½ cup	3.0	160	17%
pistachio				
mix only	1 serving	0.5	100	5%
prepared w/2% milk	½ cup	3.0	160	17%
vanilla				
mix only	1 serving	–	90	–
prepared w/2% milk	½ cup	2.5	150	15%
(McCormick/Schilling) pie glaze mix for				
blueberries	2 oz	–	60	–
peaches	2 oz	–	70	–
strawberries	2 oz	–	70	–
(Nabisco) My-T-Fine/mix only				
butterscotch	1 serving	–	80	–
chocolate	1 serving	–	90	–
chocolate almond	1 serving	1.0	90	10%
chocolate fudge	1 serving	–	90	–
lemon	1 serving	–	80	–
vanilla	1 serving	–	80	–
(Royal) mix only				
cook & serve				
banana cream	1 serving	–	80	–
butterscotch	1 serving	–	90	–
chocolate	1 serving	–	90	–
dark 'n sweet	1 serving	–	90	–
vanilla	1 serving	–	80	–
instant				
regular				
banana cream	1 serving	–	90	–
butterscotch	1 serving	–	90	–
cherry vanilla	1 serving	–	90	–
chocolate	1 serving	–	100	–
chocolate almond	1 serving	1.0	120	8%
chocolate chocolate chip	1 serving	1.0	110	8%
chocolate peanut butter	1 serving	1.0	110	8%
dark 'n sweet	1 serving	–	110	–

Food and Description	Amount	Fat Grams	Total Calories	% Fat Calories
lemon	1 serving	–	90	–
pistachio	1 serving	1.0	90	10%
strawberry	1 serving	–	100	–
toasted coconut	1 serving	2.0	100	18%
vanilla	1 serving	–	90	–
vanilla chocolate chip	1 serving	1.0	90	10%
sugar-free				
chocolate	1 serving	–	45	–
pistachio	1 serving	–	40	–
vanilla	1 serving	–	40	–
PIEROGI/POTATO DUMPLING (*See* FROZEN ENTRÉE/DINNER)				
PIGEON (*See* SQUAB)				
PIGEON PEA				
dried/mature/shelled				
boiled	½ cup	–	100	–
raw	½ cup	1.5	350	4%
fresh				
cooked	½ cup	1.0	90	10%
raw	½ cup	1.5	350	4%
shelled				
boiled-drained	½ cup	1.5	120	11%
raw	½ cup	2.0	155	12%
seeds/immature				
boiled-drained	½ cup	1.0	85	11%
raw	20 seeds	<1.0	10	18%
PIGNOLA (*See* PINE NUT)				
PIG'S FEET (*See* PORK; PORK DINNER/ENTRÉE)				
PIKE (*See also* PIKE ROE)				
northern				
cooked-dry heat	3 oz	1.0	95	9%
raw	3 oz	1.0	75	12%
walleye				
cooked-dry heat	3 oz	1.0	100	9%
raw	3 oz	1.0	79	11%
PIKE ROE				
northern/raw	3 oz	1.7	110	14%
PILAF (*See* RICE DISH; PASTA ENTRÉE/DINNER)				
PIMIENTO/canned				
(Dromedary)	1 oz	–	10	–
(Dunbar's)	½ oz	–	4	–
generic				
diced or sliced	4 oz	–	30	–
whole	1 medium	–	11	–
(S&W) whole	2¼ oz	–	20	–
PIÑA COLADA (*See* COCKTAIL)				
PINE NUT				
dried				
pignola	1 oz	14.0	146	86%

Food and Description	Amount	Fat Grams	Total Calories	% Fat Calories
piñon	1 oz	17.0	161	95%
jarred				
(Progresso) pignoli nuts	1 oz	13.0	170	69%
PINEAPPLE				
can or cup				
(Del Monte)				
chunks				
in heavy syrup	½ cup	–	90	–
in juice	½ cup	–	70	–
crushed				
in heavy syrup	½ cup	–	90	–
in juice	½ cup	–	70	–
diced/in light syrup/fruit cup	3½ oz	–	70	–
sliced				
in heavy syrup	2 slices	–	90	–
in juice	2 slices	–	60	–
spears or wedges/in juice	½ cup	–	70	–
tidbits/in juice				
canned	½ cup	–	70	–
fruit cup	4¼ oz	–	60	–
(Dole)				
chunks				
in clarified juice	½ cup	–	60	–
in heavy syrup	½ cup	–	90	–
coarse-cut crushed				
in juice	½ cup	–	70	–
crushed				
in extra heavy syrup	½ cup	–	110	–
in heavy syrup	½ cup	–	90	–
in juice	½ cup	–	70	–
cubes				
in extra heavy syrup	½ cup	–	200	–
in light syrup	½ cup	–	80	–
pieces				
in light syrup	½ cup	–	80	–
sliced				
in clarified juice	2 slices	–	60	–
in heavy syrup	2 slices	–	90	–
52 slices/in heavy syrup	2 slices	–	90	–
90 slices/in light syrup	3½ slices	–	60	–
100-110 slices/in heavy syrup	4 slices	–	90	–
66 slices				
in clarified juice	2½ slices	–	60	–
in heavy syrup	2½ slices	–	90	–
tidbits				
in clarified juice	½ cup	–	60	–
in heavy syrup	½ cup	–	90	–
in light syrup	½ cup	–	80	–

Food and Description	Amount	Fat Grams	Total Calories	% Fat Calories
(Empress)				
chunks	½ cup	–	70	–
crushed	½ cup	–	70	–
sliced	½ cup	–	70	–
generic/sliced or chunks				
in heavy syrup	1 slice	–	45	–
in juice	1 slice	<1.0	35	3%
	1 cup	0.5	150	3%
in water	1 slice	<1.0	19	6%
	1 cup	<1.0	79	6%
(S&W) Hawaiian/sliced/in syrup	2 slices	–	90	–
candied				
(S&W) glacé				
slices				
green	1 piece	–	180	–
natural	1 piece	–	180	–
red	1 piece	–	180	–
wedges				
natural	5 pieces	–	80	–
tri-color	5 pieces	–	80	–
fresh	1 slice	<1.0	42	8%
	1 cup	0.7	77	8%
(Chiquita)	1 cup	1.0	90	10%
(Del Monte)	½ cup	–	52	–
	2 slices	–	90	–
(Dole)	2 slices	1.0	90	10%
frozen/generic/chunks				
sweetened	½ cup	–	104	–
unsweetened	3.5 oz	<1.0	50	9%

PINEAPPLE JUICE/JUICE BLEND (*See also* FRUIT PUNCH; PINEAPPLE JUICE DRINK)

Food and Description	Amount	Fat Grams	Total Calories	% Fat Calories
bottled, boxed, or canned				
(Del Monte)	6 fl oz	–	80	–
	8 fl oz	–	110	–
	11.5 fl oz	–	190	–
(Dole)				
Juice Cooler	8.45 fl oz	–	130	–
100% juice				
bottled				
pineapple-orange	10 fl oz	–	150	–
pineapple-orange-banana	10 fl oz	–	160	–
pineapple-passion-banana	10 fl oz	–	160	–
canned				
pineapple	8 fl oz	–	120	–
pineapple-grapefruit	6 fl oz	–	100	–
pineapple-orange	6 fl oz	–	100	–
pineapple-orange-banana	6 fl oz	–	100	–

Food and Description	Amount	Fat Grams	Total Calories	% Fat Calories
refrigerated				
pineapple	8 fl oz	–	130	–
pineapple-orange	8 fl oz	–	120	–
pineapple-orange-banana	4 fl oz	–	70	–
	8 fl oz	–	130	–
pineapple-orange-berry	8 fl oz	–	130	–
pineapple-orange-guava	8 fl oz	–	120	–
pineapple-orange-strawberry	8 fl oz	–	130	–
pineapple-passion-banana	8 fl oz	–	120	–
unfrozen juice concentrate				
reconstituted	6 fl oz	–	80	–
	8 fl oz	–	110	–
single strength	6 fl oz	–	80	–
	8 fl oz	–	110	–
generic	8 fl oz	–	140	–
(Kern's) pineapple-orange-passion fruit	11.5 fl oz	–	210	–
(Knudsen) Thirst Quencher/ pineapple-coconut	8 fl oz	–	130	–
(Minute Maid) drink box	8.45 fl oz	–	130	–
(Mott's) pineapple-orange	10 fl oz	–	170	–
(S&W)	6 fl oz	–	90	–
	8 fl oz	–	110	–
individual serving	12 fl oz	–	180	–
(Seneca)	8 fl oz	–	130	–
frozen				
(Dole) prepared				
100% pineapple juice	8 fl oz	–	130	–
pineapple-grapefruit	8 fl oz	–	130	–
pineapple-orange	8 fl oz	–	120	–
pineapple-orange-banana	8 fl oz	–	130	–
pineapple-orange-berry	8 fl oz	–	130	–
pineapple-orange-guava	8 fl oz	–	120	–
pineapple-orange-strawberry	8 fl oz	–	130	–
pineapple-passion-banana	8 fl oz	–	120	–
pineapple-strawberry	8 fl oz	–	130	–
generic/frozen concentrate				
prepared	8 fl oz	<1.0	130	1%
undiluted	6 oz	<1.0	385	1%
(Welch's) pineapple-banana/prepared	8 fl oz	–	130	–
PINEAPPLE JUICE DRINK (*See also* FRUIT PUNCH; PINEAPPLE JUICE/JUICE BLEND)				
(Dole) pineapple-pink grapefruit	6 fl oz	–	100	–
	8 fl oz	–	130	–
	10 fl oz	–	160	–
PINK BEAN				
canned				
(Goya)				
habichuelas rosadas/Spanish style	½ cup	0.5	80	9%
original	½ cup	0.5	80	9%

Food and Description	Amount	Fat Grams	Total Calories	% Fat Calories
dried				
boiled	½ cup	0.5	125	4%
raw	½ cup	1.0	360	3%
PIÑON/PINYON (*See* PINE NUT)				
PINTO BEAN (*See also* PINTO BEAN DISH)				
canned				
(Bush's)	½ cup	–	60	–
(Eden)	½ cup	–	100	–
(Gebhardt)	½ cup	0.5	110	4%
generic	½ cup	–	93	–
(Goya) Spanish style	½ cup	0.5	110	4%
(Green Giant)	½ cup	0.5	110	4%
(Hain)	½ cup	1.0	110	8%
(Joan of Arc)	½ cup	0.5	110	4%
(Luck's) seasoned w/pork				
regular	7 oz	3.0	200	14%
	½ cup	4.0	140	26%
w/onions	½ cup	3.0	150	18%
(Progresso)	½ cup	1.0	130	7%
(Sun-Vista)	½ cup	0.5	80	6%
(Trappey's)				
hearty Texas	½ cup	2.0	110	16%
jalapinto	½ cup	1.0	90	10%
original	½ cup	1.0	90	10%
dried/raw				
(Arrowhead Mills)	¼ cup	0.5	150	3%
(Bean Cuisine)	½ cup	1.0	115	8%
generic				
cooked	½ cup	0.5	133	3%
raw	½ cup	1.0	325	3%
sprouted/mature seeds				
boiled-drained	½ cup	0.5	25	18%
raw	½ cup	1.0	65	14%
PINTO BEAN DISH (*See also* PINTO BEAN)				
(Luck's) pinto & great northern beans/ seasoned w/pork	½ cup	2.0	130	14%
PISTACHIO				
(Alma) extra jumbo				
natural	1 oz	14.0	160	79%
red	1 oz	14.0	160	79%
(Ann's House Of Nuts) natural	1 oz	14.0	160	79%
(Dole) dry-roasted				
shelled	1 oz	14.0	163	77%
unshelled	1 oz	7.0	90	70%
(Fisher) red	1 oz	15.0	170	79%
generic				
dried	1 oz	13.7	164	75%
	1 cup	61.9	739	75%

Food and Description	Amount	Fat Grams	Total Calories	% Fat Calories
dry roasted	1 oz	15.0	172	79%
	1 cup	67.6	776	78%
shelled	1 oz	15.0	168	80%
unshelled	1 oz	7.0	84	75%
(Lance)	1⅛ oz	7.0	90	70%
	¼ cup	7.0	100	63%
(Planters) dry-roasted shelled				
Munch 'N Go	2 oz	29.0	330	79%
regular	1 oz	14.0	160	79%
unshelled				
red/salted	1 oz	14.0	160	79%
uncolored	½ cup	14.0	160	79%
	1 oz	14.0	160	79%
	2.25 oz	16.0	190	76%

PITA BREAD (*See* BREAD)
PITANGA/BRAZILIAN CHERRY/SURINAM CHERRY

fresh	2 pieces	<1.0	5	11%
	1 cup	0.7	57	11%
	1 lb	1.6	132	11%

PIZZA (*See also* FROZEN ENTREE/DINNER; VEGETARIAN FOODS; individual FAST FOOD listings.)
■ **(ACT II)**

pizza pocket/pepperoni	1 pizza	20.0	400	45%

■ **(Bacino's)**

America's heart healthy pizza	8 oz	10.7	318	30%

■ **(Celentano)**
pizza

9-slice	2.7 oz	4.0	150	24%
thick-crust	4.3 oz	11.0	290	34%

■ **(Celeste)**

garlic & herb bread pizza	1 pizza	8.0	260	28%
Italian bread pizza				
deluxe	1 pizza	11.0	290	34%
pepperoni	1 pizza	13.0	320	37%
zesty four-cheese	1 pizza	12.0	300	36%
original				
cheese	¼ pizza	16.0	320	45%
deluxe	¼ pizza	18.0	350	46%
four-cheese	¼ pizza	16.0	330	44%
pepperoni	¼ pizza	20.0	350	51%
suprema	⅕ pizza	16.0	290	50%
Pizza For One				
cheese	1 pizza	25.0	540	42%
deluxe	1 pizza	29.0	540	48%
four-cheese				
hot & zesty	1 pizza	27.0	530	46%
original	1 pizza	30.0	540	50%

Food and Description	Amount	Fat Grams	Total Calories	% Fat Calories
zesty	1 pizza	27.0	530	46%
pepperoni	1 pizza	27.0	520	47%
sausage	1 pizza	27.0	530	46%
suprema	1 pizza	23.0	480	43%
suprema vegetable w/meat	1 pizza	31.0	580	48%
■ **(Chef Boyardee)**				
boxed mix				
cheese pizza				
complete	¼ pkg	6.0	230	24%
2 complete	⅛ pkg	5.0	210	21%
pepperoni pizza				
complete	¼ pkg	9.0	250	32%
2 complete	⅛ pkg	7.0	210	30%
pizza kit/cheese/prepared	⅐ pkg	6.0	310	17%
plain pizza	¼ pkg	3.0	180	15%
sausage pizza/complete	¼ pkg	10.0	270	33%
■ **(Chicago Brother's)**				
pizza/pepperoni	⅓ pizza	15.0	420	32%
■ **(Di Giorno)**				
pizza				
cheese	⅙ pizza	10.0	340	26%
Italian sausage	⅙ pizza	13.0	370	32%
pepperoni	⅙ pizza	16.0	390	37%
supreme	⅙ pizza	15.0	380	36%
3 meat	⅙ pizza	16.0	390	37%
vegetable	⅛ pizza	7.0	240	26%
■ **(Graindance)**				
pizza/cheese w/whole wheat crust	¼ pizza	8.0	190	38%
■ **(Healthy Choice)**				
French bread pizza				
cheese	5.6 oz	4.0	310	12%
deluxe	6.3 oz	6.0	330	16%
Italian sausage	6.3 oz	5.0	330	14%
pepperoni	6 oz	9.0	360	23%
■ **(Hormel)**				
Quick Meal				
pepperoni	1 pizza	14.0	380	33%
pizza nuggets	5 nuggets	9.0	210	39%
■ **(Jack's)**				
pizza				
bacon cheeseburger	¼ pizza	18.0	360	45%
double cheese	¼ pizza	19.0	380	45%
original	¼ pizza	15.0	330	48%
pepperoni & mushroom	¼ pizza	16.0	340	42%
sausage	¼ pizza	14.0	320	39%
sausage & pepperoni	¼ pizza	19.0	370	46%
supreme	¼ pizza	18.0	370	44%

Food and Description	Amount	Fat Grams	Total Calories	% Fat Calories
■ (Jaclyn's)				
fat-free pizza	⅛ pizza	–	120	–
■ (Jeno's)				
Crisp 'n Tasty Pizza				
Canadian-style bacon	1 pizza	18.0	430	38%
cheese	1 pizza	19.0	450	38%
combination	1 pizza	28.0	520	48%
hamburger	1 pizza	23.0	480	43%
pepperoni	1 pizza	26.0	500	47%
sausage	1 pizza	27.0	510	48%
supreme	1 pizza	28.0	520	48%
three meat	1 pizza	26.0	500	47%
microwave pizza for one				
cheese	1 pizza	11.0	240	42%
combination	1 pizza	18.0	310	52%
pepperoni	1 pizza	16.0	280	51%
sausage	1 pizza	16.0	280	51%
■ (John's)				
pizza				
cheese 3-pack	1 pizza	12.0	300	36%
golden topping	½ pizza	11.0	240	41%
sausage				
deluxe	½ pizza	13.0	260	45%
regular	½ pizza	13.0	260	45%
3-pack	1 pizza	12.0	300	36%
■ (Kid Cuisine)				
pizza				
cheese	8 oz	11.0	430	23%
hamburger	8.3 oz	11.0	400	25%
■ LEAN CUISINE (See Stouffer's in this section)				
■ LUNCHABLES (See Oscar Mayer in this section)				
■ (Mama Rosa's) combo/8 pack	1 pizza	12.0	320	34%
■ (Marie Callender's)				
pizza				
chicken & broccoli	½ pizza	15.0	350	39%
classic 5-meat combo	½ pizza	17.0	370	41%
deluxe	½ pizza	23.0	380	63%
easy cheese	½ pizza	25.0	410	55%
pepperoni	½ pizza	29.0	440	59%
primavera	½ pizza	15.0	350	39%
sausage & pepperoni	½ pizza	28.0	430	59%
sliced tomato & mozzarella	½ pizza	15.0	350	39%
■ (Michelina's)				
Krisp 'n Flaky Crust Pizza				
cheese	1 pizza	22.0	420	47%
combination	1 pizza	24.0	430	50%
Mexican style	1 pizza	21.0	400	47%
pepperoni	1 pizza	24.0	440	49%

Food and Description	Amount	Fat Grams	Total Calories	% Fat Calories
sausage	1 pizza	20.0	420	43%
supreme	1 pizza	24.0	440	49%
■ (Micro Magic)				
deep dish pizza				
combination	1 pizza	28.0	520	48%
pepperoni	1 pizza	32.0	560	51%
sausage	1 pizza	29.0	530	49%
■ (Mr. P's Pizza)				
pizza				
combination (7.2 oz)	½ pizza	13.0	260	45%
golden topping (6.8 oz)	½ pizza	11.0	240	41%
hamburger (7.6 oz)	½ pizza	12.0	260	42%
pepperoni (7 oz)	½ pizza	13.0	250	47%
sausage (7.2 oz)	½ pizza	13.0	260	45%
■ (Oscar Mayer) Lunchables				
fun pack				
mozzarella/fruit punch	1 pkg	17.0	480	32%
pepperoni/orange	1 pkg	17.0	480	32%
regular				
pepperoni/mozzarella	1 pkg	15.0	330	41%
2-cheese	1 pkg	13.0	330	35%
■ (Pappalo's)				
deep-dish pizza				
pepperoni	⅕ pizza	14.0	340	37%
sausage	⅕ pizza	13.0	330	35%
sausage & pepperoni	⅕ pizza	14.0	330	38%
supreme	⅕ pizza	14.0	340	37%
three-cheese	¼ pizza	12.0	370	29%
For One pizza				
deep-dish				
pepperoni	1 pizza	26.0	600	39%
sausage & pepperoni	1 pizza	27.0	610	40%
supreme	1 pizza	27.0	610	40%
three-cheese	1 pizza	20.0	540	33%
regular				
pepperoni	1 pizza	27.0	570	43%
sausage & pepperoni	1 pizza	27.0	570	43%
supreme	1 pizza	27.0	560	43%
three-cheese	1 pizza	20.0	500	36%
pizzeria-style crust				
pepperoni				
9" pizza	½ pizza	19.0	440	39%
12" pizza	½ pizza	17.0	380	40%
sausage				
9" pizza	½ pizza	18.0	420	39%
12" pizza	½ pizza	16.0	370	39%
sausage & pepperoni				
9" pizza	½ pizza	19.0	430	40%

Food and Description	Amount	Fat Grams	Total Calories	% Fat Calories
12" pizza	½ pizza	17.0	380	40%
supreme				
9" pizza	⅓ pizza	13.0	290	40%
12" pizza	½ pizza	17.0	380	38%
three-cheese				
9" pizza	½ pizza	15.0	400	34%
12" pizza	½ pizza	12.0	340	32%
■ (Pepperidge Farm)				
Croissant Crust Pizza				
cheese	1 pizza	20.0	390	46%
deluxe	1 pizza	27.0	450	54%
pepperoni	1 pizza	23.0	420	49%
■ (Prezzo Giusto)				
5" deep-dish pizza				
cheese	1 pizza	15.0	420	32%
pepperoni	1 pizza	20.0	470	38%
pepperoni & sausage	1 pizza	20.0	470	38%
■ (Red Baron)				
deep-dish single-serve pizza				
cheese	1 pizza	26.0	500	47%
cheese deluxe	1 pizza	23.0	460	45%
meat trio	1 pizza	26.0	490	48%
pepperoni	1 pizza	31.0	530	53%
sausage	1 pizza	29.0	520	50%
supreme	1 pizza	28.0	490	51%
original				
Canadian bacon	¼ pizza	17.0	380	40%
four-cheese	¼ pizza	21.0	430	44%
hamburger	⅕ pizza	17.0	340	45%
Mexican supreme	⅕ pizza	24.0	430	50%
pepperoni	¼ pizza	24.0	450	48%
pepperoni deluxe	⅕ pizza	18.0	340	48%
sausage	⅕ pizza	18.0	350	46%
sausage & mushroom	⅕ pizza	18.0	350	46%
sausage & pepperoni	⅕ pizza	20.0	370	49%
special deluxe	⅕ pizza	18.0	340	48%
supreme	⅕ pizza	18.0	350	46%
Sunrise Singles				
bacon scramble	1 pizza	24.0	420	51%
cheesey scramble	1 pizza	19.0	350	49%
ham scramble	1 pizza	19.0	370	46%
huevos rancheros	1 pizza	18.0	350	46%
sausage gravy	1 pizza	17.0	340	45%
sausage scramble	1 pizza	21.0	380	50%
Western scramble	1 pizza	21.0	380	50%
■ (Schwan's)				
deep-dish single-serve pizza				
cheese	1 pizza	26.0	510	47%

Food and Description	Amount	Fat Grams	Total Calories	% Fat Calories
Mexican style	1 pizza	25.0	440	51%
pepperoni	1 pizza	31.0	530	53%
sausage	1 pizza	29.0	520	50%
supreme	1 pizza	28.0	490	51%
Special Recipe Pizza				
Canadian bacon	⅓ pizza	23.0	430	48%
cheese	⅓ pizza	25.0	440	51%
hamburger	¼ pizza	21.0	360	53%
pepperoni	⅓ pizza	29.0	480	54%
sausage	¼ pizza	24.0	380	57%
sausage & pepperoni	¼ pizza	24.0	390	55%
supreme	¼ pizza	25.0	420	54%
■ (Spanky's)				
pizza				
cheese/7-oz pizza	1 pizza	6.0	390	14%
deluxe/2-pizza pkg	⅕ pizza	10.0	290	31%
pepperoni				
7-oz pizza	1 pizza	15.0	460	29%
30-oz pizza	½ pizza	9.0	320	25%
sausage & pepperoni combo/7-oz pizza	1 pizza	15.0	450	30%
■ (Stouffer's)				
French bread pizza				
bacon cheddar/11⅜-oz pizza	½ pizza	22.0	440	45%
cheese/10⅜-oz pizza	½ pizza	14.0	350	36%
cheeseburger/11⅞-oz pizza	½ pizza	26.0	440	53%
deluxe/12⅜-oz pizza	½ pizza	22.0	440	45%
double cheese/11¾-oz pizza	½ pizza	19.0	420	41%
pepperoni /11¼-oz pizza	½ pizza	20.0	420	43%
pepperoni & mushroom/12¼-oz pizza	½ pizza	21.0	430	44%
sausage/12-oz pizza	½ pizza	20.0	420	43%
sausage & pepperoni/12.5-oz pizza	½ pizza	25.0	490	46%
vegetable deluxe/12.75-oz pizza	½ pizza	17.0	400	38%
white/10⅛-oz pizza	½ pizza	28.0	490	51%
Lean Cuisine French bread pizza				
cheese	6 oz	8.0	350	21%
deluxe	6⅛ oz	6.0	330	16%
pepperoni	5¼ oz	7.0	330	19%
■ (Tombstone)				
double top pizza				
pepperoni w/double cheese	⅙ pizza	20.0	350	51%
sausage & pepperoni	⅙ pizza	20.0	360	50%
sausage w/double cheese	⅙ pizza	19.0	350	49%
lower fat pizza				
light				
supreme	⅕ pizza	9.0	270	30%
vegetable	⅕ pizza	7.0	240	26%
original				
Canadian style bacon/12" pizza	¼ pizza	15.0	360	38%

Food and Description	Amount	Fat Grams	Total Calories	% Fat Calories
cheese/9" pizza	½ pizza	19.0	420	41%
cheese & hamburger				
9" pizza	⅓ pizza	25.0	310	73%
12" pizza	⅕ pizza	16.0	320	45%
cheese & pepperoni				
9" pizza	⅓ pizza	19.0	340	50%
12" pizza	⅕ pizza	18.0	340	48%
cheese & sausage				
9" pizza	⅓ pizza	16.0	310	46%
12" pizza	⅕ pizza	16.0	320	45%
cheese, sausage, & mushroom/ 12" pizza	⅕ pizza	16.0	320	45%
deluxe				
9" pizza	⅓ pizza	16.0	320	45%
12" pizza	⅕ pizza	16.0	320	45%
extra cheese/12" pizza	¼ pizza	17.0	370	41%
pepperoni & sausage				
9" pizza	⅓ pizza	21.0	360	53%
12" pizza	⅕ pizza	18.0	340	48%
supreme/12" pizza	⅕ pizza	17.0	330	46%
Special Order				
four-cheese/12" pizza	⅕ pizza	19.0	400	43%
four-meat				
9" pizza	⅓ pizza	20.0	400	45%
12" pizza	⅕ pizza	18.0	350	46%
pepperoni				
9" pizza	⅓ pizza	21.0	400	47%
12" pizza	⅕ pizza	19.0	360	48%
super supreme				
9" pizza	⅓ pizza	21.0	400	47%
12" pizza	⅕ pizza	18.0	350	46%
three-sausage				
9" pizza	⅓ pizza	19.0	390	44%
12" pizza	⅕ pizza	17.0	340	45%
thin-crust pizza				
Italian style				
four-meat combo	¼ pizza	25.0	410	55%
Italian sausage	¼ pizza	24.0	400	54%
pepperoni	¼ pizza	27.0	420	58%
supreme	¼ pizza	24.0	400	54%
three-cheese	¼ pizza	22.0	380	52%
Mexican style supreme				
taco	¼ pizza	23.0	380	54%
Tombstone for one				
½ less fat				
cheese	1 pizza	10.0	360	25%
pepperoni	1 pizza	13.0	400	29%
supreme	1 pizza	13.0	400	29%

Food and Description	Amount	Fat Grams	Total Calories	% Fat Calories
vegetable	1 pizza	10.0	360	25%
regular				
cheese & pepperoni	1 pizza	35.0	580	54%
extra cheese	1 pizza	30.0	540	50%
Italian sausage	1 pizza	33.0	560	53%
sausage & pepperoni	1 pizza	37.0	590	56%
supreme	1 pizza	34.0	570	54%
■ (Tony's)				
French bread pizza				
cheese	1 pizza	9.0	310	23%
pepperoni	1 pizza	15.0	380	36%
sausage	1 pizza	15.0	380	36%
supreme	1 pizza	16.0	380	38%
garlic bread/4 cheese	1 pizza	26.0	450	52%
Italian Style Pastry Crust				
Canadian bacon	⅓ pizza	19.0	370	46%
extra cheese	⅓ pizza	20.0	380	47%
hamburger	⅓ pizza	22.0	400	50%
pepperoni	⅓ pizza	27.0	450	54%
pepperoni & mushroom	⅓ pizza	24.0	420	51%
pepperoni & sausage	⅓ pizza	25.0	430	52%
sausage	⅓ pizza	24.0	420	51%
sausage & pepperoni	⅓ pizza	26.0	440	53%
supreme	⅓ pizza	25.0	430	52%
taco style	⅓ pizza	25.0	430	52%
personal pizza				
Canadian style bacon	1 pizza	29.0	580	45%
cheese	1 pizza	29.0	570	46%
pepperoni	1 pizza	37.0	650	51%
sausage	1 pizza	37.0	650	51%
sausage & pepperoni	1 pizza	37.0	650	51%
supreme	1 pizza	38.0	660	52%
taco	1 pizza	39.0	670	52%
Pizza d'Primo				
4-cheese	⅓ pizza	14.0	380	33%
meat trio	⅓ pizza	17.0	420	36%
sausage	⅓ pizza	17.0	420	36%
sausage & pepperoni	⅓ pizza	19.0	430	40%
super pepperoni	⅓ pizza	18.0	430	38%
supreme	⅓ pizza	15.0	340	40%
Pizza Pockets				
meat trio	1 pocket	15.0	320	42%
pepperoni	1 pocket	17.0	350	44%
sausage	1 pocket	15.0	320	42%
sausage & pepperoni	1 pocket	18.0	350	43%
supreme	1 pocket	15.0	310	44%
vegetable	1 pocket	10.0	270	33%

Food and Description	Amount	Fat Grams	Total Calories	% Fat Calories
■ (Totino's)				
Party Pizza				
bacon	½ pizza	20.0	370	49%
Canadian style bacon	½ pizza	15.0	320	42%
cheese				
family size	⅓ pizza	16.0	360	40%
regular	½ pizza	14.0	320	39%
combination				
family size	¼ pizza	16.0	300	48%
regular	½ pizza	21.0	390	48%
hamburger	½ pizza	18.0	350	46%
pepperoni				
family size	⅓ pizza	22.0	410	48%
regular	½ pizza	21.0	380	50%
sausage				
family size	¼ pizza	16.0	300	48%
regular	½ pizza	20.0	380	47%
supreme	½ pizza	20.0	380	47%
three-meat	½ pizza	19.0	360	48%
zesty Italiano	½ pizza	21.0	390	48%
zesty Mexican style	½ pizza	19.0	370	46%
Pizza For One/microwave				
cheese	1 pizza	11.0	240	41%
combination	1 pizza	18.0	310	52%
pepperoni	1 pizza	16.0	280	51%
sausage	1 pizza	16.0	280	51%
supreme	1 pizza	17.0	290	53%
zesty Mexican style	1 pizza	16.0	280	51%
Pizza Pops				
Italian sausage	1 pizza	15.0	310	44%
Italian sausage & pepperoni	1 pizza	17.0	320	48%
pepperoni	1 pizza	16.0	320	45%
supreme	1 pizza	15.0	300	45%
Pizza Rolls				
combination	10 rolls	17.0	370	41%
hamburger & cheese	10 rolls	14.0	350	36%
nacho cheese & beef	10 rolls	16.0	340	42%
pepperoni & cheese	10 rolls	17.0	360	43%
sausage & cheese	10 rolls	16.0	350	41%
sausage & mushroom	10 rolls	14.0	330	38%
spicy Italian style	10 rolls	18.0	370	44%
three-cheese	10 rolls	15.0	360	38%
three-meat	10 rolls	15.0	340	40%
Select Pizza				
sausage & pepperoni	⅓ pizza	19.0	360	48%
supreme	⅓ pizza	18.0	340	48%
three-cheese	⅓ pizza	14.0	300	42%
two-cheese & Canadian style bacon	⅓ pizza	14.0	310	41%

Food and Description	Amount	Fat Grams	Total Calories	% Fat Calories
two-cheese & pepperoni	⅓ pizza	20.0	360	50%
two-cheese & sausage	⅓ pizza	19.0	360	48%
■ **(Weight Watchers)**				
pizza				
deluxe combo	6.57 oz	11.0	380	26%
extra cheese	5.74 oz	12.0	390	28%
pepperoni	5.56 oz	12.0	390	28%
pocket pizza deluxe sandwich	5 oz	7.0	300	21%
■ **(Wolfgang Puck)**				
pizza				
barbecue chicken	½ pizza	11.0	340	29%
cheeseless fat-free grilled vegetable	½ pizza	–	200	–
four cheeses	½ pizza	15.0	360	38%
pepperoni & mushroom	½ pizza	15.0	390	35%
sausage & herb	½ pizza	18.0	380	43%
PIZZA CRUST				
(Boboli) Italian bread shell/prebaked/ready to use				
12" size/single or family pack	⅛ shell	3.0	160	17%
thin crust	⅕ shell	3.5	150	21%
twin pack	½ shell	3.0	160	17%
(Chef Boyardee) Quick & Easy mix	⅓ pkg	1.5	150	9%
(Earth Grains) brown 'n serve pizza round	1 round	4.0	210	17%
(Jiffy) mix	0.81 oz	2.0	90	20%
(Mama Mary's) fresh baked gourmet/ 12" dia	1 slice	4.0	148	24%
(Martha White) mix				
deep dish/crust only	1 slice	<1.0	110	4%
regular/crust only	1 slice	2.0	100	18%
(Mia) chilled/precooked	⅙ crust	1.0	150	6%
(Pillsbury) refrigerated	¼ crust	2.5	180	13%
(Ragu) Pizza Quick/mix only	⅓ cup	1.0	130	7%
(Robin Hood) mix/prepared	¼ crust	2.0	160	11%
(Totino's)	¼ crust	7.0	180	35%
PIZZA SAUCE (*See also* SAUCE)				
(Borden) traditional	¼ cup	–	20	–
(Contadina)				
chunky				
basic	¼ cup	–	30	–
mushroom	¼ cup	–	30	–
3 cheese	¼ cup	0.5	35	17%
regular				
Italian cheese	¼ cup	1.0	30	30%
original	¼ cup	0.5	25	18%
pepperoni flavored	¼ cup	1.0	30	30%
squeeze				
Italian cheese	¼ cup	1.5	40	34%
original	¼ cup	1.5	35	39%

Food and Description	Amount	Fat Grams	Total Calories	% Fat Calories
(Progresso)	¼ cup	1.0	35	26%
(Ragu) Pizza Quick				
chunky mushroom	¼ cup	1.5	40	34%
chunky tomato	¼ cup	1.5	50	27%
garlic & basil	¼ cup	1.5	40	34%
100% natural	¼ cup	1.0	30	30%
pepperoni flavored	¼ cup	2.0	60	30%
traditional	¼ cup	1.5	40	34%
PLANTAIN/BAKING BANANA/COOKING BANANA				
cooked/sliced	1 cup	<1.0	180	3%
raw				
sliced	½ cup	<1.0	90	3%
whole	1 medium	1.0	220	4%
PLUM				
canned				
generic/purple				
in extra heavy syrup				
w/liquid	1 cup	–	265	–
w/o liquid	½ cup	–	135	–
in heavy syrup				
w/liquid	1 cup	–	230	–
w/o liquid	½ cup	–	115	–
in juice				
w/liquid	1 cup	–	145	–
w/o liquid	½ cup	–	75	–
in light syrup				
w/liquid	1 cup	–	160	–
w/o liquid	½ cup	–	80	–
in water				
w/liquid	1 cup	–	105	–
w/o liquid	½ cup	–	50	–
(S&W) whole purple/in heavy syrup	½ cup	–	130	–
(Solo) prune/plum filling	2 Tbs	–	70	–
(Stokely) in light syrup	½ cup	–	100	–
fresh/raw				
sliced	½ cup	–	90	–
whole	1 medium	<1.0	36	13%
PLUM FILLING (See PRUNE/PLUM FILLING)				
POI	½ cup	–	135	–
POKEBERRY/fresh				
cooked	½ cup	–	16	–
raw	½ cup	–	20	–
POLENTA				
chilled				
(Melissa's)	4 oz	–	100	–
mix				
(Fantastic Foods) Polenta Fantastica				
mix only	⅜ cup	5.0	260	17%

Food and Description	Amount	Fat Grams	Total Calories	% Fat Calories
prepared	1 cup	5.0	260	17%
(Golden Pheasant) mix only	3.5 oz	1.5	370	4%
POLISH SAUSAGE (See SAUSAGE)				
POLLACK/POLLOCK (See also SEAFOOD ENTRÉE/DINNER)				
Alaskan/walleye				
cooked-dry heat	3 oz	1.0	100	9%
raw	3 oz	0.7	70	9%
Atlantic/raw	3 oz	1.0	80	10%
POMEGRANATE/fresh	1 medium	0.5	104	4%
POMPANO/Florida				
breaded & fried	3 oz	17.0	270	57%
cooked-dry heat	3 oz	10.0	180	50%
raw	3 oz	8.0	140	51%
POP (See COCKTAIL MIXER; SOFT DRINK; SPORTS DRINK)				
POP TART (See PASTRY, TOASTER)				
POPCORN (See also POPCORN BARS & CAKES)				
(NOTE: Unless stated otherwise, data are for popped corn.)				
(ACT I) microwave				
butter	3 cups	8.0	140	51%
extra butter	3 cups	10.0	160	56%
(Act II)				
frozen				
butter flavored	3 cups	10.0	190	47%
real butter	3 cups	8.0	140	51%
microwave				
butter				
96% fat-free				
popped	1 cup	–	20	–
unpopped	3 Tbs	1.5	120	11%
regular	3 cups	8.0	140	51%
caramel	3 cups	14.0	280	45%
50% less salt				
natural	3 cups	3.0	100	27%
regular	3 cups	3.0	100	27%
natural	3 cups	8.0	140	51%
sour cream & onion	3 cups	8.0	150	48%
tangy ranch	3 cups	8.0	140	51%
white cheddar cheese	3 cups	9.0	160	51%
(America's Best)				
air-popped	5 cups	0.5	100	5%
unpopped	2 Tbs	0.5	100	5%
(Arrowhead Mills) unpopped	¼ cup	2.5	180	13%
(Bag O'Beans)				
Apache red				
air-popped	1 cup	<1.0	27	17%
oil-popped	1 cup	1.4	33	38%
Hopi				
air-popped	1 cup	<1.0	27	17%

Food and Description	Amount	Fat Grams	Total Calories	% Fat Calories
oil-popped	1 cup	1.4	33	38%
Kiowa black				
air-popped	1 cup	<1.0	27	17%
oil-popped	1 cup	1.4	33	38%
Painted Desert				
air-popped	1 cup	<1.0	27	17%
oil-popped	1 cup	1.4	33	38%
Paiute pearl				
air-popped	1 cup	<1.0	27	17%
oil-popped	1 cup	1.4	33	38%
Zuni				
air-popped	1 cup	<1.0	27	17%
oil-popped	1 cup	1.4	33	38%
(Bearitos) microwave				
all natural buttery	1 cup	4.0	60	60%
	1 bag	31.0	420	66%
lite buttery	1 cup	1.0	30	30%
	1 bag	9.0	230	35%
(Betty Crocker) Pop Secret				
By Your Request				
butter	1 cup	<1.0	20	19%
	6 cups	2.5	120	19%
cheddar cheese	1 cup	2.0	30	60%
	5 cups	10.0	150	60%
nacho cheese	1 cup	2.0	30	60%
	5 cups	10.0	150	60%
natural	1 cup	<1.0	20	19%
	6 cups	2.5	120	19%
jumbo pop/butter	1 cup	2.5	40	56%
Movie Theater/butter	1 cup	2.5	40	56%
pop chips				
butter	1 oz	3.0	120	23%
cheddar cheese	1 oz	3.0	120	23%
original	1 oz	3.0	120	23%
sour cream & onion	1 oz	3.5	120	26%
regular				
butter				
light	1 cup	1.0	25	36%
	6 cups	5.0	130	35%
original	1 cup	2.5	35	64%
	4 cups	10.0	150	60%
buttery burst				
light	1 cup	1.0	25	36%
	6 cups	5.0	130	35%
original	1 cup	2.5	35	64%
	4 cups	10.0	150	60%
natural				

Food and Description	Amount	Fat Grams	Total Calories	% Fat Calories
light	1 cup	1.0	25	36%
	6 cups	5.0	130	35%
original	1 cup	2.5	35	64%
	4 cups	10.0	150	60%
(Black Jewel) microwaveable				
hulless	1¼ cups	8.0	150	48%
(Blue Heaven) microwaveable				
blue corn	2 cups	8.0	130	55%
(Borden) ready to eat				
butter-flavored	1 oz	10.0	150	60%
Cracker Jack				
fat-free	1 cup	–	110	–
nutty deluxe	1 cup	6.0	130	42%
original	⅔ cup	2.5	120	19%
tender eating				
baby rice popcorn	1 oz	13.0	170	69%
baby white popcorn	1 oz	13.0	170	69%
yellow popcorn	1 oz	13.0	170	69%
(Cape Cod)				
all natural	3.5 cups	9.0	160	51%
old-fashioned butter	3 cups	10.0	170	53%
white cheddar	2.3 cups	12.0	170	64%
(Chester's)				
microwave				
butter	5 cups	12.0	200	54%
natural	5 cups	12.0	200	54%
prepopped				
butter	3 cups	12.0	160	68%
cheese	3 cups	13.0	190	68%
flamin' hot	3 cups	9.0	170	48%
triple mix	1½ cups	7.0	140	45%
(Crunch & Munch) buttery popcorn w/peanuts				
almond	½ cup	3.0	130	21%
caramel	⅔ cup	3.0	140	26%
maple walnut	⅔ cup	4.0	140	34%
toffee				
original	⅔ cup	4.0	140	34%
	1.25 oz	4.0	160	23%
reduced fat	⅔ cup	2.5	140	16%
	1.25 oz	2.5	150	15%
(Estee) caramel	1 cup	1.5	120	11%
(Featherweight) microwaveable				
lite butter	1 bag	6.0	210	26%
lite natural	1 bag	2.0	160	11%
(Fit Foods) ready to eat	1 oz	–	120	–
decadent caramel	1 oz	–	120	–
(Frookie) Nature's Popcorn				
butter flavor	½ oz	3.0	70	39%

Food and Description	Amount	Fat Grams	Total Calories	% Fat Calories
original	½ oz	2.0	70	26%
sour cream & chives	½ oz	3.0	70	39%
white cheddar	½ oz	3.0	80	34%
generic				
air-popped/no butter added	1 cup	–	30	–
caramel-coated				
plain	1 oz	3.0	122	22%
w/peanuts	1.5 oz	5.0	180	25%
oil-popped/no butter added	1 cup	3.0	55	49%
regular				
white/no butter added	4 cups	0.6	77	7%
yellow/no butter added	4 cups	0.8	77	9%
syrup-coated	1 cup	1.0	135	7%
(Greenfield) caramel/fat-free	⅔ cup	–	100	–
(HBO) microwaveable/unpopped				
butter	3 Tbs	12.0	170	64%
movie butter	3 Tbs	12.0	170	64%
(Healthy Choice) microwaveable				
butter				
popped	1 cup	–	20	–
unpopped	3 Tbs	2.5	130	17%
natural				
popped	1 cup	–	20	–
unpopped	3 Tbs	2.5	130	17%
(Jiffy Pop)				
bag				
butter				
light	3 cups	3.0	70	39%
regular	3 cups	5.0	90	50%
glazed clusters	1 oz	2.0	120	15%
microwaveable				
butter	3 cups	7.0	140	45%
regular	3 cups	7.0	140	45%
pan				
butter	4 cups	6.0	130	42%
regular	4 cups	6.0	130	42%
(Jolly Time) microwaveable				
butter				
light				
popped	1 cup	0.8	20	38%
	4 cups	5.0	120	38%
unpopped	2 Tbs	5.0	120	38%
regular	3 cups	5.0	90	50%
cheddar cheese	3 cups	11.0	180	55%
natural				
light	3 cups	2.0	70	26%
regular	3 cups	7.0	120	53%

Food and Description	Amount	Fat Grams	Total Calories	% Fat Calories
original				
popped	1 cup	2.0	35	51%
	4 cups	9.0	140	58%
unpopped	2 Tbs	9.0	140	58%
(Krun-Chee's) ready to eat				
cheese-flavored	1¾ cups	13.0	170	69%
(Lance)				
cheese	⅝ oz	5.0	90	45%
plain	½ oz	2.5	70	32%
	1 oz	5.0	130	35%
white cheddar cheese	⅝ oz	8.0	100	72%
	⅞ oz	11.0	150	66%
	1½ oz	18.0	250	65%
(Lapida's Popcorn Co.) ready to eat				
caramel	2 cups	4.5	140	29%
herb corn	2 cups	11.0	170	37%
(Laura Scudder's) ready to eat				
tender baby white	1 oz	13.0	170	69%
white	1 oz	11.0	160	62%
(Louise's) fat-free				
apple cinnamon	1 oz	–	100	–
buttery toffee	1 oz	–	100	–
caramel	1 oz	–	100	–
(Newman's Own) Oldstyle Picture Show				
butter				
light	3 cups	3.0	90	30%
natural	3 cups	8.0	150	48%
natural				
light	3 cups	3.0	90	30%
regular	3⅓ cups	1.0	80	11%
no salt	3 cups	8.0	150	48%
plain	3⅓ cups	1.0	80	11%
(Old Vienna)				
butter	1 oz	10.0	160	56%
cheese	1 oz	10.0	160	56%
(Orville Redenbacher's) unpopped				
hot air	2 Tbs	1.0	90	10%
microwaveable				
butter				
no salt added	2 Tbs	12.0	175	62%
regular	2 Tbs	12.0	170	64%
caramel	2 Tbs	10.0	180	50%
cheddar cheese	2 Tbs	9.0	145	43%
herb & garlic	2 Tbs	13.0	175	67%
movie theater				
butter	2 Tbs	13.0	180	65%
light	2 Tbs	5.0	110	41%
plain	2 Tbs	13.0	175	67%

Food and Description	Amount	Fat Grams	Total Calories	% Fat Calories
natural				
light	2 Tbs	5.0	110	41%
no salt added	2 Tbs	12.0	175	62%
regular	2 Tbs	11.0	154	60%
plain	2 Tbs	6.0	120	45%
Redenbudders golden cheddar	2 Tbs	13.0	170	69%
smart pop	2 Tbs	3.0	95	28%
zesty	2 Tbs	13.0	180	65%
regular				
original	2 Tbs	1.0	90	10%
white	2 Tbs	1.0	90	10%
(Pillsbury) microwaveable				
butter	3 cups	13.0	210	56%
original	3 cups	13.0	210	56%
salt-free	3 cups	7.0	170	37%
Pop Secret (See Betty Crocker in this section)				
(Poppycock) ready to eat				
porpcorn, pecans, & almonds	½ cup	10.0	180	50%
(Pops-Rite)				
butter	3 cups	5.0	90	50%
natural	3 cups	5.0	90	50%
(Schwan's) microwaveable/unpopped				
natural lite	3 Tbs	5.0	130	35%
w/butter	3 Tbs	12.0	180	60%
(Smartfood)				
butter	3 cups	9.0	150	54%
cheddar cheese	2 cups	12.0	190	57%
(Ultra Slim Fast)				
butter flavored	4⅓ cups	3.5	130	24%
caramel	½ cup	1.5	120	11%
(Vic's) Corn Popper/ready to eat				
butter				
low-fat	3 cups	1.5	120	11%
regular	2½ cups	7.0	150	42%
caramel				
fat-free	1 cup	–	110	–
lite	1 cup	2.0	110	16%
regular	¾ cup	4.0	130	28%
cheese				
white				
lite	2½ cups	6.0	130	42%
regular	2 cups	13.0	180	65%
yellow				
lite	2½ cups	7.0	140	45%
regular	1½ cups	14.0	190	66%
white				
lite				
full salt	2¾ cups	3.0	130	21%

Food and Description	Amount	Fat Grams	Total Calories	% Fat Calories
½ salt	2¾ cups	3.0	130	21%
low-fat	3½ cups	1.0	110	8%
regular				
full salt	2½ cups	6.0	150	36%
½ salt	2½ cups	6.0	150	36%
white CDR/low-fat	3½ cups	2.5	110	20%
(Weaver's) Mrs Weaver's home-popped	3 cups	8.0	140	51%
(Weight Watchers)	1 pkg	1.0	100	9%
microwaveable	1 pouch	1.0	90	10%
ready to eat				
butter	0.66 oz	2.5	90	25%
butter toffee	0.9 oz	2.5	110	20%
caramel	0.9 oz	1.0	100	9%
white cheddar	0.66 oz	4.0	90	40%
(Wise) ready to eat				
buttery cheddar	1 oz	11.0	160	62%
hot cheese flavored	1 oz	9.0	150	54%
tender eating baby	1 oz	13.0	170	69%
white cheddar cheese	1 oz	11.0	160	62%
(Wise Choice) ready to eat/reduced fat				
baby white	1 oz	6.0	140	39%
butter-flavored	1 oz	5.0	140	32%
POPCORN BARS & CAKES (See also RICE CAKES)				
(Betty Crocker) Pop Secret popcorn bars				
caramel w/chocolate-flavored topping	1 bar	2.5	80	28%
(Hain)				
butter				
mini	7 cakes	–	60	–
regular	1 cake	1.0	45	20%
caramel/mini	5 cakes	–	60	–
lightly salted/mini	7 cakes	–	50	–
mild cheddar/mini	6 cakes	2.0	70	26%
nacho cheese/regular	1 cake	1.0	45	20%
plain/regular	1 cake	–	35	–
white cheddar/regular	1 cake	1.0	45	20%
(Konriko) popcorn cakes				
butter	1 cake	–	40	–
lightly salted	1 cake	–	40	–
(Orville Redenbacher's)				
apple cinnamon/mini	11 cakes	<1.0	100	5%
butter				
mini	13 cakes	2.0	100	18%
regular	3 cakes	2.0	110	16%
caramel				
mini	11 cakes	<1.0	100	5%
regular	2 cakes	<1.0	85	5%
honey nut/mini	11 cakes	<1.0	100	5%

Food and Description	Amount	Fat Grams	Total Calories	% Fat Calories
white cheddar cheese				
mini	13 cakes	1.5	100	14%
regular	3 cakes	2.0	110	16%
(Quaker)				
butter				
mini	6 cakes	–	50	–
regular	1 cake	–	35	–
caramel				
mini	5 cakes	–	50	–
regular	1 cake	–	50	–
Monterey jack				
mini	6 cakes	–	50	–
regular	1 cake	–	40	–
white cheddar				
mini	6 cakes	–	50	–
regular	1 cake	–	40	–
POPCORN OIL (See OIL)				
POPPY SEED (See also POPPY SEED FILLING)				
	1 tsp	1.0	15	60%
	1 Tbs	4.0	50	72%
POPPY SEED FILLING				
(Solo)	2 Tbs	4.0	140	26%
POPSICLE (See FRUIT ICES, BARS, & POPS; ICE CREAM BARS, SANDWICHES, & FROZEN NOVELTIES)				
PORGY				
beaded & fried	3 oz	13.0	246	48%
cooked-dry heat	3 oz	8.7	172	46%

PORK (See also BACON; HAM; LUNCHEON MEAT; PORK DINNER/ENTRÉEE; SAUSAGE)

(NOTE: The information listed under Today's Leaner Pork was provided by the National Pork, Livestock, and Meat Board. Following this is nutritional information provided by the United States Department of Agriculture. "Lean" means pork trimmed of separable fat before cooking. "Lean & fat" means untrimmed and cooked or eaten as purchased. Prime cuts have the most fat; choice cuts less; and select cuts the least. In most cases, 4 ounces of raw pork yields approximately 3 ounces cooked. Serving amounts do not include bone.)

■ TODAY'S LEANER PORK

(Note: Unless otherwise stated, meat has been trimmed of all separable fat and roasted.)

blade steak	3 oz	10.7	193	50%
center loin chop	3 oz	6.9	165	38%
center rib chop	3 oz	8.3	179	43%
loin chop	3 oz	6.6	173	34%
loin roast	3 oz	6.0	165	33%
rib chop	3 oz	8.3	186	41%
rib roast	3 oz	8.6	182	43%
ribs (country style)	3 oz	12.6	210	54%
sirloin chop	3 oz	5.7	164	31%
sirloin roast	3 oz	8.7	184	43%
tenderloin	3 oz	4.0	139	26%

Food and Description	Amount	Fat Grams	Total Calories	% Fat Calories
top loin chop	3 oz	6.6	165	36%
■ PORK CUTS/FRESH				
backfat/raw	1 oz	24.0	230	94%
	3.5 oz	84.5	812	94%
backribs/lean & fat/roasted	3 oz	23.0	315	66%
	7.7 oz	58.5	815	65%
belly/raw	1 oz	14.0	150	84%
	1 lb	225.5	2350	86%
center loin/bone in				
chop				
lean				
braised	3 oz	6.5	175	33%
broiled	3 oz	6.0	170	32%
pan-fried	3 oz	8.0	200	36%
lean & fat				
braised	3 oz	11.0	210	47%
broiled	3 oz	10.0	205	44%
pan-fried	3 oz	13.0	235	50%
roast/roasted				
lean	3 oz	7.0	170	37%
lean & fat	3 oz	10.5	200	47%
composite cuts				
loin & shoulder blade				
lean/cooked	3 oz	7.0	180	35%
lean & fat/cooked	3 oz	11.0	215	46%
ground				
cooked	3 oz	16.0	250	58%
	1 lb	59.0	930	57%
raw	4 oz	22.0	300	66%
leg				
rump half				
lean				
roasted	3 oz	6.5	175	33%
roasted/chopped or diced	1 cup	10.0	280	32%
lean & fat				
roasted	3 oz	11.0	215	46%
roasted/chopped or diced	1 cup	17.5	340	46%
shank half				
lean				
roasted	3 oz	8.0	185	39%
roasted/chopped or diced	1 cup	13.0	290	40%
lean & fat				
roasted	3 oz	15.5	245	57%
roasted/chopped or diced	1 cup	24.5	390	57%
whole				
lean				
roasted	3 oz	7.5	180	37%
roasted/chopped or diced	1 cup	11.5	285	36%

Food and Description	Amount	Fat Grams	Total Calories	% Fat Calories
lean & fat				
roasted	3 oz	13.5	230	53%
roasted/chopped or diced	1 cup	21.5	370	52%
loin				
blade/bone-in/chop				
lean				
braised	3 oz	10.0	190	47%
broiled	3 oz	10.5	200	47%
pan-fried	3 oz	11.5	205	50%
roasted	3 oz	11.0	210	47%
lean & fat				
braised	3 oz	19.5	275	64%
broiled	3 oz	19.0	275	62%
pan-fried	3 oz	21.0	290	65%
roasted	3 oz	19.0	275	62%
center rib				
chop/bone-in				
lean				
braised	3 oz	7.5	175	39%
broiled	3 oz	7.0	190	33%
pan-fried	3 oz	9.0	185	44%
lean & fat				
braised	3 oz	12.0	215	50%
broiled	3 oz	12.0	225	48%
pan-fried	3 oz	13.5	225	54%
chop/boneless				
lean				
braised	3 oz	8.0	180	40%
broiled	3 oz	7.5	185	36%
pan-fried	3 oz	9.5	190	45%
lean & fat				
braised	3 oz	12.5	215	52%
broiled	3 oz	12.0	220	49%
pan-fried	3 oz	14.0	235	54%
roast/bone-in				
lean/roasted	3 oz	9.0	190	43%
lean & fat/roasted	3 oz	12.0	220	49%
roast/boneless				
lean/roasted	3 oz	7.5	185	36%
lean & fat/roasted	3 oz	11.5	215	48%
ribs/country style				
lean				
braised	3 oz	10.0	200	45%
roasted	3 oz	11.0	210	47%
lean & fat				
braised	3 oz	16.5	250	59%
roasted	3 oz	19.0	280	61%

Food and Description	Amount	Fat Grams	Total Calories	% Fat Calories
whole				
lean				
braised	3 oz	7.0	175	36%
broiled	3 oz	7.5	180	38%
roasted	3 oz	7.0	180	35%
lean & fat				
braised	3 oz	11.0	210	47%
broiled	3 oz	11.0	210	52%
roasted	3 oz	11.0	210	52%
shoulder				
arm picnic				
lean				
braised	3 oz	9.5	215	40%
braised/chopped or diced	1 cup	22.0	490	40%
roasted	3 oz	10.0	195	45%
roasted/chopped or diced	1 cup	22.0	435	46%
lean & fat				
braised	3 oz	18.0	280	58%
braised/chopped or diced	1 cup	28.5	445	58%
roasted	3 oz	18.5	270	62%
roasted/chopped or diced	1 cup	29.5	430	62%
Boston blade				
roast				
lean				
raw	1 lb	30.5	555	49%
roasted	3 oz	11.0	200	50%
lean & fat				
raw	1 lb	44.5	705	57%
roasted	3 oz	14.5	230	57%
steak				
lean				
braised	3 oz	12.0	235	47%
broiled	3 oz	9.5	195	44%
lean & fat				
braised	3 oz	16.5	270	55%
broiled	3 oz	12.5	220	51%
whole				
lean				
roasted	3 oz	10.5	200	47%
roasted/chopped or diced	1 cup	16.5	315	47%
lean & fat				
roasted	3 oz	16.5	250	59%
roasted/chopped or diced	1 cup	26.0	395	59%
sirloin				
chop/bone in				
lean				
braised	3 oz	7.0	170	37%
broiled	3 oz	7.5	180	37%

Food and Description	Amount	Fat Grams	Total Calories	% Fat Calories
lean & fat				
braised	3 oz	11.5	210	49%
broiled	3 oz	12.0	220	49%
chop/boneless				
lean				
braised	3 oz	5.0	150	30%
broiled	3 oz	5.0	165	27%
lean & fat				
braised	3 oz	6.5	160	37%
broiled	3 oz	6.0	180	30%
roast/bone in				
lean				
raw	1 lb	19.0	450	38%
roasted	3 oz	8.0	185	39%
lean & fat				
raw	1 lb	32.5	600	49%
roasted	3 oz	12.0	225	48%
roast/boneless	3 oz	5.5	165	30%
lean				
raw	1 lb	22.5	610	33%
roasted	3 oz	6.0	170	32%
lean & fat				
raw	1 lb	26.5	650	37%
roasted	3 oz	7.0	180	35%
spareribs/lean & fat				
braised	3 oz	23.5	340	62%
raw	1 lb	48.5	700	62%
tenderloin				
lean				
broiled	3 oz	4.5	160	25%
raw	1 lb	13.5	545	22%
roasted	3 oz	3.5	140	23%
lean & fat				
broiled	3 oz	6.0	170	32%
roasted	3 oz	4.5	150	27%
top loin				
chop/boneless				
lean				
braised	3 oz	6.5	170	34%
broiled	3 oz	6.0	175	31%
pan-fried	3 oz	8.0	190	38%
lean & fat				
braised	3 oz	10.0	200	45%
broiled	3 oz	8.5	195	41%
pan-fried	3 oz	11.5	220	47%
roast/boneless				
lean/roasted	3 oz	5.5	165	30%

Food and Description	Amount	Fat Grams	Total Calories	% Fat Calories
lean & fat				
raw	1 lb	31.0	690	40%
roasted	3 oz	9.0	195	42%
■ **PORK CUTS, ORGAN & OTHER/FRESH**				
brain/braised	3 oz	4.5	120	33%
	13.5 oz	18.0	530	31%
chitterlings/chitlins/simmered	3 oz	23.0	260	80%
	6 oz	46.0	520	80%
ear/simmered	1 ear	–	185	–
	15 oz	–	700	–
feet/simmered	2.5 oz	8.0	140	51%
	5 oz	16.0	275	52%
heart				
braised	1 heart	5.0	190	24%
braised/chopped or diced	1 cup	5.5	215	23%
jowl/raw	4 oz	75.0	740	91%
kidney				
braised	3 oz	3.0	130	21%
braised/chopped or diced	1 cup	5.0	215	22%
liver/braised	3 oz	2.5	140	16%
lung/braised	3 oz	2.0	85	21%
pancreas/braised	3 oz	–	190	–
salt pork/cured/raw	1 oz	22.0	215	92%
	8 oz	174.0	1700	92%
spleen/braised	3 oz	2.0	130	14%
stomach/raw	4 oz	–	180	–
tail				
raw	4 oz	35.0	430	73%
simmered	3 oz	28.0	340	74%
tongue/braised	3 oz	14.5	230	57%
PORK & BEANS (*See* BEANS, BAKED & VARIETY)				
PORK ENTRÉE/DINNER (*See also* ASIAN FOOD; FROZEN ENTRÉE/DINNER)				
(Armour Star) pork brains in milk gravy	⅔ cup	5.0	150	30%
(Delores)				
pickled pork rinds	2 oz	3.0	60	30%
pig's feet	2 oz	6.0	90	60%
(Grandad's) real bacon rinds	½ oz	1.5	60	23%
homemade/USDA Standard Home Recipe				
ham croquette	~2 oz	9.8	165	54%
pickled pig's feet	1 oz	4.0	60	60%
	1 lb	67.5	925	66%
(Hormel)				
pickled pig's feet	2 oz	6.0	80	68%
pickled pork hocks	2 oz	8.0	110	65%
pickled pork tidbits	2 oz	8.0	100	72%
(Schwan's) frozen				
center cut pork loin chops	1 chop	5.0	140	42%
chopped pork fritter	1 fritter	10.0	220	41%

Food and Description	Amount	Fat Grams	Total Calories	% Fat Calories
pork spareribs	5 oz	18.0	310	16%
PORK FAT (See LARD)				
PORK RINDS (See PORK ENTRÉE DINNER; SNACKS)				
PORK SAUSAGE (See SAUSAGE)				
POT PIE (See BEEF DISH/ENTRÉE; CHICKEN ENTRÉE/DINNER; FROZEN ENTRÉE/ DINNER; TURKEY ENTRÉE/DINNER; VEGETARIAN FOODS)				
POTATO (See also POTATO DISH/ENTRÉE; SWEET POTATO; YAM)				
canned				
(Bush's Best)				
diced	½ cup	–	40	–
sliced	½ cup	–	40	–
whole	½ cup	–	40	–
(Del Monte) new				
sliced	⅔ cup	–	60	–
whole w/liquid	~2 medium	–	60	–
generic/w/o skin	½ cup	–	54	–
(S&W)	½ cup	–	60	–
(Seneca)	5.8 oz	–	80	–
(Veg All)	½ cup	–	60	–
flakes/granules				
(Betty Crocker) Potato Buds				
cheddar cheese				
mix only	⅓ cup	3.0	120	23%
prepared				
reduced fat recipe	⅔ cup	6.0	160	34%
regular recipe	⅔ cup	10.0	190	47%
original				
mix only	⅓ cup	–	80	–
prepared				
reduced fat recipe	⅔ cup	4.0	120	30%
regular recipe	⅔ cup	8.0	160	45%
sour cream 'n chive				
mix only	⅓ cup	3.5	120	26%
prepared				
reduced fat recipe	⅔ cup	7.0	160	39%
regular recipe	⅔ cup	11.0	190	52%
generic/mix only				
flakes	1 cup	–	164	–
granules	1 cup	1.0	704	1%
(Hungry Jack) flakes/mashed/prepared	½ cup	7.0	140	45%
(Idaho Spuds) flakes/prepared	½ cup	7.0	140	45%
(Idahoan) mix only				
cheddar/spicy	⅙ pkg	1.0	90	10%
real	⅓ cup	1.0	80	11%
fresh				
baked				
in microwave				
w/skin	1 large	–	212	–

Food and Description	Amount	Fat Grams	Total Calories	% Fat Calories
w/o skin	1 large	–	156	–
in oven				
skin only	1 medium	–	115	–
w/skin	~7 oz	–	220	–
w/o skin	~5.5 oz	–	145	–
boiled				
w/skin	½ cup	–	68	–
w/o skin	½ cup	–	67	–
raw				
w/skin	1 medium	–	110	–
w/o skin	1 medium	–	88	–
	~4.75 oz	–	116	–
frozen				
(C&W) whole red	2 large or 3 small	–	60	–
POTATO CHIPS & SNACKS				
(Borden)				
Calypso/sweet & spicy Caribbean	1 oz	10.0	160	56%
Curlie/plain	1 oz	10.0	150	60%
home fries	1 oz	10.0	150	60%
Krunchers				
jalapeño	1 oz	8.0	140	51%
mesquite barbecue	1 oz	8.0	140	51%
original	1 oz	9.0	150	54%
New York Deli				
jalapeño	1 oz	8.0	140	51%
plain	1 oz	10.0	150	60%
original				
BBQ	1 oz	10.0	160	56%
hot	1 oz	10.0	150	60%
lightly salted	1 oz	10.0	150	60%
onion & garlic	1 oz	10.0	150	60%
salt & vinegar	1 oz	10.0	150	60%
Ranch Fries				
no salt added	1 oz	10.0	150	60%
plain	1 oz	10.0	150	60%
Ridgies				
plain	1 oz	10.0	150	60%
super crispy	1 oz	10.0	150	60%
sour cream & onion/ridged	1 oz	10.0	150	60%
Texas BBQ	1 oz	10.0	150	60%
(Cape Cod)				
no salt	1 oz	10.0	150	60%
original	1 oz	8.0	150	48%
sea salt & vinegar	1 oz	8.0	150	48%
select	1 oz	6.0	130	42%
sour cream & chive	1 oz	9.0	150	54%
(Cottage Fries) no salt added	1 oz	10.0	150	60%

Food and Description	Amount	Fat Grams	Total Calories	% Fat Calories
(Deli Style)				
mesquite Bar-B-Q	1 oz	8.0	150	48%
regular	1 oz	8.0	150	48%
sour cream & onion	1 oz	8.0	150	48%
(Durkee) shoestring potato sticks	1 oz	9.0	160	51%
(Eagle)				
Hawaiian Kettle/extra crunchy	1 oz	8.0	150	48%
Idaho Russet dark & crunchy	1 oz	7.0	140	45%
ripples				
cheddar & sour cream/crispy cooked	1 oz	11.0	160	62%
mesquite BBQ	1 oz	10.0	160	56%
plain	1 oz	10.0	150	60%
sour cream & onion	1 oz	10.0	160	56%
thins				
crispy cooked	1 oz	8.0	150	48%
Louisiana BBQ/crispy cooked	1 oz	8.0	150	48%
mesquite BBQ	1 oz	10.0	160	56%
no salt	1 oz	10.0	150	60%
plain	1 oz	10.0	150	60%
sour cream & onion	1 oz	10.0	160	56%
spicy fiesta	1 oz	9.0	160	51%
(Fit Foods) baked potato chips				
BBQ	1 oz	–	100	–
original	1 oz	–	100	–
sour cream & chives	1 oz	–	100	–
(Frito Lay)				
Lay's baked potato crisps				
BBQ	1 oz	1.5	110	12%
original	1 oz	1.5	110	12%
Lay's potato chips				
Bar B Q	1 oz	10.0	150	60%
cheddar cheese	1 oz	10.0	150	60%
Flamin' Hot	1 oz	9.0	150	54%
Italian cheese	1 oz	9.0	150	54%
jalapeno 'n cheddar	1 oz	9.0	150	54%
KC Masterpiece BBQ	1 oz	9.0	150	54%
original	1 oz	10.0	150	60%
salt & vinegar	1 oz	10.0	160	56%
sour cream & onion	1 oz	9.0	160	51%
tangy ranch	1 oz	9.0	160	51%
unsalted	1 oz	10.0	160	56%
wavy au gratin	1 oz	10.0	160	56%
wavy original	1 oz	10.0	160	56%
Ruffles				
cheddar & sour cream	1 oz	10.0	160	56%
mesquite grille B-B-Q	1 oz	9.0	150	54%
original	1 oz	10.0	150	60%
ranch	1 oz	9.0	150	54%

Food and Description	Amount	Fat Grams	Total Calories	% Fat Calories
reduced fat	1 oz	6.0	130	42%
sour cream & onion	1 oz	10.0	150	60%
generic/potato sticks	1 oz	9.0	148	55%
	1 cup	12.0	190	57%
(Health Valley) Hot Potatoes				
mesquite	1½ cups	–	110	–
spicy pizza	1½ cups	–	110	–
zesty ranch	1½ cups	–	110	–
(Keebler) potato snack chips				
Ripplin's				
barbecue	12 chips	9.0	150	54%
original	12 chips	11.0	160	62%
ranch	12 chips	9.0	150	54%
Tato Skins				
baked potato	18 chips	8.0	150	48%
cheese n' bacon	18 chips	9.0	150	54%
sour cream n' onion	18 chips	10.0	150	60%
(Kelly's)				
Bar-B-Q	1 oz	9.0	150	54%
crunchy	1 oz	9.0	150	54%
rippled	1 oz	9.0	150	54%
sour cream n' onion	1 oz	9.0	150	54%
unsalted	1 oz	9.0	150	54%
(Kettle Chips)				
lightly salted	1 oz	9.0	150	54%
low-fat oven-baked	1 oz	1.5	120	9%
New York cheddar w/herbs	1 oz	9.0	150	54%
(Lance)				
BBQ				
big bag	1 oz	10.0	160	56%
value size	1.5 oz	16.0	230	43%
vending pkg	⅞ oz	9.0	140	58%
	1 oz	10.0	160	62%
Cajun				
value size	1.5 oz	15.0	230	59%
vending pkg	1 oz	10.0	150	60%
mesquite				
value size	1.5 oz	15.0	230	59%
vending pkg	1 oz	10.0	150	60%
plain				
big bag	1 oz	10.0	160	56%
value size	1.5 oz	15.0	240	56%
vending pkg	1 oz	10.0	160	56%
ripple				
plain				
big bag	1 oz	10.0	160	56%
value size	1.5 oz	15.0	230	59%
vending pkg	1 oz	11.0	160	62%

Food and Description	Amount	Fat Grams	Total Calories	% Fat Calories
sour cream & onion	1 oz	10.0	160	62%
salt & vinegar				
value size	1.5 oz	16.0	240	60%
vending pkg	1 oz	10.0	160	62%
sour cream & onion				
big bag	1 oz	11.0	160	62%
value size	1.5 oz	16.0	240	60%
vending pkg	1 oz	10.0	160	62%
(Laura Scudder)				
Bar-B-Q	1 oz	10.0	150	60%
for dips	1 oz	10.0	150	60%
Hawaiian	1 oz	9.0	150	54%
natural style	1 oz	10.0	150	60%
plain	1 oz	10.0	150	60%
sour cream & onion	1 oz	9.0	150	54%
(Louise's) potato chips				
Maui onion/fat-free	1 oz	–	110	–
mesquite BBQ				
fat-free	1 oz	–	110	–
"1g"	1 oz	1.0	110	8%
70% less fat	1 oz	2.5	110	20%
no salt/fat-free	1 oz	–	110	–
original				
fat-free	1 oz	–	110	–
"1g"	1 oz	1.0	110	8%
70% less fat	1 oz	2.5	110	20%
(Michael Season's)				
Bakes				
cheddar	1.1 oz	2.0	120	15%
original	1.1 oz	2.0	120	15%
sour cream & green onion	1.1 oz	2.0	120	15%
chips/40% less fat				
honey barbeque	1 oz	6.0	140	39%
lightly salted	1 oz	6.0	130	42%
unsalted	1 oz	6.0	130	42%
yogurt & green onion	1 oz	6.0	130	42%
(Mother's) Potato Snaps				
BBQ	22 pieces	4.0	120	30%
original	22 pieces	4.5	120	34%
salt & vinegar	22 pieces	3.5	120	26%
sour cream & onion	22 pieces	4.0	120	30%
(Nabisco) Mr Phipps Tater Crisps				
bar-b-que	12 crisps	4.0	130	28%
original	23 crisps	4.5	120	34%
sour cream 'n onion	22 crisps	4.0	130	28%
(O'Boises)				
cheddar flavor	1 oz	10.0	150	60%
original	1 oz	9.0	150	54%

Food and Description	Amount	Fat Grams	Total Calories	% Fat Calories
sour cream & onion	1 oz	9.0	150	54%
(O'Grady's)				
au gratin	1 oz	8.0	150	48%
hearty seasoning	1 oz	8.0	140	51%
plain	1 oz	9.0	150	54%
(Old Dutch Foods)				
au gratin	1 oz	8.0	150	48%
BBQ	1 oz	8.0	140	51%
dill	1 oz	8.0	150	48%
onion & garlic	1 oz	9.0	150	54%
original	1 oz	9.0	150	54%
ripple	1 oz	9.0	150	54%
sour cream & onion	1 oz	10.0	150	54%
(Old Vienna)				
Missouri dairy sour cream & onion	1 oz	9.0	150	54%
original/Heartland Pride	1 oz	11.0	180	55%
Ozark hickory	1 oz	10.0	170	53%
Riplets				
grilled steak & onion	1 oz	9.0	150	54%
Heartland Pride	1 oz	10.0	150	60%
red hot	1 oz	9.0	150	54%
Wisconsin cheddar & sour cream	1 oz	10.0	150	60%
(Pacific Grain) French baked potato snacks				
BBQ	1 oz	–	110	–
original	1 oz	–	110	–
ranch	1 oz	–	110	–
Pik-Nik (*See* S&W in this section)				
(Poore Brothers)				
bar-b-que	1 oz	8.0	140	51%
Cajun	1 oz	8.0	140	51%
dill pickle	1 oz	8.0	140	51%
jalapeño	1 oz	8.0	140	51%
original				
regular	1 oz	10.0	150	60%
unsalted	1 oz	8.0	140	51%
Parmesan & garlic	1 oz	8.0	140	51%
salt & vinegar	1 oz	7.0	130	48%
sour cream & onion	1 oz	8.0	140	51%
(Pringle's) potato crisps				
regular				
BBQ				
light	1 oz	6.0	130	42%
regular	1 oz	10.0	150	60%
right	1 oz	7.0	140	45%
Cheez-ums/regular	1 oz	10.0	150	60%
original				
light	1 oz	6.0	130	42%
regular	1 oz	11.0	160	62%

Food and Description	Amount	Fat Grams	Total Calories	% Fat Calories
right	1 oz	7.0	140	45%
ranch				
light	1 oz	6.0	130	42%
regular	1 oz	10.0	150	60%
right	1 oz	7.0	140	45%
sour cream 'n onion				
light	1 oz	6.0	130	42%
regular	1 oz	10.0	160	56%
right	1 oz	7.0	140	45%
Ridges				
cheddar & sour cream	1 oz	10.0	150	60%
mesquite BBQ	1 oz	10.0	150	60%
original	1 oz	10.0	150	60%
rippled original	1 oz	11.0	160	62%
Ruffles (*See* Frito Lay in this section)				
(S&W) Pik-Nik				
Fabulous Fries	⅔ cup	9.0	150	54%
Ketchup 'n Fries	⅔ cup	10.0	160	56%
shoestring potatoes				
50% less salt	¾ cup	12.0	165	65%
regular	1.75 oz	18.0	280	58%
Santa Fe BBQ	⅔ cup	12.0	180	60%
sour cream & cheddar	⅔ cup	13.0	180	65%
(Snyder's)				
BBQ	1 oz	10.0	150	60%
cheddar bacon	1 oz	10.0	150	60%
Coney Island	1 oz	10.0	150	60%
grilled steak & onion	1 oz	10.0	150	60%
hot Buffalo wings	1 oz	10.0	150	60%
kosher dill	1 oz	10.0	150	60%
no salt	1 oz	10.0	150	60%
original	1 oz	10.0	150	60%
salt & vinegar	1 oz	10.0	150	60%
sausage pizza	1 oz	10.0	150	60%
sour cream & onion				
no salt	1 oz	10.0	150	60%
regular	1 oz	10.0	150	60%
	1 oz	10.0	150	60%
Tato Skins (*See* Keebler in this section)				
(Weaver's)	1 oz	9.0	150	54%
(Westbrae)				
original				
no salt	1 oz	8.0	150	48%
salted	1 oz	10.0	150	60%
ripple	1 oz	8.0	150	48%
(Wise)				
regular				
BBQ	1 oz	10.0	150	60%

Food and Description	Amount	Fat Grams	Total Calories	% Fat Calories
hot	1 oz	11.0	160	62%
New York Deli	1 oz	11.0	160	62%
onion-garlic	1 oz	10.0	150	60%
plain	1 oz	10.0	150	60%
Ridgies				
BBQ	1 oz	10.0	150	60%
original	1 oz	10.0	150	60%
plain	1 oz	10.0	150	60%
sour cream & onion	1 oz	11.0	160	62%
rippled	1 oz	10.0	150	60%

POTATO DISH/ENTRÉE (See also FROZEN ENTRÉE/DINNER; SEASONINGS; VEGETARIAN FOODS)

■ **CANNED OR JARRED**

Food and Description	Amount	Fat Grams	Total Calories	% Fat Calories
(Dinty Moore)				
canned sliced potatoes & beef	7.5 oz	9.0	230	31%
generic				
canned potato salad/homestyle	½ cup	11.0	170	58%
(Hormel)				
au gratin potatoes & bacon	7.5 oz	14.0	250	50%
scalloped potatoes & ham	7.5 oz	16.0	260	55%
(Read) potato salad				
German style	½ cup	3.0	120	23%
homestyle	½ cup	11.0	170	58%
(Reesur's) potato salad	½ cup	15.0	250	54%
■ **FROZEN OR REFRIGERATED**				
(Brighton's) baked potatoes				
broccoli & cheese	10.2 oz	12.0	337	32%
cheese sauce/bacon	9.5 oz	13.0	352	33%
cheese sauce/ham	10.2 oz	12.0	347	31%
classic combination	9.6 oz	13.0	326	36%
generic				
cottage cut potatoes				
cooked in oven	10 pieces	4.0	109	33%
French-fried/heated	10 pieces	4.0	109	33%
fried in vegetable oil	10 pieces	8.0	158	46%
hash browns				
plain	½ cup	9.0	170	48%
w/butter	3.5 oz	9.0	180	43%
potato puffs	1 puff	0.8	16	45%
scalloped potatoes & ham				
plain	½ cup	6.0	123	44%
w/cheese	½ cup	9.6	177	49%
(Golden) potato pancakes	1 pancake	3.0	70	39%
(Gorton's)				
potato crisp fillets	2 fillets	19.0	300	57%
potato sticks	6 sticks	16.0	270	53%
(Heinz) deep fries				
crinkle cut	3 oz	6.0	150	36%

Food and Description	Amount	Fat Grams	Total Calories	% Fat Calories
hash brown/onion	3 oz	7.0	110	57%
regular	3 oz	6.0	160	34%
shoestring	3 oz	10.0	200	45%
(Inland Valley)				
fajita fries	1 cup	7.0	140	45%
mashed homestyle	⅔ cup	7.0	160	39%
munch skin meals	2 topped skins	15.0	250	54%
potato stix	3 oz	10.0	170	53%
seasoned crisscut fries	3 oz	2.0	180	10%
Simply Shred				
O'Brien	1 cup	–	60	–
regular	1 cup	–	70	–
Tasty Q's	1 cup	7.0	160	39%
Tater Puffs	10 pieces	7.0	160	39%
(J.R. Simplot)				
crinkle cut	3 oz	5.0	120	38%
hash brown shreds	3 oz	–	60	–
mashed singles	1 scoop	–	90	–
Performers 101's	1 patty	8.0	130	55%
regular cut	3 oz	4.0	120	30%
seasoned crisp				
lattice cuts	3 oz	9.0	170	48%
original	3 oz	8.0	150	48%
sour cream & chive	3 oz	7.0	140	45%
tater loops	3 oz	7.0	150	42%
shoestrings	3 oz	6.0	140	39%
skincredible				
lattice cuts	3 oz	10.0	230	39%
loops	3 oz	6.0	150	36%
tater gems	10 gems	10.0	170	53%
(Larry's) stuffed potatoes				
cheddar cheese	1 potato	9.0	160	51%
combination	1 potato	8.0	160	45%
sour cream & chives	1 potato	8.0	150	48%
(Mrs. T's) pierogies				
potato & cheese	3 pieces	2.6	180	13%
potato & onion	3 pieces	2.0	180	10%
(Micromagic)				
skinny fries	3.5 oz	9.0	210	39%
tater sticks	4 oz	16.0	260	55%
(Oh Boy!)				
cheddar cheese	6 oz	4.0	130	28%
real bacon	6 oz	3.0	120	23%
sour cream, onion, & chives	6 oz	2.5	140	16%
(Ore Ida)				
baked/topped/broccoli & cheese	6 oz	4.0	150	24%
cheddar browns	1 patty	2.0	80	23%

Food and Description	Amount	Fat Grams	Total Calories	% Fat Calories
cottage fries	3 oz	4.0	130	38%
Crispers!	3 oz	13.0	220	59%
Crispy Crowns	3 oz	11.0	190	53%
Crispy Crunchies	3 oz	8.0	160	45%
deep fries				
crinkle cut	3 oz	6.0	160	34%
regular cut	3 oz	7.0	160	39%
fast fries				
ranch flavor	3 oz	7.0	150	39%
regular	3 oz	6.0	150	36%
French fries				
country	3 oz	3.5	120	26%
golden crinkles	3 oz	3.5	140	23%
golden fries	3 oz	3.5	120	26%
pixie crinkles	3 oz	5.0	130	35%
shoestrings	3 oz	6.0	150	36%
steak	3 oz	3.0	110	25%
waffle	3 oz	7.0	150	42%
golden patties	1 patty	9.0	160	51%
golden twirls	3 oz	6.0	150	36%
hash browns				
country style	1 cup	–	60	–
microwave	4 oz	12.0	220	49%
shredded	1 patty	–	70	–
Southern style	¾ cup	–	80	–
toaster	3.5 oz	11.0	190	52%
mashed potatoes	⅔ cup	2.5	90	25%
potatoes O'Brien	¾ cup	–	60	–
Snackin' Fries				
extra zesty	5 oz	21.0	340	56%
regular	5 oz	20.0	340	53%
Tater Tots				
Hot Tots	3 oz	7.0	160	39%
microwave	3.5 oz	8.0	180	40%
regular	3 oz	8.0	160	42%
w/onion	3 oz	7.0	150	36%
twice-baked				
butter flavor	5 oz	8.0	200	36%
cheddar cheese	5 oz	8.0	190	38%
sour cream & chives	5 oz	7.0	190	33%
Wedges home style	3 oz	8.0	110	25%
Zesties!	3 oz	8.0	160	45%
(Simply Potatoes)				
au gratin	¼ pkg	8.0	130	55%
hash browns				
plain	⅕ pkg	–	100	–
onion	⅕ pkg	–	120	–
Southwestern style	⅕ pkg	–	100	–

Food and Description	Amount	Fat Grams	Total Calories	% Fat Calories
mashed	⅕ pkg	2.0	90	20%
scalloped	⅕ pkg	5.0	100	45%
(Weight Watchers)				
broccoli & cheese	10 oz	6.0	230	23%
■ HOMEMADE				
USDA Standard Home Recipe				
hash brown potatoes	½ cup	10.0	165	55%
mashed potatoes				
made w/whole milk	½ cup	0.6	81	7%
made w/whole milk & butter	½ cup	4.0	94	38%
potato pancakes/made w/butter & milk	1 pancake	12.6	495	23%
potato salad				
made w/mayonnaise	½ cup	10.0	179	50%
made w/mustard	½ cup	6.0	120	45%
potatoes au gratin	½ cup	9.0	160	51%
potatoes O'Brien/made w/bread crumbs & butter	½ cup	1.0	79	11%
scalloped potatoes				
made w/butter	½ cup	4.5	105	39%
made w/cheese	½ cup	9.5	175	49%
■ MICROWAVE CONTAINER				
(Hormel)				
scalloped potatoes & ham				
micro cup meal	1 cup	16.0	260	55%
10.5-oz container	1 cup	23.0	360	58%
(Lunch Bucket)				
scalloped flavored w/ham	1 container	7.0	170	37%
■ MIX				
(Betty Crocker)				
cheddar classics				
cheddar & bacon				
mix only	½ cup	1.5	100	14%
prepared	½ cup	6.0	150	36%
cheddar & sour cream				
mix only	⅔ cup	1.5	120	11%
prepared	½ cup	6.0	170	32%
three cheese				
mix only	½ cup	1.5	100	14%
prepared	½ cup	6.0	150	36%
white cheddar				
mix only	½ cup	2.0	110	16%
prepared	½ cup	6.0	150	36%
Hamburger Helper				
potato stroganoff				
mix	⅔ cup	2.0	120	15%
prepared	1 cup	12.0	270	40%
potatoes au gratin				
mix	⅔ cup	2.5	120	19%

Food and Description	Amount	Fat Grams	Total Calories	% Fat Calories
prepared	1 cup	14.0	290	43%
homestyle potatoes				
American cheese				
mix only	⅔ cup	1.5	100	14%
prepared	½ cup	6.0	150	36%
broccoli au gratin				
mix only	⅔ cup	1.5	100	14%
prepared	½ cup	6.0	150	36%
cheddar cheese				
mix only	⅔ cup	2.0	100	18%
prepared	½ cup	7.0	160	39%
cheesy scalloped				
mix only	⅔ cup	2.0	100	18%
prepared	½ cup	6.0	150	36%
Potato Buds				
cheddar cheese				
mix only	⅓ cup	3.0	120	23%
prepared				
reduced fat recipe	⅔ cup	6.0	160	34%
regular recipe	⅔ cup	10.0	190	47%
original				
mix only	⅓ cup	–	80	–
prepared				
reduced fat recipe	⅔ cup	4.0	120	30%
regular recipe	⅔ cup	8.0	160	45%
sour cream 'n chive				
mix only	⅓ cup	3.5	120	26%
prepared				
reduced fat recipe	⅔ cup	7.0	160	39%
regular recipe	⅔ cup	11.0	190	52%
Potato Shakers				
crispy cheddar fries				
mix only	2 tsp	1.0	25	36%
prepared				
low-fat recipe	7 fries	2.5	110	20%
regular recipe	7 fries	5.0	130	35%
original				
mix only	3 tsp	0.5	30	15%
prepared				
low-fat recipe	¾ cup	1.5	130	10%
regular recipe	¾ cup	4.5	150	27%
Parmesan				
mix only	3 tsp	1.0	30	30%
prepared				
low-fat recipe	¾ cup	2.0	130	14%
regular recipe	¾ cup	5.0	150	30%
seasoned fries				
mix only	3 tsp	–	20	–

Food and Description	Amount	Fat Grams	Total Calories	% Fat Calories
prepared				
low-fat recipe	7 fries	2.5	100	23%
regular recipe	7 fries	4.0	120	30%
zesty cheddar				
mix only	3 tsp	1.5	30	45%
prepared				
low-fat recipe	¾ cup	2.5	130	17%
regular recipe	¾ cup	5.0	160	28%
Potatoes Express				
broccoli au gratin				
mix only	½ cup	1.0	100	9%
prepared	⅔ cup	4.0	130	28%
cheddar cheese				
mix only	½ cup	1.0	100	9%
prepared	⅔ cup	4.0	140	26%
Specialty Potatoes				
au gratin				
mix only	½ cup	1.5	100	14%
prepared				
low-fat recipe	½ cup	1.5	110	12%
regular recipe	½ cup	6.0	150	36%
cheddar 'n bacon				
mix only	½ cup	1.5	100	14%
prepared	½ cup	6.0	160	34%
hash brown				
mix only	½ cup	–	130	–
prepared	½ cup	8.0	200	36%
julienne				
mix only	½ cup	1.0	90	10%
prepared	½ cup	6.0	140	39%
scalloped				
8.25-oz box				
mix only	½ cup	1.5	110	12%
prepared	½ cup	6.0	160	34%
5- or 20-oz box				
mix only	½ cup	1.0	90	10%
prepared	½ cup	7.0	160	39%
scalloped potatoes 'n ham				
mix only	½ cup	1.5	100	14%
prepared	½ cup	7.0	160	39%
smoky cheddar				
mix only	½ cup	1.0	100	9%
prepared	½ cup	6.0	150	36%
sour cream 'n chive				
mix only	½ cup	1.5	100	14%
prepared	½ cup	7.0	160	39%
Twice-Baked/cheddar & bacon				
mix only	⅓ cup	2.5	110	20%

Food and Description	Amount	Fat Grams	Total Calories	% Fat Calories
prepared	⅔ cup	11.0	210	47%
(Good Harvest) mix only				
country French	½ cup	1.0	100	9%
southern Italian	½ cup	0.5	110	4%
vegetable & herb	½ cup	0.5	110	4%
(Idohoan) prepared				
au gratin	½ cup	5.0	130	35%
hash brown				
quick one-pan	½ cup	7.0	140	45%
regular	½ cup	7.0	140	45%
mashed/cheddar	½ cup	5.0	140	32%
scalloped				
sour cream & chives	½ cup	5.0	130	35%
traditional	½ cup	7.0	140	45%
(Manischewitz) potato pancake/mix only	3 Tbs	1.0	80	11%
(Panni) mix only				
Bavarian potato dumpling	½ pkg	–	80	–
Bavarian potato pancake	½ pkg	–	50	–
POTATO PANCAKE (See POTATO DISH/ENTRÉE)				
POTATO SNACKS (See POTATO CHIPS & SNACKS)				
POTATO SOUP (See SOUP)				
POTATO STARCH				
(Manischewitz)	½ cup	–	285	–
POTTED MEAT (See LUNCHEON MEAT; LUNCHEON MEAT SPREAD)				
POULTRY SEASONING (See also SEASONINGS)				
	1 tsp	–	5	–
POUT, OCEAN				
raw	3 oz	1.0	70	13%
PRESERVES (See JAM/JELLY/PRESERVES)				
PRETZEL				
(Bakers Best) soft/frozen				
Dutch twists	2.5 oz twist	1.0	180	5%
(Barbara's Bakery)				
Bavarian				
no salt added	2 pretzels	<1.0	110	4%
regular	2 pretzels	<1.0	110	4%
honey sweet	2 pretzels	<1.0	110	4%
minis				
no salt added	17 pretzels	<1.0	110	4%
regular	17 pretzels	<1.0	110	4%
(Borden)				
fat-free				
thins	6 pieces	–	100	–
ultra thin	8 pieces	–	100	–
low-fat mini				
cheddar	21 pieces	1.5	110	12%
mustard & honey	21 pieces	1.5	110	12%
(Cape Cod) no-fat multigrain	30 pretzels	–	110	–

Food and Description	Amount	Fat Grams	Total Calories	% Fat Calories
(Delicious) sticks or twists	1 oz	1.0	110	8%
(Eagle)				
low-fat				
mini bites	¾ cup	1.0	110	8%
pretzel sticks	46 sticks	1.0	110	8%
thin twists	1 oz	1.0	110	8%
no-fat				
sourdough Bavarian				
no salt added	1 oz	–	110	–
plain	1 oz	–	110	–
thin twists	1 oz	–	100	–
(Estee)				
nuggets				
original	30 nuggets	1.5	120	11%
ranch	23 nuggets	2.0	130	14%
unsalted				
Dutch	2 pretzels	1.0	130	7%
original	23 pretzels	1.0	120	8%
(Featherweight) unsalted	23 pretzels	1.0	120	8%
(Good Health) peanut butter-filled	8 pieces	6.0	140	39%
(Gus) soft baked/frozen				
sticks	1 pretzel	1.0	210	4%
twists	1 pretzel	1.0	210	4%
(Keebler)				
butter				
braids	22 pretzels	1.0	100	9%
knots	7 pretzels	1.0	100	9%
mini knots	18 pretzels	1.0	100	9%
traditional				
Bavarian	3 pretzels	2.0	120	15%
knots	7 pretzels	1.0	110	8%
(Lance)	1¼ oz	1.0	140	6%
(Laura Scudder's)				
Bavarian	1 oz	1.0	110	8%
sticks	1 oz	1.0	110	8%
twists	1 oz	1.0	110	8%
(Louise's) fat-free sourdough	1 oz	–	90	–
(Michael Season's) O.G.'s Organic				
honey mustard nuggets	1 oz	<1.0	120	3%
lightly salted				
mini	1 oz	<1.0	110	3%
sticks	1 oz	<1.0	110	3%
twists	1 oz	<1.0	110	3%
sesame garlic nuggets	1 oz	1.0	120	8%
unsalted				
mini	1 oz	<1.0	110	3%
twists	1 oz	<1.0	110	3%
Mister Salty (See Nabisco in this section)				

Food and Description	Amount	Fat Grams	Total Calories	% Fat Calories
(Mrs. Manischewitz) Bagel Pretzel				
everything onion	4 pretzels	–	110	–
garlic	4 pretzels	–	110	–
onion	4 pretzels	–	110	–
original	4 pretzels	–	110	–
(Nabisco)				
Mr. Phipps Pretzel Chips				
fat-free	16 pieces	–	100	–
lower sodium	16 pieces	2.5	120	19%
original	16 pieces	2.5	120	19%
Mister Salty				
chips	1 oz	2.5	110	16%
Dutch	1 oz	1.0	120	8%
fat-free				
chips	1 oz	–	100	–
regular	1 oz	–	110	–
sticks or twists	1 oz	–.	110	–
mini	1 oz	1.0	110	8%
(Newman's Own)				
Bavarian	1 pretzel	–	90	–
rounds				
regular	1 oz	1.0	110	8%
salt & pepper	1 oz	1.0	110	8%
sticks	1 oz	1.0	110	8%
(Pepperidge Farm) snack sticks	9 sticks	3.0	130	21%
(Planter's) twists	1 oz	0.5	100	5%
	1.5 oz	1.0	160	6%
(Pocket Pretzels) peanut butter-filled	1 oz	4.0	126	29%
(Quinlan)				
beer	2 pieces	2.0	110	16%
logs	8 pieces	1.5	110	12%
mini	1 oz	2.0	110	16%
nuggets	17 pieces	2.0	110	16%
rods	3 pieces	1.5	110	12%
sourdough/fat-free				
no salt added	1 pretzel	–	80	–
regular	1 pretzel	–	80	–
sticks	1 oz	1.0	110	8%
thins				
party	1 oz	<1.0	110	4%
plain	1 oz	1.5	160	8%
sourdough	1 oz	–	100	–
tiny thins				
cheese	1 oz	1.0	110	8%
party	28 pieces	2.0	110	16%
plain	1 oz	2.0	110	16%
ultra thin	8 pieces	1.0	110	8%

Food and Description	Amount	Fat Grams	Total Calories	% Fat Calories
(Rokeach)				
Dutch	1 oz	–	110	–
no salt	1 oz	–	110	–
party canister	1 oz	1.0	110	8%
(Rold Gold)				
fat-free				
sourdough	1 oz	–	80	–
sticks	1 oz	–	110	–
thins	1 oz	–	110	–
tinys	1 oz	–	100	–
regular				
Bavarian	1 oz	2.0	110	16%
rods	1 oz	1.5	110	14%
sticks	1 oz	1.0	110	8%
tiny twist	1 oz	1.0	110	8%
twists	1 oz	1.0	110	8%
(Seyfert's) butter/rods	1 oz	1.0	110	8%
(Snyder's)				
buttermilk ranch	1 oz	5.0	130	35%
cheddar cheese	1 oz	7.0	160	39%
honey mustard & onion	1 oz	7.0	140	45%
logs	1 oz	–	110	–
minis	1 oz	–	110	–
nibblers	1 oz	–	110	–
oat bran	1 oz	1.0	120	8%
old fashioned hard	1 oz	–	110	–
Old Tyme				
regular	1 oz	–	118	–
unsalted	1 oz	–	110	–
rods	1 oz	–	110	–
sourdough				
regular	1 oz	–	100	–
unsalted	1 oz	–	110	–
stix	1 oz	–	110	–
very thins	1 oz	–	110	–
(SuperPretzel) soft-baked/frozen				
pretzels				
bites	5 bites	–	110	–
original	1 pretzel	–	170	–
Softstix				
cheddar	2 stix	2.0	110	16%
nacho	2 stix	2.0	110	16%
pizza	2 stix	2.0	110	16%
(Tastykake) Tasty Twists	7 pretzels	6.0	130	42%
	1 bag	9.0	200	41%
(Ultra Slim Fast)	1 oz	1.5	110	12%
(Weight Watchers) Smart Snackers				
oat bran pretzel nuggets	1.5 oz	2.5	170	13%

Food and Description	Amount	Fat Grams	Total Calories	% Fat Calories
PRICKLY PEAR	1 medium	0.5	42	11%
PROSCIUTTO (*See* SAUSAGE)				
PRUNE (*See also* PRUNE/PLUM FILLING)				
canned				
generic/in heavy syrup	5 medium	<1.0	90	2%
	1 cup	<1.0	240	2%
(S&W) in heavy syrup	8 pieces	–	210	–
dried				
(Del Monte) uncooked				
pitted	2 oz	–	140	–
unpitted	2 oz	–	120	–
(Dole)	2 oz	1.0	140	6%
generic				
cooked				
sweetened	1 cup	<1.0	225	2%
unsweetened	1 cup	<1.0	294	2%
uncooked/pitted	10 medium	<1.0	201	2%
(Mariani)				
large	¼ cup	1.0	140	6%
pitted	¼ cup	1.0	140	6%
(Sun Sweet)				
bite-size breakfast	¼ cup	–	140	–
medium	¼ cup	–	140	–
orange essence/pitted	6 medium	–	100	–
pitted	¼ cup	–	140	–
PRUNE JUICE/bottled or canned				
(Del Monte) unsweetened	8 fl oz	–	170	–
(Mott's)				
country style	6 fl oz	–	130	–
unsweetened	6 fl oz	–	130	–
(S&W) unsweetened	8 fl oz	–	180	–
(Seneca)	8 fl oz	–	180	–
(Sun Sweet)				
regular	8 fl oz	–	180	–
w/prune pulp	8 fl oz	–	170	–
PRUNE/PLUM FILLING				
(Solo)	2 Tbs	–	70	–
PUDDING & MOUSSE (*See also* CUSTARD; PIE FILLING & GLAZE)				
■ **HOMEMADE**				
(Note: Unless otherwise stated, homemade puddings were prepared with whole milk.)				
USDA Standard Home Recipe				
apple brown betty	1 cup	7.6	325	21%
blancmange	~4.5 oz	5.0	150	30%
bread pudding w/raisins	1 cup	16.0	495	29%
chocolate				
prepared w/2% milk	½ cup	4.0	205	18%
prepared w/whole milk	½ cup	5.0	220	20%
corn	½ cup	5.0	130	35%

Food and Description	Amount	Fat Grams	Total Calories	% Fat Calories
Indian pudding/baked	½ cup	4.5	120	34%
mousse/chocolate	½ cup	30.0	447	60%
rice pudding w/raisins	½ cup	4.0	220	16%
tapioca	½ cup	5.0	190	23%
vanilla	½ cup	4.0	130	31%
Yorkshire				
prepared w/skim milk	~3.5 oz	4.0	90	40%
prepared w/whole milk	~3.5 oz	5.0	105	43%
▧ MIX (Note: Unless stated otherwise, 1 serving of mix = the amount in ½ cup prepared.)				
(D-Zerta)				
chocolate				
mix only	1 serving	–	20	–
prepared w/skim milk	½ cup	–	60	–
(Jeli-O) pudding & pie filling				
Americana pudding & custard				
custard				
mix only	1 serving	–	80	–
prepared w/2% milk	½ cup	2.5	140	16%
rice pudding				
mix only	1 serving	–	100	–
prepared w/2% milk	½ cup	2.5	160	14%
tapioca pudding				
mix only	1 serving	–	80	–
prepared w/2% milk	½ cup	2.5	140	16%
cook & serve				
original				
banana cream				
mix only	1 serving	–	80	–
prepared w/2% milk	½ cup	2.5	140	16%
butterscotch				
mix only	1 serving	–	90	–
prepared w/2% milk	½ cup	2.5	160	14%
chocolate				
mix only	1 serving	–	90	–
prepared w/2% milk	½ cup	2.5	150	15%
chocolate fudge				
mix only	1 serving	–	90	–
prepared w/2% milk	½ cup	2.5	150	15%
coconut cream				
mix only	1 serving	2.5	90	25%
prepared w/2% milk	½ cup	5.0	150	30%
flan				
mix only	1 serving	–	80	–
prepared w/2% milk	½ cup	2.5	140	16%
lemon				
mix only	1 serving	–	50	–
prepared w/sugar egg yolks, & water	½ cup	2.0	140	13%

Food and Description	Amount	Fat Grams	Total Calories	% Fat Calories
milk chocolate				
mix only	1 serving	–	90	–
prepared w/2% milk	½ cup	2.5	150	15%
vanilla				
mix only	1 serving	–	80	–
prepared w/2% milk	½ cup	2.5	140	16%
sugar-free/reduced calorie				
chocolate				
mix only	1 serving	–	30	–
prepared w/2% milk	½ cup	2.5	90	25%
vanilla				
mix only	1 serving	–	20	–
prepared w/2% milk	½ cup	2.5	80	28%
instant				
fat-free/sugar-free/reduced calorie				
banana				
mix only	1 serving	–	25	–
prepared w/skim milk	½ cup	–	70	–
butterscotch				
mix only	1 serving	–	25	–
prepared w/skim milk	½ cup	–	70	–
chocolate				
mix only	1 serving	–	35	–
prepared w/skim milk	½ cup	–	80	–
chocolate fudge				
mix only	1 serving	–	35	–
prepared w/skim milk	½ cup	–	80	–
pistachio				
mix only	1 serving	–	30	–
prepared w/skim milk	½ cup	–	70	–
vanilla				
mix only	1 serving	–	25	–
prepared w/skim milk	½ cup	–	70	–
original				
banana cream				
mix only	1 serving	–	90	–
prepared w/2% milk	½ cup	2.5	150	15%
butter pecan				
mix only	1 serving	0.5	100	5%
prepared w/2% milk	½ cup	3.0	160	17%
butterscotch				
mix only	1 serving	–	90	–
prepared w/2% milk	½ cup	2.5	150	15%
chocolate				
mix only	1 serving	–	100	–
prepared w/2% milk	½ cup	2.5	160	14%

Food and Description	Amount	Fat Grams	Total Calories	% Fat Calories
chocolate fudge				
mix only	1 serving	–	100	–
prepared w/2% milk	½ cup	3.0	160	17%
coconut cream				
mix only	1 serving	2.0	100	18%
prepared w/2% milk	½ cup	4.5	160	25%
French vanilla				
mix only	1 serving	–	90	–
prepared w/2% milk	½ cup	2.5	150	15%
lemon				
mix only	1 serving	–	90	–
prepared w/2% milk	½ cup	2.5	150	15%
milk chocolate				
mix only	1 serving	0.5	100	5%
prepared w/2% milk	½ cup	3.0	160	17%
pistachio				
mix only	1 serving	0.5	100	5%
prepared w/2% milk	½ cup	3.0	160	17%
vanilla				
mix only	1 serving	–	90	–
prepared w/2% milk	½ cup	2.5	150	15%
(Knorr) Alsa International Desserts/mix only				
dark chocolate	¼ pkg	4.0	80	45%
milk chocolate	¼ pkg	4.0	80	45%
white chocolate	¼ pkg	3.5	70	45%
(Lundberg) Elegant Rice Pudding/mix only				
cinnamon raisin	½ cup	–	70	–
coconut	½ cup	2.0	70	26%
honey almond	½ cup	0.5	70	6%
(Nabisco) My-T-Fine/prepared				
butterscotch	½ cup	–	90	–
chocolate	½ cup	–	90	–
chocolate almond	½ cup	1.0	100	9%
chocolate fudge	½ cup	–	100	–
lemon	½ cup	–	90	–
tapioca	½ cup	–	80	–
vanilla	½ cup	–	90	–
(Royal) mix only (Note: 1 serving of mix = the amount of mix in 1 serving prepared.)				
cook & serve				
banana cream	1 serving	–	80	–
butterscotch	1 serving	–	90	–
chocolate	1 serving	–	90	–
dark 'n sweet	1 serving	–	90	–
vanilla	1 serving	–	80	–
instant				
regular				
banana cream	1 serving	–	90	–
butterscotch	1 serving	–	90	–

Food and Description	Amount	Fat Grams	Total Calories	% Fat Calories
cherry vanilla	1 serving	–	90	–
chocolate	1 serving	–	100	–
chocolate almond	1 serving	1.0	120	8%
chocolate chocolate chip	1 serving	1.0	110	8%
chocolate peanut butter	1 serving	1.0	110	8%
dark 'n sweet	1 serving	–	110	–
lemon	1 serving	–	90	–
pistachio	1 serving	1.0	90	10%
strawberry	1 serving	–	100	–
toasted coconut	1 serving	–	90	–
vanilla	1 serving	–	90	–
vanilla chocolate chip	1 serving	1.0	90	10%
sugar-free				
chocolate	1 serving	–	45	–
pistachio	1 serving	–	40	–
vanilla	1 serving	–	40	–
(SnackWell's) prepared				
devil's food	½ cup	–	100	–
double fudge	½ cup	–	100	–
lemon	½ cup	–	90	–
pistachio	½ cup	–	90	–
vanilla	½ cup	–	90	–
■ READY TO SERVE				
(Del Monte) pudding cup				
fat-free				
chocolate	3.5 oz	–	90	–
vanilla	3.5 oz	–	90	–
original				
banana	3.5 oz	3.0	120	23%
butterscotch	3.5 oz	3.0	120	23%
chocolate	3.5 oz	4.0	130	28%
chocolate fudge	3.5 oz	4.0	130	28%
tapioca	3.5 oz	3.0	120	23%
vanilla	3.5 oz	3.0	120	23%
generic/can or cup				
banana	½ cup	4.0	150	24%
butterscotch	½ cup	4.0	150	24%
chocolate	½ cup	4.0	190	19%
egg custard	½ cup	6.0	140	39%
fudge	½ cup	4.0	190	19%
lemon	½ cup	2.0	170	11%
rice	½ cup	3.0	150	18%
tapioca	½ cup	4.0	140	26%
vanilla	½ cup	4.0	150	24%
(Hunt's)				
pudding				
banana	½ cup	6.0	160	34%
butterscotch	½ cup	6.0	150	36%

Food and Description	Amount	Fat Grams	Total Calories	% Fat Calories
chocolate/fat-free	½ cup	<1.0	90	4%
chocolate marshmallow	½ cup	6.0	155	35%
lemon	½ cup	3.0	160	17%
tapioca				
fat-free	½ cup	<1.0	90	4%
regular	½ cup	6.0	150	36%
vanilla/fat free	½ cup	<1.0	90	4%
Pudding Snack				
banana	1 snack	7.0	170	37%
chocolate				
fat-free	1 snack	–	100	–
regular	1 snack	5.0	160	28%
chocolate-caramel swirl	1 snack	5.0	160	28%
chocolate-vanilla swirl				
fat-free	1 snack	–	100	–
regular	1 snack	5.0	160	28%
tapioca	1 snack	4.0	140	26%
vanilla	1 snack	5.0	160	28%
vanilla-chocolate swirl				
fat-free	1 snack	–	100	–
regular	1 snack	5.0	160	28%
Snack Pack				
chocolate	1 snack	6.0	170	32%
chocolate caramel swirl	1 snack	6.0	170	32%
chocolate fudge	1 snack	6.0	170	32%
chocolate caramel swirl	1 snack	6.0	170	32%
chocolate peanut milk chocolate swirl	1 snack	5.5	165	32%
s'mores swirl	1 snack	5.5	155	32%
vanilla	1 snack	6.0	165	32%
(Musselman's)				
banana	4 oz	5.0	150	30%
butterscotch	4 oz	7.0	170	37%
chocolate	4 oz	7.0	180	35%
chocolate fudge	4 oz	8.0	180	40%
rice	4 oz	3.0	120	23%
tapioca	4 oz	6.0	140	39%
vanilla	4 oz	7.0	170	37%
(Rice Dream) Dream Pudding/nondairy				
banana/fat-free	4 oz	–	120	–
butterscotch/fat-free	4 oz	–	120	–
carob/fat-free	4 oz	–	130	–
chocolate/fat-free	4 oz	–	170	–
coconut	4 oz	2.0	150	12%
lemon/fat-free	4 oz	–	120	–
(Rich's)				
butterscotch	3 oz	6.0	140	39%
chocolate	3 oz	7.0	140	45%
vanilla	3 oz	6.0	140	39%

Food and Description	Amount	Fat Grams	Total Calories	% Fat Calories
(Swiss Miss)				
pudding/fat-free				
chocolate	½ cup	<1.0	100	3%
chocolate fudge	½ cup	<1.0	100	3%
tapioca	½ cup	<1.0	100	3%
vanilla	½ cup	<1.0	100	3%
vanilla-chocolate parfait	½ cup	<1.0	100	3%
pudding snack				
butterscotch	1 snack	5.5	160	31%
chocolate	1 snack	6.0	170	32%
chocolate caramel swirl	1 snack	6.0	170	32%
chocolate fudge	1 snack	5.5	175	28%
chocolate vanilla parfait	1 snack	6.0	165	33%
chocolate vanilla swirl	1 snack	6.0	170	32%
milk chocolate fudge parfait	1 snack	6.0	165	33%
tapioca	1 snack	4.0	140	26%
vanilla	1 snack	5.5	160	31%
vanilla-chocolate parfait	1 snack	6.0	165	33%
PUMMELO/POMELO				
fresh				
sections	1 cup	–	70	–
whole	1 medium	–	230	–
PUMPKIN				
canned				
(Comstock)	½ cup	–	50	–
(Del Monte)	½ cup	–	35	–
(Festal)	½ cup	1.0	40	23%
(Libby's) solid pack	½ cup	0.5	60	8%
(Stokely)	½ cup	–	40	–
fresh				
boiled-mashed	1 cup	–	48	–
raw/cubed	1 cup	–	30	–
PUMPKIN BUTTER				
(Smucker's)	1 tsp	–	12	–
PUMPKIN FLOWER				
cooked	½ cup	<1.0	10	45%
raw	½ cup	<1.0	5	90%
PUMPKIN LEAVES/cooked	½ cup	<1.0	7	64%
PUMPKIN PIE SPICE (See also SEASONINGS)				
	1 tsp	–	6	–
PUMPKIN SEEDS				
dried/hulled	1 oz	13.0	155	75%
	1 cup	63.0	747	76%
kernels/roasted				
(David)	¼ cup	13.0	160	73%
generic	1 oz	12.0	150	72%
	1 cup	95.6	1185	72%

Food and Description	Amount	Fat Grams	Total Calories	% Fat Calories
whole/roasted	1 oz	5.5	127	39%
	1 cup	12.0	285	38%
PUNCH (See FRUIT PUNCH; SOFT DRINK; SOFT DRINK MIX)				
PURPLE HULL PEA				
canned (Allens Fresh)	½ cup	0.5	100	5%
frozen (Frosty Acres)	3.3 oz	–	130	–
PURSLANE				
boiled	½ cup	–	10	–
raw	1 cup	–	7	–

Q

Food and Description	Amount	Fat Grams	Total Calories	% Fat Calories
QUAIL/raw				
breast meat only	~2 oz	1.7	69	22%
meat & skin-raw	~4 oz	13.0	210	56%
meat only	~3 oz	4.0	123	29%
QUICHE (See EGG DISH/MEAL)				
QUINCE/fresh	1 medium	–	53	–
QUINOA (See also FLOUR; PASTA; QUINOA SEED)				
whole grain/dry				
(Eden)	½ cup	4.0	200	9%
generic	1 oz	1.6	106	14%
	1 cup	10.0	637	14%
QUINOA SEED				
(Arrowhead Mills)	¼ cup	2.0	140	13%

R

Food and Description	Amount	Fat Grams	Total Calories	% Fat Calories
RABBIT				
domesticated/meat only				
roasted	3 oz	5.5	130	38%

Food and Description	Amount	Fat Grams	Total Calories	% Fat Calories
roasted/chopped or diced	1 cup	9.0	220	37%
stewed	3 oz	7.0	175	36%
stewed/chopped or diced	1 cup	12.0	290	37%
wild/meat only				
stewed	3 oz	3.0	150	18%
stewed/chopped or diced	1 cup	5.0	245	18%
RACCOON/meat only				
roasted	3 oz	12.5	220	51%
roasted/chopped or diced	1 cup	20.0	355	51%
RADICCHIO/raw/shredded	½ cup	–	5	–
RADISH				
dried				
Chinese	¼ cup	–	75	–
daikon	¼ cup	–	75	–
fresh				
Black	1 oz	–	5	–
Chinese				
cooked-drained/sliced	½ cup	–	15	–
raw				
sliced	½ cup	–	10	–
whole	1 medium	–	60	–
daikon				
cooked-drained/sliced	½ cup	–	15	–
raw				
sliced	½ cup	–	10	–
whole	1 medium	–	60	–
red/raw	10 pieces	–	7	–
	½ cup	–	13	–
(Dole)	7 medium	–	20	–
white icicle/raw				
sliced	½ cup	–	7	–
whole	1 medium	–	2	–
RADISH LEAVES	1 oz	–	15	–
RADISH SPROUTS	½ cup	0.5	8	56%
RAISIN (*See also* SNACK MIX)				
(Del Monte)				
golden	¼ cup	–	120	–
natural	¼ cup	–	120	–
yogurt raisin snack bag				
strawberry	0.9 oz	3.0	110	25%
vanilla yogurt	0.9 oz	3.0	110	25%
(Dole)				
dark/seedless	½ cup	–	250	–
golden	½ cup	–	250	–
generic				
dark				
ground/uncooked				
loose	1 cup	–	578	–

Food and Description	Amount	Fat Grams	Total Calories	% Fat Calories
packed	1 cup	<1.0	780	1%
seedless				
loose	1 cup	0.5	435	1%
packed	1 cup	1.0	495	1%
w/seeds				
loose	1 cup	1.0	430	2%
packed	1 cup	1.0	490	2%
golden/seedless				
loose	1 cup	0.5	438	1%
packed	1 cup	1.0	498	1%
(S&W)				
dark/seedless	¼ cup	–	130	–
golden/seedless	¼ cup	–	130	–
(Sun Maid)				
dark/seedless				
regular	¼ cup	–	130	–
golden w/seeds	½ cup	–	250	–
muscat	½ cup	1.0	270	3%
snack box	1.5 oz	–	130	–
RASPBERRY (See also BERRIES, MIXED)				
canned/generic				
in heavy syrup	1 cup	<1.0	234	2%
in water	1 cup	2.0	110	16%
fresh				
black	1 cup	2.0	100	18%
red	1 cup	0.7	61	10%
(Dole)	1 cup	–	45	–
frozen				
(Big Valley)	3.5 oz	<1.0	55	8%
(Birds Eye) in lite syrup	½ cup	1.0	100	9%
(C&W) red/sweetened	1 cup	–	50	–
generic				
sweetened	1 cup	<1.0	255	2%
	10 oz	<1.0	290	2%
unsweetened	3.5 oz	<1.0	50	9%
RASPBERRY JUICE/JUICE BLEND (See also FRUIT PUNCH; LEMONADE; SOFT DRINK; SOFT DRINK MIX)				
bottled, boxed, or canned				
(Chiquita) 100% juice/Polynesian Passion	8 fl oz	–	120	–
(Dole) country raspberry 100% juice blend				
bottled	8 fl oz	–	140	–
	10 fl oz	–	180	–
refrigerated	4 fl oz	–	70	–
	8 fl oz	–	140	–
(Knudsen)				
raspberry float	8 fl oz	–	140	–

Food and Description	Amount	Fat Grams	Total Calories	% Fat Calories
raspberry-peach (Smucker's)	8 fl oz	–	115	–
juice	8 fl oz	–	120	–
juice sparkler	10 fl oz	–	130	–
fresh/black	4 fl oz	–	50	–
frozen/prepared				
(Dole) country raspberry 100% juice blend	8 fl oz	–	140	–
generic	6 fl oz	–	90	–

RASPBERRY JUICE DRINK (See also FRUIT PUNCH; LEMONADE; SOFT DRINK; SOFT DRINK MIX; TEA)

bottled, boxed, or canned

(Betty Crocker) Squeezit	6.76 fl oz	–	110	–
(Dole) Raspberry-Lemon Splash	8 fl oz	–	120	–
juice drink	16 fl oz	–	250	–
frozen				
(Dole) Raspberry-Lemon Splash juice drink	8 fl oz	–	120	–
(Seneca) raspberry-cranapple juice cocktail	8 fl oz	–	140	–

RAVIOLI (See BEEF DISH/ENTRÉE; FROZEN ENTRÉE/DINNER; PASTA ENTRÉE/ DINNER; VEGETARIAN FOODS)

RED BEAN (See also BEANS, BAKED & VARIETY; RICE DISH)

canned

(Bush's Best)	½ cup	–	70	–
generic	½ cup	–	100	–
(Green Giant) dry beans in brine	½ cup	0.5	100	5%
(Hunt's) small	½ cup	0.5	90	5%
(Joan of Arc) dry beans in brine	½ cup	0.5	100	5%
(Van Camp's)	1 cup	1.0	195	5%
dry				
(Bean Cuisine)	½ cup	1.0	115	8%

RED BEAN SOUP (See SOUP)

REFRIED BEANS (See MEXICAN FOOD)

RELISH (See CHUTNEY; CORN DISH; PICKLE RELISH)

RENNIN PRODUCTS	1 tablet	–	1	–
	1 pkg	–	12	–

RHUBARB

fresh

cooked-sweetened	1 cup	–	280	–
raw/diced	½ cup	–	13	–
frozen				
generic/cooked w/sugar	1 cup	–	278	–

RICE (See also ASIAN FOOD; RICE DISH)

(A Taste of Thai) prepared

brown jasmine	½ cup	–	220	–
coconut ginger	½ cup	1.0	325	3%
garlic basil	½ cup	1.0	270	3%

Food and Description	Amount	Fat Grams	Total Calories	% Fat Calories
soft jasmine	½ cup	–	160	–
(Arrowhead Mills) dry				
basmati/long-grain	¼ cup	1.0	150	6%
brown				
long-grain	¼ cup	1.0	150	6%
medium-grain	¼ cup	1.0	160	6%
quick				
regular	⅓ cup	1.0	150	6%
Spanish	⅓ cup	1.0	150	6%
vegetable	⅓ cup	1.0	150	6%
wild	⅓ cup	1.0	140	6%
short-grain	¼ cup	1.0	170	5%
(Colavita) arborio/dry	1 ounce	–	100	–
(Fantastic Foods) Elegant Grains/dry				
arborio	¼ cup	–	210	–
basmati				
brown	¼ cup	1.5	170	8%
white	¼ cup	–	180	–
jasmine				
brown	¼ cup	1.5	170	8%
white	¼ cup	–	170	–
wild	¼ cup	–	140	–
generic				
brown				
long-grain				
cooked	½ cup	0.9	108	7%
dry	½ cup	2.7	342	7%
medium-grain				
cooked	½ cup	<1.0	109	6%
dry	½ cup	2.5	343	6%
glutinous				
cooked	½ cup	<1.0	117	1%
dry	½ cup	0.5	342	1%
white				
long-grain				
instant				
cooked	½ cup	<1.0	180	3%
dry	½ cup	<1.0	230	2%
parboiled				
cooked	½ cup	<1.0	100	2%
dry	½ cup	0.5	340	1%
regular				
cooked	½ cup	<1.0	131	2%
dry	½ cup	<1.0	338	1%
raw	1 cup	0.7	672	1%
medium-grain				
cooked	½ cup	<1.0	133	1%
dry	½ cup	0.5	350	1%

Food and Description	Amount	Fat Grams	Total Calories	% Fat Calories
raw	1 cup	0.8	708	1%
short-grain				
cooked	½ cup	<1.0	133	1%
dry	½ cup	0.5	358	1%
raw	1 cup	0.8	726	1%
wild				
cooked	½ cup	<1.0	83	3%
dry	½ cup	<1.0	285	3%
raw	4 oz	<1.0	400	1%
(Mahatma)				
brown/dry	1 oz	–	110	–
instant				
cooked, w/o butter or margarine	½ cup	–	110	–
dry	1 oz	–	110	–
white /dry	1 oz	–	100	–
(Minute)				
brown/instant whole grain				
dry	½ cup	1.5	170	8%
prepared, w/o butter or margarine	⅔ cup	1.5	170	8%
white				
boil-in-bag				
dry	½ bag	–	190	–
prepared, w/o butter or margarine	1 cup	–	190	–
original				
dry	½ cup	–	170	–
prepared, w/o butter or margarine	¾ cup	–	170	–
premium long-grain				
dry	½ cup	–	170	–
prepared, w/o butter or margarine	1 cup	–	170	–
(MJB) brown				
quick/cooked	½ cup	1.0	110	8%
(New Frontier)				
Ultra Roast				
cooked	1 serving	0.9	111	7%
dry	3.5 oz	3.0	395	7%
wild				
cooked	½ cup	1.0	110	3%
dry	½ cup	1.0	280	2%
(S&W) dry				
brown				
long-grain	¼ cup	1.0	150	6%
quick	½ cup	1.0	150	6%
white/long-grain	¼ cup	–	25	–
wild	½ cup	1.0	110	8%
(Success)				
brown				
boil-in-bag/prepared	½ cup	1.0	150	6%
10-minute/prepared	½ cup	1.0	190	5%

Food and Description	Amount	Fat Grams	Total Calories	% Fat Calories
white/natural long-grain				
precooked/prepared	½ cup	–	190	–
(Texmati)				
brown	¼ cup	1.0	170	5%
Jasmati	¼ cup	–	150	–
Kasmati	¼ cup	0.5	150	3%
light brown	¼ cup	1.0	170	5%
risotto	¼ cup	–	150	–
Royal Blend	¼ cup	–	160	–
white/long-grain	¼ cup	0.5	150	3%
(Uncle Ben's)				
brown				
cooked	⅔ cup	1.0	140	6%
dry	1.6 oz	1.0	158	6%
fast cooking/dry	1.6 oz	1.0	158	6%
white				
aromatic/cooked	½ cup	–	100	–
boil-in-bag				
cooked	½ cup	–	90	–
dry	1 oz	–	90	–
converted				
cooked	⅔ cup	–	120	–
dry	1.2 oz	<1.0	123	3%
Rice-in-an-Instant	1.1 oz	<1.0	110	2%
wild/combinations				
brown & wild/fast-cooking				
long-grain & wild				
fast-cooking	1 oz	<1.0	100	4%
original				
cooked	½ cup	–	100	–
dry	1 oz	<1.0	105	4%
(Vita Fiber) rice grain	1 oz	6.0	100	54%
RICE BRAN (*See also* CEREAL)				
crude	½ cup	8.5	130	59%
RICE BRAN OIL				
generic	1 Tbs	14.0	120	100%
(Hollywood)	1 Tbs	14.0	120	100%
RICE CAKES (*See also* POPCORN BARS & CAKES)				
■ MINI				
(Hain)				
Mini-Munchies				
banana split	5 cakes	–	60	–
chocolate mint	5 cakes	–	60	–
peach cobbler	5 cakes	–	60	–
peanut butter	5 cakes	1.0	50	18%
strawberry cheesecake	5 cakes	–	60	–
original				
apple cinnamon	6 cakes	–	60	–

Food and Description	Amount	Fat Grams	Total Calories	% Fat Calories
barbecue	5 cakes	3.0	70	39%
caramel	5 cakes	–	60	–
cheese	6 cakes	2.5	70	32%
honey nut	5 cakes	<1.0	60	8%
nacho	5 cakes	2.0	70	26%
plain/no salt	5 cakes	–	60	–
ranch	6 cakes	3.5	80	39%
teriyaki	6 cakes	0.5	60	8%
white cheddar	6 cakes	3.0	70	39%
(Hollywood)				
apple cinnamon	~5 cakes	<1.0	50	9%
cheese	~5 cakes	2.0	60	30%
honey nut	~5 cakes	1.0	60	15%
plain	~5 cakes	<1.0	50	9%
(Pacific Rice) Mini Crispys				
apple spice	2 cakes	–	30	–
barbecue	2 cakes	–	30	–
honey sesame	1 cake	–	12	–
teriyaki	1 cake	–	12	–
(Pritikin)				
apple crisp	5 cakes	–	50	–
(Quaker)				
apple cinnamon	5 cakes	–	50	–
banana nut crunch	5 cakes	–	50	–
caramel corn	5 cakes	–	50	–
cinnamon crunch	5 cakes	–	50	–
honey nut	5 cakes	–	50	–
Monterey jack	6 cakes	–	50	–
white cheddar	6 cakes	–	50	–
(Roman Meal)				
apple	8 cakes	–	50	–
caramel	8 cakes	–	50	–
honey nut	8 cakes	–	50	–
(Too Good To Be True)				
apple cinnamon	5 cakes	0.5	60	8%
white cheddar	5 cakes	1.0	60	15%
■ REGULAR SIZE				
(Hain)				
butter flavor	1 cake	2.0	45	40%
5-grain	1 cake	–	50	–
plain				
no salt added	1 cake	–	40	–
regular	1 cake	–	40	–
sesame				
no salt	1 cake	<1.0	40	11%
regular	1 cake	<1.0	40	11%
white cheddar	1 cake	2.0	45	40%

Food and Description	Amount	Fat Grams	Total Calories	% Fat Calories
(Lundberg)				
organic				
brown rice	1 cake	–	60	–
mochi/sweet	1 cake	–	60	–
premium				
brown rice	1 cake	–	60	–
buckwheat	1 cake	–	60	–
mochi/sweet	1 cake	–	60	–
rye	1 cake	–	60	–
sesame	1 cake	–	60	–
wild rice	1 cake	–	60	–
(Pacific Grain)				
apple cinnamon	1 cake	–	30	–
cheddar	1 cake	–	35	–
toasted brown	1 cake	–	35	–
(Pritikin)				
multigrain				
regular	1 cake	–	35	–
unsalted	1 cake	–	35	–
plain				
regular	1 cake	–	35	–
unsalted	1 cake	–	35	–
sesame				
low-sodium	1 cake	–	35	–
unsalted	1 cake	–	35	–
(Quaker)				
apple cinnamon	1 cake	–	50	–
banana nut crunch	1 cake	–	50	–
blueberry crunch	1 cake	–	50	–
cinnamon crunch	1 cake	–	50	–
salt-free	1 cake	–	35	–
salted	1 cake	–	35	–
strawberry crunch	1 cake	–	50	–
(Westbrae Natural)				
double sesame	1 cake	<1.0	30	15%
sesame garlic	1 cake	<1.0	30	15%
teriyaki	1 cake	<1.0	30	15%

RICE DISH (*See also* ASIAN FOOD; FROZEN ENTRÉE/DINNER; MEXICAN FOOD)

■ **CANNED**

Food and Description	Amount	Fat Grams	Total Calories	% Fat Calories
(Old El Paso) Spanish rice	1 cup	1.0	130	7%
(Van Camp's) Spanish rice	1 cup	4.0	160	23%
■ **FROZEN**				
(Birds Eye) International Rice Recipes				
French style	½ cup	3.0	170	16%
Italian style	3.3 oz	1.0	120	8%
Spanish style	3.3 oz	–	110	–
(Green Giant) Rice & Vegetable Combinations				
rice medley	1 pkg	3.0	240	11%

Food and Description	Amount	Fat Grams	Total Calories	% Fat Calories
rice 'n broccoli	1 pkg	12.0	320	34%
rice pilaf	1 pkg	3.0	230	12%
white & wild rice	1 pkg	5.0	250	18%
(King's Hawaiian)				
teriyaki rice bowl	1 cup	3.5	210	15%
■ MICROWAVE CONTAINER				
(Chef Boyardee) microwave bowl				
rice w/beef & vegetables	1 bowl	7.0	250	25%
rice w/chicken & vegetables	1 bowl	6.0	220	25%
■ MIX				
(Casbah) pilaf				
original				
mix only	2 oz	–	90	–
prepared	1 cup	<1.0	200	2%
nutted				
mix only	2 oz	2.5	220	10%
prepared	1 cup	2.5	220	10%
Spanish				
mix only	2 oz	0.5	200	2%
prepared	1 cup	0.5	200	2%
(Fantastic Foods)				
quick pilaf				
brown rice w/miso				
mix only	½ cup	3.0	250	11%
prepared	1 cup	3.0	250	11%
Spanish brown rice				
mix only	½ cup	2.0	240	8%
prepared	1 cup	2.0	240	8%
rice & beans				
Bombay curry	1 pkg	3.0	260	10%
Cajun	1 pkg	1.5	240	6%
Caribbean black beans	1 pkg	1.5	230	6%
Northern Italian	1 pkg	1.5	240	6%
Szechuan	1 pkg	2.0	210	9%
Tex-Mex	1 pkg	2.0	270	7%
(Farm House) mix only				
beans & rice				
w/Mexican pinto beans	⅓ cup	1.0	190	5%
w/red beans	⅓ cup	1.0	180	5%
w/Spanish black beans	⅓ cup	1.0	200	5%
broccoli au gratin	⅓ cup	2.0	210	9%
chicken	⅓ cup	1.5	180	8%
herb & butter	⅓ cup	2.0	210	9%
long grain & wild	⅓ cup	2.0	200	9%
Mexican	⅓ cup	1.0	180	5%
rice pilaf	⅓ cup	1.0	200	5%
Spanish rice	⅓ cup	1.5	180	8%

Food and Description	Amount	Fat Grams	Total Calories	% Fat Calories
(Golden Grain)				
Rice-A-Roni				
fast-cooking/prepared				
broccoli cheese	1 cup	12.0	300	36%
chicken flavor	1 cup	6.5	250	23%
Oriental style	1 cup	10.0	290	31%
Spanish	1 cup	5.5	250	20%
original/prepared				
beef & mushroom	1 cup	6.0	290	19%
beef flavor				
⅓ less salt	1 cup	5.0	280	16%
regular	1 cup	9.5	320	27%
broccoli au gratin				
⅓ less salt	1 cup	11.0	320	31%
regular	1 cup	17.0	370	41%
chicken & broccoli	1 cup	7.5	290	23%
chicken & mushroom	1 cup	14.0	360	35%
chicken & vegetables	1 cup	7.0	290	22%
chicken flavor				
⅓ less salt	1 cup	5.0	280	16%
regular	1 cup	9.5	320	27%
fried rice				
⅓ less salt	1 cup	3.5	260	12%
regular	1 cup	11.0	320	31%
herb & butter	1 cup	9.0	310	26%
long grain & wild rice	1 cup	8.5	290	26%
long grain & wild pilaf	1 cup	5.5	240	21%
Long Grain & Wild Rice				
chicken w/almonds	1 cup	8.5	290	26%
Oriental stir-fry	1 cup	5.5	290	17%
red beans & rice	1 cup	7.0	280	23%
rice pilaf	1 cup	9.0	310	26%
Spanish rice	1 cup	8.0	270	27%
stroganoff	1 cup	14.5	360	36%
white cheddar & herbs	1 cup	14.0	340	37%
(Good Harvest) Creative Sides/mix only				
Mediterranean rice pilaf	⅓ cup	2.0	160	11%
savory black beans & rice	⅓ cup	0.5	160	3%
Spanish style rice	⅓ cup	1.0	160	6%
spicy red beans & rice	⅓ cup	1.0	160	6%
tomato/wild mushroom risotto	⅓ cup	0.5	160	3%
(Kashi) 7 whole grain & sesame pilaf/cooked	½ cup	3.0	170	26%
(Knorr) Italian Rice/mix only				
basmati rice pilaf/tomato & herbs	¼ pkg	0.5	150	3%
jasmine rice pilaf/lemon & hebs	¼ pkg	1.0	130	7%
	⅓ cup	2.0	270	7%
rice medley & carrots	¼ pkg	0.5	90	5%

Food and Description	Amount	Fat Grams	Total Calories	% Fat Calories
risotto				
broccoli au gratin	⅓ cup	2.5	260	9%
Milanese	¼ pkg	0.5	130	3%
	⅓ cup	1.0	280	3%
mushrooms	¼ pkg	0.5	140	3%
	⅓ cup	1.0	300	3%
onion & herbs	¼ pkg	0.5	150	3%
	⅓ cup	1.0	310	3%
primavera	¼ pkg	0.5	140	3%
(Konriko) wild pecan rice	⅕ box	1.0	160	6%
(Lipton) mix only				
Golden Sauté				
beef flavor	½ cup	4.0	230	16%
chicken broccoli	½ cup	4.5	260	15%
chicken flavor	½ cup	5.0	240	14%
herb & butter	½ cup	5.0	240	19%
onion mushroom	½ cup	4.0	240	15%
Oriental fried rice	½ cup	1.0	240	4%
rice Oriental	½ cup	4.5	240	17%
savory herb	½ cup	4.5	240	17%
Spanish	½ cup	4.5	250	16%
Rice & Beans				
Cajun	½ cup	1.0	260	3%
Rice & Sauce				
alfredo broccoli	½ cup	4.5	250	16%
beef broccoli	½ cup	1.0	230	4%
Cajun beans	¼ pkg	<1.0	123	4%
cheddar broccoli	½ cup	3.0	250	11%
chicken	¼ pkg	1.0	125	7%
chicken broccoli	¼ pkg	2.0	130	14%
chicken risotto	½ cup	2.0	230	8%
creamy chicken	¼ pkg	2.0	140	13%
herb & butter	¼ pkg	2.0	125	14%
long grain				
mushrooms	½ pkg	<1.0	125	4%
original	¼ pkg	–	120	–
medley	½ cup	2.0	240	8%
Oriental	½ cup	1.0	230	4%
pilaf	¼ pkg	<1.0	120	4%
Spanish	¼ pkg	<1.0	120	4%
(Luzianne) dinner kit/mix only				
étouffée	¼ box	1.0	200	5%
gumbo	⅕ box	1.0	160	6%
jambalaya	⅕ box	1.0	160	6%
shrimp Creole	⅕ box	0.5	150	3%
(Mahatma) mix only				
black bean	2 oz	1.5	200	7%

Food and Description	Amount	Fat Grams	Total Calories	% Fat Calories
jambalaya	2 oz	1.0	190	5%
red bean	2 oz	1.5	200	7%
Spanish	2 oz	1.0	180	5%
yellow	2 oz	–	190	–
(Mayacamas) Just Enough				
chicken w/broccoli	1 cup	–	100	–
rice jalapeño	1 cup	–	130	–
(Minute) long grain & wild rice				
mix only	⅓ box	0.5	230	2%
prepared, w/o butter or margarine	1 cup	0.5	230	2%
(MJB) prepared				
fried rice Oriental	½ cup	1.0	110	8%
herb & butter	½ cup	1.0	100	9%
Mexican style	½ cup	–	120	–
rice pilaf	½ cup	1.0	110	8%
savory beef	½ cup	1.0	100	9%
savory chicken	½ cup	1.0	100	9%
(Near East) rice pilaf/prepared				
barley	1 cup	4.0	220	16%
beef flavor	1 cup	4.5	220	18%
brown rice	1 cup	5.0	220	20%
chicken flavor	1 cup	4.5	220	18%
curry	1 cup	4.0	220	16%
garden vegetable bean & rice	1 cup	5.0	270	17%
lentil	1 cup	4.0	210	17%
long grain & wild rice	1 cup	4.5	220	18%
Mediterranean black bean & rice	1 cup	5.0	270	17%
Mediterranean chicken				
wheat	1 cup	4.5	220	18%
w/wild rice	1 cup	4.0	220	16%
red beans & rice	1 cup	3.5	220	14%
rice pilaf	1 cup	4.5	220	18%
Spanish rice	1 cup	6.0	230	23%
toasted almond	1 cup	6.0	230	23%
tomato herb bean & rice	1 cup	5.0	270	17%
(Old El Paso)				
Mexican rice				
cheesy				
mix only	½ cup	3.5	420	8%
prepared	4 oz	3.5	420	8%
regular				
mix only	½ cup	2.0	410	4%
prepared	4 oz	2.0	410	4%
Spanish rice				
mix only	½ cup	2.0	410	4%
prepared	4 oz	3.0	410	4%

Food and Description	Amount	Fat Grams	Total Calories	% Fat Calories
(Pritikin)				
Mexican	⅓ cup	2.0	200	9%
Oriental	⅓ cup	1.5	190	7%
(Quick Pilaf) prepared				
miso				
w/butter	½ cup	5.5	134	34%
w/o butter	½ cup	1.0	105	9%
Spanish				
w/butter	½ cup	5.0	135	33%
w/o butter or salt	½ cup	<1.0	100	6%
Rice-A-Roni (See (Golden Grain) in this section)				
(Spice Islands) Quick Meal/prepared				
chicken rice pilaf	1 pkg	1.5	180	8%
curry rice	1 pkg	2.5	190	12%
hearty lentils & wild rice	1 pkg	2.5	200	11%
Oriental rice & vegetables	1 pkg	2.5	180	13%
rice & country vegetables	1 pkg	0.5	170	3%
rice & spicy black beans	1 pkg	–	100	–
rice & spicy red beans	1 pkg	0.5	110	4%
wild rice & vegetables	1 pkg	–	160	–
(Success) prepared				
beef Oriental	½ cup	–	100	–
broccoli & cheese	½ cup	–	120	–
brown & wild	½ cup	–	120	–
chicken	½ cup	–	100	–
pilaf	½ cup	–	120	–
Spanish	½ cup	–	110	–
(Suzi Wan) prepared, w/o butter or margarine				
chicken flavor				
w/broccoli	½ cup	1.0	120	8%
w/vegetables	½ cup	1.0	120	8%
dinner recipe				
sweet & sour	½ cup	1.0	130	7%
teriyaki	½ cup	1.0	120	8%
(Uncle Ben's)				
Country Inn/mix only				
fast cooking				
broccoli almondine	1.2 oz	1.5	125	11%
creamy chicken & mushroom	1.2 oz	3.0	140	19%
creamy chicken & wild rice	1.3 oz	1.5	135	10%
green bean & almondine casserole	1.2 oz	2.0	130	14%
homestyle chicken & vegetables	1.2 oz	3.0	140	19%
original recipe				
broccoli rice au gratin	1.1 oz	2.0	115	16%
chicken stock rice	1.1 oz	1.0	125	7%
chicken w/wild rice	1.1 oz	<1.0	110	7%
herbed rice au gratin	1.1 oz	1.5	120	11%
rice Florentine	1.1 oz	1.5	120	11%

Food and Description	Amount	Fat Grams	Total Calories	% Fat Calories
Spanish tomato & herb	2.5 oz	1.0	240	4%
vegetable pilaf	1.1 oz	1.0	115	8%
long grain & wild/mix only				
butter & herb	2 oz	2.0	200	9%
chicken & herb	2 oz	1.5	200	7%
chicken stock	1.3 oz	2.0	135	13%
garden vegetable	1.3 oz	1.0	130	7%
vegetable & herb	2 oz	1.5	200	7%
Specialty Blend				
multigrain				
mix only	¼ cup	1.0	160	6%
prepared	1 cup	1.0	160	6%
pilaf				
mix only	¼ cup	0.5	170	3%
prepared	1 cup	0.5	170	3%
rice trio				
mix only	¼ cup	1.0	160	6%
prepared	1 cup	1.0	160	6%
(Vigo) mix only				
black beans & rice	⅓ cup	0.5	190	2%
pinto beans & rice	⅓ cup	2.0	200	9%
red beans & rice	⅓ cup	–	190	–
Santa Fe beans & rice	⅓ cup	2.0	200	9%
yellow rice	⅓ cup	1.0	190	5%
(Wick Fowler's) Rice Kit/mix only				
Cajun	1 serving	1.0	120	8%
jalapeño	1 serving	1.0	130	7%
ranchero	1 serving	1.0	110	8%
(Zatarain's)				
gumbo w/rice				
mix only	3 Tbs	–	150	–
prepared	1 cup	–	150	–
New Orleans jambalaya				
mix	3 Tbs	–	150	–
prepared	1 cup	–	150	–
RICE DRINK				
(Don Jose) Hor Chata nondairy	6 oz	4.0	120	30%
(Grainaissance) Amazake				
almond	8 fl oz	4.0	200	18%
apricot	8 fl oz	–	160	–
cocoa-almond	8 fl oz	3.0	200	14%
mocha java	8 fl oz	2.0	180	10%
sesame	8 fl oz	1.0	200	5%
vanilla pecan	8 fl oz	4.0	200	18%
(Rice Dream)				
chocolate	8 fl oz	2.5	160	14%
original	8 fl oz	2.0	130	14%

Food and Description	Amount	Fat Grams	Total Calories	% Fat Calories
vanilla				
enriched	8 fl oz	2.0	120	15%
regular	8 fl oz	2.0	130	14%
RICE FLOUR (See FLOUR)				
RICE FROZEN DESSERT				
(Rice Dream)				
Dream Bar				
chocolate/chocolate	1 bar	15.0	270	50%
nutty	1 bar	18.0	260	62%
strawberry/carob	1 bar	11.0	190	52%
vanilla/carob	1 bar	11.0	200	50%
nondairy dessert				
carob chip	½ cup	6.0	130	42%
lemon	½ cup	5.0	130	35%
mint carob chip	½ cup	6.0	130	42%
Neapolitan	½ cup	5.0	130	35%
vanilla	½ cup	5.0	130	35%
RICE NOODLE (See ASIAN FOOD)				
RICE POLISH/stirred & spooned into cup	1 cup	13.0	278	42%
RICE PUDDING (See PUDDING & MOUSSE)				
RICE SYRUP (See also PANCAKE & WAFFLE SYRUP)				
(Lundberg) Sweet Dreams	1 Tbs	<1.0	40	7%
RIGATONI (See PASTA; PASTA ENTRÉE/DINNER)				
ROAST BEEF (See BEEF, LUNCHEON MEAT)				
ROAST BEEF HASH (See BEEF DISH/ENTRÉE)				
ROAST BEEF SPREAD (See LUNCHEON MEAT SPREAD)				
ROASTING BAGS, SEASONED (See SEASONINGS)				
ROCKFISH				
Pacific/mixed species				
cooked	3 oz	2.0	110	16%
raw	3 oz	1.0	80	11%
ROLL (See also CROISSANT; PASTRY; SCONE)				
▉ **BROWN & SERVE**				
(Arnold) Francisco				
sourdough	1 roll	1.0	80	11%
(Country Hearth) krusty				
Italian	1 roll	4.0	170	21%
plain	1 roll	4.0	170	21%
generic				
cloverleaf	1 roll	1.9	84	20%
(Pepperidge Farm)				
bakery/French	½ roll	2.0	180	10%
European Bake Shoppe				
club	1 roll	1.5	120	11%
French	1 roll	2.5	240	9%
hearth	3 rolls	2.0	150	12%
(Roman Meal)	2 rolls	2.0	140	13%

Food and Description	Amount	Fat Grams	Total Calories	% Fat Calories
(Wonder) Rolls du Jour				
crusty Italian	1 roll	1.0	80	11%
gem style	1 roll	2.0	80	23%
petite French	1 roll	2.0	230	8%
w/buttermilk	1 roll	2.0	80	23%
■ FROZEN				
(Cole's)				
garlic	1 roll	5.0	100	45%
generic/dough, baked				
Parker House	1 roll	1.0	75	12%
(Mama Bella) garlic dinner	1 roll	4.0	130	28%
(Pepperidge Farm)				
garlic & cheese	1 roll	5.0	130	35%
(Rhodes) bread dough, baked				
cinnamon roll	1 roll	10.0	240	38%
lite white	1 roll	–	84	–
Texas dinner				
wheat	1 roll	3.0	140	19%
white	1 roll	3.0	150	18%
white dinner	1 roll	2.0	100	18%
(Sara Lee) food service				
hard				
light rye	1 roll	1.0	80	11%
malt rye	1 roll	1.0	80	11%
sandwich kaiser	¼" roll	4.0	170	21%
white/assorted	1 roll	2.0	80	23%
soft				
butterfly	1 roll	3.0	90	30%
cloverleaf	1 roll	3.0	90	30%
crescent	1 roll	5.0	100	5%
finger	3 rolls	5.0	170	27%
Parker House	3 rolls	5.0	170	27%
sesame seed	1 roll	3.0	70	39%
white	1 roll	2.0	90	20%
■ HEAT & SERVE				
(Pepperidge Farm) bakery				
butter crescent	1 roll	5.0	110	41%
golden twist	1 roll	4.0	110	33%
■ HOMEMADE				
USDA Standard Home Recipe				
cloverleaf/2½" dia	1 roll	3.0	120	23%
dinner/soft white	1 roll	3.0	120	23%
popover	1 roll	3.7	90	37%
■ MIX				
(Dromedary) mix only				
date nut	1 roll	7.0	200	32%
hot	1 roll	0.5	100	5%

Food and Description	Amount	Fat Grams	Total Calories	% Fat Calories
generic				
popover/prepared	1 roll	5.0	170	26%
(Pillsbury)				
hot roll				
mix only	¼ cup	1.0	110	17%
prepared	1 roll	3.0	130	21%
■ READY TO SERVE				
(Arnold)				
Arnold				
deli onion	1 roll	2.0	170	11%
dinner				
plain				
12 per pkg	2 rolls	2.5	110	20%
24 per pkg	2 rolls	2.0	110	16%
w/sesame seeds	2 rolls	2.5	110	20%
hamburger				
8 per pkg	1 roll	2.0	130	14%
12 per pkg	1 roll	2.0	120	15%
hot dog				
New England style	1 roll	2.0	110	16%
regular				
8 per 11-oz pkg	1 roll	2.0	100	18%
8 per 12-oz pkg	1 roll	2.0	110	16%
12 per pkg	1 roll	2.0	110	16%
kaiser sandwich				
w/sesame seeds	1 roll	3.5	140	23%
potato				
dinner	1 roll	1.5	110	12%
hot dog	1 roll	2.0	120	15%
Italian	1 roll	3.5	280	11%
plain	1 roll	2.0	150	12%
premium steak	1 roll	2.5	170	13%
sesame	1 roll	3.0	150	18%
soft sandwich				
plain	1 roll	3.0	140	19%
sesame				
8 per pkg	1 roll	3.5	140	23%
12 per pkg	1 roll	3.0	130	21%
August Brothers				
dinner				
wheat	1 roll	2.0	100	18%
white				
10 per pkg	1 roll	2.0	90	20%
16-oz pkg	1 roll	1.0	90	10%
hamburger				
wheat	1 roll	2.0	130	14%
white	1 roll	2.5	140	16%
kaiser	1 roll	2.0	160	11%

Food and Description	Amount	Fat Grams	Total Calories	% Fat Calories
onion	1 roll	2.0	160	11%
sesame	1 roll	2.5	170	13%
steak	1 roll	2.5	170	13%
sub	1 roll	2.5	170	13%
Bran'nola				
bun	1 roll	1.5	130	10%
dinner/white	1 roll	1.0	70	13%
hot dog	1 roll	1.5	110	12%
Francisco				
French				
6" roll	1 roll	1.5	160	8%
mini	1 roll	1.0	110	8%
kaiser	1 roll	2.0	170	11%
sourdough	1 roll	1.0	90	10%
steak	1 roll	2.0	170	11%
super sub loaf	1-oz slice	0.5	70	6%
3" roll	1 roll	1.0	90	10%
Levy Old Country				
egg twist	1 roll	4.0	170	21%
kaiser	1 roll	2.0	170	11%
onion	1 roll	3.0	160	17%
sub	1 roll	1.5	140	10%
(Awrey's)				
dinner	1 roll	1.0	60	15%
Black Forest	1 roll	1.0	50	18%
cracked wheat	1 roll	1.0	50	18%
crusty	1 roll	1.0	70	13%
poppy seed	1 roll	1.0	60	15%
sesame seed	1 roll	1.0	60	15%
sandwich/oat bran	1 roll	2.0	120	15%
(Brownberry)				
Brownberry				
hot dog				
sliced	1 roll	2.0	110	16%
wheat	1 roll	2.0	110	16%
sandwich				
potato	1 roll	2.5	150	15%
wheat	1 roll	2.0	130	14%
white	1 roll	2.5	140	16%
Francisco International				
dinner	1 roll	1.0	120	8%
French/6" roll	1 roll	1.0	170	5%
kaiser	1 roll	1.0	170	5%
Hearth				
assorted	1 roll	1.5	120	11%
kaiser	1 roll	2.5	150	15%
National/white sandwich				
plain	1 roll	2.5	140	16%

Food and Description	Amount	Fat Grams	Total Calories	% Fat Calories
w/sesame seeds	1 roll	3.0	140	19%
(Circle S) steak	1 roll	3.0	150	18%
(Colombo)				
49er				
sour	1 roll	<1.0	90	5%
sweet	1 roll	2.0	95	19%
Luigi/twin pack	1 roll	1.5	145	9%
steak				
sour	1 roll	2.0	200	9%
sweet	1 roll	3.0	200	14%
(Earth Grains)				
French	1 roll	1.0	100	9%
kaiser	1 roll	2.0	190	10%
onion	1 roll	2.0	190	10%
submarine	½ roll	1.0	180	5%
generic				
cloverleaf	1 roll	1.6	83	17%
cracked wheat	1 roll	<1.0	95	8%
dinner/white				
hard	1 roll	1.6	156	9%
soft	1 roll	2.0	85	21%
egg	1 roll	2.0	110	16%
French	1 roll	1.0	130	7%
hamburger				
multigrain	1 roll	2.0	115	16%
reduced calorie	1 roll	1.0	85	11%
white	1 roll	2.0	125	14%
hard	1 roll	2.0	170	11%
hot cross bun	1 roll	4.0	200	18%
hot dog				
multigrain	1 roll	2.0	115	16%
reduced calorie	1 roll	1.0	85	11%
regular	1 roll	2.0	125	14%
kaiser	1 roll	2.0	170	11%
oat bran	1 roll	2.0	80	23%
potato roll	1 roll	2.0	130	14%
rye	1 roll	1.0	80	11%
sourdough	1 roll	1.0	130	7%
whole wheat	1 roll	1.0	93	10%
(Hollywood) dark	1 roll	–	40	–
(Holsum) hamburger	1 roll	2.0	120	15%
(Home Pride) dinner				
wheat	1 roll	1.0	70	13%
white	1 roll	2.0	80	23%
(Lewis) Italian crispy dinner	1 roll	2.0	100	18%
(King's Hawaiian)				
honey wheat	1 roll	3.0	90	30%
regular	1 roll	2.0	80	23%

Food and Description	Amount	Fat Grams	Total Calories	% Fat Calories
(Martin's)				
Big Marty				
poppy	1 roll	3.0	180	15%
sesame	1 roll	3.0	180	15%
dinner	1 roll	1.0	90	10%
hoagie				
plain	1 roll	4.0	250	14%
sesame	1 roll	4.0	250	14%
long	1 roll	1.5	140	10%
party	3 rolls	1.5	140	10%
potato/sliced	1 roll	1.0	90	30%
sandwich	1 roll	2.0	140	13%
whole wheat	1 roll	2.0	160	11%
(Oroweat)				
health nut	1 roll	3.0	160	17%
master's best/winter wheat	1 roll	4.0	160	23%
(Pepperidge Farm)				
bakery				
dinner				
country style classic	1 roll	3.0	150	18%
hearty potato classic	1 roll	2.5	80	28%
finger				
w/poppy seeds	3 rolls	4.5	150	27%
w/sesame seeds	3 rolls	4.5	150	27%
frankfurter				
Dijon	1 roll	3.0	140	19%
side-sliced	1 roll	2.5	140	16%
top-sliced	1 roll	2.5	140	16%
hamburger/sliced	1 roll	2.5	130	17%
hoagie				
deli classic soft	1 roll	4.5	200	20%
multigrain	1 roll	4.5	200	20%
Parker House	3 rolls	4.5	150	27%
party	5 rolls	4.5	170	24%
sandwich				
hearty	1 roll	5.0	230	20%
multigrain	1 roll	3.0	150	18%
onion/sliced	1 roll	3.0	150	18%
potato	1 roll	4.0	160	23%
sliced w/sesame seeds	1 roll	3.0	140	19%
sourdough	1 roll	3.5	170	19%
European Bake Shoppe/French style				
plain	1 roll	1.0	100	9%
seven grain	1 roll	2.0	80	23%
sourdough	1 roll	1.0	100	9%
food service				
frankfurter				
Dijon	1 roll	3.0	140	19%

Food and Description	Amount	Fat Grams	Total Calories	% Fat Calories
side-sliced	1 roll	2.5	140	16%
hamburger	1 roll	2.5	130	17%
hoagie (bulk)	1 roll	4.5	200	20%
sandwich				
bun tray	1 roll	7.0	160	39%
5" roll	1 roll	5.0	230	20%
onion w/poppy seeds	1 roll	2.5	140	16%
w/sesame seeds	1 roll	3.0	140	19%
(Rainbo) hog dog/white	1 roll	1.5	100	14%
(Roman Meal)				
dinner	2 rolls	3.0	150	18%
hamburger	1 roll	2.0	120	15%
hot dog	1 roll	2.0	110	16%
sandwich	1 roll	3.0	185	15%
(Wonder)				
country grain hot	1 roll	1.0	100	9%
dinner	1 roll	1.0	80	11%
hamburger				
light	1 roll	1.0	80	11%
regular	1 roll	2.0	110	16%
hoagie	1 roll	7.0	400	16%
hot dog				
bun	1 roll	2.0	110	16%
roll	1 roll	2.0	80	11%
pan	1 roll	1.0	80	11%
■ REFRIGERATED				
(Pillsbury)				
crescent				
cheese	2 rolls	12.0	210	51%
plain	2 rolls	11.0	200	50%
dinner/butterflake	1 roll	5.0	130	35%
ROOT BEER (See SOFT DRINK)				
ROSE APPLE/fresh	3.5 oz	<1.0	25	11%
ROSELLE/raw	½ cup	–	15	–
ROSEMARY/dried	1 tsp	–	4	–
ROTINI (See PASTA; PASTA ENTRÉE/DINNER)				
ROUGHY (See ORANGE ROUGHY; SEAFOOD ENTRÉE/DINNER)				
RUM (See LIQUOR, DISTILLED)				
RUTABAGA/fresh				
boiled-drained				
cubed	½ cup	–	30	–
mashed	½ cup	–	40	–
raw	½ cup	–	25	–
RYE (See also FLOUR; CEREAL; LIQUOR, DISTILLED)				
(Arrowhead Mills)				
flakes/rolled	⅓ cup	0.5	110	4%
whole-grain	¼ cup	1.0	160	6%
generic/whole-grain	1 cup	4.0	565	6%

S

Food and Description	Amount	Fat Grams	Total Calories	% Fat Calories
SABLEFISH				
raw	3 oz	13.0	165	71%
smoked	3 oz	17.0	220	70%
SAFFLOWER MARGARINE/SPREAD (*See* MARGARINE, MARGARINE SPREAD, & SPRAY)				
SAFFLOWER MEAL	1 oz	0.7	97	6%
SAFFLOWER OIL (*See* OIL)				
SAFFLOWER SEEDS				
kernels/dried	1 oz	11.0	150	66%
SAFFRON				
dried	1 tsp	–	2	–
SAGE				
ground	1 tsp	–	4	–
SALAD DRESSING (*See also* MAYONNAISE/MAYONNAISE-TYPE DRESSING)				
■ **HOMEMADE**				
USDA Standard Home Recipe				
cooked/made w/margarine	1 Tbs	2.0	25	72%
French	1 Tbs	10.0	90	100%
vinegar & oil	1 Tbs	8.0	70	100%
■ **MIX** (Note: Unless otherwise stated, mixes were prepared as directed on package.)				
(Andre Prost) A Taste of Thai				
spicy peanut	2 Tbs	1.5	40	34%
(Good Seasons)				
cheese garlic				
mix only	⅛ pkg	–	5	–
prepared	2 Tbs	15.0	140	96%
farm-style buttermilk				
mix only	⅟₁₆ pkg	–	10	–
prepared	2 Tbs	12.0	120	90%
garlic & herbs				
mix only	⅛ pkg	–	5	–
prepared	2 Tbs	15.0	140	96%
gourmet Caesar				
mix only	⅛ pkg	–	15	–
prepared	2 Tbs	16.0	150	96%
honey mustard				
fat-free				
mix only	⅛ pkg	–	20	–
prepared	2 Tbs	–	20	–

Food and Description	Amount	Fat Grams	Total Calories	% Fat Calories
regular				
mix only	⅛ pkg	–	15	–
prepared	2 Tbs	15.0	150	90%
Italian				
creamy/fat-free				
mix only	⅛ pkg	–	10	–
prepared	2 Tbs	–	20	–
mild				
mix only	⅛ pkg	–	10	–
prepared	2 Tbs	15.0	150	90%
regular				
fat-free				
mix only	⅛ pkg	–	10	–
prepared	2 Tbs	–	10	–
reduced calorie				
mix only	⅛ pkg	–	5	–
prepared	2 Tbs	5.0	50	90%
regular				
mix only	⅛ pkg	–	5	–
prepared	2 Tbs	15.0	140	96%
zesty				
reduced calorie				
mix only	⅛ pkg	–	5	–
prepared	2 Tbs	5.0	50	90%
regular				
mix only	⅛ pkg	–	5	–
prepared	2 Tbs	15.0	140	96%
Mexican spice				
mix only	⅛ pkg	–	10	–
prepared	2 Tbs	15.0	140	96%
Oriental sesame				
mix only	⅛ pkg	–	15	–
prepared	2 Tbs	16.0	150	96%
ranch				
reduced calorie				
mix only	⅟₁₆ pkg	–	10	–
prepared	2 Tbs	4.5	60	68%
regular				
mix only	⅟₁₆ pkg	–	5	–
prepared	2 Tbs	12.0	120	90%
zesty herb/fat-free				
mix only	⅛ pkg	–	10	–
prepared	2 Tbs	–	20	–
(Hain) fat-free				
Caesar				
mix only	1 tsp	–	10	–
prepared	2 Tbs	–	10	–

Food and Description	Amount	Fat Grams	Total Calories	% Fat Calories
(Hidden Valley)				
bacon				
mix only	1/16 pkg	–	10	–
prepared	2 Tbs	12.0	120	90%
blue cheese				
mix only	1/16 pkg	–	100	–
prepared	2 Tbs	12.0	120	90%
honey Dijon				
mix only	1/16 pkg	–	15	–
prepared	2 Tbs	12.0	120	90%
original				
buttermilk				
mix only	1/16 pkg	–	–	–
prepared	2 Tbs	11.0	110	90%
low-fat				
mix only	1/16 pkg	–	10	–
prepared	2 Tbs	1.0	30	30%
milk				
mix only	1/16 pkg	–	5	–
prepared	2 Tbs	12.0	120	90%
reduced calorie				
mix only	1/16 pkg	–	5	–
prepared	2 Tbs	6.0	70	77%
ranch Italian				
mix only	1/16 pkg	–	15	–
prepared	2 Tbs	14.0	140	90%
(Lawry's) mix only				
Caesar	1 pkg	3.0	75	36%
Italian				
regular	1 pkg	<1.0	45	4%
w/cheese	1 pkg	2.0	75	24%
(Macayamas) mix only (Note: 1 serving of mix = the amount in 1 Tbs prepared.)				
buttermilk herb	1 serving	<1.0	8	56%
cheese & garlic	1 serving	<1.0	12	38%
garlic-lemon-dill	1 serving	<1.0	8	56%
Italian supreme	1 serving	<1.0	8	56%
(Weight Watchers) mix only (Note: 1 serving of mix = the amount in 2 Tbs prepared.)				
blue cheese	1 serving	–	10	–
French	1 serving	–	–	–
Italian				
creamy	1 serving	–	5	–
regular	1 serving	–	–	–
Russian	1 serving	–	–	–
Thousand Island	1 serving	–	–	–
⊠ READY TO USE				
(Andre Prost) A Taste of Thai				
Mexican chipotle	1½ Tbs	9.0	100	81%
spicy peanut	¼ cup	8.0	120	60%

Food and Description	Amount	Fat Grams	Total Calories	% Fat Calories
(Annie's) wild herbal organics				
balsamic	2 Tbs	10.0	100	90%
cilantro & lime	2 Tbs	10.0	100	90%
cowgirl ranch	2 Tbs	8.0	90	80%
gingerly	2 Tbs	10.0	100	90%
shiitake & sesame	2 Tbs	13.0	120	98%
vinaigrette				
ginger & chamomile	2 Tbs	13.0	130	90%
honey & turmeric	2 Tbs	15.0	170	79%
raspberry	2 Tbs	9.0	110	74%
yogurt/no-fat	2 Tbs	–	20	–
(Arcobasso's)				
bleu vinaigrette	2 Tbs	12.0	120	90%
creamy Caesar	2 Tbs	18.0	180	90%
creamy Italian	2 Tbs	16.0	160	90%
poppy seed	2 Tbs	18.0	180	90%
ranch	2 Tbs	12.0	120	90%
(Ayla's) fat-free				
creamy dill	2 Tbs	–	15	–
French	2 Tbs	–	10	–
garlic & onion	2 Tbs	–	10	–
Italian				
creamy	2 Tbs	–	15	–
regular	2 Tbs	–	10	–
Russian	2 Tbs	–	10	–
spicy Indonesian	2 Tbs	2.5	35	64%
(Bernstein's)				
bistro-style blue cheese	2 Tbs	–	20	–
Caesar	2 Tbs	10.0	100	90%
cheese fantastico				
light	2 Tbs	1.0	30	30%
regular	2 Tbs	10.0	100	90%
country cafe Dijon & honey	2 Tbs	–	45	–
country herb ranch	2 Tbs	–	30	–
French vinaigrette	2 Tbs	10.0	100	90%
Parmesan garlic ranch	2 Tbs	1.0	45	50%
Rio Grande Thousand Island	2 Tbs	–	40	–
Roquefort	2 Tbs	14.0	130	97%
wine country Italian	2 Tbs	11.0	110	91%
(Bertolli) olive oil				
creamy	2 Tbs	12.0	120	90%
original	2 Tbs	16.0	160	90%
zesty	2 Tbs	14.0	140	90%
(Brianna's) homestyle				
blush wine vinaigrette	2 Tbs	6.0	100	54%
poppy seed	2 Tbs	10.0	130	69%
real French vinaigrette	2 Tbs	10.0	130	69%

Food and Description	Amount	Fat Grams	Total Calories	% Fat Calories
(Cardini's)				
Italian	2 Tbs	14.0	130	97%
lime dill	2 Tbs	15.0	140	96%
original Caesar	2 Tbs	8.0	80	90%
summer honey mustard	2 Tbs	13.0	140	84%
(Cook's Classics)				
apple honey mustard	2 Tbs	9.0	100	81%
Caesar	2 Tbs	13.0	120	98%
Dijon	2 Tbs	–	6	–
garlic lover's	2 Tbs	10.5	100	95%
Italian garlic gusto	2 Tbs	–	12	–
vinaigrette	2 Tbs	9.0	90	90%
(Dorothy Lynch) homestyle/ reduced calorie	2 Tbs	–	60	–
(Estee)				
blue cheese	2 Tbs	–	15	–
creamy French	2 Tbs	–	10	–
creamy garlic	2 Tbs	–	10	–
Italian				
creamy	2 Tbs	–	15	–
regular	2 Tbs	–	5	–
Thousand Island	2 Tbs	–	10	–
(Featherweight)				
creamy Dijon	2 Tbs	0.5	15	30%
French	2 Tbs	–	10	–
Italian	2 Tbs	–	5	–
(Gardini's)				
herb poppy seed	2 Tbs	1.0	27	30%
honey mustard	2 Tbs	13.0	140	84%
Italian	2 Tbs	14.0	130	97%
original Caesar	2 Tbs	8.0	80	90%
Parmesan ranch	2 Tbs	1.0	21	43%
pesto pasta	2 Tbs	14.0	140	90%
zesty garlic	2 Tbs	13.0	120	98%
(Girard's)				
Caesar	2 Tbs	16.0	150	96%
fat-free	2 Tbs	–	20	–
light	2 Tbs	7.0	80	79%
champagne				
light	2 Tbs	5.0	60	75%
regular	2 Tbs	15.0	140	96%
chardonnay	2 Tbs	11.0	110	90%
chenin blanc	2 Tbs	12.0	110	98%
cilantro	2 Tbs	12.0	120	90%
French				
old San Francisco	2 Tbs	12.0	130	83%
regular	2 Tbs	13.0	120	98%
honey Dijon peppercorn	2 Tbs	13.0	150	78%

Food and Description	Amount	Fat Grams	Total Calories	% Fat Calories
Italian				
old Venice	2 Tbs	13.0	130	90%
Romano cheese	2 Tbs	12.0	120	90%
Parisian	2 Tbs	17.0	160	96%
Parmesan peppercorn	2 Tbs	17.0	160	96%
poppy seed	2 Tbs	13.0	150	78%
rancho California	2 Tbs	16.0	150	96%
raspberry				
fat-free	2 Tbs	–	70	–
regular	2 Tbs	12.0	160	68%
red wine vinegar & oil	2 Tbs	13.0	140	84%
seafood Louie dressing	2 Tbs	17.0	170	90%
spinach	2 Tbs	12.0	140	77%
sweet slaw dressing	2 Tbs	14.0	170	74%
vinaigrette				
balsamic/fat-free	2 Tbs	–	35	–
Greek	2 Tbs	11.0	100	99%
red wine/fat-free	2 Tbs	–	40	–
(Hain)				
Dijon	2 Tbs	13.0	130	90%
Italian				
creamy	2 Tbs	16.0	180	80%
regular	2 Tbs	–	35	–
old-fashioned buttermilk	2 Tbs	14.0	140	58%
poppy seed ranchers	2 Tbs	14.0	140	58%
Thousand Island	2 Tbs	9.0	110	74%
vinaigrette				
raspberry	2 Tbs	–	12	–
white wine	2 Tbs	–	25	–
(Henri's)				
chef's ranch house				
light	2 Tbs	4.0	80	45%
regular	2 Tbs	14.0	140	90%
cucumber & onion/light	2 Tbs	4.0	70	51%
French				
hearty	2 Tbs	12.0	140	77%
original				
light	2 Tbs	4.0	80	45%
regular	2 Tbs	12.0	120	90%
sweet & saucy	2 Tbs	12.0	140	77%
Parmesan ranch/lite	2 Tbs	4.0	70	51%
tas-tee dressing				
private blend/light	2 Tbs	4.0	60	60%
regular	2 Tbs	8.0	100	72%
Thousand Island/light	2 Tbs	4.0	60	60%
(Herb Magic)				
creamy cucumber	2 Tbs	–	15	–
Italian	2 Tbs	–	10	–

Food and Description	Amount	Fat Grams	Total Calories	% Fat Calories
sweet & sour	2 Tbs	–	35	–
vinaigrette	2 Tbs	–	10	–
zesty tomato	2 Tbs	–	15	–
(Hidden Valley)				
blue cheese/fat-free	2 Tbs	–	20	–
coleslaw/fat-free	2 Tbs	–	35	–
creamy Parmesan/fat-free	2 Tbs	–	30	–
French/low-fat	2 Tbs	1.0	35	26%
honey Dijon/fat-free	2 Tbs	–	35	–
original ranch				
low-fat	2 Tbs	3.0	40	68%
reduced calorie	2 Tbs	7.0	80	95%
Parmesan Italian/fat-free	2 Tbs	–	20	–
ranch Italian /reduced calorie	2 Tbs	5.0	50	90%
Thousand Island/low-fat	2 Tbs	1.0	35	26%
(Hollywood)				
Caesar	1 Tbs	7.0	70	90%
Dijon vinaigrette	1 Tbs	6.0	60	90%
Italian				
cheese	1 Tbs	8.0	80	90%
creamy	1 Tbs	9.0	90	90%
regular	1 Tbs	9.0	90	90%
poppy seed	1 Tbs	8.0	75	70%
Thousand Island ranchers	1 Tbs	6.0	60	90%
(Ken's Steak House)				
Caesar w/imported anchovies	2 Tbs	6.0	70	77%
creamy Parmesan w/ peppercorns	2 Tbs	10.0	100	90%
cucumber w/chives	2 Tbs	–	30	–
honey Dijon	2 Tbs	–	40	–
honey mustard vinaigrette	2 Tbs	10.0	100	90%
raspberry walnut	2 Tbs	6.0	80	68%
sun-dried tomato	2 Tbs	–	60	–
(Kozlowski Farms)				
sesame seed	2 Tbs	0.5	15	30%
south of the border	2 Tbs	–	10	–
zesty herb	2 Tbs	–	10	–
(Kraft)				
bacon & tomato				
deliciously right/reduced calorie	2 Tbs	5.0	60	75%
regular	2 Tbs	14.0	140	90%
blue cheese				
fat-free	2 Tbs	–	50	–
roka	2 Tbs	7.0	90	70%
Caesar				
deliciously right/reduced calorie	2 Tbs	5.0	60	75%
ranch	2 Tbs	15.0	140	96%
regular	2 Tbs	13.0	130	90%

Food and Description	Amount	Fat Grams	Total Calories	% Fat Calories
Catalina				
fat-free	2 Tbs	–	45	–
w/honey	2 Tbs	12.0	140	77%
Catalina French				
deliciously right/reduced calorie	2 Tbs	4.0	80	45%
regular	2 Tbs	11.0	140	71%
coleslaw	2 Tbs	12.0	150	72%
creamy garlic	2 Tbs	11.0	110	90%
French style				
deliciously right/reduced calorie	2 Tbs	3.0	50	54%
fat-free	2 Tbs	–	50	–
regular	2 Tbs	12.0	120	90%
honey Dijon				
fat-free	2 Tbs	–	50	–
regular	2 Tbs	15.0	150	90%
Italian				
creamy				
deliciously right/reduced calorie	2 Tbs	5.0	50	90%
regular	2 Tbs	11.0	110	90%
regular				
deliciously right/reduced calorie	2 Tbs	7.0	70	90%
fat-free	2 Tbs	–	10	–
house	2 Tbs	12.0	120	90%
oil-free/fat-free	2 Tbs	–	5	–
presto	2 Tbs	15.0	140	96%
zesty	2 Tbs	11.0	110	90%
ranch				
buttermilk	2 Tbs	16.0	150	96%
cucumber				
deliciously right/reduced calorie	2 Tbs	5.0	60	75%
regular	2 Tbs	15.0	150	90%
peppercorn				
fat-free	2 Tbs	–	50	–
regular	2 Tbs	18.0	170	95%
regular				
deliciously right/reduced calorie	2 Tbs	11.0	110	90%
fat-free	2 Tbs	–	50	–
regular	2 Tbs	18.0	170	95%
sour cream & onion	2 Tbs	18.0	170	95%
red wine vinegar/fat-free	2 Tbs	–	15	–
Russian	2 Tbs	10.0	130	69%
salsa				
ranch	2 Tbs	13.0	130	90%
zesty garden	2 Tbs	6.0	70	77%
Thousand Island				
deliciously right/reduced calorie	2 Tbs	4.0	70	51%
fat-free	2 Tbs	–	45	–
regular	2 Tbs	10.0	110	82%

Food and Description	Amount	Fat Grams	Total Calories	% Fat Calories
w/bacon	2 Tbs	12.0	120	90%
(Lawry's)				
Caesar				
creamy	2 Tbs	14.0	130	97%
regular	2 Tbs	13.0	130	90%
Italian	2 Tbs	14.0	140	90%
red wine vinaigrette	2 Tbs	7.0	90	70%
San Francisco w/Romano cheese	2 Tbs	13.0	120	98%
(Life) all natural				
avocado w/tofu	1 Tbs	7.0	70	90%
creamy egg salad/egg-free	1 Tbs	4.0	40	90%
garlic w/tofu	1 Tbs	7.0	70	90%
tofu	1 Tbs	7.0	75	84%
(Litehouse)				
bleu				
chunky	2 Tbs	16.0	150	96%
lite	2 Tbs	7.0	70	90%
Caesar				
fat-free	2 Tbs	–	15	–
lite	2 Tbs	8.0	80	90%
regular	2 Tbs	12.0	120	90%
dilly dip	2 Tbs	16.0	150	96%
French				
country herb	2 Tbs	10.0	110	82%
fat-free	2 Tbs	–	25	–
lite	2 Tbs	0.5	25	18%
regular	2 Tbs	10.0	110	90%
honey Dijon/fat-free	2 Tbs	–	35	–
honey mustard	2 Tbs	13.0	130	90%
hot bacon	2 Tbs	1.0	60	15%
Italian				
creamy	2 Tbs	13.0	120	98%
traditional	2 Tbs	14.0	130	97%
poppy seed	2 Tbs	12.0	130	83%
ranch				
jalapeño	2 Tbs	12.0	120	90%
peppercorn	2 Tbs	10.0	100	90%
regular				
fat-free	2 Tbs	–	15	–
country	2 Tbs	13.0	120	98%
lite	2 Tbs	5.0	60	75%
regular	2 Tbs	13.0	120	98%
Roquefort	2 Tbs	14.0	130	97%
sour cream & chives	2 Tbs	14.0	130	97%
Thousand Island	2 Tbs	13.0	120	98%
vinaigrette				
raspberry/fat-free	2 Tbs	–	15	–
regular/fat-free	2 Tbs	–	5	–

Food and Description	Amount	Fat Grams	Total Calories	% Fat Calories
(Maple Grove Farms)				
Caesar/lite	2 Tbs	5.0	70	64%
honey Dijon/fat-free	2 Tbs	–	45	–
pesto Parmesan	2 Tbs	5.0	70	64%
(Marie's)				
creamy blue cheese/low-fat	2 Tbs	2.0	45	40%
Italian/fat-free	2 Tbs	–	8	–
red wine vinaigrette/fat-free	2 Tbs	–	10	–
Marzetti (See (T. Marzetti) in this section)				
(Nabisco) Grey Poupon				
country French	2 Tbs	11.0	120	83%
honey Dijon mustard	2 Tbs	12.0	130	83%
Italian vinaigrette	2 Tbs	8.0	80	90%
(Nasoya) vegi dressings				
Italian/creamy	2 Tbs	5.0	60	75%
sesame garlic	2 Tbs	5.0	60	75%
Thousand Island	2 Tbs	4.0	60	60%
(Newman's Own)				
Caesar	2 Tbs	16.0	150	96%
Italian	2 Tbs	16.0	150	96%
(Old Dutch) sweet & sour	2 Tbs	–	50	–
(Oriental Chef)				
honey orange	2 Tbs	6.0	80	68%
original French	2 Tbs	6.0	80	68%
snappy ginger	2 Tbs	8.0	80	90%
tangy soy	2 Tbs	8.0	70	100%
(Ott's)				
buttermilk ranch	2 Tbs	14.0	140	90%
Italian	2 Tbs	18.0	180	90%
original				
fat-free	2 Tbs	–	35	–
reduced calorie	2 Tbs	1.5	50	27%
regular	2 Tbs	6.0	80	68%
poppy seed				
fat-free	2 Tbs	–	45	–
regular	2 Tbs	7.0	90	70%
(Peggy Jane's)				
fruit salad	2 Tbs	4.0	70	51%
garden herb	2 Tbs	8.0	90	80%
ground peppercorn	2 Tbs	17.0	160	96%
honey mustard	2 Tbs	12.0	120	90%
Oriental chicken salad	2 Tbs	12.0	130	83%
poppy seed	2 Tbs	9.0	120	68%
raspberry low-fat	2 Tbs	2.0	50	36%
roasted garlic Caesar	2 Tbs	15.0	140	96%
sesame	2 Tbs	10.0	120	75%
sun-dried tomato	2 Tbs	9.0	100	81%

Food and Description	Amount	Fat Grams	Total Calories	% Fat Calories
(Pfeiffer)				
blue cheese	2 Tbs	17.0	160	96%
buttermilk & herb	2 Tbs	20.0	180	100%
Caesar				
house	2 Tbs	16.0	150	96%
light	2 Tbs	1.0	20	45%
regular	2 Tbs	16.0	150	96%
coleslaw	2 Tbs	13.0	130	90%
French				
regular				
light	2 Tbs	2.0	40	45%
regular	2 Tbs	13.0	150	78%
California				
fat-free	2 Tbs	–	45	–
regular	2 Tbs	12.0	140	77%
honey Dijon				
fat-free	2 Tbs	–	60	–
regular	2 Tbs	13.0	140	84%
Italian				
creamy	2 Tbs	16.0	150	96%
regular				
fat-free	2 Tbs	–	15	–
gusto	2 Tbs	13.0	120	98%
light	2 Tbs	5.0	60	75%
regular	2 Tbs	12.0	120	90%
ranch				
Dijon	2 Tbs	18.0	170	95%
garden	2 Tbs	19.0	180	95%
peppercorn				
fat-free	2 Tbs	–	30	–
regular	2 Tbs	19.0	180	95%
regular				
fat-free	2 Tbs	–	30	–
light	2 Tbs	8.0	90	80%
regular	2 Tbs	20.0	180	100%
red wine vinegar & oil				
light	2 Tbs	1.0	20	45%
regular	2 Tbs	14.0	130	97%
Russian	2 Tbs	14.0	140	90%
spring garden	2 Tbs	15.0	160	84%
sweet & sour	2 Tbs	13.0	160	73%
Thousand Island				
fat-free	2 Tbs	–	40	–
light	2 Tbs	5.0	70	64%
regular	2 Tbs	14.0	140	90%
(Pritikin)				
Dijon balsamic vinaigrette	2 Tbs	–	30	–
French style	2 Tbs	–	35	–

Food and Description	Amount	Fat Grams	Total Calories	% Fat Calories
honey Dijon	2 Tbs	–	45	–
honey French	2 Tbs	–	40	–
Italian	2 Tbs	–	20	–
raspberry	2 Tbs	–	45	–
(Richelieu) western				
fat-free	2 Tbs	–	45	–
reduced calorie	2 Tbs	2.0	70	26%
regular	2 Tbs	10.0	140	64%
(S&W) vintage lites				
balsamic vinegar	2 Tbs	–	35	–
mango key lime	2 Tbs	–	30	–
Oriental rice wine vinegar	2 Tbs	–	30	–
raspberry blush vinegar	2 Tbs	–	40	–
red wine vinegar w/herbs	2 Tbs	–	40	–
white wine vinegar w/ herbs	2 Tbs	–	40	–
(Seven Seas)				
blue cheese/chunky	2 Tbs	7.0	90	70%
Caesar				
creamy	2 Tbs	15.0	140	96%
viva	2 Tbs	12.0	120	90%
Green Goddess	2 Tbs	13.0	120	98%
herbs & spices	2 Tbs	12.0	120	90%
Italian				
creamy				
reduced calorie	2 Tbs	5.0	60	75%
regular	2 Tbs	12.0	110	98%
regular/fat-free	2 Tbs	–	10	–
two cheese	2 Tbs	7.0	70	90%
viva				
reduced calorie	2 Tbs	4.0	45	80%
regular	2 Tbs	11.0	110	90%
w/olive oil	2 Tbs	5.0	50	90%
ranch				
fat-free	2 Tbs	–	50	–
reduced calorie	2 Tbs	9.0	100	90%
regular	2 Tbs	16.0	150	96%
red wine vinegar	2 Tbs	–	15	–
red wine vinegar & oil				
reduced calorie	2 Tbs	5.0	60	75%
regular	2 Tbs	11.0	110	90%
Russian/viva	2 Tbs	16.0	150	96%
(T. Marzetti)				
House Dressing				
Caesar				
fat-free	2 Tbs	–	20	–
olde world	2 Tbs	16.0	150	96%
coleslaw/fat-free	2 Tbs	–	45	–
honey Dijon/fat-free	2 Tbs	–	60	–

Food and Description	Amount	Fat Grams	Total Calories	% Fat Calories
honey French/fat-free	2 Tbs	–	35	–
Italian				
fat-free	2 Tbs	–	15	–
olde Venice	2 Tbs	13.0	130	90%
peppercorn ranch/fat-free	2 Tbs	–	30	–
poppy seed/fat-free	2 Tbs	–	60	–
raspberry/fat-free	2 Tbs	–	70	–
teriyaki stir-fry	2 Tbs	1.5	80	17%
Thousand Island/fat-free	2 Tbs	–	35	–
vinaigrette				
lemon Dijon/fat-free	2 Tbs		35	–
red wine/fat-free	2 Tbs	–	40	–
wild raspberry	2 Tbs	12.0	150	72%
pourable dressing/bottled				
blue cheese				
light	2 Tbs	6.0	80	68%
regular	2 Tbs	17.0	160	96%
buttermilk & herb	2 Tbs	20.0	180	100%
Caesar				
house	2 Tbs	16.0	150	96%
ranch	2 Tbs	20.0	190	95%
regular	2 Tbs	16.0	150	96%
celery seed	2 Tbs	13.0	160	73%
Dijon				
fat-free	2 Tbs	–	60	–
honey	2 Tbs	13.0	140	84%
ranch	2 Tbs	18.0	170	95%
French				
California				
fat-free	2 Tbs	–	45	–
light	2 Tbs	6.0	80	68%
regular	2 Tbs	13.0	160	73%
country	2 Tbs	15.0	160	84%
regular/light	2 Tbs	2.0	40	45%
Italian	2 Tbs	12.0	120	90%
creamy	2 Tbs	16.0	150	96%
gusto	2 Tbs	13.0	120	98%
regular				
fat-free	2 Tbs	–	15	–
light	2 Tbs	5.0	60	75%
Romano	2 Tbs	17.0	160	96%
Parmesan pepper	2 Tbs	17.0	160	96%
poppy seed				
fat-free	2 Tbs	–	60	–
regular	2 Tbs	13.0	160	73%
ranch				
regular				
fat-free	2 Tbs	–	30	–

Food and Description	Amount	Fat Grams	Total Calories	% Fat Calories
light	2 Tbs	8.0	90	80%
regular	2 Tbs	20.0	180	100%
garden	2 Tbs	19.0	180	95%
peppercorn				
fat-free	2 Tbs	–	30	–
regular	2 Tbs	19.0	180	95%
style	2 Tbs	13.0	160	73%
raspberry vinegar	2 Tbs	11.0	120	83%
red wine vinegar & oil				
light	2 Tbs	1.0	20	45%
regular	2 Tbs	14.0	130	97%
sweet & saucy	2 Tbs	12.0	140	77%
sweet & sour				
fat-free	2 Tbs	–	50	–
light	2 Tbs	6.0	100	54%
regular	2 Tbs	13.0	160	73%
Thousand Island				
fat-free	2 Tbs	–	40	–
light	2 Tbs	5.0	70	64%
regular	2 Tbs	14.0	140	90%
produce dressing/refrigerated jar				
bacon spinach salad	2 Tbs	2.0	80	23%
blue cheese				
chunky				
light	2 Tbs	7.0	80	79%
regular	2 Tbs	16.0	150	96%
honey French	2 Tbs	13.0	160	73%
sour cream	2 Tbs	18.0	170	95%
buttermilk Parmesan pepper	2 Tbs	18.0	170	95%
buttermilk veggie dip	2 Tbs	18.0	170	95%
Caesar				
classic ranch	2 Tbs	20.0	190	95%
Romano cheese	2 Tbs	16.0	150	96%
celery seed/crispy	2 Tbs	13.0	160	73%
cracked peppercorn	2 Tbs	14.0	140	90%
creamy garlic Italian	2 Tbs	17.0	160	96%
creamy tomato	2 Tbs	17.0	160	90%
Dijon honey mustard	2 Tbs	13.0	140	84%
Dutch sweet 'n sour	2 Tbs	13.0	160	73%
honey French				
light	2 Tbs	4.0	80	45%
regular	2 Tbs	14.0	160	79%
old-fashioned poppy seed	2 Tbs	11.0	140	71%
potato salad dressing	2 Tbs	13.0	140	84%
ranch				
buttermilk				
light	2 Tbs	9.0	90	90%
regular	2 Tbs	20.0	180	100%

Food and Description	Amount	Fat Grams	Total Calories	% Fat Calories
buttermilk bacon	2 Tbs	19.0	180	95%
buttermilk Parmesan	2 Tbs	17.0	160	90%
honey dijon	2 Tbs	15.0	150	90%
slaw dressing				
original				
fat-free	2 Tbs	–	45	–
light	2 Tbs	7.0	100	63%
regular	2 Tbs	16.0	170	85%
southern	2 Tbs	11.0	150	66%
Thousand Island	2 Tbs	15.0	150	90%
(Walden Farms) fat-free				
bleu cheese	2 Tbs	–	25	–
Caesar	2 Tbs	–	25	–
French	2 Tbs	–	30	–
honey Dijon vinaigrette	2 Tbs	–	25	–
Italian				
creamy w/Parmesan	2 Tbs	–	45	–
regular				
no sugar added	2 Tbs	–	–	–
regular	2 Tbs	–	10	–
sodium-free	2 Tbs	–	10	–
w/sun-dried tomato	2 Tbs	–	15	–
ranch				
regular	2 Tbs	–	25	–
w/sun-dried tomato	2 Tbs	–	25	–
Russian	2 Tbs	–	30	–
Thousand Island	2 Tbs	–	20	–
vinaigrette				
balsamic	2 Tbs	–	15	–
cranberry	2 Tbs	–	20	–
raspberry	2 Tbs	–	20	–
(Weight Watchers) Salad Celebrations				
French	2 Tbs	–	40	–
honey Dijon	2 Tbs	–	45	–
Italian				
creamy	2 Tbs	–	30	–
regular	2 Tbs	–	10	–
ranch	2 Tbs	–	35	–
(Western) original				
fat-free	2 Tbs	–	45	–
regular	2 Tbs	12.0	150	72%
(Wish Bone)				
Caesar				
lite	2 Tbs	8.0	100	72%
w/olive oil	2 Tbs	9.5	100	86%
chunky blue cheese				
fat-free	2 Tbs	–	35	–
lite	2 Tbs	7.0	80	79%

Food and Description	Amount	Fat Grams	Total Calories	% Fat Calories
regular	2 Tbs	17.0	170	90%
creamy roasted garlic				
fat-free	2 Tbs	–	40	–
regular	2 Tbs	13.0	140	84%
French				
deluxe	2 Tbs	11.0	120	83%
lite	2 Tbs	2.0	50	36%
sweet 'n spicy				
fat-free	2 Tbs	–	30	–
regular	2 Tbs	12.0	130	83%
honey Dijon				
fat-free	2 Tbs	–	45	–
lite	2 Tbs	5.0	60	75%
regular	2 Tbs	10.0	130	69%
Italian				
classic house	2 Tbs	14.0	140	90%
creamy				
fat-free	2 Tbs	–	35	–
lite	2 Tbs	3.5	60	53%
regular	2 Tbs	10.0	100	90%
olive oil	2 Tbs	6.0	70	77%
regular				
fat-free	2 Tbs	–	15	–
lite	2 Tbs	0.5	15	30%
regular	2 Tbs	9.0	100	81%
robusto	2 Tbs	10.0	100	90%
olive oil vinaigrette	2 Tbs	5.0	60	75%
ranch				
fat-free	2 Tbs	–	40	–
lite	2 Tbs	8.0	100	72%
regular	2 Tbs	17.0	160	96%
Russian	2 Tbs	6.0	110	49%
Santa Fe	2 Tbs	15.0	150	90%
Sierra	2 Tbs	16.0	150	96%
Thousand Island				
fat-free	2 Tbs	–	35	–
lite	2 Tbs	5.0	80	56%
regular	2 Tbs	12.0	130	83%
SALAD GREENS, MIXED				
(Dole)				
Salad in-a-Minute/includes dressing				
Caesar	3.5 oz	14.0	170	74%
Oriental	3.5 oz	7.0	110	57%
spinach	3.5 oz	9.0	180	45%
salad mix				
classic	3.5 oz	1.0	25	36%
coleslaw blend	3.5 oz	0.5	30	15%
French blend	3.5 oz	0.5	25	18%

Food and Description	Amount	Fat Grams	Total Calories	% Fat Calories
(Et Tu Caesar) salad kit w/dressing & croutons				
Caesar				
Greek	1 serving	9.0	120	68%
Italian	1 serving	10.0	130	69%
light	1 serving	6.0	93	58%
original	1 serving	12.0	140	77%
spinach/classic	1 serving	12.0	180	60%

SALAD TOPPINGS & MIXES (*See also* BACON BITS, CHIPS, & PIECES; CROUTONS; SEASONINGS)

Food and Description	Amount	Fat Grams	Total Calories	% Fat Calories
(Betty Crocker) Suddenly Salad				
Caesar				
mix only	⅔ cup	1.0	170	5%
prepared				
low-fat recipe	¾ cup	3.0	190	14%
regular recipe	¾ cup	10.0	250	36%
classic pasta				
mix only	¾ cup	1.0	170	5%
prepared				
low-fat recipe	¾ cup	3.0	180	15%
regular recipe	¾ cup	7.0	220	29%
creamy macaroni				
mix only	⅓ cup	1.0	140	6%
prepared				
low-fat recipe	¾ cup	1.5	210	6%
regular recipe	¾ cup	20.0	320	56%
garden Italian/98% fat-free				
mix only	½ cup	1.0	130	7%
prepared	¾ cup	1.0	130	7%
ranch & bacon				
mix only	¾ cup	1.0	150	6%
prepared				
low-fat recipe	¾ cup	2.0	180	10%
regular recipe	¾ cup	19.0	320	53%
(Hidden Valley) Salad Crispins				
bac'n & onion	1 Tbs	1.0	35	26%
cheddar & onion	1 Tbs	1.0	35	26%
Italian Parmesan	1 Tbs	1.0	35	26%
ranch	1 Tbs	1.0	35	26%
sour cream & herb	1 Tbs	1.0	35	26%
(McCormick/Schilling) Salad Toppins				
garden	1⅓ Tbs	1.0	30	30%
Oriental	1⅓ Tbs	2.0	40	45%
original	1⅓ Tbs	1.5	35	39%
(Pepperidge Farm) Salad Toppers				
bacon cheddar	1 Tbs	2.0	35	51%
Caesar salad bar mix	1 Tbs	2.0	35	51%
cinnamon raisin	1 Tbs	2.0	35	51%
garlic Italian	1 Tbs	1.5	35	39%

Food and Description	Amount	Fat Grams	Total Calories	% Fat Calories
(Produce Partners)				
bacon crumbles	1 Tbs	1.5	30	45%
salad crunchies	1 Tbs	1.0	30	30%
(Salad Nibbler) crouton topping				
buttermilk ranch	1 oz	5.0	130	35%
seasoned cheddar	1 oz	6.0	130	42%
SALAMI (*See* LUNCHEON MEAT; SAUSAGE)				
SALMON (*See also* SALMON SPREAD; SEAFOOD ENTRÉE/DINNER)				
canned				
(Bumble Bee)				
pink	¼ cup	5.0	90	50%
red	¼ cup	7.0	110	57%
(Deming's) Alaska				
keta	½ cup	5.0	140	32%
pink	½ cup	6.0	140	39%
red	½ cup	9.0	170	48%
(Featherweight) pink	¼ cup	5.0	90	50%
(Chicken Of The Sea) chunk style/ skinless-boneless	¼ cup	2.0	60	30%
generic				
Atlantic				
drained	3 oz	2.8	173	15%
solids & liquid	8 oz	6.0	268	20%
	15 oz	12.0	500	22%
chum	3 oz	4.7	120	35%
(Libby's)				
pink				
boneless	⅓ cup	2.0	70	26%
w/bones	¼ cup	5.0	90	50%
red/sockeye	¼ cup	7.0	110	57%
(S&W) red/sockeye	¼ cup	7.0	110	57%
	3.75 oz	11.0	190	52%
fresh				
Atlantic				
cooked-dry heat	3 oz	7.0	155	41%
raw	3 oz	5.5	120	41%
chinook/lox				
raw	3 oz	9.0	155	29%
smoked	3 oz	3.7	100	33%
chum/keta/raw	3 oz	3.0	100	27%
coho				
cooked-moist heat	3 oz	6.5	160	36%
raw	3 oz	5.0	125	36%
pink				
cooked-dry heat	3 oz	4.0	130	27%
raw	3 oz	3.0	100	27%
red/sockeye				
cooked-dry heat	3 oz	9.0	185	44%

Food and Description	Amount	Fat Grams	Total Calories	% Fat Calories
raw	3 oz	7.0	143	44%
frozen				
(Healthy Desire) salmon burgers	1 burger	1.2	100	11%
smoked				
chinook	3 oz	3.7	100	33%
generic	3 oz	8.0	150	48%
(Lascco) sliced/refrigerated	3 oz pkg	6.0	120	45%
SALMON SPREAD				
(Vita) smoked	¼ cup	5.0	180	25%
SALSA (See also MEXICAN FOOD/SAUCE)				
(Robert Rothchild Berry Farm)				
basil raspberry	1.1 oz	–	40	–
hot raspberry	1.1 oz	–	40	–
raspberry	1.1 oz	–	40	–
SALSIFY				
fresh/sliced				
cooked-drained	½ cup	–	46	–
raw	½ cup	–	55	–
SALT (See also SEASONINGS)				
(Durkee)				
seasoned				
lite	½ tsp	–	–	–
regular	½ tsp	–	–	–
unseasoned	½ tsp	–	–	–
(Hain) sea salt				
iodized	1 tsp	–	–	–
plain	1 tsp	–	–	–
Generic				
iodized	any amount	–	–	–
kosher	any amount	–	–	–
plain	any amount	–	–	–
seasoned	1 tsp	–	2-10	–
(McCormick/Schilling)				
Salt 'n Spice	¼ tsp	–	–	–
SALT PORK (See PORK)				
SALT SUBSTITUTE (See also SEASONINGS)				
(Durkee) seasoned	½ tsp	–	–	–
(Estee) Salt It	⅛ tsp	–	–	–
(Featherweight)				
plain	¼ tsp	–	–	–
seasoned	¼ tsp	–	–	–
Generic				
seasoned	1 tsp	–	2	–
seasoned/no salt	1 tsp	–	4	–
unseasoned	1 tsp	–	–	–
(Health Valley) Instead of Salt	1 tsp	–	–	–
(Lawry's)				
plain	1 tsp	–	10	–

Food and Description	Amount	Fat Grams	Total Calories	% Fat Calories
seasoned	1 tsp	–	3	–
(McCormick/Schilling) Salt-Less				
seasoned	¼ tsp	–	–	–
unseasoned	¼ tsp	–	–	–
(Morton)				
plain	1 tsp	–	<1	–
seasoned	1 tsp	–	4	–
SANDWICH (See BREAKFAST SANDWICH; FROZEN ENTRÉE/DINNER; HAMBURGER; VEGETARIAN FOODS; Individual FAST FOOD listings)				
SANDWICH SPREAD (See also LUNCHEON MEAT SPREAD)				
(Best Foods)	1 Tbs	5.0	50	90%
(Hellman's)	1 Tbs	5.0	50	90%
(Kraft) Sandwich Spread & Burger Sauce	1 Tbs	5.0	50	90%
SAPODILLO				
tropical American	1 medium	1.9	140	12%
	1 cup	2.0	178	10%
SAPOTE/fresh	1 medium	1.5	300	5%
SARDINE				
(Del Monte) in tomato sauce/ including sauce	½ fish	4.0	80	45%
(Empress) Norway/boneless & skinless				
in olive oil	3.8 oz	38.0	420	81%
in soy oil	4.4 oz	45.0	500	81%
generic				
canned				
Atlantic/in soy oil w/bone	2 pieces	2.8	50	50%
	3.2 oz	11.0	192	52%
Pacific/in tomato sauce w/bone	~13 oz	44.0	658	60%
(S&W)				
Norwegian brisling/drained	1.86 oz	13.0	160	73%
skinless-boneless	1.69 oz	6.0	100	54%
(Underwood)				
in mustard sauce	3.73 oz	12.0	180	60%
in soy oil	2.96 oz	16.0	220	65%
in tomato sauce	3.73 oz	11.0	180	55%
(Viking's Delight) brisling/in olive oil				
drained	3.75 oz	20.0	260	69%
undrained	3.75 oz	42.0	460	82%
SAUCE (See also ASIAN FOOD/SAUCES & SEASONINGS; BARBECUE SAUCE; GRAVY; MARINADE; MEXICAN FOOD; PASTA ENTRÉE/DINNER; SEASONINGS; SOUP, TOMATO; TOMATO SAUCE)				
■ **HOMEMADE**				
USDA Standard Home Recipe				
clam	½ cup	22.0	275	72%
white				
medium	1 cup	31.0	405	69%
thick	1 cup	39.0	495	71%
thin	1 cup	22.0	305	65%

Food and Description	Amount	Fat Grams	Total Calories	% Fat Calories
■ MIX				
(Andre Prost) A Taste of Thai/mix only				
peanut sauce	¼ envelope	1.5	45	30%
tangy hot sweet & sour sauce	¼ envelope	–	45	–
(Betty Crocker) prepared				
Hamburger Helper sloppy joe sauce				
BBQ	¼ cup	–	80	–
pepperoni pizza	¼ cup	–	45	–
sloppy joes	¼ cup	–	50	–
taco	¼ cup	–	45	–
Recipe Sauce				
Alfredo	½ cup	20.0	220	82%
creamy broccoli	½ cup	20.0	210	86%
pepper steak	½ cup	1.5	50	27%
sweet & sour	½ cup	–	160	–
(De Boles) elbow style pasta & cheese sauce				
mix only	½ cup	3.5	200	16%
prepared	¾ cup	9.5	250	34%
(Durkee) mix only				
à la king	½ pkg	4.0	60	60%
burrito	⅒ pkg	1.0	35	26%
cheese	½ pkg	1.5	25	54%
chicken				
cacciatore	⅒ pkg	–	10	–
Mexican salsa	⅒ pkg	–	10	–
mushroom	⅛ pkg	–	15	–
sweet & sour	⅑ pkg	–	20	–
enchilada	⅛ pkg	–	10	–
fish				
lemon pepper dill	⅙ pkg	0.5	20	23%
tomato basil	⅐ pkg	–	15	–
hollandaise	⅒ pkg	–	10	–
nacho cheese	⅕ pkg	2.0	25	72%
sloppy joe	⅙ pkg	–	20	–
spaghetti	⅕ pkg	–	15	–
American-style	⅙ pkg	–	15	–
family	⅒ pkg	–	20	–
w/mushrooms	⅕ pkg	–	15	–
zesty	⅕ pkg	–	20	–
white	¼ pkg	0.5	20	23%
(French's) mix only				
cheese	¼ pkg	0.5	25	18%
enchilada	⅐ pkg	–	15	–
hollandaise	⅒ pkg	–	10	–
sloppy joe	⅙ pkg	–	20	–
spaghetti				
all-American	⅕ pkg	–	20	–

Food and Description	Amount	Fat Grams	Total Calories	% Fat Calories
Italian	⅕ pkg	–	15	–
mushroom	⅕ pkg	1.0	20	45%
thick	⅙ pkg	–	10	–
stroganoff	¼ pkg	2.0	45	40%
zesty pasta	⅕ pkg	–	20	–
generic				
bearnaise/prepared w/milk & butter	1 cup	68.0	700	87%
cheese sauce				
mix only	1.2 oz	9.0	158	51%
prepared w/milk	1 cup	17.0	307	50%
curry sauce				
mix only	1 oz	6.5	121	48%
prepared w/milk	1 cup	14.7	270	49%
hollandaise/prepared				
made w/butter & water	1 cup	19.7	237	75%
made w/vegetable oil, milk, & butter	1 cup	68.0	703	87%
stroganoff				
mix only	1.6 oz	4.0	161	22%
prepared w/milk & water	1 cup	10.7	271	36%
sweet & sour/prepared	1 cup	–	295	–
teriyaki				
mix only	1 pkg	1.0	30	30%
prepared	1 Tbs	<1.0	8	7%
	1 cup	1.0	131	7%
(Hunt's) Manwich/mix only	1 serving	–	25	–
(Knorr) mix only				
Classic Sauce				
bearnaise	⅕ pkg	0.5	20	23%
bourguignonne	⅙ pkg	1.0	40	23%
chicken Dijon	⅙ pkg	1.0	30	30%
curry	⅕ pkg	1.5	30	45%
demi-glace	⅕ pkg	1.0	30	30%
goulash	1⅓ Tbs	1.0	35	26%
hollandaise	⅕ pkg	1.0	20	45%
lemon dill	⅕ pkg	1.0	30	30%
mushroom	⅕ pkg	1.0	20	45%
mustard herb	¼ pkg	1.5	40	34%
Newburg	⅕ pkg	0.5	20	23%
peppercorn	⅕ pkg	1.0	25	36%
sauerbraten	⅙ pkg	1.0	35	26%
white	⅑ pkg	1.0	25	36%
pasta sauce				
Alfredo	⅙ pkg	1.5	35	39%
carbonara	⅙ pkg	2.0	30	60%
creamy pesto	⅕ pkg	1.0	30	30%
four cheese	⅙ pkg	2.0	30	60%
garlic herb	⅙ pkg	2.0	35	51%

Food and Description	Amount	Fat Grams	Total Calories	% Fat Calories
parma rosa	⅓ pkg	1.0	30	30%
pesto	⅓ pkg	0.5	15	30%
(Lawry's) mix only				
pasta sauce				
Alfredo	1 pkg	13.0	225	52%
pesto	2 tsp	2.0	20	90%
rich & thick	1 pkg	2.0	145	12%
w/mushrooms	1 pkg	1.5	145	9%
stroganoff	1 pkg	<1.0	125	2%
(Mayacamas) mix only				
gourmet sauce				
Alfredo	1 Tbs	<1.0	8	56%
bearnaise	1 Tbs	<1.0	6	75%
curry	1 Tbs	<1.0	6	75%
demi-glace	1 Tbs	<1.0	6	75%
hollandaise	1 Tbs	<1.0	6	75%
honey mustard	1 Tbs	<1.0	6	75%
pesto				
creamy	1 Tbs	<1.0	8	56%
tomato	1 Tbs	<1.0	8	56%
white	1 Tbs	<1.0	6	75%
pasta sauce				
Alfredo	1 Tbs	<1.0	8	56%
basil butter	1 Tbs	<1.0	8	56%
cheddar cheese	1 Tbs	<1.0	8	56%
creamy clam	1 Tbs	<1.0	6	75%
creamy Italian	1 Tbs	<1.0	8	56%
marinara	1 Tbs	<1.0	6	75%
mushroom	1 Tbs	<1.0	6	75%
Skillet Pasta Mix				
black olive pesto	1½ Tbs	<1.0	55	8%
garden skillet	1½ Tbs	<1.0	55	8%
green olive pesto	1½ Tbs	<1.0	55	8%
seafood skillet	1½ Tbs	<1.0	50	9%
spicy skillet	1½ Tbs	<1.0	55	8%
(McCormick/Schilling) mix only				
chicken sauce blend				
barbecue	1 Tbs	–	25	–
cacciatore	2 tsp	–	20	–
curry	4 tsp	1.5	40	34%
Dijon	5 tsp	1.5	40	34%
l'orange	4 tsp	–	40	–
Mexican	2 tsp	–	25	–
Parmesan	4 tsp	1.0	40	23%
piccata	4 tsp	–	25	–
Southwest style	2 tsp	–	20	–
stir-fry	2 tsp	–	20	–

Food and Description	Amount	Fat Grams	Total Calories	% Fat Calories
sweet & sour	4 tsp	–	30	–
teriyaki	1 Tbs	1.0	40	23%
McCormick Collection				
Alfredo pasta	5 tsp	2.5	40	56%
bearnaise	1 tsp	–	10	–
country Dijon	5 tsp	2.0	45	40%
dill & lemon	5 tsp	2.5	45	50%
hollandaise	2 tsp	–	15	–
hunter	1 Tbs	–	30	–
pepper medley	1 Tbs	1.5	30	45%
pesto pasta	1 Tbs	–	10	–
primavera pasta	1 Tbs	1.0	25	36%
white	2 tsp	0.5	20	23%
white clam pasta	2 tsp	–	20	–
(Old Bay) mix only				
crab classic	1 Tbs	1.0	30	30%
dash o'lemon	¼ tsp	–	–	–
salmon classic	5 tsp	1.5	40	34%
seas'n easy				
garlic & herb	1 Tbs	–	25	–
lemon dill	1 Tbs	–	30	–
seafood marinara	1 Tbs	–	25	–
tuna classic	1 Tbs	1.0	30	30%
(Produce Partners) nacho cheese/ mix only	5 tsp	3.0	60	45%
(Spice Islands) mix only				
Alfredo	½ pkg	2.5	45	50%
garlic & herb	¼ pkg	–	15	–
pesto	¼ pkg	0.5	15	30%
primavera	⅕ pkg	1.5	30	45%
tomato pesto	¼ pkg	–	15	–
Weight Watchers) lemon butter/mix only	¼ pkg	–	5	–
■ READY TO USE				
A.1.) steak sauce				
bold	1 Tbs	–	20	–
original	1 Tbs	–	15	–
thick & hearty	1 Tbs	–	25	–
Andre Prost) A Taste of Thai				
chili sauce				
green	1 tsp	–	10	–
red	1 tsp	–	10	–
garlic chili pepper	1 tsp	–	–	–
mole fiesta	1 Tbs	1.5	35	39%
peanut (satay)	2 Tbs	3.0	50	54%
seasoning fish	1 Tbs	–	15	–
tomatillo chile	1 tsp	–	2	–
(Armour Star) sloppy joe/meatless	¼ cup	–	30	–

Food and Description	Amount	Fat Grams	Total Calories	% Fat Calories
(Aunt Millie's) spaghetti sauce				
family style				
chunky tomato & Italian spice	½ cup	1.5	90	15%
w/ground beef	½ cup	2.5	100	23%
w/sliced mushrooms	½ cup	1.0	80	11%
marinara	½ cup	2.5	70	32%
meatless/traditional				
meat-flavored	½ cup	3.0	80	34%
mushroom	½ cup	2.0	70	26%
regular	½ cup	0.5	70	6%
sweet pepper & Italian sausage	½ cup	2.0	60	30%
(Aunt Penny's)				
hollandaise	2 Tbs	4.0	45	80%
white sauce	¼ cup	6.0	90	60%
(Barilla) pasta sauce				
marinara	½ cup	4.0	80	45%
mushroom & garlic	½ cup	3.5	80	39%
spicy pepper	½ cup	3.5	80	39%
tomato & basil	½ cup	2.5	70	32%
(Bennett's)				
cocktail sauce	¼ cup	2.0	80	23%
hot seafood sauce	2 Tbs	–	50	–
(Campbell's)				
nacho cheese sauce	¼ cup	7.0	100	63%
spaghetti sauce				
extra garlic & onion	½ cup	1.0	100	9%
Italian style	½ cup	1.5	120	11%
mushroom	½ cup	1.0	100	10%
mushroom & garlic	½ cup	1.0	90	10%
traditional	½ cup	1.5	120	11%
Summer Chef cooking sauce				
creamy mushroom & herb	½ cup	9.0	110	74%
Oriental sweet & sour	½ cup	1.0	110	8%
(Chun King)				
hot teriyaki sauce	1 Tbs	–	17	–
soy sauce	1 Tbs	–	10	–
(Classico) pasta sauce				
d'Abruzzi/Italian sausage & fennel	½ cup	5.0	90	50%
di Capri/sun-dried tomatoes	½ cup	4.0	80	45%
di Firenze/spinach & cheese	½ cup	4.5	80	51%
di Florentine/spinach & cheese	½ cup	4.5	80	51%
di Genoa/tomato & pesto	½ cup	6.0	90	60%
di Milano/zucchini & Parmesan cheese	½ cup	2.5	70	32%
di Napoli/tomato & basil	½ cup	1.0	50	18%
di Parma/tomato & four cheeses	½ cup	4.0	70	51%
di Roma arrabbiata/spicy red pepper	½ cup	2.5	60	38%
di Salerno/tomato, sweet peppers & onion	½ cup	4.0	70	51%

Food and Description	Amount	Fat Grams	Total Calories	% Fat Calories
di Sicilia/w/pizza taste	½ cup	1.0	50	18%
di Sorrento/tomato, onion, & garlic	½ cup	4.0	80	45%
(Contadina)				
Italian cooking sauce				
cacciatore	½ cup	1.5	70	19%
garden vegetable	½ cup	1.5	70	19%
mushroom & garlic	½ cup	1.5	70	19%
three cheeses & herbs	½ cup	2.5	90	25%
pasta sauce				
Alfredo	½ cup	38.0	400	86%
garden vegetable	½ cup	–	40	–
marinara	½ cup	4.0	80	45%
pesto w/basil	¼ cup	30.0	310	87%
sweet & sour	2 Tbs	1.0	40	23%
(Crosse & Blackwell) mint	1 tsp	–	5	–
(Del Monte)				
chili sauce	1 Tbs	–	20	–
pasta sauce/d'Italia				
classic marinara	½ cup	1.5	50	27%
four cheese	½ cup	2.0	60	30%
spicy red pepper	½ cup	1.5	50	27%
tomato & basil	½ cup	1.5	50	27%
seafood cocktail sauce	¼ cup	–	100	–
sloppy joe sauce				
hickory flavor	¼ cup	–	60	–
original recipe	¼ cup	–	50	–
spaghetti sauce				
garden style	½ cup	1.0	60	15%
garlic & herb	½ cup	1.5	60	23%
Italian herb	½ cup	1.0	60	15%
tomato basil	½ cup	1.0	60	15%
traditional	½ cup	1.0	80	11%
w/garlic & onion	½ cup	1.0	70	13%
w/green peppers & mushrooms	½ cup	1.0	70	13%
w/meat	½ cup	1.5	70	19%
w/mushrooms	½ cup	1.5	80	17%
(Digiorno) pasta sauce				
Alfredo				
reduced fat	¼ cup	10.0	170	53%
regular	¼ cup	22.0	230	86%
chunky tomato w/basil/light	½ cup	–	70	–
four cheese	¼ cup	19.0	200	86%
marinara	½ cup	4.5	100	41%
olive oil & garlic w/grated cheeses	¼ cup	36.0	370	88%
pesto	¼ cup	31.0	320	87%
plum tomato & mushroom	½ cup	–	70	–
traditional meat	½ cup	6.0	120	45%

Food and Description	Amount	Fat Grams	Total Calories	% Fat Calories
(Durkee) Famous Sandwich & Salad Sauce	1 Tbs	6.0	60	90%
(Eden) organic				
pasta sauce	½ cup	2.5	80	28%
soy sauce/shoyu				
reduced sodium	½ tsp	–	2	–
regular	½ tsp	–	2	–
(Enrico's) organic pasta sauce				
bountiful basil	½ cup	–	50	–
garlic lovers	½ cup	–	50	–
hot & spicy arabiati	½ cup	1.8	60	27%
Italian style	½ cup	4.0	55	65%
mushroom				
regular	½ cup	1.0	60	15%
w/fresh mushrooms	½ cup	1.0	60	15%
no salt added	½ cup	1.0	60	15%
peppers w/mushrooms	½ cup	1.5	70	19%
tomato basil	½ cup	2.0	65	28%
traditional	½ cup	1.0	60	15%
(Escoffier)				
Diable	1 Tbs	–	20	–
Robert	1 Tbs	–	20	–
(Five Brothers) pasta sauce				
Alfredo				
regular	¼ cup	11.0	120	83%
w/mushrooms	¼ cup	7.0	80	79%
garden vegetable primavera	½ cup	3.0	70	39%
marinara w/Burgundy wine	½ cup	4.0	80	45%
sautéed mushroom	½ cup	4.0	90	40%
summer tomato basil	½ cup	2.0	60	30%
(Francesco Rinaldi) pasta sauce				
chunky garden				
mushroom & peppers	½ cup	2.0	80	23%
tomato & garlic	½ cup	2.0	80	23%
Neapolitan	½ cup	2.5	80	28%
spaghetti/plain	½ cup	4.0	90	40%
(French's) Worcestershire sauce				
original	1 Tbs	–	10	–
smoky	1 Tbs	–	10	–
generic				
cheese/canned	2 oz	4.0	60	60%
clam				
red	¼ cup	1.5	40	34%
white	¼ cup	4.8	60	72%
cream/white	½ cup	9.0	118	69%
soy sauce				
shoyu	1 Tbs	–	9	–
	¼ cup	–	30	–

Food and Description	Amount	Fat Grams	Total Calories	% Fat Calories
tamari	1 Tbs	–	11	–
	¼ cup	–	35	–
tartar sauce	1 Tbs	8.0	75	96%
(Girard's) Seafood Shop				
cocktail	2 Tbs	1.0	90	10%
tartar sauce	2 Tbs	15.0	140	96%
(Golden Dipt)				
cooking sauce				
creole	2 Tbs	1.0	25	36%
lemon butter dill				
fat-free	2 Tbs	–	35	–
regular	2 Tbs	10.0	120	75%
scampi/garlic-herb	2 Tbs	25.0	240	94%
seafood cocktail				
extra hot	¼ cup	–	100	–
original	¼ cup	–	110	–
tartar sauce	2 Tbs	15.0	160	84%
(Gold's) rib sauce	2 Tbs	–	60	–
(Great Impressions)				
horseradish	2 Tbs	14.0	140	90%
seafood				
creole	1 Tbs	–	20	–
dipping	1 Tbs	–	17	–
Polynesian	1 Tbs	<1.0	40	11%
(Green Giant) sloppy joe				
sauce only	¼ cup	–	50	–
w/meat	1 sandwich	11.0	200	50%
(Hain) pasta sauce				
marinara	½ cup	1.0	40	23%
mushroom	½ cup	1.0	40	23%
(Healthy Choice) pasta sauce				
flavored w/meat	½ cup	1.0	50	18%
garlic & herbs	½ cup	<1.0	50	9%
garlic & onion/extra chunky	½ cup	–	40	–
Italian vegetable/extra chunky	½ cup	–	40	–
mushroom				
extra chunky	½ cup	–	40	–
original	½ cup	<1.0	50	9%
mushroom & sweet peppers/ super chunky	½ cup	–	45	–
super tomato, mushroom, & garlic	½ cup	–	45	–
traditional	½ cup	<1.0	50	9%
vegetable primavera/super chunky	½ cup	–	45	–
(Heinz)				
chili sauce	1 Tbs	–	15	–
Heinz 57 steak sauce				
hickory smoke	1 Tbs	–	10	–
regular	1 Tbs	–	10	–

Food and Description	Amount	Fat Grams	Total Calories	% Fat Calories
horseradish	1 Tbs	7.0	75	84%
seafood	¼ cup	–	60	–
Worcestershire	1 tsp	–	–	–
(Hormel)				
Not-So-Sloppy Joe Sauce	¼ cup	–	70	–
(House Of Tsang)				
Oriental cooking sauce				
Bangkok padang	1 Tbs	2.5	45	50%
classic stir fry	1 Tbs	1.0	25	–
hoisin	1 tsp	–	15	–
Hong Kong BBQ	1 tsp	–	10	–
Korean teriyaki	1 Tbs	0.5	30	15%
Mandarin marinade	1 Tbs	–	18	–
Saigon sizzle	1 Tbs	1.0	40	23%
spicy brown bean	1 tsp	–	15	–
sweet & sour concentrate	1 tsp	–	10	–
sweet & sour stir fry	1 Tbs	–	35	–
Szechuan spicy stir fry	1 Tbs	0.5	20	23%
soy sauce				
dark	1 Tbs	–	17	–
ginger-flavored	1 Tbs	–	20	–
light	1 Tbs	–	5	–
low-sodium				
ginger-flavored	1 Tbs	–	10	–
mushroom-flavored	1 Tbs	–	10	–
regular	1 Tbs	–	5	–
(Hunt's)				
Chicken Sensations cooking sauce				
BBQ flavor	1 Tbs	2.7	35	69%
Italian garlic	1 Tbs	2.7	30	81%
lemon herb	1 Tbs	2.7	30	81%
Southwestern	1 Tbs	2.5	30	75%
Manwich				
barbecue	¼ cup	<1.0	60	3%
bold	¼ cup	1.0	65	14%
original	¼ cup	0.5	35	13%
spaghetti sauce				
classic Italian				
garlic & onion	½ cup	2.0	50	36%
Parmesan	½ cup	2.0	50	36%
tomato & basil	½ cup	2.0	50	36%
chunky				
Italian style vegetables	½ cup	1.0	65	14%
marinara	½ cup	1.5	60	23%
tomato, garlic, & onion	½ cup	1.0	60	15%
homestyle				
flavored w/meat	½ cup	2.5	60	38%

Food and Description	Amount	Fat Grams	Total Calories	% Fat Calories
mushroom	½ cup	2.5	60	38%
traditional	½ cup	2.5	60	38%
Italian sausage	½ cup	2.7	80	30%
Italian style cheese & garlic	½ cup	2.5	65	35%
old country				
flavored w/meat	½ cup	2.6	60	39%
garlic & herbs	½ cup	2.7	65	37%
Italian style vegetables	½ cup	2.5	65	35%
mushroom	½ cup	2.7	55	44%
traditional	½ cup	2.7	55	44%
original				
flavored w/meat	½ cup	2.5	65	35%
mushroom	½ cup	2.5	65	35%
tradtional	½ cup	2.5	65	35%
steak sauce	1 Tbs	–	10	–
(Jake's) World Famous				
cocktail	¼ cup	0.5	45	10%
tartar sauce	2 Tbs	15.0	140	96%
(Just Rite) hot dog	¼ cup	3.0	50	54%
(Kaukauna) nacho cheese	1 oz	6.0	80	68%
(Kikkoman)				
soy sauce				
lite	1 Tbs	–	12	–
milder	1 Tbs	–	12	–
regular	1 Tbs	–	18	–
stir-fry	1 Tbs	–	18	–
sweet & sour	1 Tbs	–	16	–
teriyaki				
baste & glaze	1 Tbs	–	27	–
regular	1 Tbs	–	18	–
(Knorr) grilling & broiling sauce				
spicy plum	⅛ bottle	–	60	–
(Kraft)				
Kraft				
horseradish				
cream style	1 tsp	–		–
mustard	1 tsp	–		–
prepared	1 tsp	–		–
sandwich spread & burger sauce				
reduced fat	1 Tbs	2.5	35	64%
regular	1 Tbs	5.0	50	90%
sweet 'n sour	2 Tbs	0.5	80	6%
tartar sauce/nonfat	2 Tbs	–	25	–
Sauceworks				
cocktail	¼ cup	0.5	60	9%
horseradish	1 tsp	1.5	20	68%
sweet 'n sour	2 Tbs	–	60	–

Food and Description	Amount	Fat Grams	Total Calories	% Fat Calories
tartar sauce				
natural lemon & herb flavor	2 Tbs	16.0	150	96%
regular	2 Tbs	10.0	100	90%
(La Choy)				
bead molasses	1 Tbs	–	50	–
brown gravy	¼ cup	–	275	–
plum	1 Tbs	–	25	–
soy sauce/lite	1 Tbs	–	15	–
stir-fry				
Mandarin soy sauce	½ cup	–	70	–
sweet & sour	½ cup	–	140	–
Szechwan	½ cup	–	80	–
teriyaki	½ cup	–	95	–
sweet & sour				
duck sauce	2 Tbs	–	60	–
original	2 Tbs	–	60	–
teriyaki				
lite	1 Tbs	–	18	–
original	1 Tbs	–	16	–
(Lea & Perrins)				
steak				
garlic peppercorn	1 Tbs	–	25	–
private label	1 Tbs	–	15	–
sweet & spicy	1 Tbs	–	25	–
Worcestershire				
original	1 tsp	–	5	–
white wine	1 tsp	–	–	–
(Libby's) sloppy joe	⅓ cup	–	45	–
(Litehouse)				
barbecue	2 Tbs	–	35	–
salsa	2 Tbs	–	10	–
seafood cocktail	2 Tbs	–	25	–
stir-fry	2 Tbs	–	45	–
tartar sauce	2 Tbs	14.0	130	97%
(Maull's) steak				
mild	1 Tbs	–	20	–
original	1 Tbs	–	20	–
(Merkt's) cheese				
cheddar	2 Tbs	7.0	90	70%
mild nacho	2 Tbs	7.0	90	70%
(Millina's Finest) fat-free organic pasta sauce				
garlic garlic	½ cup	–	40	–
hot n spicy	½ cup	–	48	–
sweet pepper & onion	½ cup	–	41	–
tomato & basil	½ cup	–	45	–
zesty basil	½ cup	–	45	–
(Monterey Pasta Co.) sun-dried tomato pesto	¼ cup	26.0	260	90%

Food and Description	Amount	Fat Grams	Total Calories	% Fat Calories
(Muir Glen) organic low-fat pasta sauce				
chunky style	½ cup	2.0	80	23%
mushroom & green pepper	½ cup	2.5	90	25%
Romano cheese	½ cup	2.5	90	25%
(Newman's Own) pasta sauce				
mushroom	½ cup	2.0	60	30%
plain	½ cup	2.0	60	30%
Socarooni	½ cup	2.0	60	30%
(Old Bay)				
cocktail	¼ cup	0.5	110	4%
tartar sauce	2 Tbs	12.0	130	83%
(Prego) pasta sauce				
fresh mushroom	½ cup	5.0	150	30%
mushroom & dried onion/extra chunky	½ cup	6.0	120	45%
mushroom & extra spice/extra chunky	½ cup	4.0	120	30%
mushroom & green pepper/extra chunky	½ cup	4.0	100	36%
mushroom supreme/extra chunky	½ cup	4.5	130	31%
traditional				
flavored w/meat	½ cup	6.0	160	34%
regular	½ cup	6.0	150	36%
vegetable supreme/extra chunky	½ cup	3.0	90	30%
(Prince) pasta sauce				
marinara/traditonal	½ cup	0.5	50	9%
meatless				
chunky				
meat-flavored	½ cup	3.0	90	30%
mushroom	½ cup	1.5	70	19%
regular	½ cup	1.5	70	19%
traditional	½ cup	0.5	50	9%
(Pritikin) spaghetti sauce				
chunky garden style	½ cup	0.5	50	9%
marinara	½ cup	–	60	–
original	½ cup	0.5	60	8%
(Progresso)				
pasta sauce				
Alfredo/authentic	½ cup	27.0	310	78%
creamy clam	½ cup	6.0	100	54%
marinara	½ cup	4.5	90	45%
marinara/authentic	½ cup	5.0	100	45%
meat flavored	½ cup	4.5	100	45%
red clam	½ cup	3.0	80	34%
rock lobster	½ cup	7.0	100	63%
white clam	½ cup	9.0	120	68%
white clam/authentic	½ cup	7.0	90	70%
pizza sauce	¼ cup	1.0	35	26%
spaghetti sauce				
mushroom	½ cup	4.5	100	45%
original	½ cup	4.5	100	45%

Food and Description	Amount	Fat Grams	Total Calories	% Fat Calories
(Ragu)				
Chicken Tonight simmer sauce				
chicken cacciatore	½ cup	1.5	80	17%
country French chicken	½ cup	11.0	130	76%
creamy chicken primavera				
plain	½ cup	6.0	90	60%
w/mushrooms	½ cup	9.0	110	74%
herbed chicken w/wine	½ cup	6.0	80	68%
sweet & sour chicken	½ cup	–	120	–
pasta sauce				
gardenstyle				
garden combination/chunky	½ cup	4.0	120	30%
green & red pepper/chunky	½ cup	4.0	120	30%
mushroom/super	½ cup	4.0	120	30%
mushroom & green pepper/chunky	½ cup	4.0	120	30%
mushroom & onion/chunky	½ cup	4.0	120	30%
tomato, garlic & onion/chunky	½ cup	4.0	120	30%
vegetable primavera/super	½ cup	4.0	110	33%
hearty				
flavored w/sautéed beef	½ cup	4.5	130	31%
Italian tomato	½ cup	3.0	120	23%
Parmesan	½ cup	4.0	120	30%
sautéed onion & garlic	½ cup	5.0	130	35%
sautéed onion & mushroom	½ cup	4.0	110	33%
light				
chunky mushroom	½ cup	–	50	–
garden harvest	½ cup	–	50	–
no sugar added	½ cup	1.5	60	23%
tomato & herb	½ cup	–	50	–
Pizza Toss/herbs & olive oil w/tomatoes & garlic	½ cup	8.0	70	100%
spaghetti sauce/Old World style				
flavored w/meat	½ cup	5.0	90	50%
marinara	½ cup	5.0	90	50%
mushroom	½ cup	3.5	80	39%
traditional	½ cup	3.5	80	39%
(Rese) mint/w/leaves	1 Tbs	–	50	–
(S&W) cooking sauce				
herb & garlic Italian tomato	1 Tbs	1.0	15	60%
mesquite	1 Tbs	–	10	–
Oriental stir-fry	1 Tbs	–	20	–
seafood cocktail	1 Tbs	–	20	–
Southwestern fajitas	1 Tbs	–	10	–
steakhouse chili	1 Tbs	–	15	–
teriyaki				
lite	1 Tbs	–	25	–
regular	1 Tbs	–	25	–
Sauceworks (See (Kraft) in this section)				

Food and Description	Amount	Fat Grams	Total Calories	% Fat Calories
(Sinatra's) Gourmet Italian Pasta Sauce				
Alfredo	¼ cup	14.0	160	79%
marinara				
Milano style	½ cup	3.0	60	45%
tomato basil	½ cup	3.0	70	39%
w/mushrooms	½ cup	3.0	50	54%
Marsala	¼ cup	9.0	100	81%
pesto	¼ cup	14.0	160	79%
scampi	¼ cup	9.0	100	81%
(Snow's)				
Welsh rarebit cheese	½ cup	11.0	170	58%
Newburg w/sherry	⅓ cup	8.0	120	60%
(Tabasco) chili recipe/7 spice	½ cup	0.5	50	9%
(Texas Best)				
hot	1 tsp	–	–	–
steak	1 Tbs	–	15	–
(Trio's) pasta sauce				
Alfredo/light	½ cup	8.0	160	45%
pesto	¼ cup	33.0	310	96%
thick & chunky tomato	½ cup	–	60	–
(Uncle Ben's) marinade & sauce				
Cantonese orange ginger	1 Tbs	–	25	–
Chinese black bean	1 Tbs	0.5	15	30%
French four peppercorn	1 Tbs	0.5	15	30%
Jamaican island	1 Tbs	1.0	15	60%
Japanese roasted garlic	1 Tbs	–	10	–
Thai peanut satay	1 Tbs	1.0	25	36%
(Westbrae) pasta sauce				
marinara	½ cup	<1.0	40	11%
primavera				
no salt	½ cup	–	40	–
regular	½ cup	3.0	60	45%
(Wing Tip) chicken wing/Buffalo style	1 Tbs	0.5	5	90%
SAUERKRAUT/canned or jarred				
(Bush's Best)				
Bavarian kraut	½ cup	–	60	–
deli style kraut	½ cup	–	20	–
shredded kraut	½ cup	–	20	–
(Claussen)	¼ cup	–	5	–
(Del Monte)	2 Tbs	–	–	–
(Eden)	½ cup	–	25	–
(Hebrew National)				
gallon kraut	½ cup	–	25	–
regular	2 Tbs	–	50	–
(Libby's)				
Bavarian w/caraway seeds	2 Tbs	–	15	–
crispy	2 Tbs	–	5	–

Food and Description	Amount	Fat Grams	Total Calories	% Fat Calories
(Rosoff's)	½ cup	1.0	50	18%
(S&W)	2 Tbs	–	5	–
	½ cup	–	25	–
(Schorr's) new kraut	½ cup	1.0	50	18%
(Seneca)				
Bavarian	1 oz	–	10	–
original	1 oz	–	5	–
(Stokely)				
Bavarian	½ cup	–	30	–
shredded & chopped	½ cup	–	20	–
(Vlasic) old fashioned	1 oz	–	4	–
SAUERKRAUT JUICE/canned				
(S&W)	10 fl oz	–	35	–

SAUSAGE (See also FRANKFURTER; LUNCHEON MEAT; SAUSAGE DISH; SAUSAGE STICK)

Food and Description	Amount	Fat Grams	Total Calories	% Fat Calories
▣ **(Aidells)**				
smoked chicken & apple	1 link	16.0	210	69%
▣ **(Armour/Armour Star)**				
Vienna sausage				
in BBQ sauce	3 sausages	14.0	160	81%
in beef stock	3 sausages	16.0	170	77%
in hot sauce	3 sausages	15.0	170	81%
smoked	3 sausages	16.0	170	85%
25% less fat	3 sausages	11.0	130	78%
▣ **(Ball Park)**				
bratwurst	1 bratwurst	17.0	190	80%
knockwurst	¼ pound	32.0	340	85%
▣ **(Bilinski's)**				
chicken & spinach w/garlic & fennel	1 link	3.0	100	27%
▣ **(Bob Evans)**				
country lite	3 links	8.0	120	60%
original	3 links	16.0	190	76%
▣ **(Bridgford)**				
pepperoni	1 oz	12.0	130	83%
pepperoni stick	1.5 oz	14.0	170	74%
salami/hard	1 oz	12.0	130	83%
summer	2 oz	17.0	190	80%
▣ **(Butterball)**				
turkey sausage				
bratwurst	1 link	10.0	170	53%
breakfast				
links	2 links	5.0	90	50%
original	3 links	9.0	120	68%
Italian				
hot	1 link	10.0	170	53%
sweet	1 link	10.0	170	53%
Polish	1 link	10.0	170	53%
salami	1 oz	4.0	60	60%

Food and Description	Amount	Fat Grams	Total Calories	% Fat Calories
■ **(Eckrich)**				
Little Smokies & Sauce				
hickory & brown sugar				
plain	6 links	15.0	170	79%
w/1½ Tbs sauce	6 links	15.0	220	61%
hot & spicy				
plain	6 links	15.0	170	79%
w/1½ Tbs sauce	6 links	15.0	225	60%
Polska kielbasa/Lean Supreme	2 oz	5.0	100	45%
smoked/Lean Supreme				
regular	2 oz	5.0	100	45%
3 pepper	2 oz	5.0	100	45%
■ **(Galileo)**				
pepperoni/pizza-size	9 slices	13.0	140	84%
salami/Italian dry				
light	5 slices	4.0	60	60%
thin sliced	5 slices	8.0	110	65%
whole	1 oz	10.0	120	75%
summer/smoked	2 oz	16.0	190	76%
■ **GENERIC**				
beerwurst/beer salami				
beef	1 oz	6.8	75	81%
pork	1 oz	4.0	55	66%
Berliner/beef & pork	1 oz	4.9	65	68%
blood	1 oz	9.8	107	82%
bratwurst/pork, cooked	1 oz	7.0	85	74%
	3-oz link	22.0	256	77%
chorizo	~2-oz link	23.0	273	76%
honey roll/beef	1 oz	3.0	52	52%
Italian/pork/cooked	3 oz	21.0	268	71%
kielbasa				
pork or beef	1 oz	7.7	88	79%
skinless	1 oz	16.0	180	80%
knockwurst/pork & beef	3 oz	16.0	210	69%
mortadella/beef & pork	1 oz	7.0	88	72%
pepperoni/pork & beef	1 oz	12.0	135	80%
	~9 oz	110.0	1248	79%
Polish/pork	1 oz	8.0	92	78%
10" long/1.5" dia	1 sausage	6.5	74	79%
pork				
brown & serve/link/~1 oz	1 link	5.0	50	90%
country style/cooked				
links/0.5 oz each	1 link	8.0	96	75%
patties/1 oz each	1 patty	8.0	100	72%
fresh/cooked				
link	1 oz	11.0	118	84%
patty	1 oz	8.0	100	72%

Food and Description	Amount	Fat Grams	Total Calories	% Fat Calories
raw				
links/1 oz each	1 link	11.0	118	84%
patties/2 oz each	1 patty	23.0	238	87%
smoked links				
4" long/1⅛" dia	1 link	22.6	265	73%
2" long/¾" dia	1 link	5.0	62	73%
pork & beef				
fresh, cooked				
links/2" long/¾" dia	1 link	5.0	55	82%
patties/~1 oz each	1 patty	10.0	110	82%
luncheon/pork & beef	~1 oz	4.8	60	72%
salami				
cooked				
beef	1 oz	5.9	74	72%
beef & pork	1 oz	5.7	71	72%
turkey	2 oz	7.8	111	63%
dry or hard/pork	1 oz	7.0	85	74%
salt pork/raw	1 oz	22.8	212	97%
summer				
beef	~1 oz	7.6	86	80%
cervelat	1 oz	8.5	98	78%
Thuringer	1 oz	8.5	98	78%
turkey	1 oz	3.5	52	61%
Vienna/canned				
beef	1 sausage	4.0	45	80%
chicken	7 sausages	28.0	315	80%
pork	1 sausage	4.0	45	80%
■ (Healthy Choice)				
low-fat sausage				
links	2 links	1.5	50	27%
patties	2 patties	1.5	50	27%
Polska kielbasa	1 link	3.0	100	27%
■ (Hebrew National)				
kishka	2 oz	11.0	160	62%
knocks/beef	3 oz	25.0	260	87%
Polish/beef	1 link	22.0	240	83%
salami/beef				
lite/reduced fat	2 oz	8.0	110	57%
midget/bullet stubbie	2 oz	14.0	170	74%
regular	2 oz	14.0	170	74%
■ (Hickory Farms)				
salami				
dry or hard	1 oz	10.0	120	75%
Genoa	1 oz	10.0	110	82%
■ (Hillshire Farm)				
beef & cheddar/Flavorseal	2 oz	15.0	190	71%

Food and Description	Amount	Fat Grams	Total Calories	% Fat Calories
bratwurst				
beer	2 oz	17.0	190	81%
fresh	2 oz	17.0	190	81%
fully cooked	2 oz	16.0	170	85%
light	2 oz	11.0	150	66%
plain	2 oz	17.0	190	81%
smoked	2 oz	17.0	190	81%
spicy	2 oz	17.0	180	85%
cheddarwurst				
bun size	2 oz	18.0	200	81%
lite	2.7 oz	15.0	190	71%
original	2 oz	17.0	190	81%
country recipe/Flavorseal	2 oz	16.0	180	80%
hot				
cheddar hots/80% fat free	2 oz	12.0	150	72%
Hot Links				
beef	2 oz	17.0	190	81%
lite	2 oz	15.0	190	71%
Italian				
hot				
light	2 oz	11.0	150	66%
regular	2 oz	17.0	180	85%
mild				
light	2 oz	11.0	150	66%
regular	2 oz	17.0	190	81%
Italian dry	~1 oz	7.0	90	70%
knockwurst	2 oz	16.0	180	80%
Mexican-style				
lower fat	2 oz	11.0	150	66%
original	2 oz	17.0	190	81%
pepperoni	~1 oz	10.0	110	82%
Polska kielbasa				
bun size	2 oz	16.0	180	80%
80% fat free	2 oz	10.0	130	69%
Flavorseal				
beef	2 oz	17.0	190	81%
lite	2 oz	11.0	130	73%
mild	2 oz	17.0	190	81%
regular	2 oz	17.0	190	81%
turkey	2 oz	5.0	90	50%
lite	2.7 oz	15.0	190	71%
Lit'l Polskas	2 oz	16.0	180	80%
lower fat	2 oz	11.0	150	66%
original	2 oz	17.0	190	81%
salami/hard	~1 oz	9.0	100	90%
smoked				
bun size				
beef	2 oz	16.0	180	80%

Food and Description	Amount	Fat Grams	Total Calories	% Fat Calories
regular	2 oz	16.0	180	80%
80% fat free	2 oz	10.0	130	69%
Flavorseal				
beef	2 oz	16.0	180	80%
hot	2 oz	16.0	180	80%
Italian	2 oz	18.0	200	81%
lite	2 oz	11.0	130	73%
regular	2 oz	17.0	190	81%
turkey	2 oz	15.0	190	71%
Lit'l Smokies				
beef	2 oz	16.0	180	80%
cheddar	2 oz	16.0	180	80%
light	2 oz	8.0	120	60%
original	2 oz	16.0	180	80%
original	2 oz	18.0	190	85%
summer				
beef	2 oz	17.0	190	81%
light	2 oz	12.0	150	72%
original	2 oz	16.0	180	80%
w/cheese	2 oz	18.0	200	81%
yard-o-beef	2 oz	17.0	190	81%
■ (Hormel)				
breakfast/Little Sizzlers/cooked				
brown 'n serve				
links	3 links	22.0	230	86%
patties	2 patties	18.0	190	85%
links	3 links	20.0	210	86%
patties	2 patties	23.0	250	83%
pork/hot & spicy	3 links	20.0	210	86%
pepperoni				
Leoni	1 oz	13.0	140	84%
pillow pack	1 oz	13.0	140	84%
Rosa Grande	1 oz	13.0	140	84%
chunk/6-oz pkg	1 oz	13.0	140	84%
sliced/3.5-oz pkg	15 slices	13.0	140	84%
twin/5-oz pkg	1 oz	13.0	140	84%
pickled				
hot	6 links	11.0	140	71%
smoked	6 links	11.0	140	71%
prosciutto				
primissimo	1 oz	4.5	70	58%
Spiral Cure 81	3 oz	9.0	150	54%
salami				
Genoa				
Di Lusso	1 oz	9.0	120	68%
San Remo	1 oz	9.0	120	68%
sandwich maker	1 oz	11.0	120	83%

Food and Description	Amount	Fat Grams	Total Calories	% Fat Calories
hard				
homeland	1 oz	10.0	110	82%
pillow pack	4 slices	10.0	120	75%
sandwich maker	1 oz	10.0	110	82%
smoked/Light & Lean 97				
smoked dinner links	2 oz	2.0	60	30%
summer/Old Smokehouse				
1.5-lb pkg	1 oz	10.0	110	82%
2.15-lb pkg	1 oz	10.0	110	82%
3-lb pkg	1 oz	10.0	110	82%
Vienna				
chicken	2 oz	10.0	110	82%
original	2 oz	13.0	140	84%
■ (Jimmy Dean)				
links/heat & serve				
beef	3 links	18.0	200	81%
lite/turkey & pork				
hot	2.5 oz	14.0	180	70%
regular	2.5 oz	14.0	180	70%
sage	2.5 oz	14.0	180	70%
patties	2 patties	28.0	290	87%
pork				
country mild	2 oz	24.0	250	86%
extra mild	2 oz	24.0	250	86%
hot	3 links	19.0	200	86%
	2 oz	24.0	250	86%
Italian	2 oz	24.0	250	86%
maple-flavored	3 links	19.0	200	86%
regular	2 oz	24.0	250	86%
	3 links	19.0	200	86%
	2 oz	24.0	250	86%
sage	2 oz	24.0	250	86%
■ (Johnsonville)				
(Note: All portions are cooked unless stated otherwise.)				
Beer City Grillers	1 link	27.0	310	
Better w/cheddar				
light	1 link	9.0	140	58%
regular	1 link	22.0	240	83%
bratwurst				
beef				
raw	1 link	27.0	330	74%
smoked	1 link	22.0	240	83%
beer 'n bratwurst				
cheesy	1 link	27.0	310	78%
regular	1 link	27.0	300	81%
burger	1 patty	20.0	230	78%
bun bratz				
3-oz patties	1 patty	20.0	230	78%

Food and Description	Amount	Fat Grams	Total Calories	% Fat Calories
4-oz patties	1 patty	27.0	310	78%
German	1 link	27.0	300	81%
original	1 link	27.0	300	81%
smoked				
light	1 link	9.0	140	58%
regular	1 link	22.0	240	83%
breakfast				
country/apple 'n cinnamon	3 links	18.0	200	81%
hot 'n zesty	3 links	18.0	200	81%
original				
link	3 links	18.0	200	81%
patty	2 patties	18.0	210	77%
sage 'n pepper	3 links	18.0	200	81%
skillet cheddars	3 links	17.0	200	77%
smoky bacon flavored	3 links	18.0	200	81%
Vermont maple syrup				
link	3 links	18.0	200	81%
patty	2 patties	18.0	210	77%
chorizo	1 link	20.0	220	82%
hot links				
light	1 link	9.0	140	58%
regular	1 link	22.0	220	82%
Irish O'Garlic	1 link	27.0	300	81%
Italian				
bun Italian				
4-oz patties	1 patty	27.0	310	78%
3-oz patties	1 patty	20.0	230	78%
hot	1 link	27.0	300	81%
Italia	1 link	20.0	220	82%
Italian sausage burger	1 patty	20.0	230	78%
Italianti	1 link	27.0	300	81%
mild	1 link	27.0	300	81%
Now That's Italian	1 link	27.0	310	78%
Old World				
hot	1 link	27.0	300	81%
mild	1 link	27.0	300	81%
sweet	1 link	27.0	300	81%
kielbasa	2 oz	18.0	200	81%
knackwurst	1 link	22.0	240	83%
Polish				
light	1 link	9.0	140	58%
regular	1 link	27.0	300	81%
summer				
beef recipe				
regular	2 oz	15.0	180	75%
sliced	13 slices	15.0	180	75%
garlic recipe				
regular	2 oz	15.0	180	75%

Food and Description	Amount	Fat Grams	Total Calories	% Fat Calories
sliced	13 slices	15.0	180	75%
Old World recipe	2 oz	16.0	190	76%
original recipe				
regular	2 oz	15.0	180	75%
sliced	13 slices	15.0	180	75%
Swisswurst	1 link	22.0	240	83%
Texas Hot Stuff	1 link	27.0	300	81%
■ (Jones Dairy Farm)				
all natural				
brown & serve light	1 link	4.0	60	60%
golden brown	1 patty	15.0	155	87%
beef	1 link	6.0	75	72%
mild	2 links	18.0	190	85%
pork/light	1 link	4.0	55	65%
spicy	2 links	18.0	190	85%
little	3 links	17.0	190	81%
pork				
light	1 link	5.0	70	64%
regular	1 link	14.0	140	90%
■ (Kahn's)				
bratwurst	1 sausage	17.0	190	81%
kielbasa/bun size Polska	1 sausage	17.0	190	81%
salami				
beef				
8-oz pkg	1 slice	6.0	70	77%
family pack	1 slice	5.0	60	75%
cooked/8-oz pkg	1 slice	4.0	60	60%
cotto/family pack	1 slice	3.0	45	60%
■ (Libby's)				
Vienna				
chicken	3 links	8.0	100	72%
meat/regular or w/BBQ sauce	3 links	12.0	130	83%
■ (Louis Rich)				
turkey sausage				
Polska kielbasa	2 oz	4.5	80	51%
smoked				
hot	2.5 oz	8.0	120	60%
original	2 oz	5.0	80	56%
	2.5 oz	8.0	120	60%
w/cheese	2 oz	5.0	90	50%
salami				
cooked/chunk specialty	2 oz	9.0	120	68%
cooked/sliced	1 slice	2.5	40	56%
cotto/sliced	1 slice	2.5	40	56%
■ (Mr. Turkey)				
turkey salami				
regular	2 oz	7.0	100	63%

Food and Description	Amount	Fat Grams	Total Calories	% Fat Calories
variety pack	1 slice	3.0	50	54%
■ (Oscar Mayer)				
New England	2 slices	2.5	60	38%
pepperoni	15 slices	13.0	140	84%
pork links/cooked	2 links	16.0	180	80%
salami				
cotto				
beef	2 slices	7.0	90	70%
pork, chicken, & beef	2 slices	9.0	110	74%
for beer	3 slices	9.0	110	74%
Genoa	3 slices	9.0	100	81%
hard				
Deli-Thin	4 slices	11.0	130	76%
regular	3 slices	9.0	100	81%
Machiaeh/beef	2 slices	10.0	120	75%
smoked				
beef smokies	1 link	11.0	120	83%
cheese smokies	1 link	12.0	130	83%
links sausage	1 link	12.0	130	83%
little cheese	6 links	16.0	180	80%
little links sausage	6 links	16.0	170	85%
summer/Thuringer cervelat				
beef	2 slices	12.0	140	77%
other	2 slices	13.0	140	84%
■ (Perdue)				
turkey sausage				
breakfast				
links	1 link	4.0	40	90%
patties	1 patty	3.0	61	44%
Italian/2-oz link	1 link	6.0	94	57%
■ (Reser's)				
hunter's	2 oz	10.0	140	64%
salami/cooked	2 oz	11.0	140	71%
summer/reduced fat	2 oz	11.0	140	71%
Thuringer/smoked/reduced fat	2 oz	12.0	150	72%
■ (Schwan's)				
bratwurst	1 link	23.0	270	77%
Polish	1 link	24.0	270	80%
pork				
links	3 links	32.0	340	85%
patties	1 patty	22.0	230	86%
summer	2 oz	13.0	160	73%
■ (Swift)				
Premium Brown 'N Serve/frozen				
country recipe				
links				
lite	2 links	11.0	120	83%

Food and Description	Amount	Fat Grams	Total Calories	% Fat Calories
regular	1 link	12.0	130	83%
patties	1 patty	12.0	130	83%
hot	3 links	15.0	180	75%
maple-flavored				
lite	1 link	5.0	60	75%
regular	1 link	12.0	120	90%
microwave links				
lite	1 link	6.0	90	60%
regular	1 link	12.0	120	90%
original				
links				
lite	3 links	8.0	120	60%
regular	3 links	12.0	140	77%
patties	1 patty	12.0	120	90%
smoke-flavored	1 link	11.0	120	83%
w/bacon	1 link	11.0	120	83%
w/ham	1 link	13.0	130	90%
■ (The Turkey Store)				
turkey sausage				
bratwurst	3 oz	10.0	160	56%
breakfast links				
apple cinnamon	2 oz	11.0	140	71%
hot	2 oz	11.0	140	71%
maple syrup	2 oz	11.0	140	71%
mild	2 oz	11.0	140	71%
w/smoked bacon	1 oz	11.0	130	76%
breakfast patties				
apple cinnamon	1.3 oz	12.0	160	68%
hot	2.3 oz	12.0	150	72%
maple syrup	2.3 oz	12.0	160	68%
mild	2.3 oz	12.0	150	72%
w/smoked bacon	2.3 oz	12.0	150	72%
Italian				
hot	3 oz	9.0	140	58%
sweet	3 oz	9.0	140	58%
sweet w/cheese	3 oz	9.0	140	58%
Mexican w/jalapeño cheese	3 oz	9.0	140	58%
Polish	3 oz	9.0	140	58%
smoked	3 oz	9.0	140	58%

SAUSAGE DISH (See also BREAKFAST SANDWICH; FROZEN DINNER/ENTRÉE; SAUSAGE)

(Mary Kitchen) sausage hash	1 cup	27.0	410	59%

SAUSAGE STICK (See also BEEF JERKY, STICKS, & STRIPS)

(Bridgford)				
pepperoni	1 oz	12.0	140	77%
pepperoni & cheese	1.5 oz	14.0	170	74%
(Eagle) beef pepperoni	1.25 oz	11.0	150	66%

Food and Description	Amount	Fat Grams	Total Calories	% Fat Calories
(Slim Jim)				
nacho/Super Slim	0.31 oz	3.0	40	68%
smoked				
Big Slim	0.52 oz	7.0	80	79%
Giant Slim	1.1 oz	16.0	180	80%
Jumbo Slim	1 oz	12.0	150	72%
Super Slim	0.7 oz	10.0	110	82%
spicy	0.31 oz	4.0	50	72%
tabasco	0.31 oz	4.0	50	72%
SAUSAGE SUBSTITUTE (See VEGETARIAN FOODS)				
SAVORY/ground	1 tsp	–	4	–
SCALLION/GREEN ONION/SPRING ONION (See also ONION)				
fresh				
chopped	½ cup	–	15	–
(Dole)	1 Tbs	–	2	–
w/tops	5 large	–	10	–
SCALLOP (See also SCALLOP, IMITATION; SEAFOOD ENTRÉE/DINNER)				
fresh				
breaded & fried/~½ oz each	2 scallops	3.0	67	40%
raw	3 oz	0.6	75	7%
frozen				
(Contessa)	4 oz	–	90	–
(Crystal Isle)	3 oz	1.0	150	6%
(Louis Kemp) scallop delights/bay style	½ cup	–	80	–
(Mrs. Paul's) real bay scallops	12 pieces	8.0	200	36%
SCALLOP, IMITATION	3 oz	<1.0	85	5%
SCONE (See also ROLL)				
(Health Valley) Healthy Scones/fat-free				
apple kiwi	1 scone	–	180	–
cinnamon raisin	1 scone	–	180	–
cranberry orange	1 scone	–	180	–
mountain blueberry	1 scone	–	180	–
pineapple banana	1 scone	–	180	–
homemade/USDA Standard Home Recipe				
apricot	1 scone	7.0	230	27%
cheese	1 scone	9.0	185	44%
plain	1 scone	7.0	180	35%
(Krusteaz) scone & shortcake mix				
mix only	¼ cup	1.5	80	17%
prepared	1 scone	2.0	180	10%
SCOTCH (See LIQUOR, DISTILLED)				
SCOTCH BROTH (See SOUP)				
SCRAPPLE				
generic	1 oz	4.0	61	59%
(Jones Dairy Farm) country style	2 oz	8.0	120	60%
SCROD (See SEAFOOD ENTRÉE/DINNER)				
SCUP/raw	3 oz	2.0	90	20%

Food and Description	Amount	Fat Grams	Total Calories	% Fat Calories
SEA BASS (*See also* SEAFOOD ENTRÉE/DINNER)				
fresh				
breaded & fried	3 oz	7.0	176	36%
cooked-dry heat	3 oz	2.0	105	17%
raw	3 oz	1.7	82	19%
frozen				
(Mirabel) Chilean/boneless-skinless	4 oz	21.0	250	76%
SEA SALT	1 tsp	–	–	–
SEA TROUT/raw	3 oz	3.0	88	31%
SEA VEGETABLE (*See* SEAWEED)				
SEAFOOD CHOWDER (*See* SOUP)				
SEAFOOD ENTRÉE/DINNER (*See also* FROZEN ENTRÉE/DINNER; PASTA ENTRÉE/DINNER; individual listings)				
■ **CANNED**				
generic/crab cakes	4.5 oz	13.0	252	46%
(Gorton's)				
cod cakes	4 oz	0.5	100	5%
crunchy fried clams	3 oz	17.0	260	59%
■ **FROZEN**				
(Arctic Ice) herb & garlic	2 pieces	16.0	280	51%
(Contessa)				
shrimp				
cooked				
shell on	3 oz	–	60	–
shelled	3 oz	–	40	–
uncooked	4 oz	–	80	–
shrimp & linguini	2 cups	3.0	300	9%
shrimp stir-fry	2¼ cup	–	150	–
(Fisher Boy)				
jumbo butterfly shrimp	3 oz	9.0	200	41%
quik stix				
original	6 sticks	8.0	170	42%
taco & salsa	8 sticks	13.0	210	56%
(Fishery Products International)				
shrimp scampi	3 oz	19.0	220	78%
(Frionor U.S.A.)				
Alaska pollack				
Batter Dipt Puf!	3 oz	7.0	160	39%
Easy Grill/lemon pepper Puf!	4.2 oz	1.5	80	17%
English cut/raw/unbreaded	4 oz	1.0	90	10%
fillettes/seasoned/crunchy	3 oz	1.0	120	8%
	4 oz	1.0	160	6%
fish sticks/precooked/breaded	4 oz	10.0	210	43%
FishFries Puf!				
country style	3.7 oz	1.0	120	8%
lite 'n crunchy	3.75 oz	3.0	160	17%
potato crunch	3.9 oz	17.0	250	57%

Food and Description	Amount	Fat Grams	Total Calories	% Fat Calories
Santa Fe style	3.75 oz	1.0	160	6%
Southern cornmeal	3.75 oz	4.0	160	23%
Nuggets Puf!				
lite 'n crunchy	4 oz	4.0	180	20%
oven crispy crunchy	4 oz	11.0	210	47%
	5 oz	14.0	265	47%
rectangles/precooked/breaded	3 oz	7.0	150	42%
	3.6 oz	9.0	180	45%
	4 oz	10.0	200	45%
Rectangles Puf!				
pollock 'n cheese/oven crispy	3.6 o.z	11.0	240	41%
precooked/breaded	3 oz	7.0	150	42%
raw/breaded	3 oz	1.0	120	8%
squares/fully cooked	2.5 oz	7.0	140	45%
Tail-r-Cut Puf!/golden broil	4.5 oz	8.0	160	45%
Wedges Puf!				
English style batter dipt	4 oz	11.0	200	50%
lite 'n crunchy	3.6 oz	3.0	140	19%
oven crispy	3 oz	6.0	140	39%
	3.6 oz	8.0	170	42%
catfish				
fillets	4 oz	1.5	100	14%
fillettes/Southern cornmeal	2.75 oz	3.0	120	23%
	4 oz	5.0	170	26%
FishFries Puf!/Southern cornmeal	3.75 oz	4.0	160	23%
Nuggets Puf!	4 oz	10.0	230	39%
clam strips/prefried/breaded	4 oz	18.0	350	46%
cod fillet				
Batter Dipt Puf!	2 oz	7.0	120	53%
	3 oz	10.0	180	50%
Easy Grill/lemon pepper Puf!	4.2 oz	2.0	100	18%
English cut/raw/unbreaded	4 oz	0.5	70	6%
fillettes				
gourmet/raw/breaded	3 oz	0.5	100	5%
	4 oz	1.0	130	7%
seasoned/crunchy	3 oz	1.0	110	8%
	4 oz	1.0	150	6%
tender crisp	3 oz	1.0	100	9%
	4 oz	1.0	130	7%
fish sticks/precooked/breaded				
minced	4 oz	10.0	210	43%
regular	4 oz	11.0	210	47%
Nordic cut/raw/unbreaded	4.22 oz	0.5	75	6%
Nuggets Puf!/oven crispy crunchy				
Bunch 'O Crunch	3.5 oz	13.0	240	49%
minced	4 oz	11.0	210	47%
regular	5 oz	19.0	350	49%

Food and Description	Amount	Fat Grams	Total Calories	% Fat Calories
raw				
breaded	3 oz	0.4	90	4%
	4 oz	0.5	110	4%
unbreaded	4 oz	1.0	90	10%
rectangles/precooked/breaded				
minced	3 oz	7.0	160	39%
regular	3 oz	7.0	140	45%
	3.6 oz	8.0	170	42%
	4 oz	9.0	190	43%
Rectangles Puf!				
precooked/breaded	3 oz	7.0	160	39%
raw/breaded	3 oz	1.0	120	8%
squares/raw/breaded	4 oz	1.5	120	11%
Squares Puf! /raw/breaded	4 oz	1.5	160	8%
Sticks Puf!/oven crispy crunchy				
Bunch 'O Crunch	3 oz	12.0	230	47%
Tail-r-Cut Puf!				
golden broil	3 oz	6.0	120	45%
	4.5 oz	8.0	160	45%
raw/breaded	4 oz	1.5	160	8%
	5.3 oz	2.0	220	8%
Wedges Puf!				
English style batter dipt.	3 oz	9.0	160	51%
	4 oz	12.0	210	51%
oven crispy	2 oz	7.8	150	47%
	3 oz	10.0	190	47%
crab/stuffed/in natural shell	3 oz	5.0	140	32%
fish cake				
Neptune burger	3 oz	6.0	150	36%
regular	4 oz	9.0	220	8%
flounder				
stuffed/fancy				
w/broccoli, cheese, & lobster	9 oz	13.0	270	43%
w/crabmeat	9 oz	13.0	260	45%
fillets/raw/breaded	4 oz	1.5	140	10%
	5 oz	2.0	170	10%
haddock fillet				
raw/unbreaded	4 oz	1.0	90	10%
Rectangles Puf!				
precooked/breaded	3 oz	7.0	170	37%
raw/breaded	3 oz	1.0	120	8%
Squares Puf!/raw/breaded	4 oz	1.5	180	8%
Tail-r-Cut Puf!/raw/breaded	4 oz	1.0	140	6%
	5.3 oz	2.0	240	8%
salmon				
fillets/boned-skinless	4 oz	11.0	190	52%
Kiev style w/hollandaise sauce filling	6 oz	22.0	370	54%

Food and Description	Amount	Fat Grams	Total Calories	% Fat Calories
smoked/boned/sliced	2 oz	5.0	95	47%
Tail-r-Cut Puf!/Norwegian golden broil	4.5 oz	19.0	290	59%
shrimp, Norwegian/cooked & peeled	4 oz	1.0	100	9%
smelt/great silver				
Puf!/breaded/precooked	3 oz	7.0	170	37%
Wedges Puf!				
English syle batter dipt	4 oz	9.0	190	43%
oven crispy	3 oz	10.0	210	43%
	3.6 oz	12.0	250	43%
Nuggets Puf!/oven crispy crunchy	5 oz	20.0	345	52%
whiting				
Batter Dipt Puf!	2 oz	7.0	160	39%
	3 oz	10.0	180	50%
fish sticks/breaded, precooked	4 oz	12.0	220	49%
Nuggets Puf!/oven crispy crunchy	5 oz	24.0	360	60%
rectangles/breaded, precooked	3 oz	8.0	150	48%
	3.6 oz	9.0	180	45%
Rectangles Puf!				
oven crispy	3.6 oz	10.0	200	45%
raw, breaded	3 oz	2.0	130	14%
Wedges Puf!				
English style batter dipt	3 oz	8.0	150	48%
	4 oz	11.0	200	50%
oven crispy	3 oz	8.0	170	42%
	3.6 oz	10.0	200	45%
generic				
cod fillets/crunchy/microwaveable	1 fillet	22.0	330	60%
fish cakes				
bite-size	5 pieces	11.0	165	60%
large	1 piece	11.0	165	60%
fish sticks/4" x 2" x ½"	1 stick	3.0	75	36%
(Gorton's)				
fish fillets				
garlic 'n herb/crunchy breaded	2 fillets	14.0	250	50%
hot 'n spicy/crunchy breaded	2 fillets	14.0	250	50%
Italian herb/grilled	1 fillet	6.0	130	42%
lemon pepper				
crispy batter	2 fillets	16.0	250	58%
grilled	1 fillet	6.0	120	45%
plain				
crispy batter	2 fillets	21.0	290	65%
breaded/crunchy	2 fillets	14.0	250	50%
Southern-fried country style/ breaded/crunchy	2 fillets	16.0	270	53%
fish portions/value pack				
batter-dipped	1 portion	10.0	160	56%

Food and Description	Amount	Fat Grams	Total Calories	% Fat Calories
breaded/crunchy	1 portion	12.0	180	60%
fish sticks				
breaded				
crunchy	6 sticks	15.0	260	52%
regular				
115 or more per pkg	6 sticks	12.0	220	49%
20 per pkg	5 sticks	8.0	220	33%
value pack	8 sticks	12.0	220	49%
minced/crispy batter	5 sticks	20.0	290	62%
mini/value pack				
minced	13 sticks	14.0	230	55%
regular/18 per pkg	13 sticks	13.0	230	51%
haddock fillets/crispy batter	2 fillets	19.0	270	63%
pollock fillets/crispy batter	2 fillets	19.0	280	61%
shrimp				
baked scampi	6 pieces	16.0	250	58%
beer batter	6 pieces	15.0	250	54%
crunchy/microwaveable	1 pkg	16.0	300	48%
popcorn				
garlic & herb	1 ¼ cup	13.0	270	43%
plain	1 cup	16.0	260	55%
Stir-Fry Kit				
scampi	10 oz	14.0	320	39%
sweet & sour	10 oz	1.5	280	5%
teriyaki	10 oz	1.5	300	5%
(Harvest of the Sea) shrimp/cooked	½ cup	–	45	–
(Kibun & Kibun Gold)				
dill sauce & fish	10 oz	5.0	280	16%
Mediterranean fish	10 oz	1.0	230	4%
piccata	10 oz	25.0	470	48%
primavera	10 oz	19.0	360	48%
sea pasta Pacific fish & shrimp				
w/ dressing	½ pkg	9.0	210	39%
w/o dressing	½ pkg	1.0	140	6%
Sea Stix	4 oz	<1.0	110	4%
Sea Tails	4 oz	<1.0	110	4%
seafood fettucini Alfredo	10 oz	11.0	330	30%
seafood linguini	10 oz	6.0	260	21%
seafood marinara	11 oz	2.0	240	8%
seafood Newburg	10 oz	7.0	300	21%
seafood piccata	1 serving	21.0	450	42%
seafood primivera	1 serving	7.0	300	21%
(Mrs. Paul's)				
clams/real	3 oz	15.0	280	48%
cod fillets				
au natural	5 oz	2.0	110	16%
premium	1 fillet	11.0	250	40%

Food and Description	Amount	Fat Grams	Total Calories	% Fat Calories
deviled crab cakes				
miniatures	3½ oz	12.0	240	43%
regular size	1 cake	9.0	180	37%
fish cakes	2 cakes	7.0	190	40%
fish fillet sandwich w/cheese/ crispy crunchy	1 sandwich	15.0	330	41%
fish fillets				
batter dipped	2 fillets	17.0	330	37%
breaded/Healthy Treasures	4 oz	3.0	170	16%
crispy crunchy	2 fillets	12.0	240	45%
crunch batter	2 fillets	14.0	280	45%
light/in butter sauce	1 fillet	5.0	120	38%
fish portions				
battered	2 portions	19.0	300	57%
value pack	2 portions	10.0	190	47%
fish sticks				
battered	6 sticks	15.0	240	56%
crispy crunchy	6 sticks	9.0	200	41%
minced & breaded/value pack	6 sticks	11.0	210	47%
flounder fillets				
au natural	5 oz	2.0	110	16%
crunch batter	2 fillets	9.0	220	37%
premium	1 fillet	8.0	170	42%
haddock fillets				
au natural	5 oz	2.0	110	16%
crunch batter	2 fillets	5.0	190	24%
premium	1 fillet	9.0	220	25%
perch fillets/au natural	5 oz	2.0	110	16%
sole fillets				
au natural	5 oz	2.0	110	16%
premium	1 fillet	8.0	170	42%
(Ocean Supreme) gourmet breaded shrimp	5 pieces	2.5	220	10%
(Oven Poppers)				
cod stuffed w/broccoli & cheese	1 piece	6.0	150	36%
sole				
stuffed w/crab	1 piece	13.0	250	47%
stuffed w/garlic shrimp & almonds	1 piece	13.0	250	47%
(Sambrand of Iceland)	4 oz	1.0	90	10%
(Schwan's)				
blue hake				
loins	4 oz	–	70	–
portions	~3 oz	8.0	180	40%
catfish				
fingers/raw	4 oz	6.0	170	32%
fillets/oven-ready/breaded	4 oz	7.0	180	35%
clams/strips/breaded & fried	4 oz	14.0	270	47%

Food and Description	Amount	Fat Grams	Total Calories	% Fat Calories
cod				
batter crisp-breaded	2 oz	7.0	120	53%
fillets	4 oz	0.5	90	5%
nuggets/breaded	6 nuggets	11.0	200	50%
flounder				
fillets	4 oz	1.5	100	14%
oven-ready/breaded	4 oz	9.0	220	37%
haddock				
fish 'n batter	2 oz	19.0	300	57%
squares/breaded	~4 oz	8.0	200	36%
sticks/breaded	3 sticks	7.0	160	39%
halibut fillets	4 oz	4.5	130	31%
ocean perch	4 oz	2.0	90	20%
orange roughy	4 oz	1.5	80	17%
seafood legs/fancy	3.5 oz	0.5	100	5%
scrod/New England style	5 oz	13.0	230	51%
shrimp				
fantail/breaded	3.9 oz	1.5	170	8%
oven-ready/breaded	3 oz	9.0	200	41%
peeled & deveined	4 oz	0.5	60	8%
pieces/breaded	4 pieces	1.0	180	5%
(Sea Pak) shrimp				
butterfly	4 oz	1.0	140	6%
jumbo butterfly/breaded	3 oz	9.0	200	41%
popcorn	3 oz	12.0	210	51%
poppers	20 pieces	12.0	210	51%
Shrimp Sensations Oriental stir-fry	½ pkg	2.5	190	12%
(Seafood Elites) sole fillet				
w/broccoli & mozzarella	1 fillet	7.0	150	42%
w/lemon & wild rice	1 fillet	7.0	150	42%
w/spinach & cheddar	1 fillet	6.0	130	42%
(Singleton)				
popcorn shrimp	3 oz	13.0	260	45%
shrimp poppers	3 oz	9.0	260	31%
scallop poppers	3 oz	11.0	240	41%
(Swanson)				
fish & fries	6.5 oz	16.0	340	42%
fish 'n chips	10 oz	21.0	500	38%
(Tyson) fish & chips kit				
2 pieces fish & chips				
plain	4 oz	33.0	550	54%
w/2 tsp malt vinegar	4 oz	33.0	550	54%
w/2 tsp malt vinegar & 2 Tbs tartar sauce	4 oz	37.0	600	56%
(Van de Kamp's)				
cod fillets/lightly breaded	1 fillet	10.0	220	41%
fish fillets				
battered	1 fillet	11.0	180	55%

Food and Description	Amount	Fat Grams	Total Calories	% Fat Calories
breaded	2 fillets	19.0	280	61%
crisp & healthy/breaded	2 fillets	2.5	150	15%
fish 'n fries/breaded	1 pkg	18.0	380	43%
fish nuggets/battered	8 pieces	18.0	280	58%
fish portions				
battered	2 pieces	22.0	350	57%
breaded	3 pieces	21.0	330	57%
fish sticks				
battered	6 sticks	16.0	260	55%
breaded				
regular	6 sticks	17.0	290	53%
snack pack	6 sticks	14.0	260	48%
value pack	6 sticks	14.0	260	48%
crisp & healthy/breaded	6 sticks	3.0	180	15%
mini/breaded	13 sticks	14.0	250	50%
flounder fillets				
lightly breaded	1 fillet	11.0	230	43%
natural	1 fillet	2.0	110	16%
haddock fillets				
battered	2 fillets	16.0	260	55%
breaded	2 fillets	17.0	280	55%
lightly breaded	1 fillet	10.0	220	41%
halibut fillets/battered	3 fillets	21.0	300	63%
perch fillets/battered	2 fillets	20.0	300	60%
shrimp/breaded				
butterfly	7 shrimp	14.0	280	45%
popcorn	20 shrimp	13.0	270	43%
whole	7 shrimp	10.0	240	38%
sole fillets				
lightly breaded	1 fillet	11.0	220	45%
natural	1 fillet	1.5	110	12%

■ HOMEMADE

USDA Standard Home Recipe (Note: Homemade dishes were not made with low-fat substitute ingredients.The amount of fat and calories may vary, depending on the type and amount of certain ingredients used.)

Food and Description	Amount	Fat Grams	Total Calories	% Fat Calories
clam fritter/~1.5 oz	1 fritter	6.0	124	44%
crab				
deviled	½ cup	12.0	185	58%
stuffed	½ cup	4.0	86	42%
crab cake/fried in margarine/~4 oz	1 cake	11.0	205	48%
fish cake/fried	1 regular or 5 bite-size	5.0	105	43%
fish loaf	~5 oz	5.6	186	27%
jambalaya	1 cup	6.7	250	24%
lobster Newburg	~6.5 oz	35.0	455	69%
oyster stew	1 cup	15.0	233	58%
oysters Rockefeller	4 oysters	2.7	90	27%

ood and Description	Amount	Fat Grams	Total Calories	% Fat Calories
paella w/saffron rice, seafood, & vegetables	~8 oz	11.0	350	28%
salmon cake	3.5 oz	15.0	248	54%
salmon casserole	1 cup	35.0	555	57%
salmon patty	3.5 oz	12.0	239	45%
salmon-rice loaf	6 oz	8.0	212	34%
seafood Creole w/rice	1 cup	8.7	300	26%
seafood curry	3/5 cup	11.5	232	45%
seafood gumbo	5 oz	1.0	48	19%
seafood salad	3½ oz	10.0	160	56%
shrimp salad	¾ cup	12.0	210	51%
tuna patty	3 oz	3.0	80	34%

MIX (Note: The amount of fat and calories in dishes prepared from boxed mixes may ary slightly depending on the fat and calorie content of the seafood used in preparation.)

Betty Crocker) Tuna Helper				
au gratin				
mix only	½ cup	4.0	190	19%
prepared	1 cup	12.0	300	36%
cheesy noodles				
mix only	⅔ cup	4.0	170	21%
prepared	1 cup	12.0	290	37%
creamy broccoli				
mix only	⅔ cup	5.0	190	24%
prepared	1 cup	13.0	310	38%
creamy noodles				
mix only	¾ cup	6.0	190	28%
prepared	1 cup	14.0	310	41%
fettuccine Afredo				
mix only	1 cup	4.0	180	20%
prepared	1 cup	16.0	340	42%
garden cheddar				
mix only	⅔ cup	4.0	190	19%
prepared	1 cup	12.0	310	35%
pasta salad				
mix only	⅓ cup	0.5	120	4%
prepared				
low-fat recipe	⅓ cup	1.5	230	6%
regular recipe	⅔ cup	27.0	380	64%
tetrazzini				
mix only	½ cup	3.0	180	15%
prepared	1 cup	12.0	310	35%
tuna pot pie				
mix only	½ cup	20.0	340	53%
prepared	⅕ pie	24.0	440	49%
tuna Romanoff				
mix only	⅔ cup	3.0	210	13%
prepared	1 cup	8.0	280	26%

Food and Description	Amount	Fat Grams	Total Calories	% Fat Calorie
SEASONINGS (*See also* ASIAN FOOD/SAUCES & SEASONINGS; BAKE & FRY MIX; GRAVY; MEXICAN FOOD; SAUCE; individual listings)				
(NOTE: Unless stated otherwise, data are for seasoning or seasoning mix only.)				
(Ac'cent)				
flavor enhancer	⅛ tsp	–	–	–
Sa-son				
con ajo cebolla	¼ tsp	–	–	–
con azafran	¼ tsp	–	–	–
con culantro	¼ tsp	–	–	–
original	¼ tsp	–	–	–
(Andre Prost) A Taste Of Thai				
chorizo ancho seasoning	1 Tbs	–	5	–
green curry				
base mix	1 tsp	1.5	15	90%
dinner kit	3.5 oz	7.0	91	69%
lemon grass hearts	1 piece	–	–	–
mussaman curry				
base mix	1 tsp	1.5	20	68%
dinner kit	3.5 oz	6.0	102	53%
panang curry				
base mix	1 tsp	2.0	25	72%
dinner kit	3.5 oz	8.0	105	69%
red chili peppers/minced	1 tsp	–	–	–
red curry				
base mix	1 tsp	1.5	20	68%
dinner kit	3.5 oz	7.0	94	67%
spicy chicken & rice dinner mix	¼ pkg	–	15	–
Thai peanut bake seasoning mix	¼ pkg	1.5	45	30%
yellow curry				
base mix	1 tsp	3.0	30	90%
dinner kit	3.5 oz	9.0	113	72%
(Betty Crocker) Potato Shakers				
crispy cheddar fries	3 tsp	1.0	25	36%
original	3 tsp	0.5	30	15%
Parmesan	3 tsp	1.0	30	30%
seasoned fries	3 tsp	–	20	–
zesty cheddar	3 tsp	1.5	30	45%
(Borden)				
Soup Starter				
beef barley vegetable	⅛ pkg	0.5	100	5%
beef vegetable	⅛ pkg	0.5	90	5%
chicken & rice				
quick cook	¼ container	–	50	–
regular	⅛ pkg	0.5	70	6%
chicken noodle				
quick cook	¼ container	1.0	80	11%
regular	⅛ pkg	–	80	–
chicken w/white & wild rice	⅛ pkg	–	70	–

Food and Description	Amount	Fat Grams	Total Calories	% Fat Calories
ground beef vegetable				
quick cook	¼ container	0.5	80	6%
regular	⅛ pkg	0.5	80	6%
hearty chicken vegetable	⅛ pkg	–	70	–
Stew Starter/hearty beef	⅐ pkg	–	80	–
(Chi-Chi's) seasoning mix	1 tsp	–	10	–
(Durkee)				
garlic bread sprinkles	½ tsp	–	–	–
roasting bag				
au jus	⅛ pkg	–	10	–
barbecue chicken	⅙ pkg	–	30	–
beef stew	⅒ pkg	–	15	–
chicken	⅙ pkg	–	20	–
country chicken	⅙ pkg	1.5	35	39%
lemon butter fish	¼ pkg	0.5	30	15%
meat loaf	⅛ pkg	–	15	–
onion pot roast	⅙ pkg	–	25	–
pork	⅙ pkg	–	25	–
pot roast	⅙ pkg	–	15	–
spareribs	⅐ pkg	–	25	–
Swiss steak	⅑ pkg	–	10	–
seasoning packet				
beef fajita/"easy"	⅙ pkg	–	15	–
beef stew	⅑ pkg	–	–	–
beef teriyaki/"easy"	⅕ pkg	1.0	30	30%
burrito	⅒ pkg	1.0	35	26%
chicken cacciatore/"easy"	⅒ pkg	–	10	–
chicken mushroom/"easy"	⅛ pkg	–	15	–
fried rice	¼ pkg	–	15	–
ground beef	¼ pkg	–	25	–
Italian meatball	⅛ pkg	–	20	–
lemon pepper dill fish/"easy"	⅙ pkg	0.5	20	9%
meat loaf	⅑ pkg	–	20	–
Mexican salsa chicken/"easy"	⅒ pkg	–	10	–
pasta slad	⅙ pkg	–	10	–
sloppy joe	⅙ pkg	–	20	–
spaghetti	⅕ pkg	–	15	–
American style	⅙ pkg	–	15	–
family	⅒ pkg	–	20	–
w/mushrooms	⅕ pkg	–	15	–
zesty	⅕ pkg	–	20	–
stroganoff	⅛ pkg	–	10	–
sweet & sour chicken/"easy"	⅑ pkg	–	20	–
tomato basil fish/"easy"	⅐ pkg	–	15	–
(French's)				
roasting bag				
au jus	⅛ pkg	<1.0	10	45%
chicken	⅕ pkg	<1.0	25	18%

Food and Description	Amount	Fat Grams	Total Calories	% Fat Calories
lemon butter fish	¼ pkg	<1.0	25	18%
meatloaf	⅙ pkg	<1.0	25	18%
onion pot roast	⅛ pkg	<1.0	18	25%
pork	⅙ pkg	<1.0	25	18%
pot roast	⅛ pkg	<1.0	18	25%
Swiss steak	⅙ pkg	<1.0	20	23%
seasonings				
beef stew	⅑ pkg	–	5	–
Chili-O				
mild	⅕ pkg	0.5	30	15%
onion	⅕ pkg	–	40	–
original	⅕ pkg	–	30	–
Texas style	⅓ pkg	1.0	45	20%
fajita	⅕ pkg	1.0	82	11%
meat marinade	⅛ pkg	–	10	–
meat loaf	⅛ pkg	–	20	–
sloppy joe	⅛ pkg	–	16	–
spaghetti				
Italian	⅕ pkg	–	16	–
mushroom	⅕ pkg	1.0	20	45%
thick	⅕ pkg	–	10	–
stroganoff	¼ pkg	2.0	45	40%
zesty pasta	⅕ pkg	–	20	–
(Golden Dipt)				
Oven Easy				
Cajun style	¼ cup	3.0	90	30%
lemon & pepper	¼ cup	1.5	80	17%
shrimp & seafood	2 Tbs	2.0	70	26%
tortilla	3 Tbs	2.0	80	23%
seasonings				
all purpose seafood	½ tsp	–	–	–
blackened redfish	½ tsp	–	–	–
broiled fish	¼ tsp	–	–	–
Cajun style shrimp & crab	¼ tsp	–	2	–
lemon pepper seafood	¼ tsp	–	8	–
(Hunt's) Manwich/sloppy joe mix	⅙ pkg	<1.0	20	23%
(Knorr) recipe mix				
beef stew w/wine	⅙ pkg	1.0	40	23%
chicken Dijonne	⅙ pkg	1.0	30	30%
goulash beef stew	⅙ pkg	1.0	40	23%
sauerbraten	⅙ pkg	1.0	35	26%
(Lawry's)				
bacon onion	1 tsp	–	10	–
garlic pepper	¼ tsp	–	2	–
garlic powder w/parsley	1 tsp	–	12	–
garlic salt	1 tsp	–	4	–
lemon pepper	1 tsp	–	6	–
minced onion	1 tsp	–	7	–

Food and Description	Amount	Fat Grams	Total Calories	% Fat Calories
pinch of herbs	1 tsp	0.5	9	50%
pepper/seasoned	1 tsp	–	4	–
salt/seasoned				
hot 'n spicy	1 tsp	–	3	–
lite	1 tsp	–	8	–
plain	1 tsp	–	4	–
salt free	1 tsp	–	3	–
salt free 17	1 tsp	–	10	–
(Lipton) Recipe Secrets				
fiesta herb w/red pepper	⅓ Tbs	–	–	–
onion				
mushroom	2 Tbs	–	–	–
original	1 Tbs	–	20	–
savory herb w/garlic	1 Tbs	–	30	–
Manwich (See (Hunt's) in this section)				
(McCormick/Schilling)				
Bag 'n Season				
beef stew	1 tsp	–	15	–
Buffalo wings	1 Tbs	–	30	–
chicken	1 Tbs	–	20	–
country chicken	2 tsp	1.0	25	36%
meat loaf	2 tsp	–	15	–
pork chops	2 tsp	–	15	–
pot roast	1 tsp	–	10	–
spareribs	1 Tbs	–	30	–
Swiss steak	1 tsp	–	15	–
turkey w/gravy	1 tsp	–	15	–
gourmet spices				
arrowroot	1½ Tbs	–	40	–
beef flavor base	1 tsp	–	–	–
Bon Appetit	¼ tsp	–	–	–
char-grill seasoning	¼ tsp	–	–	–
chicken flavor base	1 tsp	2.0	35	51%
cinnamon sugar	1 tsp	–	15	–
ginger/crystallized	¼ tsp	–	–	–
lemon & pepper	¼ tsp	–	–	–
season pepper medley	¼ tsp	–	2	–
vanilla flavored powder	¼ tsp	–	2	–
vegetable delight	½ tsp	–	–	–
Grill Mates				
Montreal	¼ tsp	–	–	–
Montreal chicken & fish	¼ tsp	–	–	–
spicy Montreal steak	¼ tsp	–	–	–
International Blends				
Meditteranean rice	½ tsp	–	–	–
Szechuan	½ tsp	–	–	–
Thai	½ tsp	–	–	–

Food and Description	Amount	Fat Grams	Total Calories	% Fat Calories
rice seasonings				
Creole	⅔ Tbs	–	20	–
curry	1 Tbs	1.0	25	36%
Japanese	1½ Tbs	1.5	50	27%
saffron	1 Tbs	–	25	–
Spanish	1½ Tbs	–	45	–
Rotisserie Recipe				
herb & spice	2 tsp	–	15	–
tangy barbecue	2 tsp	–	20	–
salt-free blends				
all purpose	¼ tsp	–	–	–
garlic & herb	¼ tsp	–	–	–
lemon & pepper	¼ tsp	–	–	–
onion & herb	¼ tsp	–	–	–
spicy	¼ tsp	–	–	–
seasoning blends				
beef stew	2 tsp	–	15	–
beef stroganoff	2 tsp	–	15	–
Cajun	½ tsp	–	–	–
Caribbean jerk	¼ tsp	–	–	–
celery salt	¼ tsp	–	–	–
cheese sauce	4 tsp	2.0	40	45%
chili				
hot	¼ pkg	1.0	40	23%
mild	⅙ pkg	–	30	–
original	⅛ pkg	0.5	30	15%
citrus pepper	¼ tsp	–	–	–
Creole	¼ tsp	–	–	–
fajita	¼ tsp	–	1	–
garlic, minced-wet/California style	1 tsp	0.5	15	30%
garlic & parsley salt	¼ tsp	–	–	–
garlic bread sprinkle	½ tsp	1.0	10	90%
garlic pepper				
California style	¼ tsp	–	–	–
regular	¼ tsp	–	3	–
garlic salt				
California style	¼ tsp	–	–	–
regular	¼ tsp	–	–	–
garlic spread				
garlic & herb	½ Tbs	4.5	45	90%
regular	½ Tbs	4.0	45	80%
hamburger	¼ tsp	–	–	–
herb chicken	¼ tsp	–	–	–
homestyle	¼ tsp	–	–	–
imitation butter-flavored salt	¼ tsp	–	–	–
lemon herb	½ tsp	–	–	–
lemon pepper/California style	½ tsp	–	5	–
meat loaf	1 tsp	–	15	–

Food and Description	Amount	Fat Grams	Total Calories	% Fat Calories
meat marinade	1 tsp	–	15	–
meat tenderizer				
seasoned	¼ tsp	–	–	–
unseasoned	¼ tsp	–	–	–
mesquite chicken	¼ tsp	–	2	–
old bay	½ tsp	–	–	–
onion salt/California style	¼ tsp	–	–	–
pork seasoing	½ tsp	–	–	–
rotisserie chicken	¼ tsp	–	–	–
sloppy joe	⅛ pkg	–	15	–
Swedish meatball (1 serving = 2 tsp meat mix + 1 tsp sauce mix)	1 serving	1.0	45	20%
spice blends				
barbecue seasoning	½ tsp	–	–	–
Best O'Butter butter salt	¼ tsp	–	–	–
broiled steak seasoning	¼ tsp	–	<1	–
Chesapeake Bay seafood seasoning	¼ tsp	–	–	–
chicken seasoning	¼ tsp	–	–	–
garlic bread sprinkle	½ tsp	1.0	10	90%
lemon & herb	½ tsp	–	–	–
lemon & pepper	¼ tsp	–	–	–
Mexican seasoning	¼ tsp	–	–	–
onion salt	¼ tsp	–	–	–
Salad Supreme	¼ tsp	–	–	–
Season All				
garlic	¼ tsp	–	–	–
lite	¼ tsp	–	–	–
original	¼ tsp	–	–	–
peppered	¼ tsp	–	–	–
spicy	¼ tsp	–	2	–
Szechuan pepper	¼ tsp	–	–	–
vegetable supreme	¼ tsp	–	–	–
(Mrs. Dash)				
extra spicy	1 tsp	–	12	–
garlic & herb	1 tsp	–	12	–
lemon & herb	1 tsp	–	12	–
low pepper	1 tsp	–	12	–
original	1 tsp	–	12	–
table blend	1 tsp	–	12	–
(Molly McButter)				
cheese-flavor sprinkles	½ tsp	–	5	–
sour cream-flavor sprinkles	½ tsp	–	5	–
(NewMenu) Tofumate				
breakfast scramble	¼ pkg	–	15	–
eggless salad	¼ pkg	–	15	–
Mandarin stir-fry	¼ pkg	–	30	–
Szechwan stir-fry	¼ pkg	–	25	–
Texas taco	¼ pkg	–	15	–

Food and Description	Amount	Fat Grams	Total Calories	% Fat Calories
(Nile Spice)				
Cleopatra's Secret	⅛ tsp	–	–	–
desert spice	⅛ tsp	–	–	–
ginger curry	⅛ tsp	–	–	–
maya maize popcorn	½ tsp	–	–	–
Nile spice	⅛ tsp	–	–	–
seasoning of garlic	⅛ tsp	–	–	–
spicy lemon pepper	⅛ tsp	–	–	–
(Old El Paso) seasoning mix				
burrito	2 tsp	–	20	–
enchilada	2 tsp	–	10	–
chili	1 Tbs	0.5	25	18%
taco				
less sodium	2 tsp	–	20	–
regular	2 tsp	–	20	–
(Pancho Villa) taco seasoning mix	2 tsp	–	20	–
(Produce Partners) vegetable seasonings				
oven potato fries	1 Tbs	1.0	30	30%
potato toppers	1 Tbs	1.0	35	26%
roasted potatoes				
cheddar	1 Tbs	1.5	35	39%
Italian herb	2 tsp	1.5	30	45%
onion	2 tsp	1.0	30	30%
stir-fry	2 tsp	–	15	–
(Shake & Bake)				
Oven Fry seasoned coating mix				
chicken				
extra crispy	⅛ pouch	1.0	60	15%
homestyle	⅛ pouch	1.0	40	23%
pork/extra crispy	⅛ pouch	1.5	60	23%
Perfect Potatoes seasoning mix				
crispy cheddar	⅙ pkt	2.0	30	60%
herb & garlic	⅙ pkt	–	20	–
seasoning & coating mixture				
country mild recipe	⅛ pouch	2.0	35	51%
for chicken				
hot & spicy recipe	⅛ pouch	1.0	40	23%
original recipe	⅛ pouch	1.0	40	23%
for fish/original	⅛ pouch	1.5	70	19%
for pork				
hot & spicy recipe	⅛ pouch	0.5	45	10%
original recipe	⅛ pouch	–	40	–%
Italian herb	¼ pouch	1.0	80	11%
seasoning & coating mixture glaze				
barbecue chicken	⅛ pouch	1.0	45	20%
barbecue pork	⅛ pouch	–	35	–
honey mustard	⅛ pouch	1.0	45	20%
tangy honey	⅛ pouch	1.0	45	20%

Food and Description	Amount	Fat Grams	Total Calories	% Fat Calories
(Smart Seas)				
butter sprinkles	¾ tsp	–	–	–
cheese sprinkles	½ tsp	–	–	–
garlic w/Italian herb	½ tsp	–	–	–
garlic w/parsley	¼ tsp	–	–	–
pepper & herb	¾ tsp	–	–	–
steak spice	½ tsp	–	–	–
(Tone's) Oriental five-spice seasoning	1 tsp	–	9	–
SEAWEED				
agar				
dried	3 oz	<1.0	260	2%
(Eden)	1 Tbs	–	10	–
raw	3 oz	<1.0	23	20%
kelp/raw	3 oz	0.6	37	15%
laver/Nori				
dried	3 oz	<1.0	30	9%
(Eden) sushi nori sea vegetable	1 sheet	–	10	–
raw	3 oz	<1.0	31	15%
spirulina				
dried	3 oz	6.6	249	24%
raw	3 oz	<1.0	22	21%
wakame				
(Eden)	½ cup	–	25	–
raw	3 oz	<1.0	40	11%
SELTZER WATER (*See* SOFT DRINK; WATER)				
SEMOLINA (*See also* FLOUR)				
enriched	½ cup	0.5	310	1%
unenriched	½ cup	<1.0	110	2%
whole-grain	1 cup	2.0	600	3%
SESAME BUTTER/TAHINI				
(Arrowhead Mills) organic	2 Tbs	17.0	170	90%
(Erewhon)				
butter	2 Tbs	17.0	190	81%
tahini	2 Tbs	17.0	170	90%
(Casbah) sauce mix/prepared	¼ cup	13.0	160	73%
generic	1 oz	15.0	169	80%
paste	1 Tbs	8.0	95	76%
tahini	2 Tbs	16.0	180	80%
toasted	2 Tbs	20.0	200	90%
(Roaster Fresh)	2 Tbs	15.0	170	79%
(Westbrae) organic				
mid-Eastern	2 Tbs	19.0	220	78%
natural	2 Tbs	19.0	220	78%
raw	2 Tbs	19.0	220	78%
toasted	2 Tbs	19.0	220	78%
SESAME FLOUR (*See* FLOUR)				
SESAME SEEDS				
dried/ground	1 tsp	–	5	–

Food and Description	Amount	Fat Grams	Total Calories	% Fat Calories
kernels				
(Arrowhead Mills) mechanically hulled	¼ cup	20.0	210	86%
generic				
dried	1 Tbs	4.0	47	77%
toasted	1 oz	13.6	161	76%
	1 cup	80.0	873	83%
whole				
(Arrowhead Mills) brown	¼ cup	20.0	200	90%
generic				
dried	1 Tbs	4.5	52	78%
roasted & toasted	1 oz	13.6	161	76%
(McCormick/Schilling) untoasted	¼ tsp	0.4	5	72%
SHAD, AMERICAN				
cooked-dry heat	3 oz	15.0	215	63%
raw	3 oz	12.0	170	63%
SHALLOT				
freeze-dried	1 Tbs	–	3	–
	¼ cup	–	13	–
	1 oz	–	100	–
fresh/raw/chopped	1 Tbs	–	7	–
SHARK				
batter-dipped & fried	3 oz	11.8	194	55%
raw	3 oz	3.8	111	31%
SHEEPSHEAD				
cooked-dry heat	3 oz	1.0	107	8%
raw	3 oz	2.0	92	20%
SHELLIE BEAN				
canned	½ cup	–	37	–
sprouted				
(La Choy)	1 cup	–	10	–
SHERBET (See also FRUIT ICES, BARS, & POPS)				
(Baskin-Robbins)				
orange	½ cup	1.5	120	11%
	reg scoop	2.0	160	11%
rainbow	½ cup	1.5	120	11%
	reg scoop	2.0	160	11%
(Borden) orange	½ cup	1.0	110	8%
(Breyers)				
orange	½ cup	1.0	120	8%
rainbow	½ cup	1.0	120	8%
raspberry	½ cup	1.0	120	8%
tropical	½ cup	1.0	120	8%
(Dreyer's)				
pink lemonade	½ cup	1.5	130	10%
strawberry kiwi	½ cup	1.5	120	11%
Swiss orange	½ cup	3.0	150	18%
tangerine	½ cup	2.0	130	14%
tropical	½ cup	2.0	130	14%

Food and Description	Amount	Fat Grams	Total Calories	% Fat Calories
(Edy's)				
pink lemonade	½ cup	1.5	130	10%
strawberry kiwi	½ cup	1.5	120	11%
Swiss orange	½ cup	3.0	150	18%
tangerine	½ cup	2.0	130	14%
tropical	½ cup	2.0	130	14%
(Knudsen) 3-gallon tub				
orange	½ cup	1.0	130	7%
rainbow	½ cup	1.0	120	8%
(Pet) orange	½ cup	1.0	130	7%
(Schwan's)				
orange	½ cup	1.0	120	8%
rainbow	½ cup	1.0	120	8%
(Sealtest)				
orange	½ cup	1.0	130	7%
rainbow	½ cup	1.0	130	7%
red raspberry	½ cup	1.0	130	7%
strawberry	½ cup	1.0	130	7%

SHORTENING, VEGETABLE (*See also* FAT; LARD; OIL; SHORTENING SUBSTITUTE)
(NOTE: All brands of vegetable shortening contain the same amount of calories and fat, just as all types of vegetable oil do. Because of the flexibility manufacturers are given in rounding off nutritional data, it may appear that one product has slightly fewer calories or less fat than another, but don't be fooled: They all get 100% of their calories from fat.)

(Crisco) regular or butter flavor	1 Tbs	12.0	110	100%
	1 cup	205.0	1845	100%
generic/soybean &/or cottonseed	1 Tbs	13.0	113	100%
	1 cup	205.0	1812	100%
(Snowdrift)	1 Tbs	12.0	110	100%
(Wesson)	1 Tbs	12.0	100	100%

SHORTENING SUBSTITUTE

(Plumlife) Just Like Shortenin	1⅔ Tbs	–	70	–
(Wonderslim) fat & egg substitute	¼ cup	–	35	–

SHOYU/SOY SAUCE (*See* ASIAN FOOD/SAUCES & SEASONINGS; SAUCE)
SHRIMP (*See also* ASIAN FOOD; FROZEN ENTRÉE/DINNER; SEAFOOD ENTRÉE/ DINNER; SHRIMP, IMITATION; SHRIMP PASTE)
canned

(Crown Prince) tiny/peeled	½ can	–	60	–
generic/mixed species/drained	4 large	1.8	102	15%
	1 cup	3.0	155	17%
(S&W) deveined				
medium	¼ cup	–	45	–
small	¼ cup	–	45	–
dried	1 oz	0.8	82	9%
fresh				
breaded & fried	4 large	3.7	73	45%
	3 oz	10.0	206	44%

Food and Description	Amount	Fat Grams	Total Calories	% Fat Calories
cooked-moist heat	4 large	–	22	–
	3 oz	0.9	84	10%
raw	3 oz	1.0	90	10%
SHRIMP, IMITATION				
from surimi	3 oz	1.0	86	10%
SHRIMP PASTE	3 oz	8.0	155	47%
SHRIMP SOUP, CREAM OF (See SOUP)				
SIM-SIM (See SESAME SEED)				
SLOPPY JOE (See FROZEN ENTRÉE/DINNER; SAUCE; SEASONINGS)				
SMELT (See also SEAFOOD ENTRÉE/DINNER)				
rainbow				
breaded & fried	3 oz	10.6	214	45%
cooked-dry heat	3 oz	2.6	106	22%
raw	3 oz	2.0	83	22%
SMOKED SALMON (See SALMON; SALMON SPREAD; SEAFOOD ENTRÉE/DINNER)				
SMOKED SAUSAGE (See SAUSAGE)				
SNACK BAR (See CANDY; GRANOLA/GRANOLA-TYPE BAR)				
SNACK CAKE (See CAKE, SNACK; PASTRY; POPCORN BARS & CAKES; RICE CAKES)				
SNACK CRACKER (See CRACKER)				
SNACK MIX				
(Betty Crocker) Cheerios Snack Mix				
cheddar cheese	¾ cup	5.0	130	35%
original w/peanuts	¾ cup	5.0	140	32%
sour cream & onion	¾ cup	5.0	130	35%
(Burns & Ricker) Party Mix/fat-free	¾ cup	–	120	–
(California Naturals)				
favorite mix	2 oz	15.0	260	52%
trail mix	2 oz	11.0	240	41%
(Del Monte) trail mix	0.9 oz	6.0	110	49%
(Dole) trail mix				
California style	1.2 oz	2.5	130	17%
	2 oz	4.0	220	16%
Hawaiian style	1.2 oz	4.0	150	24%
	2 oz	6.0	250	22%
(Fisher) Fisher Favorites nut & fruit mix				
piña colada	1 oz	10.0	150	60%
raisin cranberry	1 oz	10.0	150	60%
tropical fruit	1 oz	8.0	140	51%
(Gardetto's)				
mustard pretzel mix	½ cup	5.0	140	32%
Snackens				
original	½ cup	10.0	180	50%
reduced fat	½ cup	6.0	150	36%
sour cream & onion chips & twists	½ cup	10.0	170	53%
(Hidden Trails)				
fruit & nut mix	¼ cup	4.0	130	28%
rice crackers w/nuts	⅓ cup	9.0	160	51%

Food and Description	Amount	Fat Grams	Total Calories	% Fat Calories
trail mix	3 Tbs	7.0	148	43%
(Lawry's) Flavor Tree Party Mix				
regular	¼ cup	11.0	163	61%
no salt	¼ cup	10.8	163	60%
(Michael Season's) party mix				
traditional low-fat	1 oz	1.5	120	11%
(Pepperidge Farm)				
extra nutty	½ cup	9.0	180	45%
goldfish				
original	½ cup	8.0	170	42%
zesty cheddar	½ cup	10.0	180	50%
honey mustard & onion	½ cup	10.0	180	50%
lightly seasoned	½ cup	8.0	170	42%
(Planter's)				
fruit 'n nut mix	1 oz	9.0	140	58%
heat	1 oz	8.0	140	51%
Orchard Crunch	⅓ cup	8.0	140	51%
PB&J Crisps/bite-size	12 pieces	6.0	140	39%
(Ralston) Chex Mix				
bold & zesty	½ cup	7.0	160	39%
golden cheddar cheese	½ cup	4.5	140	29%
traditional	½ cup	3.5	130	24%
(Snyder's)	1 oz	8.0	170	42%
(Sunshine) Cheez-it Party Mix	½ cup	5.0	140	32%
SNACKS (*See also* FRUIT SNACK; MEXICAN FOOD; NUTS, MIXED; POPCORN; POPCORN BARS & CAKES; POTATO CHIPS & SNACKS; PRETZELS; RICE CAKES; SNACK MIX; TORTILLA CHIPS)				
(Baken-ets)				
cracklin	1 oz	6.0	80	68%
hot n' spicy	1 oz	5.0	70	64%
regular	1 oz	5.0	80	56%
(Banquet) frozen/mozzarella cheese nuggets	2.85 oz	11.0	210	47%
(Barbara's) natural cheese puffs	¾ cup	10.0	150	60%
(Bugles)				
baked				
BBQ	1½ cups	2.5	130	17%
cheddar cheese	1½ cups	3.0	130	21%
original	1½ cups	2.5	130	17%
regular				
nacho				
regular	1⅓ cups	9.0	160	51%
SUS	1 pouch	7.0	130	48%
original				
regular	1⅓ cups	9.0	160	51%
SUS	1 pouch	7.0	130	48%
ranch	1⅓ cups	9.0	160	51%
sour cream & onion	1⅓ cups	9.0	160	51%

Food and Description	Amount	Fat Grams	Total Calories	% Fat Calories
(Cheetos)				
Cheesy Checkers	1 oz	10.0	150	60%
crunchy	1 oz	9.0	150	54%
curls	1 oz	9.0	150	54%
flamin' hot	1 oz	9.0	160	51%
Paws	1 oz	10.0	160	56%
puffed balls	1 oz	10.0	160	56%
puffs	1 oz	10.0	160	56%
Wild Fangs	1 oz	10.0	160	56%
Cornnuts (See (Frito Lay) in this section)				
(Crunch & Munch) buttery				
almond	½ cup	3.0	130	21%
caramel	⅔ cup	3.0	140	19%
maple walnut	⅔ cup	4.0	140	26%
toffee				
original	⅔ cup	4.0	140	26%
	1.25 oz	4.0	160	23%
reduced fat	⅔ cup	2.5	140	16%
	1.25 oz	2.5	150	15%
(Eagle) cheese snacks				
baked Shamu shapes	1 cup	10.0	160	56%
Cheegles				
cheese balls				
original	2½ cups	10.0	160	56%
reduced fat	2½ cups	6.0	150	36%
cheese crunch	1 cup	10.0	160	56%
(Eden)				
brown rice chips	1 oz	5.0	130	35%
sea vegetable chips	1 oz	4.0	130	28%
wasabi snack chips	1 oz	11.0	160	62%
(Estee) Snack Crisps				
apple cinnamon	1 bag	2.0	90	30%
	27 crisps	3.0	130	21%
chocolate	1 bag	2.0	90	30%
	30 crisps	3.0	130	21%
lemon	1 bag	2.0	90	30%
	30 crisps	3.0	130	21%
ranch	1 bag	2.0	90	30%
	30 crisps	3.0	130	21%
white cheddar	1 bag	2.0	90	30%
	27 crisps	3.0	130	21%
(Featherweight) cheese curls	1 oz	7.0	140	45%
(Fisher) Fisher Favorites				
honey	1 oz	13.0	170	69%
praline	1 oz	12.0	170	64%
toffee	1 oz	11.0	160	62%
(Cornnuts)				
barbecue	1 oz	4.0	120	30%

Food and Description	Amount	Fat Grams	Total Calories	% Fat Calories
nacho cheese	1 oz	4.0	120	30%
original	1 oz	4.0	120	30%
	⅓ cup	5.0	150	30%
picante	1 oz	4.0	120	30%
ranch	1 oz	4.0	120	30%
(Funyuns) onion-flavored rings	1 oz	7.0	140	45%
(Hain) carrot chips				
barbecue	1 oz	8.0	140	51%
plain				
no salt added	1 oz	9.0	150	54%
regular	1 oz	9.0	150	54%
(Health Valley) Puffs/fat-free				
caramel corn				
apple cinnamoon	1 cup	–	110	–
original	1 cup	–	110	–
green onion cheese flavor	1½ cups	–	110	–
original cheese flavor	1½ cups	–	110	–
(Keebler) Pizzarias pizza chips				
cheese flavor	14 chips	7.0	150	42%
supreme flavor	14 chips	7.0	150	42%
zesty pepperoni flavor	14 chips	7.0	150	42$
(Kraft) Handi-Snacks				
cheez 'n breadsticks	1 pkg	7.0	130	48%
cheez 'n crackers	1 pkg	8.0	130	55%
cheez 'n pretzels	1 pkg	6.0	110	49%
peanut butter 'n crackers	1 pkg	12.0	180	60%
peanut butter 'n grahamsticks	1 pkg	10.0	170	53%
(Krun-Chee's) corn snacks				
Cheez Snaps	¾ cup	10.0	160	56%
Cheeze-Eze	2½ cups	12.0	170	64%
Puffins				
butter flavored	2½ cups	12.0	180	60%
cheese flavored	2½ cups	10.0	160	56%
(Lance)				
cheese balls	1 oz	8.0	150	48%
crunchy cheese twists	1 oz	12.0	160	68%
hot fries	⅞ oz	10.0	140	64%
onion rings	⅞ oz	6.0	120	45%
	1 oz	10.0	210	43%
pork skins				
BBQ	⁷⁄₁₆ oz	4.0	60	60%
	1 oz	10.0	150	60%
plain	⁷⁄₁₆ oz	4.0	65	55%
	1 oz	10.0	150	60%
(Laura Scudder) cheese-flavored snacks				
crunchy	½ cup	11.0	150	66%
puffed	1¼ cups	9.0	150	54%

Food and Description	Amount	Fat Grams	Total Calories	% Fat Calories
(Lawry's) Flavor Tree				
Cajun hot sticks	¼ cup	9.0	133	61%
cheddar sticks	¼ cup	8.0	129	56%
honey-roasted	¼ cup	9.0	138	59%
jalapeño & cheddar	¼ cup	8.0	129	56%
oat bran	¼ cup	7.5	124	54%
sesame chips	¼ cup	9.0	163	50%
sesame sticks				
no salt	¼ cup	8.0	131	55%
regular	¼ cup	9.0	133	61%
sour cream & onion	¼ cup	8.0	127	57%
(Lite Munchies)				
Bar B Que	0.5 oz	2.0	60	30%
nacho cheese	0.5 oz	2.0	60	30%
toasted onion	0.5 oz	2.0	60	30%
(M&M★Mars) Combos				
cheddar cheese w/pretzel shell				
family pack	1 oz	5.0	130	35%
singles	1.8 oz	9.0	240	34%
chili cheese w/corn shell				
family pack	1 oz	6.0	140	39%
singles	1.7 oz	11.0	230	43%
mustard w/pretzel shell				
family pack	1 oz	4.0	130	28%
singles	1.8 oz	8.0	230	31%
nacho cheese w/pretzel shell				
family pack	1 oz	5.0	130	35%
singles	1.7 oz	8.0	230	31%
nacho cheese w/tortilla shell				
family pack	1 oz	6.0	140	39%
singles	1.7 oz	11.0	230	43%
pepperoni & cheese pizza				
family pack	1 oz	7.0	140	45%
singles	1.7 oz	11.0	240	41%
pizzeria w/pretzel shell				
family pack	1 oz	4.0	130	28%
singles	1.8 oz	8.0	230	31%
tortilla ranch flavor				
family pack	1 oz	7.0	140	45%
singles	1.7 oz	12.0	240	45%
(Max Snax) rice curls				
caramel	33 pieces	3.0	135	20%
cheese & tomato	33 pieces	5.0	160	28%
garlic & basil	35 pieces	4.0	130	26%
nacho cheddar	35 pieces	4.0	140	26%
sour cream & onion	35 pieces	5.0	140	32%
white cheddar	35 pieces	5.0	140	32%

Food and Description	Amount	Fat Grams	Total Calories	% Fat Calories
(Michael Season's)				
Shape Ups				
original	1 cup	1.0	130	7%
salsa	¾ cup	1.5	120	11%
snack chips				
oat bran	1 oz	10.0	150	60%
white cheddar	1 oz	11.0	160	62%
(Munchos)	1 oz	10.0	150	60%
(Nabisco) Zings snack chips	1 bag	11.0	240	41%
(Pacific Grain) Gourmet Puffs				
cheese	1 oz	–	110	–
ranch	1 oz	–	110	–
(Pepperidge Farm) Snack Sticks				
pretzel	9 sticks	3.0	130	21%
pumpernickel	9 sticks	6.0	150	36%
sesame	9 sticks	6.0	150	36%
three cheese	9 sticks	5.0	150	32%
(Planter's)				
Cheez Balls	1 oz	10.0	150	60%
Cheez Curls	1 oz	10.0	150	60%
	1.2 oz	12.0	180	60%
(Poppycock)	½ cup	10.0	180	50%
(Ray's) Taro Chips				
salted	1 oz	6.0	140	39%
unsalted	1 oz	6.0	140	39%
(Sargento) Mootown Snackers				
cheese & pretzels	1 unit	3.0	90	30%
cheeze & sticks	1 unit	4.0	100	36%
cookies & creme				
honey graham sticks w/sprinkles	1 unit	7.0	140	45%
vanilla sticks & chocolate fudge cream	1 unit	6.0	130	42%
(Skinny Haven) Skinny Munchies				
chocolate fudge	0.5 oz	2.0	66	27%
nacho cheese	0.5 oz	2.0	59	31%
smoky Bar B Q	0.5 oz	2.0	59	31%
toasted onion	0.5 oz	2.0	59	31%
(Spicer's) crunchy diet snacks				
barbecue	1 oz	5.0	100	45%
cheddar	1 oz	5.0	100	45%
chocolate	1 oz	4.0	100	36%
natural	1 oz	4.0	100	36%
sour cream & onion	1 oz	5.0	100	45%
(SunChips)				
French onion	1 oz	6.0	140	39%
harvest cheddar	1 oz	6.0	140	39%
original	1 oz	7.0	140	45%
(Super Snax)				
hot & spicy	½ cup	7.0	140	45%

Food and Description	Amount	Fat Grams	Total Calories	% Fat Calories
original	½ cup	5.0	140	32%
(Ultra Slim Fast) cheese curls	1 oz	3.0	110	25%
(Upper Crust) Croissant Snack Stix				
garlic	1 piece	2.0	30	60%
original	1 piece	2.0	30	60%
sesame	1 piece	2.0	30	60%
(Weight Watchers) Smart Snackers				
bar-be-que	0.5 oz	1.5	60	23%
cheese curls	0.5 oz	2.5	70	32%
pizza flavored	0.5 oz	2.0	60	30%
ranch flavored	0.5 oz	2.0	60	30%
(Wise)				
Cheese Doodles				
crunchy/Wise Choice	1 oz	4.5	130	31%
fried				
hot	1 oz	9.0	150	54%
original	1 oz	9.0	150	54%
puff/Wise Choice	1 oz	0.5	90	5%
cheese waffles	6 pieces	8.0	140	51%
corn puffs/baked	1 oz	8.0	150	48%
Doodle O's/baked cheese-flavored	1 oz	11.0	160	62%
onion-flavored rings	1 oz	6.0	140	39%
SNAIL/ESCARGOT				
canned				
(Reese) Maurice precooked/ French helix	6 pieces	1.0	45	20%
fresh				
cooked-moist heat	3 oz	1.0	230	4%
raw	3 oz	<1.0	117	4%
SNAP BEAN (See GREEN BEAN)				
SNAPPER				
cooked-dry heat	3 oz	1.5	110	12%
raw	3 oz	1.0	85	11%
SNOW PEA				
fresh/cooked	½ cup	–	35	–
frozen				
(Birds Eye) deluxe	3 oz	–	35	–
(C&W) microwaveable box				
baby pod peas	3 oz	–	40	–
baby pod peas w/water chestnuts	⅔ cup	–	40	–
(La Choy) snow pea pods	½ pkg	<1.0	35	13%
SOCKEYE (See SALMON)				
SODA (See COCKTAIL MIXER; SOFT DRINK; SPORTS DRINK)				
SOFT DRINK (See also FRUIT PUNCH; SOFT DRINK MIX; SPORTS DRINK; TEA; individual juice drink listings)				
(A&W)				
cream soda				
diet	8 fl oz	–	–	–

Food and Description	Amount	Fat Grams	Total Calories	% Fat Calories
regular	8 fl oz	–	110	–
root beer				
diet	8 fl oz	–	–	–
regular	8 fl oz	–	110	–
(Arizona) Cowboy Cocktail				
grape kiwi	8 fl oz	–	120	–
kiwi strawberry	8 fl oz	–	120	–
Mucho Mango	8 fl oz	–	100	–
strawberry punch	8 fl oz	–	120	–
(Canada Dry)				
Barrelhead root beer	8 fl oz	–	110	–
birch beer				
brown	8 fl oz	–	110	–
clear	8 fl oz	–	110	–
Black Cherry Wishnish	8 fl oz	–	130	–
Cactus Cooler soda	8 fl oz	–	110	–
California strawberry soda	8 fl oz	–	110	–
club soda				
regular	8 fl oz	–	–	–
sodium-free	8 fl oz	–	–	–
Concord grape soda	8 fl oz	–	120	–
ginger ale				
cherry				
diet	8 fl oz	–	–	–
regular	8 fl oz	–	100	–
cranberry				
diet	8 fl oz	–	–	–
regular	8 fl oz	–	90	–
golden	8 fl oz	–	100	–
lemon				
diet	8 fl oz	–	–	–
regular	8 fl oz	–	90	–
plain				
diet	8 fl oz	–	–	–
regular	8 fl oz	–	90	–
peach soda	8 fl oz	–	120	–
piña pineapple soda	8 fl oz	–	110	–
Sunripe orange soda	8 fl oz	–	140	–
Tahitian treat soda	8 fl oz	–	150	–
vanilla cream soda/brown or clear	8 fl oz	–	120	–
wild cherry soda	8 fl oz	–	110	–
(Canfield's)				
cherry fudge soda	12 fl oz	–	–	–
chocolate fudge soda	12 fl oz	–	–	–
(Coca-Cola)				
Coca-Cola				
cherry				
diet	8 fl oz	–	1	–

Food and Description	Amount	Fat Grams	Total Calories	% Fat Calories
regular	8 fl oz	–	104	–
classic				
caffeine-free	8 fl oz	–	97	–
regular	8 fl oz	–	97	–
Coke II	8 fl oz	–	105	–
Diet Coke				
caffeine-free	8 fl oz	–	1	–
regular	8 fl oz	–	1	–
Fanta				
ginger ale	8 fl oz	–	86	–
grape	8 fl oz	–	117	–
orange	8 fl oz	–	118	–
root beer	8 fl oz	–	111	–
Fresca	8 fl oz	–	3	–
Mello Yello				
diet	8 fl oz	–	3	–
regular	8 fl oz	–	119	–
Minute Maid				
berry soda	8 fl oz	–	111	–
black cherry soda	8 fl oz	–	110	–
fruit punch				
carbonated	8 fl oz	–	117	–
noncarbonated	8 fl oz	–	119	–
grape soda	8 fl oz	–	121	–
grapefruit soda	8 fl oz	–	108	–
lemonade	8 fl oz	–	106	–
orange soda				
diet	8 fl oz	–	2	–
regular	8 fl oz	–	118	–
peach soda	8 fl oz	–	110	–
pineapple soda	8 fl oz	–	109	–
raspberry soda	8 fl oz	–	111	–
strawberry soda	8 fl oz	–	122	–
Mr. Pibb				
diet	8 fl oz	–	1	–
regular	8 fl oz	–	97	–
Sprite				
diet	8 fl oz	–	3	–
regular	8 fl oz	–	96	–
Tab	8 fl oz	–	1	–
(Country Time)				
black raspberry	8 fl oz	–	110	–
lemonade				
kiwi berry	8 fl oz	–	110	–
original	8 fl oz	–	120	–
pink	8 fl oz	–	120	–
tangerine	8 fl oz	–	110	–

Food and Description	Amount	Fat Grams	Total Calories	% Fat Calories
(Crush)				
cherry	6 fl oz	–	100	–
grape	6 fl oz	–	100	–
orange				
diet	6 fl oz	–	12	–
regular	6 fl oz	–	100	–
pineapple	6 fl oz	–	100	–
strawberry	6 fl oz	–	90	–
vanilla cream	6 fl oz	–	90	–
(Diet Rite)				
black cherry soda	12 fl oz	–	–	–
cola	12 fl oz	–	–	–
fruit punch	12 fl oz	–	–	–
golden peach soda	12 fl oz	–	–	–
key lime soda	12 fl oz	–	12	–
pink grapefruit soda	12 fl oz	–	–	–
red raspberry soda	12 fl oz	–	–	–
tangerine soda	12 fl oz	–	–	–
white grape soda	12 fl oz	–	–	–
(Dr. Pepper)				
diet				
caffeine-free	12 fl oz	–	–	–
regular	12 fl oz	–	–	–
regular				
caffeine-free	12 fl oz	–	160	–
regular	12 fl oz	–	160	–
(Ginseng Up) original or cola	12 fl oz	–	150	–
(Hansen's) natural				
cherry	12 fl oz	–	120	–
orange	12 fl oz	–	130	–
raspberry	12 fl oz	–	130	–
strawberry	12 fl oz	–	130	–
(Health Valley)				
ginger ale	12 fl oz	1.0	153	6%
root beer/old fashioned	12 fl oz	1.0	120	8%
sarsaparilla	12 fl oz	1.0	153	6%
wild berry	12 fl oz	1.0	142	6%
(Hires)				
cream soda				
diet	6 fl oz	–	2	–
regular	6 fl oz	–	90	–
root beer				
diet	6 fl oz	–	2	–
regular	6 fl oz	–	90	–
(IBC)				
cream soda				
diet	12 fl oz	–	4	–
regular	12 fl oz	–	170	–

Food and Description	Amount	Fat Grams	Total Calories	% Fat Calories
root beer				
diet	12 fl oz	–	2	–
regular	12 fl oz	–	160	–
(Jolt) cola	12 fl oz	–	150	–
(Josta)	20 fl oz	–	110	–
(Kool-Aid) Bursts				
cherry	6.75 fl oz	–	100	–
grape	6.75 fl oz	–	100	–
Great Bluedini	6.75 fl oz	–	100	–
Incrediberry	6.75 fl oz	–	100	–
orange punch	6.75 fl oz	–	100	–
Pink Swimmingo	6.75 fl oz	–	100	–
Rock-A-Dile Red	6.75 fl oz	–	100	–
tropical punch	6.75 fl oz	–	100	–
(Mountain Dew)				
diet				
caffeine-free	12 fl oz	–	–	–
regular	12 fl oz	–	–	–
regular				
caffeine-free	12 fl oz	–	170	–
regular	12 fl oz	–	170	–
(Mug)				
cream soda				
diet	12 fl oz	–	5	–
regular	12 fl oz	–	170	–
root beer				
diet	12 fl oz	–	–	–
regular	12 fl oz	–	160	–
(Nehi)				
cream	8 fl oz	–	120	–
fruit punch	8 fl oz	–	120	–
ginger ale	8 fl oz	–	90	–
grape	8 fl oz	–	120	–
orange	8 fl oz	–	130	–
peach	8 fl oz	–	130	–
pineapple	8 fl oz	–	130	–
root beer	8 fl oz	–	120	–
strawberry	8 fl oz	–	120	–
(Pepsi)				
crystal	12 fl oz	–	150	–
diet				
caffeine-free	12 fl oz	–	–	–
regular	12 fl oz	–	–	–
regular				
caffeine-free	12 fl oz	–	150	–
regular	12 fl oz	–	150	–
wild cherry	12 fl oz	–	160	–
(Pirate's Keg) root beer	12 fl oz	–	170	–

Food and Description	Amount	Fat Grams	Total Calories	% Fat Calories
(Royal Crown)				
cherry cola	8 fl oz	–	110	–
cola				
diet				
caffeine-free	8 fl oz	–	–	–
regular	8 fl oz	–	–	–
regular				
caffeine-free	8 fl oz	–	110	–
regular	8 fl oz	–	110	–
(Schweppes)				
club soda				
regular	8 fl oz	–	–	–
sodium-free	8 fl oz	–	–	–
ginger ale				
grape				
diet	8 fl oz	–	2	–
regular	8 fl oz	–	100	–
plain				
diet	8 fl oz	–	–	–
regular	8 fl oz	–	90	–
raspberry				
diet	8 fl oz	–	–	–
regular	8 fl oz	–	100	–
ginger beer	8 fl oz	–	100	–
grape soda	8 fl oz	–	130	–
grapefruit soda	8 fl oz	–	110	–
lemon-lime soda	8 fl oz	–	100	–
tonic water				
citrus	8 fl oz	–	90	–
cranberry	8 fl oz	–	90	–
plain				
diet	8 fl oz	–	–	–
regular	8 fl oz	–	90	–
raspberry	8 fl oz	–	90	–
(7-Up)				
cherry				
diet	12 fl oz	–	–	–
regular	12 fl oz	–	160	–
regular				
diet	12 fl oz	–	–	–
regular	12 fl oz	–	160	–
(Shasta)				
birch beer/diet	12 fl oz	–	4	–
black cherry	12 fl oz	–	162	–
cherry cola	12 fl oz	–	140	–
citrus mist	12 fl oz	–	170	–
club soda	12 fl oz	–	–	–

Food and Description	Amount	Fat Grams	Total Calories	% Fat Calories
cola				
diet	12 fl oz	–	–	–
free	12 fl oz	–	151	–
regular	12 fl oz	–	147	–
creme	12 fl oz	–	154	–
Dr. Diablo	12 fl oz	–	140	–
fruit punch	12 fl oz	–	173	–
ginger ale	12 fl oz	–	120	–
grape	12 fl oz	–	117	–
lemon lime	12 fl oz	–	146	–
orange	12 fl oz	–	177	–
red berry	12 fl oz	–	158	–
red pop	12 fl oz	–	158	–
root beer	12 fl oz	–	154	–
strawberry	12 fl oz	–	147	–
(Sioux City) sarsaparilla				
bottled	12 fl oz	–	110	–
canned	16 fl oz	–	170	–
(Slice)				
cherry spice	12 fl oz	–	150	–
cola	12 fl oz	–	160	–
fruit punch	12 fl oz	–	190	–
grape soda	12 fl oz	–	190	–
lemon lime soda				
diet	12 fl oz	–	–	–
regular	12 fl oz	–	150	–
Mandarin orange soda				
diet	12 fl oz	–	–	–
regular	12 fl oz	–	190	–
pineapple soda	12 fl oz	–	190	–
red	12 fl oz	–	190	–
strawberry soda	12 fl oz	–	170	–
(Snapple)				
Bali blast	8 fl oz	–	120	–
cherry lime rickey	8 fl oz	–	110	–
creme d'vanilla	8 fl oz	–	130	–
French cherry	8 fl oz	–	120	–
kiwi strawberry	8 fl oz	–	130	–
passion supreme	8 fl oz	–	120	–
peach Melba	8 fl oz	–	120	–
raspberry royale	8 fl oz	–	120	–
true root beer	8 fl oz	–	110	–
(Soho)				
black cherry	12.3 fl oz	–	160	–
old-fashioned root beer	12.3 fl oz	–	140	–
purely peach	12.3 fl oz	–	160	–
really raspberry	12.3 fl oz	–	130	–

Food and Description	Amount	Fat Grams	Total Calories	% Fat Calories
(Squirt)				
orange	8 fl oz	–	100	–
original	12 fl oz	–	150	–
ruby red	8 fl oz	–	120	–
(Stewart's)				
cream ale	12 fl oz	–	180	–
country orange n' cream	12 fl oz	–	190	–
ginger beer	12 fl oz	–	200	–
root beer				
diet	12 fl oz	–	–	–
original	12 fl oz	–	160	–
(Sun Drop)				
cherry	6 fl oz	–	90	–
regular				
diet	6 fl oz	–	2	–
regular	6 fl oz	–	100	–
(Sunkist)				
cherry	8 fl oz	–	140	–
citrus				
diet	8 fl oz	–	–	–
regular	8 fl oz	–	100	–
fruit punch	8 fl oz	–	130	–
lemonade				
diet sparkling	8 fl oz	–	–	–
regular	8 fl oz	–	120	–
orange				
diet	8 fl oz	–	5	–
regular	8 fl oz	–	140	–
peach	8 fl oz	–	120	–
pineapple	8 fl oz	–	140	–
strawberry	8 fl oz	–	140	–
(TreeTop) Juice Fizz				
cola cooler	8 fl oz	–	110	–
fruit punch	8 fl oz	–	130	–
Maui magic	8 fl oz	–	120	–
purple thunder	8 fl oz	–	130	–
wild red wonder	8 fl oz	–	120	–
(Vernor's) Ginger Soda				
diet	12 fl oz	–	–	–
regular	12 fl oz	–	150	–
(Welch's) sparkling sodas				
apple	12 fl oz	–	200	–
fruit punch	12 fl oz	–	210	–
grape	12 fl oz	–	200	–
orange	12 fl oz	–	200	–
peach	12 fl oz	–	220	–
pineappple	12 fl oz	–	210	–
strawberry	12 fl oz	–	200	–

Food and Description	Amount	Fat Grams	Total Calories	% Fat Calories
(Yoo-Hoo) chocolate	12 fl oz	1.5	180	8%

SOFT DRINK MIX (*See also* FRUIT PUNCH; SOFT DRINK; SPORTS DRINK; individual fruit drink listings)

Food and Description	Amount	Fat Grams	Total Calories	% Fat Calories
(Crystal Light)				
citrus blend	⅛ tub	–	5	–
cranberry breeze	⅛ tub	–	5	–
fruit punch	⅛ tub	–	5	–
lemon-lime	⅛ tub	–	5	–
pink grapefruit	⅛ tub	–	5	–
raspberry ice	⅛ tub	–	5	–
(Kool-Aid)				
black cherry/unsweetened				
mix only	⅛ pkg	–	–	–
prepared w/sugar & water	8 fl oz	–	100	–
cherry				
sugar-free	⅛ pkg	–	5	–
sugar-sweetened	⅛ pkg	–	60	–
unsweetened				
mix only	⅛ pkg	–	–	–
prepared w/sugar & water	8 fl oz	–	100	–
grape				
sugar-free	⅛ pkg	–	5	–
sugar-sweetened	⅛ pkg	–	60	–
unsweetened				
mix only	⅛ pkg	–	–	–
prepared w/sugar & water	8 fl oz	–	100	–
Great Bluedini				
sugar-free	⅛ pkg	–	5	–
sugar-sweetened	⅛ pkg	–	60	–
unsweetened				
mix only	⅛ pkg	–	–	–
prepared w/sugar & water	8 fl oz	–	100	–
Incrediberry				
sugar-free	⅛ pkg	–	5	–
sugar-sweetened	⅛ pkg	–	60	–
unsweetened				
mix only	⅛ pkg	–	–	–
prepared w/sugar & water	8 fl oz	–	100	–
Kickin' Kiwi-Lime/unsweetened				
mix only	⅛ pkg	–	–	–
prepared w/sugar & water	8 fl oz	–	100	–
lemonade				
sugar-free	⅛ pkg	–	5	–
sugar-sweetened	⅛ pkg	–	60	–
unsweetened				
mix only	⅛ pkg	–	–	–
prepared w/sugar & water	8 fl oz	–	100	–

Food and Description	Amount	Fat Grams	Total Calories	% Fat Calories
lemon-lime/unsweetened				
mix only	⅛ pkg	–	–	–
prepared w/sugar & water	8 fl oz	–	100	–
Man-O-Mango-Berry/unsweetened				
mix only	⅛ pkg	–	–	–
prepared w/sugar & water	8 fl oz	–	100	–
Oh Yeah Orange-Pineapple/unsweetened				
mix only	⅛ pkg	–	–	–
prepared w/sugar & water	8 fl oz	–	100	–
orange				
sugar-sweetened	⅛ pkg	–	60	–
unsweetened				
mix only	⅛ pkg	–	–	–
prepared w/sugar & water	8 fl oz	–	100	–
piña pineapple				
sugar-sweetened	⅛ pkg	–	60	–
unsweetened				
mix only	⅛ pkg	–	–	–
prepared w/sugar & water	8 fl oz	–	100	–
pink lemonade/unsweetened				
mix only	⅛ pkg	–	–	–
prepared w/sugar & water	8 fl oz	–	100	–
Pink Swimmingo				
sugar-free	⅛ pkg	–	5	–
sugar-sweetened	⅛ pkg	–	60	–
unsweetened				
mix only	⅛ pkg	–	–	–
prepared w/sugar & water	8 fl oz	–	100	–
Purplesaurus Rex				
sugar-free	⅛ pkg	–	5	–
sugar-sweetened	⅛ pkg	–	60	–
unsweetened				
mix only	⅛ pkg	–	–	–
prepared w/sugar & water	8 fl oz	–	100	–
raspberry				
sugar-sweetened	⅛ pkg	–	60	–
unsweetened				
mix only	⅛ pkg	–	–	–
prepared w/sugar & water	8 fl oz	–	100	–
Rock-A-Dile Red				
sugar-free	⅛ pkg	–	5	–
sugar-sweetened	⅛ pkg	–	60	–
unsweetened				
mix only	⅛ pkg	–	–	–
prepared w/sugar & water	8 fl oz	–	100	–
strawberry				
sugar-sweetened	⅛ pkg	–	60	–

Food and Description	Amount	Fat Grams	Total Calories	% Fat Calories
unsweetened				
mix only	⅛ pkg	–	–	–
prepared w/sugar & water	8 fl oz	–	100	–
tropical punch				
sugar-free	⅛ pkg	–	5	–
sugar-sweetened	⅛ pkg	–	60	–
unsweetened				
mix only	⅛ pkg	–	–	–
prepared w/sugar & water	8 fl oz	–	100	–
SOLE (See also FROZEN ENTRÉE/DINNER; SEAFOOD ENTRÉE/DINNER)				
baked w/butter	3 oz	6.0	120	45%
cooked-dry heat	3 oz	1.0	105	91%
raw	3 oz	1.0	80	11%
SORBET (See FRUIT ICES, BARS, & POPS; SHERBET)				
SORGHUM/whole-grain	1 cup	6.0	650	8%
SORGHUM SYRUP				
cane & maple	1 Tbs	–	53	–
	1 cup	–	794	–
regular	1 Tbs	–	53	–
	1 cup	–	848	–
table blend	1 Tbs	–	59	–
	1 cup	–	941	–

SORREL (See DOCK)
SOUP
(NOTE: Unless stated otherwise, condensed soups were prepared as directed with water. If prepared with milk, whole milk was used unless noted otherwise. If you use reduced-fat, low-fat, or skim milk, refer to the Quick Reference-Milk, below, to adjust your fat and calorie data. Ready-to-serve soups were heated as directed with no added liquid.)

QUICK REFERENCE: MILK	Amount	Fat Grams	Total Calories	% Fat Calories
Skim/fat-free	¼ cup	–	23	–
	½ cup	–	45	–
1% fat/light	¼ cup	0.5	26	17%
	½ cup	1.0	55	16%
2% fat/reduced fat	¼ cup	1.0	31	29%
	½ cup	2.5	61	37%
Whole	¼ cup	2.0	38	47%
	½ cup	4.0	75	48%

■ **CANNED/CONDENSED**
(Campbell's)
American recipe/unprepared
chicken vegetable

regular	½ cup	2.0	80	23%
Southwest style	½ cup	1.5	110	12%

Food and Description	Amount	Fat Grams	Total Calories	% Fat Calories
chicken w/white & wild rice	½ cup	2.0	70	26%
double noodle	½ cup	2.5	100	23%
New England clam chowder	½ cup	2.5	100	23%
vegetable				
California style	½ cup	1.0	60	15%
hearty/w/pasta	½ cup	1.0	90	10%
vegetarian	½ cup	1.0	70	13%
vegetable beef	½ cup	2.0	80	23%
Healthy Request/unprepared				
bean w/bacon	½ cup	5.0	180	25%
bean w/ham & bacon	½ cup	2.0	150	12%
celery, cream of	½ cup	2.0	70	26%
chicken, cream of	½ cup	2.0	70	26%
chicken & broccoli, cream of	½ cup	2.5	80	28%
chicken & stars	½ cup	2.0	70	26%
creamy chicken mushroom	½ cup	9.0	130	62%
chicken noodle				
regular	½ cup	3.0	70	39%
chicken noodleo's	½ cup	3.0	80	34%
chicken w/rice	½ cup	2.5	70	32%
hearty pasta & vegetables	½ cup	1.0	90	10%
minestrone	½ cup	1.0	90	10%
mushroom, cream of	½ cup	3.0	70	39%
potato, cream of	½ cup	3.0	100	27%
split pea w/ham & bacon	½ cup	3.5	180	18%
tomato	½ cup	2.0	100	18%
vegetable				
regular	½ cup	1.0	90	10%
w/beef stock	½ cup	2.0	90	20%
original/unprepared				
asparagus, cream of	½ cup	7.0	110	57%
bean w/bacon	½ cup	5.0	180	25%
beef broth	½ cup	–	15	–
beef consommé	½ cup	–	25	–
beef noodle	½ cup	2.5	70	32%
beef w/vegetables & barley	½ cup	2.0	80	23%
black bean	½ cup	2.0	120	15%
broccoli, cream of	½ cup	6.0	100	54%
broccoli cheese	½ cup	7.0	110	57%
celery, cream of				
reduced fat	½ cup	3.5	80	39%
regular	½ cup	7.0	110	57%
cheddar cheese	½ cup	10.0	150	60%
chicken, cream of/reduced fat	½ cup	4.0	80	45%
chicken broth	½ cup	2.0	30	60%
chicken gumbo	½ cup	1.5	60	23%
chicken noodle				
creamy	½ cup	7.0	130	48%

Food and Description	Amount	Fat Grams	Total Calories	% Fat Calories
double noodle	½ cup	2.5	100	23%
homestyle	½ cup	2.5	70	32%
original	½ cup	2.0	60	30%
chicken noodleo's	½ cup	3.0	80	34%
chicken & stars	½ cup	2.0	70	26%
chicken vegetable	½ cup	2.0	80	23%
chicken w/ rice	½ cup	3.0	70	39%
chicken w/white & wild rice	½ cup	2.0	70	26%
creamy chicken mushroom	½ cup	9.0	130	62%
French onion	½ cup	2.5	70	32%
golden mushroom	½ cup	3.0	80	34%
minestrone	½ cup	2.0	100	18%
mushroom, cream of				
reduced fat	½ cup	3.5	70	45%
regular	½ cup	7.0	110	57%
New England clam chowder	½ cup	2.5	100	23%
pepper pot	½ cup	5.0	100	45%
potato, cream of	½ cup	3.0	90	30%
Scotch broth	½ cup	3.0	80	34%
shrimp, cream of	½ cup	7.0	100	63%
split pea w/ham & bacon	½ cup	3.5	180	18%
tomato				
fiesta	½ cup	–	60	–
Italian	½ cup	0.5	100	5%
regular	½ cup	2.0	100	18%
turkey noodle	½ cup	2.5	80	28%
vegetable				
hearty/w/pasta	½ cup	1.0	90	10%
regular	½ cup	1.0	90	10%
vegetarian	½ cup	1.0	70	13%
vegetable beef	½ cup	2.0	80	23%
(Doxsee) New England clam chowder/ prepared w/skim milk	1 cup	2.0	130	14%
generic				
asparagus, cream of				
prepared w/milk	1 cup	9.0	170	48%
prepared w/water	1 cup	4.0	87	41%
black bean	1 cup	1.5	116	12%
black turtle bean	1 cup	–	218	–
bean w/franks	1 cup	7.0	187	34%
beef broth/prepared w/water	1 cup	1.0	19	47%
beef consommé				
prepared w/water	1 cup	–	25	–
unprepared	10.5 oz	–	71	–
beef mushroom	1 cup	3.0	73	37%
celery, cream of				
prepared w/milk	1 cup	9.7	165	53%
prepared w/water	1 cup	5.6	90	56%

Food and Description	Amount	Fat Grams	Total Calories	% Fat Calories
unprepared	10.75 oz	14.0	219	58%
cheese				
prepared w/milk	1 cup	14.6	230	57%
prepared w/water	1 cup	10.5	155	61%
unprepared	11 oz	25.0	377	60%
chicken, cream of/prepared w/water	1 cup	5.0	110	41%
chicken broth				
prepared w/water	1 cup	1.0	39	13%
unprepared	10.75 oz	3.0	94	29%
chicken mushroom	1 cup	9.0	132	61%
chicken noodle	1 cup	1.0	53	17%
chili beef				
prepared w/water	1 cup	6.6	169	35%
unprepared	11.25 oz	16.0	411	35%
green pea				
prepared w/milk	1 cup	7.0	239	26%
prepared w/water	1 cup	2.9	164	16%
leek	1 cup	2.0	70	26%
mushroom, cream of				
prepared w/milk	1 cup	13.6	203	60%
prepared w/water	1 cup	9.0	129	63%
unprepared	10.75 oz	23.0	313	66%
mushroom barley	2 cup	2.0	73	25%
mushroom w/beef stock	1 cup	4.0	85	42%
nacho cheese/prepared w/milk	1 cup	12.0	180	60%
onion				
prepared w/water	1 cup	1.7	57	27%
unprepared	10.5 oz	4.0	138	26%
oyster stew/prepared w/milk	1 cup	9.0	140	58%
pepper pot/unprepared	10.5 oz	11.0	251	39%
Scotch broth/unprepared	10.5 oz	6.0	195	28%
shrimp, cream of				
prepared w/milk	1 cup	10.0	160	56%
unprepared	10.75 oz	13.0	219	55%
stockpot				
prepared w/water	1 cup	3.9	100	35%
unprepared	11 oz	9.0	242	34%
tomato/prepared w/water	1 cup	2.0	100	18%
vichyssoise	1 cup	6.0	148	37%
(Gorton's) New England clam chowder	½ cup	1.0	70	13%
(Jake's) clam chowder	⅔ cup	11.0	200	50%
(Pepperidge Farm) semicondensed/prepared (Note: When milk was called for in preparation, 2% milk was used.)				
bacon, lettuce, & tomato	8 oz	8.0	170	42%
black bean	8 oz	2.0	110	16%
broccoli, cream of	8 oz	6.0	130	42%
chicken curry	8 oz	7.0	150	42%
chicken w/wild rice	8 oz	3.0	80	34%

Food and Description	Amount	Fat Grams	Total Calories	% Fat Calories
consommé madrilène	8 oz	5.0	60	75%
corn chowder	8 oz	9.0	180	45%
crab	8 oz	5.0	110	41%
French onion	8 oz	4.0	80	45%
gazpacho	8 oz	4.0	90	40%
hunter's	8 oz	3.0	90	30%
lobster bisque	8 oz	11.0	190	52%
New England clam chowder	8 oz	8.0	180	40%
oyster stew	8 oz	11.0	180	55%
shiitake mushroom	8 oz	3.0	70	39%
vichyssoise	8 oz	9.0	150	54%
watercress	8 oz	4.0	100	36%
(Pritikin) condensed/prepared				
chicken & rice	1 cup	1.0	80	11%
chicken broth	1 cup	–	15	–
chicken pasta	1 cup	1.0	100	9%
lentil	1 cup	0.5	130	3%
minestrone	1 cup	1.0	90	10%
split pea	1 cup	0.5	140	3%
three bean chili	½ cup	0.5	90	5%
vegetable				
hearty	1 cup	0.5	90	5%
vegetarian	1 cup	–	100	–
vegetable broth	1 cup	–	20	–
(Rokeach) prepared				
mushroom barley	1 cup	–	85	–
split pea w/egg barley	1 cup	0.5	130	3%
(Snow's)				
New England clam chowder/prepared	½ cup	1.5	80	17%
w/whole milk	7.5 oz	6.0	140	39%
New England corn chowder/prepared w/skim milk	1 cup	2.5	140	16%
New England fish chowder/prepared w/whole milk	7.5 oz	6.0	130	42%
■ CANNED/READY TO SERVE				
(Anderson's) split pea	1 cup	–	130	–
(Andre Prost) A Taste of Thai				
chili pepper lemon grass tom yum	1 cup	2.5	45	50%
coconut ginger tom ka	1 cup	5.0	100	45%
lemon grass basil poh taek	1 cup	0.5	35	13%
(Baxters)				
asparagus, cream of	1 cup	10.0	150	60%
country garden/99% fat-free	1 cup	0.5	70	6%
lobster bisque	1 cup	6.0	120	45%
minestrone/99% fat-free	1 cup	1.0	80	11%
onion/99% fat-free	1 cup	0.5	70	6%
potato & leek/100% fat-free	1 cup	–	60	–
royal gam soup	1 cup	2.5	90	25%

Food and Description	Amount	Fat Grams	Total Calories	% Fat Calories
tomato & brown lentil/100% fat-free (Campbell's)	1 cup	–	120	–
Chunky				
beef w/country vegetables	1 cup	4.0	160	23%
chicken broccoli cheese	1 cup	12.0	200	54%
chicken corn chowder	1 cup	15.0	250	54%
chicken mushroom chowder	1 cup	12.0	210	51%
chicken noodle				
classic	1 cup	3.0	130	21%
	10.75 oz	5.0	170	26%
w/mushrooms	1 cup	5.0	140	32%
chicken rice	1 cup	4.0	130	28%
chicken vegetable	1 cup	5.0	150	30%
clam chowder				
Manhattan	1 cup	4.0	130	28%
New England	1 cup	14.0	220	57%
	10.75 oz	17.0	280	55%
hearty bean 'n ham	1 cup	2.0	190	9%
hearty vegetables w/pasta	1 cup	3.0	130	21%
minestrone	1 cup	5.0	140	32%
mushroom, cream of	1 cup	13.0	170	69%
old-fashioned chicken	1 cup	3.0	130	21%
old-fashioned potato ham chowder	1 cup	14.0	220	57%
old-fashioned vegetable beef	1 cup	5.0	150	30%
sirloin burger w/country vegetables	1 cup	9.0	190	43%
spicy chicken & vegetables	1 cup	1.0	90	10%
vegetable	10.75 oz	4.0	160	23%
Healthy Request				
hearty chicken broth	1 cup	–	20	–
hearty chicken noodle	1 cup	3.0	160	17%
hearty chicken rice	1 cup	3.0	120	23%
hearty chicken vegetable	1 cup	2.0	120	15%
hearty vegetable beef	1 cup	2.5	140	16%
New England clam chowder	1 cup	3.0	110	25%
split pea w/ham	1 cup	2.0	170	11%
turkey vegetable w/white & wild rice	1 cup	2.5	120	19%
vegetable				
hearty	1 cup	1.0	100	9%
Southwestern w/black beans & rice	1 cup	1.0	140	6%
zesty penne & vegetables	1 cup	0.5	90	5%
Home Cookin'				
chicken noodle	1 cup	3.5	100	31%
chicken vegetable	1 cup	3.5	130	24%
chicken w/egg noodles	1 cup	3.5	100	32%
country mushroom rice	1 cup	1.0	100	9%
fiesta	1 cup	2.5	130	17%
minestrone				
regular	1 cup	2.0	120	15%

Food and Description	Amount	Fat Grams	Total Calories	% Fat Calories
Tuscany style	1 cup	7.0	160	39%
mushroom, cream of	1 cup	13.0	170	69%
New England clam chowder	1 cup	16.0	210	69%
salsa bean				
tomato garden	1 cup	3.0	130	21%
vegetable				
harborside	1 cup	2.0	100	18%
Italian	1 cup	4.0	100	36%
low-sodium				
chicken noodle	1 cup	3.0	80	34%
regular/single serving				
chicken noodle	1 can	2.0	60	30%
chicken w/rice	1 can	2.0	50	36%
mushroom, cream of	1 can	8.0	100	72%
tomato	1 can	2.0	110	16%
vegetable	1 can	2.0	70	26%
vegetable beef	1 can	3.0	60	45%
(College Inn) broth				
beef	1 cup	–	16	–
chicken				
lower salt	1 cup	2.0	20	90%
regular	1 cup	3.0	35	77%
generic				
beef broth	1 cup	0.5	16	28%
	14 oz	1.0	27	33%
chicken noodle w/meatballs	1 cup	3.6	99	33%
	20 oz	8.0	227	32%
chicken vegetable				
chunky	9.5 oz	6.0	170	32%
regular	9.5 oz	4.8	167	26%
chunky turkey	1 cup	4.0	136	27%
crab	1 cup	1.5	76	18%
escarole	1 cup	2.0	27	67%
gazpacho	1 cup	2.0	57	32%
	13 oz	3.0	87	31%
lentil w/ham	1 cup	2.8	140	18%
	13 oz	6.0	320	17%
Manhattan clam chowder	1 cup	3.0	133	21%
minestrone				
regular	1 cup	2.0	80	23%
w/Italian sausage	1.5 oz	8.0	169	43%
(Gold's)				
borscht				
low-cal	1 cup	–	20	–
original	1 cup	–	100	–
schav	1 cup	–	25	–
(Gorton's)				
New England clam chowder	1 cup	6.0	140	39%

Food and Description	Amount	Fat Grams	Total Calories	% Fat Calories
(Hain)				
Healthy Naturals				
black bean	1 cup	0.5	130	3%
mushroom barley	1 cup	1.0	100	9%
vegetable broth				
no salt added	1 cup	–	45	–
regular	1 cup	–	45	–
vegetarian lentil				
no salt added	1 cup	0.5	170	3%
regular	1 cup	0.5	170	3%
vegetarian split pea				
no salt added	1 cup	0.5	110	4%
regular	1 cup	0.5	110	4%
wild rice	1 cup	2.0	80	23%
Home Style Naturals				
chicken broth	1 cup	2.0	30	60%
chicken noodle				
no salt added	1 cup	2.0	80	23%
regular	1 cup	2.0	90	20%
chunky tomato	1 cup	0.5	80	6%
minestrone	1 cup	4.0	150	24%
mushroom, cream of	1 cup	3.0	90	30%
International				
chicken burrito	1 cup	1.0	110	8%
hot & sour	1 cup	3.0	70	39%
ravioli pomodoro	1 cup	3.0	150	18%
tortellini primavera	1 cup	1.0	80	11%
(Health Valley) fat-free				
beef broth	1 cup	–	20	–
black bean & vegetable	1 cup	–	110	–
chicken broth	1 cup	–	30	–
country corn & vegetable	1 cup	–	70	–
5 bean vegetable	1 cup	–	140	–
14 garden vegetable	1 cup	–	80	–
Italian plus carotene	1 cup	–	80	–
lentil & carrots	1 cup	–	90	–
pasta Bolognese	1 cup	–	70	–
pasta cacciatore	1 cup	–	90	–
pasta fagioli	1 cup	–	80	–
pasta primavera	1 cup	–	80	–
pasta Romano	1 cup	–	140	–
real Italian minestrone	1 cup	–	80	–
rotini & vegetable	1 cup	–	20	–
split pea & carrots	1 cup	–	110	–
super broccoli carotene	1 cup	–	70	–
tomato vegetable	1 cup	–	80	–
vegetable barley	1 cup	–	90	–
vegetable power carotene	1 cup	–	70	–

Food and Description	Amount	Fat Grams	Total Calories	% Fat Calories
(Healthy Choice)				
bean & ham	1 cup	3.0	250	11%
beef & potato	1 cup	1.5	120	11%
chicken				
cream of				
w/mushrooms	1 cup	2.0	130	14%
w/vegetables	1 cup	2.0	130	14%
hearty	1 cup	2.5	130	17%
chicken corn chowder	1 cup	3.0	176	15%
chicken pasta	1 cup	3.0	120	23%
chicken w/rice	1 cup	3.0	110	25%
chili beef	1 cup	1.5	165	8%
clam chowder	1 cup	1.0	120	8%
minestrone	1 cup	1.0	110	8%
mushroom, cream of	1 cup	1.0	80	11%
lentil	1 cup	1.0	145	6%
old-fashioned chicken noodle	1 cup	2.0	140	19%
split pea & ham	1 cup	2.0	155	12%
tomato garden	1 cup	2.0	110	16%
turkey w/wild rice	1 cup	2.0	90	20%
vegetable				
country	1 cup	1.0	105	9%
garden	1 cup	1.0	120	8%
vegetable beef	1 cup	1.0	130	7%
(Manischewitz)				
borscht				
low-cal	1 cup	–	25	–
original w/beets	1 cup	–	90	–
chicken rice	1 cup	–	47	–
chicken vegetable	1 cup	–	55	–
schav	1 cup	–	12	–
split pea	1 cup	–	133	–
vegetable	1 cup	–	63	–
(Mother's) borscht				
low-cal	1 cup	–	25	–
old fashioned	1 cup	–	100	–
(Old El Paso)				
black bean w/bacon	1 cup	1.5	160	8%
chicken vegetable	1 cup	2.5	110	20%
chicken w/rice	1 cup	2.5	90	25%
garden vegetable	1 cup	2.5	110	20%
hearty beef	1 cup	2.5	120	19%
hearty chicken noodle	1 cup	3.0	110	25%
(Progresso)				
Healthy Classics				
beef barley	1 cup	2.0	140	13%
beef vegetable	1 cup	1.5	150	9%
broccoli, cream of	1 cup	3.0	90	30%

Food and Description	Amount	Fat Grams	Total Calories	% Fat Calories
chicken noodle	1 cup	2.0	80	23%
chicken rice w/vegetables	1 cup	1.5	90	15%
garlic & pasta	1 cup	1.5	100	14%
lentil	1 cup	1.5	130	10%
minestrone	1 cup	2.5	120	19%
New England clam chowder	1 cup	2.0	120	15%
split pea	1 cup	2.5	180	13%
tomato garden vegetable	1 cup	1.0	100	9%
vegetable	1 cup	1.5	80	17%
original				
bean & ham	1 cup	2.0	160	11%
beef barley	1 cup	4.0	130	28%
beef noodle	1 cup	3.5	140	23%
black bean/hearty	1 cup	1.5	170	8%
chickarina	1 cup	5.0	120	38%
chicken				
cream of	1 cup	10.0	170	53%
hearty	10.5 oz	2.5	120	19%
w/vegetables/homestyle	1 cup	2.5	100	23%
chicken & wild rice	1 cup	2.0	100	18%
chicken barley	1 cup	2.5	110	20%
chicken broth	1 cup	0.5	20	23%
chicken noodle	1 cup	2.0	80	23%
	10.5 oz	2.5	110	20%
chicken rice w/vegetables	1 cup	3.0	110	25%
	10.5 oz	4.0	130	28%
clam chowder				
Manhattan	1 cup	2.0	110	16%
New England	1 cup	10.0	180	50%
	10.5 oz	12.0	220	49%
corn chowder	1 cup	10.0	180	50%
escarole in chicken broth	1 cup	1.0	25	36%
green split pea	1 cup	3.0	170	16%
lentil	1 cup	2.0	140	13%
	10.5 oz	2.5	170	13%
lentil w/sausage	1 cup	7.0	170	37%
macaroni & bean	1 cup	4.0	160	23%
minestrone				
beef	1 cup	4.0	140	26%
chicken	1 cup	3.5	120	26%
regular	1 cup	2.5	130	17%
	10.5 oz	3.5	170	19%
zesty	1 cup	6.0	150	36%
mushroom, cream of	1 cup	8.0	140	51%
split pea w/ham	1 cup	4.0	160	23%
tomato	1 cup	2.0	90	20%
tomato beef & rotini	1 cup	4.5	140	29%

Food and Description	Amount	Fat Grams	Total Calories	% Fat Calories
tortellini				
creamy	1 cup	15.0	210	64%
in chicken broth	1 cup	2.0	80	23%
vegetable	1 cup	2.0	90	20%
pasta soup				
beef vegetable & rotini	1 cup	3.5	120	26%
broccoli & shells	1 cup	1.0	70	13%
chicken vegetables & penne	1 cup	2.5	100	23%
clam & rotini chowder	1 cup	9.0	200	41%
chicken & rotini/hearty	1 cup	2.0	90	20%
minestrone w/shells/hearty	1 cup	1.5	120	11%
penne in chicken broth/hearty	1 cup	1.0	70	13%
tomato & rotini/hearty	1 cup	1.0	90	10%
vegetable rotini/hearty	1 cup	1.0	110	8%
lentil & shells	1 cup	1.5	130	10%
meatballs & pasta pearls	1 cup	7.0	140	45%
spicy chicken & penne	1 cup	4.0	120	30%
tomato tortellini	1 cup	5.0	120	38%
(Rokeach) borscht				
diet	1 cup	–	30	–
no salt	1 cup	–	100	–
regular	1 cup	–	100	–
(Swanson) broth				
beef	1 cup	1.0	20	45%
chicken				
naturally good	1 cup	1.0	25	36%
original	1 cup	2.0	30	60%
fat-free natural goodness	1 cup	–	15	–
Oriental	1 cup	–	15	–
vegetable	1 cup	1.0	20	45%
(Weight Watchers)				
chicken & rice	10.5 oz	1.5	110	12%
chicken noodle	10.5 oz	2.0	150	12%
minestrone	10.5 oz	2.0	130	14%
vegetable	10.5 oz	1.0	130	7%
(Westbrae) Soups of the World				
Alabama black bean	1 cup	–	80	–
Great Plains savory bean	1 cup	–	70	–
Old World split pea	1 cup	–	110	–
rich Mediterranean lentil	1 cup	–	100	–
Santa Fe vegetable	1 cup	–	120	–
■ DEHYDRATED/MIX OR CUBE				
(Andre Prost) A Taste of Thai				
chili pepper/prepared	1 cup	2.0	40	45%
tangy coconut ginger/mix only	2 tsp	1.0	15	60%
(Aunt Patsy's Pantry)				
island black bean				
mix only	1 serving	<1.0	126	4%

Food and Description	Amount	Fat Grams	Total Calories	% Fat Calories
prepared	1 serving	3.5	202	16%
13-bean bouillabaisse				
mix only	1 serving	<1.0	99	5%
prepared	1 serving	3.0	174	16%
(Bag O'Beans) mix only				
lentil & pea	¼ cup	0.5	170	3%
minestrone blend	¼ cup	0.5	150	3%
(Bean Cuisine)				
Santa Fe corn chowder				
mix only	1 serving	<1.0	112	4%
prepared	1 serving	4.5	179	23%
thick as fog split pea				
mix only	1 serving	<1.0	116	4%
prepared	1 serving	4.5	189	21%
ultima pasta & fagioli				
mix only	1 serving	<1.0	117	4%
prepared	1 serving	3.0	179	15%
(Borden)				
beef bouillon/reduced sodium	1 cube	–	5	–
	1 tsp	–	5	–
chicken bouillon/reduced sodium	1 cube	–	5	–
	1 tsp	–	5	–
homestyle chickeny-flavored noodle	¼ pkt	1.5	70	19%
Ronco natural	⅛ pkg	0.5	90	5%
(Campbell's)				
noodle/prepared	1 cup	1.5	100	14%
onion/mix only	1 Tbs	–	25	–
Ramen noodle/mix only				
beef	½ block	7.0	180	35%
chicken	½ block	7.0	180	35%
Oriental	½ block	7.0	180	35%
(Fantastic Foods)				
Only a Pinch/low-sodium				
couscous w/lentils	1 pkg	1.0	220	4%
Spanish rice & beans	1 pkg	1.5	210	6%
regular				
broccoli & cheddar	1 pkg	1.5	130	10%
cha-cha chili	1 pkg	1.0	220	4%
chicken free noodle	1 pkg	0.5	140	3%
corn & potato chowder	1 pkg	1.0	170	5%
country lentil	1 pkg	1.0	230	4%
couscous w/lentils	1 pkg	1.0	230	4%
five bean	1 pkg	1.0	230	4%
Jumpin' Black Beans	1 pkg	1.0	210	4%
minestrone	1 pkg	1.0	150	6%
mushroom	1 pkg	–	120	–
split pea	1 pkg	1.0	190	5%
tomato rice Parmesano	1 pkg	2.0	200	9%

Food and Description	Amount	Fat Grams	Total Calories	% Fat Calories
vegetable barley	1 pkg	0.5	150	3%
vegetable curry noodle	1 pkg	1.0	140	6%
vegetable miso noodle	1 pkg	1.0	130	7%
vegetable tomato noodle	1 pkg	1.0	150	6%
(Featherweight)				
bouillon				
beef	1½ tsp	0.5	15	30%
chicken	1½ tsp	–	15	–
generic				
asparagus, cream of/2.2-oz pkg	1 pkg	7.0	234	27%
beef broth/cubed				
mix only	1 cube	–	8	–
prepared	1 cup	–	8	–
beef noodle/prepared	1 cup	0.8	41	17%
cauliflower/0.7-oz pkg				
mix only	1 pkg	1.7	68	23%
prepared	1 cup	1.7	68	23%
celery, cream of/0.6-oz pkg	1 pkg	1.6	63	23%
chicken, cream of/0.6-oz pkg				
mix only	1 pkg	4.0	80	35%
prepared	1 cup	5.0	107	42%
chicken broth				
consommé				
mix only	1 pkg	0.8	16	45%
prepared	1 cup	1.0	21	43%
cubed				
mix only	1 cube	–	8	–
prepared	1 cup	–	8	–
chicken rice/prepared	1 cup	1.0	60	15%
chicken vegetable/prepared	1 cup	0.8	49	15%
clam chowder/prepared				
Manhattan	1 cup	1.6	65	22%
New England	1 cup	3.7	95	35%
consommé w/gelatin/2-oz pkg				
mix only	1 pkg	–	77	–
prepared	1 cup	–	17	–
mushroom	1 cup	4.9	96	46%
onion/mix only	1 pkg	0.5	35	13%
onion mushroom/mix only	1 pkg	0.5	80	6%
oxtail/prepared	1 cup	2.6	71	32%
pea, green or split/prepared	1 cup	1.6	133	11%
tomato/0.7-oz pkg				
mix only	1 pkg	2.0	77	23%
prepared	1 cup	2.0	102	18%
tomato vegetable/1.4-oz pkg				
mix only	1 pkg	2.0	125	14%
prepared	1 cup	0.9	55	14%
vegetable, cream of/prepared	1 cup	5.7	105	49%

Food and Description	Amount	Fat Grams	Total Calories	% Fat Calories
vegetable beef/prepared	1 cup	1.0	53	17%
(G. Washington) seasoning & broth				
brown				
kosher				
mix only	1 pkg	–	48	–
prepared	1 serving	–	6	–
regular				
mix only	1 pkg	–	48	–
prepared	1 serving	–	6	–
golden				
kosher				
mix only	1 pkg	–	48	–
prepared	1 serving	–	6	–
regular				
mix only	1 pkg	–	48	–
prepared	1 serving	–	6	–
onion				
mix only	1 pkg	–	96	–
prepared	1 serving	–	12	–
vegetable				
mix only	1 pkg	–	96	–
prepared	1 serving	–	12	–
(Goodman's) prepared				
matzo ball & soup				
50% less sodium	1 cup	1.0	50	18%
regular	1 cup	1.0	40	23%
noodleman				
low-sodium	1 cup	1.0	50	18%
regular	1 cup	1.0	45	20%
onion				
low-sodium	1 cup	1.0	30	30%
regular	1 cup	1.0	30	30%
(Health Valley) mix only				
chicken flavored noodle w/vegetables	⅓ cup	–	80	–
corn chowder w/tomatoes	½ cup	–	90	–
creamy potato w/broccoli	½ cup	–	70	–
garden split pea w/carrots	½ cup	–	130	–
lentil w/couscous	⅓ cup	–	130	–
pasta Italiano	½ cup	–	140	–
spicy black bean w/couscous	⅓ cup	–	130	–
zesty black bean w/rice	⅓ cup	–	100	–
(Herb-Ox)				
bouillon cube				
beef	1 cube	–	10	–
chicken	1 cube	–	10	–
vegetable	1 cube	–	10	–
instant bouillon				
beef	1 tsp	–	10	–

Food and Description	Amount	Fat Grams	Total Calories	% Fat Calories
chicken	1 tsp	–	10	–
instant broth/seasoning				
beef				
low-sodium	1 pkg	–	15	–
regular	1 pkg	–	10	–
chicken				
low-sodium	1 pkg	–	15	–
regular	1 pkg	–	10	–
(House Of Tsang)				
Oriental noodle soup mix				
Cantonese chicken	1 container	0.5	110	4%
Mongolian beef	1 container	0.5	110	4%
spring vegetables	1 container	1.0	120	8%
velvet corn	1 container	1.5	170	8%
(Knorr)				
bouillon cube				
beef	½ cube	1.5	20	67%
chicken	½ cube	1.5	20	67%
fish	½ cube	1.0	10	90%
vegetarian vegetable	½ cube	1.0	10	90%
soup mix				
broccoli, cream of/mix only	½ pkg	3.0	60	45%
chicken flavor noodle				
mix only	⅓ pkg	1.0	90	10%
prepared	1 cup	1.0	90	10%
fine herb/mix only	⅓ pkg	5.0	100	45%
mix only	⅓ pkg	1.0	45	20%
prepared	1 cup	1.0	45	20%
French onion				
mix only	⅓ pkg	1.0	50	18%
prepared	1 cup	1.0	50	18%
hot & sour				
mix only	⅓ pkg	1.5	50	27%
prepared	1 cup	1.5	50	27%
leek/mix only	⅓ pkg	3.0	70	39%
oxtail hearty beef				
mix only	⅓ pkg	2.5	60	38%
prepared	1 cup	2.5	60	38%
snow pea, cream of/mix only	½ pkg	2.0	70	26%
spinach, cream of/mix only	⅓ pkg	2.5	70	38%
vegetable				
regular				
mix only	¼ pkg	–	30	–
prepared	1 cup	–	30	–
spring, w/herbs				
mix only	⅓ pkg	–	25	–
prepared	1 cup	–	25	–
wild mushroom, cream of/mix only	½ pkg	3.0	90	30%

Food and Description	Amount	Fat Grams	Total Calories	% Fat Calories
(Lipton)				
Cup-A-Soup/mix only				
chicken				
cream of	1 pkg	2.5	70	32%
supreme/hearty	1 pkg	4.0	90	40%
chicken noodle				
country style hearty	1 pkg	1.0	60	15%
w/chicken meat	1 pkg	1.0	50	18%
chicken vegetable	1 pkg	1.0	50	18%
chicken-flavored broth	1 pkg	1.0	20	45%
creamy broccoli & cheese	1 pkg	3.0	70	39%
creamy chicken w/vegetables	1 pkg	4.0	90	40%
green pea	1 pkg	3.5	110	29%
mushroom, cream of	1 pkg	2.0	60	30%
ring noodle	1 pkg	1.0	50	18%
tomato	1 pkg	2.0	90	20%
vegetable				
country style harvest	1 pkg	1.5	90	15%
spring	1 pkg	1.0	50	18%
Kettle Creations/prepared				
chicken 'n onion	1 cup	1.0	120	8%
chicken w/pasta & beans	1 cup	1.5	110	12%
homestyle lentil w/bow tie pasta	1 cup	1.0	130	7%
medley	1 cup	1.5	130	10%
minestrone	1 cup	1.5	110	12%
onion & rice	1 cup	1.0	120	8%
pasta & bean	1 cup	1.5	130	10%
Recipe Secrets/mix only				
herb				
golden, w/lemon	2 Tbs	0.5	35	13%
Italian, w/tomato	2 Tbs	0.5	40	11%
w/garlic/savory	1 Tbs	0.5	35	13%
mushroom/beefy	2 Tbs	–	35	–
onion				
beefy	1 Tbs	0.5	25	18%
golden	2 Tbs	1.5	60	23%
mushroom	2 Tbs	1.0	35	26%
regular	1 Tbs	–	8	–
vegetable	2 Tbs	–	30	–
Soup Secrets /mix only				
chicken/hearty	¼ cup	2.0	80	23%
chicken noodle	3 Tbs	2.5	80	28%
extra noodle	3 Tbs	1.5	90	15%
giggle noodle	2 Tbs	2.0	80	23%
noodle w/real chicken	2 Tbs	2.0	60	30%
noodle w/vegetables/hearty	3 Tbs	2.0	70	26%
noodles w/chicken broth	2 Tbs	2.0	60	30%
ring-o-noodle	2 Tbs	2.0	70	26%

Food and Description	Amount	Fat Grams	Total Calories	% Fat Calories
ruffle pasta	2 Tbs	1.0	60	15%
(MBT) Romanoff				
beef				
low-sodium	1 pkt	–	15	–
regular	1 pkt	–	15	–
chicken				
low-sodium	1 pkt	–	125	–
regular	1 pkt	–	15	–
onion broth & dip	1 pkt	–	15	–
vegetable	1 pkt	–	10	–
(Manischewitz)				
Mrs. Manischewitz's Soup Cup				
black bean	1 cup	1.0	200	5%
chicken & rice	1 cup	1.0	130	7%
lentil/hearty	1 cup	1.0	140	6%
regular/mix only				
matzo ball	1 Tbs	0.5	40	11%
minestrone	¼ pkg	–	150	–
split pea	⅕ pkg	–	110	–
vegetable w/mushroom	⅕ pkg	–	120	–
(Mayacamas)				
Instant Soupbreak/prepared				
black bean	6 oz	<1.0	75	6%
chicken leek	6 oz	<1.0	75	6%
garden pea	6 oz	<1.0	75	6%
New England clam	6 oz	<1.0	75	6%
potato leek	6 oz	<1.0	75	6%
Just Enough Cup/prepared				
cheese & broccoli	1 cup	0.5	40	11%
chicken style vermicelli	1 cup	–	60	–
tomato vermicelli	1 cup	–	110	–
regular/prepared				
avgholemono	6 oz	<1.0	60	8%
black bean	6 oz	<1.0	65	7%
cheddar cheese	6 oz	5.0	85	53%
chicken style	6 oz	<1.0	55	8%
Cockie Leekie	6 oz	5.0	95	47%
cream	6 oz	<1.0	55	8%
creamy broccoli	6 oz	<1.0	65	7%
creamy mushroom	6 oz	<1.0	55	8%
creamy tomato	6 oz	<1.0	55	8%
French onion	6 oz	<1.0	50	9%
garden pea	6 oz	<1.0	65	7%
lentil	6 oz	<1.0	65	7%
minestrone	6 oz	<1.0	70	6%
mulligatawny	6 oz	<1.0	55	8%
New England clam	6 oz	1.0	65	7%
potato leek	6 oz	1.0	60	7%

Food and Description	Amount	Fat Grams	Total Calories	% Fat Calories
Senegalese	6 oz	<1.0	55	8%
vegetable supreme	6 oz	<1.0	65	7%
(Maruchan) Instant Lunch				
beef flavor	1 container	13.0	290	40%
chicken flavor	1 container	13.0	290	40%
chicken w/mushrooms	1 container	13.0	280	42%
Oriental noodles w/shrimp	1 container	13.0	290	40%
(Mrs. Grass) mix only				
chicken w/rice	¼ pkg	1.0	80	11%
noodle				
beef flavored	¼ pkg	1.0	70	13%
chicken flavored	¼ pkt	1.5	60	23%
onion				
mushroom	⅓ pkt	1.0	60	15%
reduced sodium	¼ pkt	–	35	–
soup & dip	¼ pkt	0.5	35	13%
vegetable soup & dip	¼ pkt	–	35	–
(Nile Spice) prepared				
black bean	1 container	1.5	170	8%
chicken vegetable	1 container	1.5	110	12%
lentil	1 container	1.5	180	8%
minestrone	1 container	1.0	140	6%
red beans & rice	1 container	1.0	170	5%
split pea	1 container	2.5	210	11%
sweet corn chowder	1 container	3.0	120	23%
(Nissin) mix only				
Top Ramen				
beef				
regular				
low-fat	½ pkg	1.0	150	6%
original	½ pkg	8.0	200	36%
spicy	½ pkg	8.0	200	36%
chicken				
low-fat	½ pkg	1.0	150	6%
original	½ pkg	8.0	200	36%
chicken mushroom	½ pkg	8.0	200	36%
chicken sesame	½ pkg	8.0	200	36%
damae	½ pkg	8.0	200	36%
garden vegetable	½ pkg	8.0	200	36%
Oriental				
low-fat	½ pkg	1.0	150	6%
original	½ pkg	8.0	200	36%
pork	½ pkg	8.0	200	36%
shrimp	½ pkg	8.0	200	36%
Cup O'Noodles				
beef	1.2 oz	7.0	160	39%
	2.3 oz	12.0	290	37%
beef onion	2.3 oz	11.0	280	35%

Food and Description	Amount	Fat Grams	Total Calories	% Fat Calories
chicken				
regular	1.2 oz	7.0	160	39%
	2.3 oz	12.0	300	36%
spicy	1.2 oz	7.0	160	39%
	2.3 oz	13.0	300	39%
chicken mushroom	2.3 oz	13.0	300	39%
crab	2.3 oz	12.0	290	37%
lobster	2.3 oz	13.0	300	39%
pork	2.3 oz	12.0	290	37%
shrimp	1.2 oz	6.0	150	36%
	2.3 oz	12.0	290	37%
shrimp picante	3 oz	12.0	290	37%
vegetable/garden	2.3 oz	12.0	290	37%
(Old Bay) mix only				
crab, cream of	2 Tbs	2.5	70	32%
Maryland crab	1⅓ Tbs	–	50	–
(Produce Partners) mix only				
broccoli, cream of	1⅓ Tbs	–	35	–
cheddar cheese broccoli	2 Tbs	3.0	70	39%
French onion	1 Tbs	–	40	–
potato, cream of	1 Tbs	–	25	–
vegetable/garden	1⅓ Tbs	–	40	–
(Soup Break) instant/prepared				
black bean	6 oz	1.0	95	10%
broccoli	6 oz	1.0	80	11%
chicken leek	6 oz	2.0	85	21%
garden pea	6 oz	1.0	85	11%
New England clam	6 oz	2.0	105	17%
potato leek	6 oz	1.0	85	11%
(Steero) mix only				
bouillon cube				
beef	1 cube	–	5	–
chicken	1 cube	–	5	–
instant bouillon				
chicken				
regular	1 tsp	–	5	–
very low sodium	1 tsp	–	10	–
(Swanson) broth/mix only				
beef	1 cube	1.0	20	45%
chicken	1 cube	2.0	30	60%
Oriental	1 cube	–	15	–
vegetable	1 cube	1.0	20	45%
(Ultra Slim Fast) prepared				
creamy chicken leek	6 oz	<1.0	50	9%
creamy potato leek	6 oz	<1.0	80	6%
creamy tomato	6 oz	<1.0	60	8%
hearty onion	6 oz	<1.0	45	10%

Food and Description	Amount	Fat Grams	Total Calories	% Fat Calories
(Weight Watchers) Smart Options				
beef broth	1 pkt	–	10	–
chicken broth	1 pkt	–	10	–
(Westbrae) mix only				
brown rice	½ pkg	0.5	140	3%
buckwheat	½ pkg	0.5	140	3%
carrot	⅓ pkg	1.0	100	9%
curry	½ pkg	0.5	140	3%
5 spice	½ pkg	0.5	140	3%
green tea	½ pkg	1.0	140	6%
miso	½ pkg	0.5	140	3%
mushroom	½ pkg	0.5	140	3%
seaweed	½ pkg	0.5	140	3%
spinach	½ pkg	0.5	140	3%
(Wyler's)				
bouillon cube				
beef	1 cube	–	5	–
chicken	1 cube	–	5	–
instant bouillon				
beef	1 tsp	–	10	–
chicken				
regular	1 tsp	–	5	–
very low sodium	1 tsp	–	10	–
vegetable	1 tsp	–	5	–
instant broth				
beef	1 pkt	–	15	–
chicken				
regular	1 pkt	–	15	–
low-sodium	1 pkt	–	15	–
■ FROZEN OR REFRIGERATED				
(Schwan's)				
Boston clam chowder	1 cup	8.0	180	40%
broccoli, cream of	1 cup	10.0	180	50%
Wisconsin cheese	1 cup	10.0	210	43%
(Stock Pot)				
clam chowder/concentrated				
prepared w/whole milk	1 cup	9.5	200	43%
unprepared	⅓ cup	4.0	100	36%
seafood gumbo	1 cup	5.0	130	35%
(Tabatchnick)				
barley mushroom				
no salt	7.5 oz	–	70	–
regular	7.5 oz	–	70	–
broccoli, cream of	7.5 oz	4.0	90	40%
cabbage	7.5 oz	–	60	–
chicken				
New York	7.5 oz	–	35	–
w/dumplings	7.5 oz	2.0	70	26%

Food and Description	Amount	Fat Grams	Total Calories	% Fat Calories
corn chowder	7.5 oz	6.0	150	36%
minestrone	7.5 oz	4.0	90	40%
pea				
no salt	7.5 oz	1.5	180	8%
regular	7.5 oz	1.5	180	8%
potato				
New England	7.5 oz	6.0	150	36%
old fashioned	7.5 oz	–	70	–
spinach, cream of	7.5 oz	4.0	90	40%
vegetable				
no salt	7.5 oz	1.0	110	8%
regular	7.5 oz	1.0	110	8%
Wisconsin cheddar vegetable	7.5 oz	9.0	140	58%
Yankee bean				
regular	7.5 oz	1.5	160	8%
vegetable	10.5 oz	1.0	130	7%
■ HOMEMADE				
USDA Standard Home Recipe				
black turtle bean	1 cup	1.0	240	4%
Brunswick stew	1 cup	5.0	230	20%
corn & cheese chowder	1 cup	16.0	287	50%
gazpacho	1 cup	–	50	–
Greek	1 cup	2.5	85	27%
hot & sour	1 cup	2.0	75	24%
pasta e fagioli	1 cup	4.5	195	42%
potato	1 cup	12.0	201	54%
ratatouille	1 cup	23.0	265	78%
vegetable	1 cup	–	70	–
vegetable beef	1 cup	25.0	320	70%
won ton	1 cup	3.0	205	13%
■ MICROWAVEABLE				
(Campbell's) microwave cup/chicken	2.3 oz	13.0	310	38%
(Hormel) Micro Cup				
bean & ham	1 cup	4.0	190	19%
beef vegetable	1 cup	1.0	90	10%
broccoli cheese w/ham	1 cup	13.0	170	69%
chicken noodle	1 cup	2.5	110	20%
chicken & rice	1 cup	3.0	110	25%
New England clam chowder	1 cup	5.0	130	38%
potato cheese w/ham	1 cup	13.0	190	62%
(Knorr)				
black bean	1 pkg	1.0	190	5%
chicken vegetable	1 pkg	–	100	–
hearty lentil	1 pkg	–	220	–
navy bean	1 pkg	–	140	–
potato leek	1 pkg	–	120	–
(Luck's)				
beef vegetable	7.5 oz	–	90	–

Food and Description	Amount	Fat Grams	Total Calories	% Fat Calories
chicken vegetable	7.5 oz	–	90	–
vegetable bean	7.5 oz	–	120	–
(Lunch Bucket)				
chicken noodle	1 container	2.0	80	23%
country vegetable	1 container	0.5	60	8%
(The Spice Hunter)				
brown & wild rice amadine	1 container	3.0	180	15%
French country lentil	1 container	1.0	130	7%
Hunan noodle	1 container	1.0	110	8%
Kasba curry	1 container	2.0	190	9%
Mandarin noodle	1 container	1.0	120	8%
Mediterranean minestrone	1 container	1.0	140	6%
Savoy fettuccini	1 container	1.5	190	7%
Szechuan noodle	1 container	1.0	130	7%
SOUR CREAM (*See also* DIP; SAUCE; SEASONINGS; SOUR CREAM SUBSTITUTE)				
(Alta Dena) premium	1 Tbs	6.0	60	90%
(Breakstone)				
sour cream				
fat-free	2 Tbs	–	35	–
original	2 Tbs	5.0	60	75%
sour half & half	2 Tbs	3.5	45	70%
(Friendship)				
lite	2 Tbs	2.0	35	51%
original	2 Tbs	5.0	55	82%
generic				
cultured	1 Tbs	2.5	26	86%
	1 cup	42.0	450	84%
nondairy	1 Tbs	2.8	30	83%
	1 cup	45.0	480	84%
(Heluva Good Cheese)				
fat-free	2 Tbs	–	20	–
light	2 Tbs	3.0	40	68%
original	2 Tbs	5.0	60	75%
(Kemps)				
sour cream				
cultured	1 oz	5.0	60	75%
lite	1 oz	2.0	30	6%
regular	1 cup	42.0	450	84%
w/chives	1 oz	5.0	60	75%
Tator Topper/lite	1 oz	2.0	30	6%
(Knudsen)				
fat-free	2 Tbs	–	35	–
Hampshire	2 Tbs	6.0	60	90%
light	2 Tbs	2.5	40	56%
(Land O'Lakes)				
sour cream				
lite				
plain	2 Tbs	2.0	40	45%

Food and Description	Amount	Fat Grams	Total Calories	% Fat Calories
w/chives	2 Tbs	2.0	40	45%
no-fat	2 Tbs	–	30	–
regular	1 Tbs	3.0	30	90%
sour half & half	1 Tbs	2.0	25	72%
(Real Dairy) fat-free	2 Tbs	–	20	–
(Sealtest)				
fat-free	2 Tbs	–	35	–
light	2 Tbs	2.5	40	56%
original	2 Tbs	5.0	60	75%
SOUR CREAM SUBSTITUTE (*See also* SEASONINGS)				
(Chivo)	2 Tbs	5.0	50	90%
(Dean's) Sour Delite	2 Tbs	5.0	50	90%
(Formagg) sour cream alternative/ fat-free	2 Tbs	–	30	–
generic				
non-butterfat	1 oz	4.0	42	86%
	1 cup	39.0	417	84%
nondairy	1 oz	6.0	60	90%
	1 cup	45.0	480	84%
(IMO)				
fat-free	2 Tbs	–	20	–
original	2 Tbs	5.0	50	90%
(Land O'Lakes) light dairy blend	1 Tbs	1.0	20	45%
(Pet)	1 Tbs	2.0	25	72%
(Soymage) sour cream alternative	2 Tbs	3.0	40	68%
(Tofutti) Sour Supreme/Better Than Sour Cream	2 Tbs	5.0	50	90%
SOURSOP/fresh				
pieces	1 cup	1.0	150	6%
whole	1 medium	2.0	420	4%
SOY CHEESE (*See* CHEESE ALTERNATIVE/IMITATION)				
SOY FLOUR (*See* FLOUR)				
SOY GRANULES				
(Feam) Soya	¼ cup	–	140	–
SOY GRITS				
(Arrowhead Mills) dry	¼ cup	6.0	140	39%
SOY LECITHIN				
(Nutri Value)	1 Tbs	4.0	50	72%
SOY NUTS (*See* SOYBEAN)				
SOY PROTEIN				
concentrate	1 oz	–	92	–
isolate				
w/potassium	1 oz	1.0	96	9%
w/sodium	1 oz	1.0	96	9%
SOY SAUCE (*See* ASIAN FOOD/SAUCES & SEASONINGS; SAUCE)				
SOYBEAN				
dried				
(Arrowhead Mills)	¼ cup	8.0	170	42%

Food and Description	Amount	Fat Grams	Total Calories	% Fat Calories
generic				
boiled-drained	½ cup	8.0	150	48%
dry-roasted	½ cup	18.6	387	43%
raw	½ cup	18.5	390	43%
roasted/salted or unsalted	1 oz	6.8	129	47%
	½ cup	21.8	405	48%
roasted & toasted	1 oz	6.8	129	47%
(Nature's Select) dry-roasted	¾ oz	4.0	90	40%
green				
boiled-drained	½ cup	6.0	130	42%
raw				
shelled	½ cup	9.0	190	43%
unshelled	4 oz	4.0	90	40%
kernels/whole/roasted & toasted	1 oz	7.0	130	48%
	1 cup	26.0	490	48%
sprouted				
raw	10 sprouts	0.5	15	30%
	½ cup	2.3	45	46%
steamed	½ cup	2.0	40	45%
stir-fried in vegetable oil	3 oz	6.0	105	51%

SOYBEAN CURD (See TOFU; TOFU FROZEN DESSERTS; VEGETARIAN FOODS)
SOYBEAN OIL (See OIL)
SOYBEAN PASTE (See MISO)
SOYMILK (See also BABY/INFANT FORMULA)

Food and Description	Amount	Fat Grams	Total Calories	% Fat Calories
dry				
(Loma Linda) Soyagen/prepared				
all-purpose	¼ cup	6.0	130	42%
carob	¼ cup	6.0	130	42%
no sucrose	¼ cup	6.0	130	42%
(Worthington) Soyamel	1 oz	7.0	130	49%
liquid				
(Edensoy)				
carob	8.45 fl oz	4.0	160	23%
original				
extra	8.45 fl oz	4.0	135	27%
regular	8.45 fl oz	4.0	135	27%
vanilla				
extra	8.45 fl oz	3.0	150	18%
regular	8.45 fl oz	3.5	150	21%
generic	1 cup	4.6	80	52%
(Health Valley) Soy Moo	1 cup	–	110	–
(Vitasoy)				
creamy original	6 fl oz	<1.0	105	9%
vanilla delite	6 fl oz	4.0	150	24%
(Westsoy)				
almond				
lite 1%	6 fl oz	4.0	160	23%
natural	6 fl oz	11.0	250	40%

Food and Description	Amount	Fat Grams	Total Calories	% Fat Calories
carob/plus	8 fl oz	5.0	160	28%
cocoa-flavored/lite 1%				
plain	8 fl oz	2.0	140	13%
w/mint	6 fl oz	3.0	160	17%
creamy banana/lite 1%	6 fl oz	3.0	160	17%
malted				
plain				
lite 1%	6 fl oz	3.0	160	17%
natural	6 fl oz	11.0	270	37%
vanilla/natural	6 fl oz	11.0	250	40%
plain				
lite 1%	8 fl oz	2.0	100	18%
natural				
regular	8 fl oz	5.0	150	30%
unsweetened	8 fl oz	5.0	100	45%
plus	8 fl oz	5.0	150	30%
vanilla				
lite 1%	8 fl oz	2.0	110	16%
natural	8 fl oz	2.5	120	19%
plus	8 fl oz	5.0	150	30%
vanilla royale/lite 1%	6 fl oz	3.0	160	17%

SPAETZLE (See DUMPLING MIX)
SPAGHETTI (See PASTA)
SPAGHETTI DINNER (See FROZEN ENTRÉE/DINNER; PASTA ENTRÉE/DINNER; VEGETARIAN FOODS)
SPAGHETTI SAUCE (See SAUCE)
SPANISH FOOD (See FROZEN ENTRÉE/DINNER; MEXICAN FOOD; RICE; RICE DISH; VEGETARIAN FOODS)
SPICES (See SEASONINGS; individual listings)
SPINACH

Food and Description	Amount	Fat Grams	Total Calories	% Fat Calories
canned				
(Bush's Best) chopped	½ cup	–	25	–
(Del Monte)				
chopped	½ cup	–	30	–
no salt added	½ cup	–	30	–
whole leaf	½ cup	–	30	–
(Freshlike)				
cut	½ cup	–	20	–
w/o salt	½ cup	–	20	–
w/o salt or sugar	½ cup	–	20	–
generic	½ cup	<1.0	25	18%
(S&W)	½ cup	–	30	–
(Stokely)	½ cup	–	30	–
(Veg-All) cut	½ cup	–	20	–
fresh				
boiled	½ cup	–	21	–
raw				
chopped	½ cup	–	6	–

Food and Description	Amount	Fat Grams	Total Calories	% Fat Calories
(Dole)	3 oz	–	10	–
frozen				
(Birds Eye)				
chopped	3.3 oz	–	20	–
whole leaf	3.3 oz	–	20	–
(C&W)				
chopped	⅓ cup	–	20	–
whole leaf	⅓ cup	–	20	–
(Freshlike) cut	3.3 oz	–	20	–
generic				
chopped	1 cup	<1.0	40	11%
	10 oz	1.0	70	13%
(Green Giant)				
cut leaf	¾ cup	–	25	–
Harvest Fresh	½ cup	–	25	–
(Pictsweet) leaf	½ cup	–	20	–
(Veg-All) cut	3.3 oz	–	20	–
SPINACH, NEW ZEALAND/fresh				
boiled	½ cup	–	12	–
raw	1 lb	1.0	86	11%
SPINACH DISH (See also FROZEN ENTRÉE/DINNER; VEGETABLES, MIXED; VEGETARIAN FOODS)				
frozen				
(Green Giant)				
creamed	½ cup	3.0	80	34%
cut leaf in butter sauce	½ cup	1.5	40	34%
homemade/USDA Standard Home Recipe				
spinach quiche	~5 oz	26.0	337	69%
spinach soufflé/made w/whole milk, butter, & cheese	1 cup	18.0	218	74%
SPIRULINA (See SEAWEED)				
SPLIT PEA (See PEA)				
SPOONBREAD (See BREAD)				
SPORTS DRINK				
bottled or canned				
(All Sport)				
fruit punch	8 fl oz	–	80	–
grape	8 fl oz	–	80	–
lemon-lime				
lite	8 fl oz	–	–	–
regular	8 fl oz	–	70	–
orange				
lite	8 fl oz	–	–	–
regular	8 fl oz	–	70	–
(GatorAde) Thirst Quencher				
original				
citrus cooler	8 fl oz	–	50	–
cool blue raspberry	8 fl oz	–	50	–

Food and Description	Amount	Fat Grams	Total Calories	% Fat Calories
grape	8 fl oz	–	50	–
lemon ice	8 fl oz	–	50	–
lemon-lime	8 fl oz	–	50	–
orange	8 fl oz	–	50	–
tropical burst	8 fl oz	–	50	–
watermelon	8 fl oz	–	50	–
sports bottle				
cherry rush	8 fl oz	–	50	–
citrus cooler	8 fl oz	–	50	–
cool blue raspberry	8 fl oz	–	50	–
fruit punch	8 fl oz	–	50	–
lemon ice	8 fl oz	–	50	–
lemon-lime	8 fl oz	–	50	–
strawberry kiwi	8 fl oz	–	50	–
wild apple	8 fl oz	–	50	–
(La Boost)				
lemon-lime	8 fl oz	–	35	–
orange	8 fl oz	–	35	–
(Powerade)				
fruit punch	8 fl oz	–	72	–
grape	8 fl oz	–	73	–
lemon-lime	8 fl oz	–	72	–
Mountain Blast	8 fl oz	–	73	–
orange	8 fl oz	–	72	–
(10-K)				
fruit punch	8 fl oz	–	60	–
lemon-lime	8 fl oz	–	60	–
orange	8 fl oz	–	60	–
(Weider)				
Dynamic Muscle Builder	11 fl oz	<1.0	220	2%
Dynamic Weight gainer	11 fl oz	2.0	280	6%
High Energy Protein Blast	11.5 fl oz	<1.0	270	2%
Power Shake/Dutch chocolate	11 fl oz	<1.0	220	2%
mix				
(Tiger's Milk) mix only				
Breakfast Booster	2 Tbs	<1.0	70	6%
Energy Booster	3 Tbs	<1.0	120	4%
Protein Booster				
Dutch chocolate	3 Tbs	<1.0	90	5%
vanilla-orange creme	3 Tbs	<1.0	90	5%
(Weider) mix only				
Big Chocolate Malt/sugar-free	4 scoops	2.0	320	6%
Carbo Energizer/orange	4 scoops	–	230	–
Dynamic Body Shaper/ Dutch chocolate	2 scoops	<1.0	110	4%
Dynamic Muscle Builder				
natural chocolate	2 scoops	1.0	120	8%
vanilla	2 scoops	1.0	120	8%

Food and Description	Amount	Fat Grams	Total Calories	% Fat Calories
Dynamic Weight Gainer				
Dutch chocolate	4 scoops	<1.0	320	1%
peanut butter	4 scoops	2.0	330	5%
90 Plus/vanilla/sugar-free	2 scoops	–	100	–
Victory Explosive Workout/citrus	4 Tbs	–	190	–
SPOT FISH/fresh				
cooked-dry heat	3 oz	4.0	134	27%
raw	2.25-oz fillet	2.5	80	28%
	3 oz	3.0	105	26%
SPRING ONION (See SCALLION)				
SQUAB/PIGEON				
raw				
breast meat only	~4 oz	4.6	135	30%
giblets	3 oz	6.0	132	41%
meat & skin	~7 oz	47.5	590	72%
meat only	~6 oz	12.6	239	47%
SQUASH				
acorn/fresh				
baked	½ cup	–	57	–
boiled-mashed	½ cup	–	41	–
banana/fresh/baked	8 oz	1.0	145	6%
butternut				
fresh				
baked	½ cup	–	41	–
boiled-mashed	½ cup	–	50	–
frozen				
generic	½ cup	–	47	–
(Southland)	½ cup	–	45	–
cocozelle				
fresh				
boiled-drained	½ cup	–	14	–
raw/sliced	½ cup	–	9	–
frozen	½ cup	–	19	–
crookneck				
fresh				
boiled-drained	½ cup	–	18	–
raw/sliced	½ cup	–	12	–
frozen	½ cup	–	24	–
hubbard/fresh				
baked/cubed	½ cup	0.6	51	11%
boiled-mashed	½ cup	0.5	37	12%
scallop/fresh				
boiled-drained	½ cup	–	14	–
boiled-drained-mashed	½ cup	–	19	–
raw/sliced	½ cup	–	12	–
spaghetti/fresh				
boiled or baked	½ cup	–	23	–
(Nature's Pasta)	1 cup	–	20	–

Food and Description	Amount	Fat Grams	Total Calories	% Fat Calories
summer/all varieties/fresh				
boiled/sliced	½ cup	–	18	–
raw/sliced	½ cup	–	13	–
winter/all varieties				
fresh				
baked/cubed	½ cup	0.6	39	14%
boiled-mashed	½ cup	0.6	39	14%
frozen				
(Birds Eye)	½ cup		45	–
zucchini				
canned				
(Del Monte) w/Italian style tomato sauce	½ cup	–	30	–
(Progresso) Italian style	½ cup	2.0	40	45%
fresh				
boiled-drained	½ cup	–	14	–
raw	½ cup	–	9	–
frozen				
(Big Valley) sliced	3.5 oz	–	12	–
(C&W) sliced	3.3 oz	–	16	–
generic	½ cup	–	19	–
(Ore Ida) breaded	3 oz	8.0	150	48%
(Stilwell) Qwik Krisp	6 pieces	11.0	190	52%
(Southland) sliced	3.2 oz	–	15	–
SQUASH SEEDS				
dried/hulled	1 oz	13.0	155	75%
	1 cup	63.0	747	76%
kernels/roasted	1 oz	12.0	148	73%
	1 cup	95.6	1184	73%
whole/roasted	1 oz	5.5	127	39%
	1 cup	12.0	285	38%
SQUID				
dried	3 oz	4.6	260	16%
fresh				
breaded & fried	3 oz	6.0	149	36%
raw	3 oz	1.0	78	12%
frozen				
(Fiesta Del Mar) ras calimari	4 oz	2.0	110	16%
pickled	1 oz	–	23	–
SQUIRREL				
raw	3 oz	3.0	105	26%
roasted	3 oz	3.0	115	23%
roasted/chopped or diced	½ cup	5.0	190	24%
STAR FRUIT/CARAMBOLA				
fresh				
cubed	½ cup	–	25	–
whole	1 medium	0.5	45	10%

Food and Description	Amount	Fat Grams	Total Calories	% Fat Calories
STEAK SAUCE (*See* SAUCE)				
STRAWBERRY (*See also* BERRIES, MIXED)				
canned				
generic/in heavy syrup	½ cup	<1.0	120	4%
freeze-dried				
(Mountain House) prepared	¼ cup	–	45	–
fresh				
(Dole)	8 berries	–	50	–
whole	1 cup	0.5	45	9%
	1 pint	1.0	97	9%
frozen				
(Big Valley)	3.5 oz	–	35	–
(Birds Eye)				
halves				
deluxe/in delicious syrup	½ cup	–	120	–
in lite syrup	½ cup	–	90	–
whole/in lite syrup	½ cup	–	80	–
(C&W) whole	⅔ cup	–	50	–
generic				
sliced/sweetened	1 cup	<1.0	245	2%
	10 oz	0.5	275	2%
whole				
sweetened	2 cup	<1.0	200	2%
unsweetened				
thawed	3.5 oz	<1.0	50	9%
unthawed	1 cup	<1.0	52	9%
STRAWBERRY DRINK (*See also* FRUIT PUNCH; LEMONADE/LEMONADE-FLAVORED DRINK; SOFT DRINK; SOFT DRINK MIX; individual juice blend listings)				
bottled, boxed, or canned				
(Betty Crocker) Squeezit/Silly Billy Strawberry	6.76 fl oz	–	110	–
(Welch's)	11.5 fl oz	–	200	–
STRAWBERRY JUICE/JUICE BLEND/JUICE DRINK (*See also* FRUIT PUNCH; SOFT DRINK MIX)				
bottled, boxed, or canned				
(Chiquita)				
Calypso breeze/strawberry kiwi	8 fl oz	–	120	–
	8.45 fl oz	–	130	–
light strawberry guava	8 fl oz	–	35	–
liquid concentrate/unprepared	1.6 fl oz	–	120	–
(Kern's)				
strawberry-banana nectar	11.5 fl oz	–	220	–
strawberry-guava juice blend	8 fl oz	–	105	–
(Knudsen)				
strawberry float	8 fl oz	–	140	–
strawberry juice	8 fl oz	–	140	–
(Libby's)				
Juicy Juice/strawberry pouch	4.23 fl oz	–	60	–

Food and Description	Amount	Fat Grams	Total Calories	% Fat Calories
nectar	8 fl oz	–	150	–
(TreeTop) strawberry, orange, banana	8 fl oz	–	120	–
STUFFING/DRESSING				
(Arnold)				
cornbread	2 cups	4.0	250	14%
herb seasoned	2 cups	3.0	240	11%
sage & onion	2 cups	3.0	240	11%
seasoned	2 cups	3.0	250	11%
unspiced	2 cups	3.0	250	11%
(Brownberry)				
cornbread	2 cups	3.5	250	13%
herb seasoned	1 cup	2.5	200	11%
sage & onion	2 cups	3.5	240	13%
unseasoned bread cubes	2 cups	3.0	240	11%
(Golden Grains) prepared				
chicken	½ cup	9.0	180	40%
corn bread	½ cup	9.0	180	40%
herb & butter	½ cup	9.0	180	40%
w/wild rice	½ cup	9.0	180	40%
(Good Harvest) mix only				
Cajun rice	½ cup	2.0	130	14%
San Francisco sourdough	½ cup	2.0	110	16%
Santa Fe	½ cup	1.5	110	12%
wild trio	½ cup	2.5	140	16%
(Kellogg's) Croutettes stuffing mix	1 cup	–	120	–
(Oroweat) dressing				
cornbread	⅓ cup	1.0	110	8%
seasoned	⅓ cup	1.0	110	8%
(Pepperidge Farms) prepared				
Distinctive				
apples & raisin	½ cup	1.5	140	10%
classic chicken	½ cup	1.5	130	10%
country garden herb	½ cup	5.0	150	30%
harvest vegetable & almond	½ cup	3.0	140	19%
wild rice & mushroom	½ cup	6.0	170	32%
original				
cornbread	¾ cup	2.0	170	11%
country style	¾ cup	1.5	140	10%
cube	¾ cup	1.5	140	10%
herb seasoned	¾ cup	1.5	170	8%
sage & onion/for turkey	½ cup	1.5	170	8%
(Sara Lee) food service/ Original Stuffins	1 stuffin	17.0	330	46%
(Shelton's) dressing				
cornbread				
mix only	1 serving	1.0	130	7%
prepared	1 serving	10.0	230	39%

Food and Description	Amount	Fat Grams	Total Calories	% Fat Calories
Stove Top)				
flexible serving				
chicken				
mix only	½ cup	3.0	120	23%
prepared	½ cup	8.0	170	42%
cornbread				
mix only	½ cup	2.5	110	20%
prepared	½ cup	8.0	160	45%
homestyle herb				
mix only	½ cup	3.0	120	23%
prepared	½ cup	8.0	170	42%
microwave				
chicken				
mix only	⅙ box	3.5	130	24%
prepared	½ cup	7.0	160	39%
homestyle cornbread				
mix only	⅙ box	3.5	120	26%
prepared	½ cup	7.0	160	39%
original				
beef				
mix only	⅙ box	1.0	110	8%
prepared	½ cup	9.0	180	45%
chicken				
lower sodium				
mix only	⅙ box	1.0	110	8%
prepared	½ cup	9.0	180	45%
regular				
mix only	⅙ box	1.0	110	8%
prepared	½ cup	9.0	170	48%
cornbread				
mix only	⅙ box	1.0	110	8%
prepared	½ cup	8.0	170	40%
long grain & wild rice				
mix only	⅙ box	1.0	110	8%
prepared	½ cup	9.0	180	45%
mushroom & onion				
mix only	⅙ box	1.5	110	12%
prepared	½ cup	9.0	180	45%
pork				
mix only	⅙ box	1.0	110	8%
prepared	½ cup	9.0	170	48%
San Francisco style				
mix only	⅙ box	1.0	110	8%
prepared	½ cup	9.0	170	48%
savory herbs				
mix only	⅙ box	1.0	110	8%
prepared	½ cup	9.0	170	48%

Food and Description	Amount	Fat Grams	Total Calories	% Fat Calories
turkey				
mix only	⅛ box	1.0	110	8%
prepared	½ cup	9.0	170	48%
STURGEON				
cooked-dry heat	3 oz	4.0	115	31%
raw	3 oz	3.0	90	30%
smoked	3 oz	3.7	147	23%
steamed	3 oz	4.8	135	32%
SUCCOTASH (See also VEGETABLES, MIXED)				
canned				
generic				
w/cream-style corn	½ cup	0.7	102	6%
w/whole kernel corn	½ cup	0.6	81	7%
(Libby)	½ cup	1.0	80	11%
(S & W) country	½ cup	1.0	80	11%
(Seneca)	½ cup	0.5	90	5%
(Stokely)	½ cup	–	90	–
frozen				
generic	10 oz	2.5	265	8%
(Hanover)	½ cup	–	80	–
(Pictsweet)	3.3 oz	1.0	100	9%
homemade/USDA Standard Home Recipe	½ cup	–	110	–
SUCKER, WHITE				
cooked-dry heat	3 oz	2.0	101	18%
raw	3 oz	2.0	79	22%
SUET, BEEF	1 Tbs	13.0	121	100%
SUGAR				
brown				
firmly packed	1 tsp	–	18	–
	1 Tbs	–	52	–
	1 cup	–	821	–
loosely packed	1 cup	–	541	–
maple	1 Tbs	–	52	–
	1 oz	–	99	–
turbinado				
(Hain)	1 Tbs	–	50	–
white				
cubed	1 cube	–	25	–
granulated	1 tsp	–	15	–
	1 Tbs	–	46	–
	1 cup	–	770	–
powdered 10-X confectioner's				
flavored				
(Domino)				
chocolate	¼ cup	–	110	–
lemon	¼ cup	–	110	–
strawberry	¼ cup	–	110	–

Food and Description	Amount	Fat Grams	Total Calories	% Fat Calories
regular/generic	1 tsp	–	10	–
	1 Tbs	–	31	–
	1 cup	–	462	–
SUGAR APPLE/SWEETSOP				
fresh				
pulp	1 cup	0.8	235	3%
whole	1 medium	0.5	145	3%
SUGAR SUBSTITUTE				
(Equal)	1 pkt	–	–	–
	¼ tsp	–	–	–
(Estee)	1 pkt	–	10	–
	1 tsp	–	15	–
(Fruit Source) sweetener & fat replacer	1 tsp	–	15	–
generic/fructose	1 tsp	–	12	–
(NutraSweet)	1 tsp	–	–	–
	1 pkt	–	4	–
(Sprinkle Sweet)	1 tsp	–	2	–
(Sucaryl)	1 tsp	–	–	–
(Sugar Twin)				
brown sugar	1 tsp	–	2	–
regular	1 tsp	–	2	–
	1 pkt	–	3	–
(Superose)	1 pkt	–	–	–
(Sweet*10)	⅛ tsp	–	–	–
(SweetLite)	1 tsp	–	12	–
(SweetMate)	1 pkt	–	3	–
(Sweet'N Low)				
liquid	10 drops	–	–	–
powder				
brown sugar	⅒ tsp	–	2	–
regular	1 packet	–	4	–
	1 tsp	–	12	–
tablet	1 tablet	–	–	–
(Weight Watchers) Sweetner	1 gm	–	5	–
SUMMER SAUSAGE (See SAUSAGE)				
SUN-DRIED TOMATO (See TOMATO)				
SUNFISH/PUMPKINSEED				
fresh				
cooked-dry heat	3 oz	0.5	97	5%
raw	3 oz	0.5	76	6%
SUNFLOWER SEED BUTTER				
(Erewhon)	2 Tbs	18.0	200	81%
generic	1 Tbs	8.0	93	78%
	1 oz	13.6	165	74%
(Hain)	2 Tbs	15.0	180	75%
SUNFLOWER SEED FLOUR (See FLOUR)				
SUNFLOWER SEEDS/NUTS				
(Arrowhead Mills) shelled	¼ cup	15.0	180	75%

Food and Description	Amount	Fat Grams	Total Calories	% Fat Calories
(David)				
shelled kernels	¼ cup	17.0	200	77%
unshelled seeds	¼ cup	15.0	190	71%
(Fisher)				
oil-roasted	1 oz	15.0	170	79%
salted in shell				
shelled kernels	1 oz	14.0	160	79%
unshelled seeds	1 oz	15.0	170	79%
(Frito-Lay)	⅓ cup	8.0	140	51%
generic				
dried	1 oz	14.0	162	78%
	1 cup	71.0	821	78%
dry-roasted	1 oz	14.0	165	76%
	1 cup	64.0	745	77%
oil-roasted	1 oz	16.0	175	82%
	1 cup	77.5	830	84%
oil-roasted/toasted	1 oz	16.0	176	82%
	1 cup	76.0	829	83%
(Lance)				
shelled kernels/roasted	1⅛ oz	16.0	190	76%
	¼ cup	17.0	210	73%
unshelled seeds	⅔ cup	13.0	160	73%
	1⅞ oz	14.0	170	74%
(Laura Scudder's)				
dry-roasted	1 oz	8.5	144	53%
oil-roasted	1 oz	17.0	190	81%
roasted in shell	1 oz	7.0	86	73%
(Planters)				
dry-roasted				
shelled kernels	¼ cup	17.0	190	81%
unshelled seeds				
original	¾ cup	15.0	160	84%
plain				
Munch 'N Go	0.75 oz	11.0	120	83%
regular	3.25 oz	20.0	230	78%
honey-roasted/shelled kernels	1.7 oz	22.0	280	71%
oil-roasted/shelled kernels				
BBQ				
Munch 'N Go	¼ cup	17.0	200	77%
regular	1.7 oz	25.0	290	78%
plain				
regular	1.7 oz	25.0	290	78%
	2 oz	29.0	340	77%
Munch 'N Go	¼ cup	17.0	200	77%
salted/shelled kernels	1 oz	14.0	170	74%

SURIMI (*See also* CRAB, IMITATION; SEAFOOD ENTRÉE/DINNER; SHRIMP, IMITATION)

	3 oz	0.8	84	9%

Food and Description	Amount	Fat Grams	Total Calories	% Fat Calories
SUSHI (*See* ASIAN FOOD)				
SWAMP CABBAGE				
fresh/boiled	½ cup	–	10	–
SWEET & SOUR SAUCE (*See* ASIAN FOOD/SAUCES & SEASONINGS; SAUCE)				
SWEET POTATO (*See also* SWEET POTATO LEAVES; YAM)				
canned				
generic				
mashed	1 cup	0.5	258	2%
pieces	1 cup	<1.0	183	3%
w/syrup	1 cup	<1.0	212	2%
(Joan of Arc)				
candied	½ cup	–	240	–
in heavy syrup	½ cup	–	130	–
in light syrup	½ cup	–	110	–
(Princella)				
candied	½ cup	–	240	–
in heavy syrup	½ cup	–	130	–
in light syrup	½ cup	–	110	–
in pineapple-orange sauce	½ cup	–	210	–
in water	½ cup	–	90	–
(Royal Prince)				
candied	½ cup	–	240	–
in heavy syrup	½ cup	–	130	–
in light syrup	½ cup	–	100	–
dried/generic				
flakes				
mix only	½ cup	<1.0	228	2%
prepared w/water	1 cup	<1.0	242	2%
fresh				
baked-mashed	½ cup	<1.0	103	4%
boiled-mashed/no skin	½ cup	0.5	172	3%
raw				
whole/5" long/~2" dia	1 potato	<1.0	135	3%
pieces	½ cup	1.0	118	5%
frozen/generic/baked	½ cup	<1.0	88	5%
SWEET POTATO DISH				
frozen				
(Birds Eye) specialty classic/ candied sweet potatoes	5 oz	9.0	220	37%
(Ore-Ida) sweet potatoes w/candied sauce	5 pieces	–	170	–
(Mrs. Paul's)				
candied sweet potatoes	4 oz	–	170	–
candied sweets 'n apples	4 oz	–	160	–
homemade/USDA Standard Home Recipe				
candied sweet potatoes w/butter & brown sugar	~3.5 oz	3.0	145	19%

Food and Description	Amount	Fat Grams	Total Calories	% Fat Calories
SWEET POTATO LEAVES/fresh				
cooked	½ cup	–	11	–
	4 oz	<1.0	40	7%
raw/chopped	½ cup	–	6	–
SWEET ROLL (*See* PASTRY)				
SWEETBREADS (*See* individual meat listings)				
SWEETENER, ARTIFICIAL (*See* SUGAR SUBSTITUTE)				
SWISS CHARD (*See* CHARD)				
SWORDFISH				
fresh				
breaded & fried	3 oz	12.0	207	52%
cooked-dry heat	3 oz	4.0	132	27%
raw	3 oz	3.0	103	26%
frozen				
(Stilwell's FanSea) steaks/raw	4 oz	6.0	140	39%

SYRUP (*See* CANE SYRUP; CORN SYRUP; ICE CREAM TOPPING; MAPLE SYRUP; PANCAKE & WAFFLE SYRUP; RICE SYRUP; SORGHUM SYRUP)

T

Food and Description	Amount	Fat Grams	Total Calories	% Fat Calories
TABASCO SAUCE (*See* SAUCE)				
TABOULI/TABOULE/TABOULY				
mix				
(Casbah) prepared	⅔ cup	<1.0	90	5%
(Fantastic Foods) tabouli salad				
mix only	¼ cup	0.5	120	11%
prepared	~½ cup	0.5	120	11%
(Near East) wheat salad/prepared	⅔ cup	3.0	120	23%
TACO SAUCE (*See* SAUCE)				
TAHINI (*See* SESAME BUTTER)				
TAMALE (*See* MEXICAN FOOD; FROZEN ENTRÉE/DINNER)				
TAMARIND/fresh	1 medium	–	5	–
TANGELO/fresh	1 medium	–	39	–
TANGELO JUICE/fresh	8 fl oz	–	100	–
TANGERINE (*See also* MANDARIN ORANGE)				
canned				
in juice	½ cup	–	46	–
in syrup	½ cup	–	76	–
fresh/whole	1 medium	–	37	–

Food and Description	Amount	Fat Grams	Total Calories	% Fat Calories
(Dole)	2 medium	–	70	–
TANGERINE JUICE				
canned				
sweetened	8 fl oz	–	125	–
unsweetened	8 fl oz	–	107	–
fresh	8 fl oz	–	108	–
frozen concentrate				
prepared	8 fl oz	–	114	–
undiluted	6 oz	<1.0	345	1%
TANGERINE JUICE DRINK (See also TEA)				
(Fruitopia) tangerine wavelength	8 fl oz	–	119	–
TAPIOCA (See also PUDDING)				
generic				
pearl/dry	⅓ cup	–	174	–
starch	3 oz	–	300	–
(Minute)	1½ tsp	–	20	–
	3.5 oz	–	352	–
TARO				
chips (See also SNACKS)	10 chips	6.0	110	49%
leaves				
raw	½ cup	–	12	–
steamed	½ cup	<1.0	17	27%
root/fresh/sliced				
cooked	½ cup	–	94	–
raw	½ cup	–	56	–
shoots/fresh/sliced				
cooked	½ cup	–	10	–
raw	½ cup	–	5	–
Tahitian/fresh/sliced				
cooked	½ cup	<1.0	30	15%
raw	½ cup	1.0	25	36%
TARRAGON/ground	1 tsp	–	5	–
TARTAR SAUCE (See SAUCE)				
TEA				
bags				
(Bigelow)				
herbal				
almond orange	1 bag	–	–	–
apple orchard	1 bag	–	–	–
chamomile	1 bag	–	–	–
chamomile-mint	1 bag	–	–	–
cranapple	1 bag	–	–	–
fruit & almond	1 bag	–	–	–
I Love Lemon	1 bag	–	–	–
mint medley	1 bag	–	–	–
orange & spice	1 bag	–	–	–
raspberry royale	1 bag	–	–	–
red raspberry	1 bag	–	–	–

Food and Description	Amount	Fat Grams	Total Calories	% Fat Calories
sweet dreams	1 bag	–	–	–
take a break	1 bag	–	–	–
regular				
Chinese fortune	1 bag	–	–	–
cinnamon stick	1 bag	–	–	–
Constant Comment/orange spice	1 bag	–	–	–
Earl Gray				
decaffeinated	1 bag	–	–	–
regular	1 bag	–	–	–
English teatime	1 bag	–	–	–
lemon lift				
decaffeinated	1 bag	–	–	–
regular	1 bag	–	–	–
plantation mint	1 bag	–	–	–
(Celestial Seasonings)				
herbal				
almond sunset	1 bag	–	3	–
Bengal spice	1 bag	–	5	–
chamomile	1 bag	–	2	–
cinnamon apple spice	1 bag	–	–	–
cinnamon rose	1 bag	–	–	–
country peach spice	1 bag	–	3	–
cranberry cove	1 bag	–	2	–
Emperor's choice	1 bag	–	4	–
ginseng plus	1 bag	–	3	–
Grandma's tummy mint	1 bag	–	2	–
harvest spice	1 bag	–	5	–
lemon mist	1 bag	–	3	–
lemon zinger	1 bag	–	5	–
Mandarin orange spice	1 bag	–	5	–
mellow mint	1 bag	–	2	–
mint magic	1 bag	–	1	–
orange zinger	1 bag	–	5	–
peppermint	1 bag	–	2	–
raspberry patch	1 bag	–	4	–
red zinger	1 bag	–	4	–
sleepytime	1 bag	–	–	–
spearmint	1 bag	–	5	–
strawberry fields	1 bag	–	4	–
Sunburst C	1 bag	–	3	–
tropical escape	1 bag	–	1	–
wild forest blackberry	1 bag	–	–	–
regular				
cinnamon Vienna	1 bag	–	2	–
Earl Gray extraordinary	1 bag	–	3	–
English breakfast	1 bag	–	3	–
lemon	1 bag	–	7	–
mint	1 bag	–	4	–

Food and Description	Amount	Fat Grams	Total Calories	% Fat Calories
Morning Thunder	1 bag	–	3	–
orange spice				
decaffeinated	1 bag	–	7	–
regular	1 bag	–	7	–
organically grown	1 bag	–	12	–
raspberry	1 bag	–	7	–
(Good Earth) original herb & tea				
caffeine-free	1 bag	–	5	–
regular	1 bag	–	–	–
(Lipton)				
cinnamon apple	1 bag	–	–	–
gentle orange	1 bag	–	–	–
green	1 bag	–	–	–
Oriental treasure	1 bag	–	–	–
plain	1 bag	–	–	–
(Luzianne)				
decaffeinated	1 bag	–	–	–
regular	1 bag	–	–	–
(Nestea)	1 bag	–	–	–
(Tetley)				
decaffeinated	1 bag	–	–	–
regular	1 bag	–	–	–
(Worthington) Natural Touch				
Kaffree/caffeine free	1 bag	–	–	–
bottled, boxed, or canned				
(Arizona) iced				
lemon				
diet	8 fl oz	–	4	–
regular	8 fl oz	–	90	–
raspberry	8 fl oz	–	90	–
(Fruitopia) iced				
Born Raspberry	8 fl oz	–	81	–
Curious Mango	8 fl oz	–	83	–
Lemon Berry Intuition	8 fl oz	–	83	–
Peaceable Peach	8 fl oz	–	81	–
(Iguana Bay) tropical iced/	6 fl oz	–	2	–
diet lemon				
(Lipton) iced/brisk				
natural lemon				
diet	12 fl oz	–	5	–
regular	12 fl oz	–	120	–
raspberry blast	12 fl oz	–	130	–
(Nestea) iced				
cool				
diet	8 fl oz	–	1.4	–
sweetened	8 fl oz	–	82	–
Earl Grey	8 fl oz	–	68	–

Food and Description	Amount	Fat Grams	Total Calories	% Fat Calories
lemon				
diet	8 fl oz	–	2.5	–
sweetened	8 fl oz	–	80	–
pitcher style				
extra sweet w/lemon	8 fl oz	–	100	–
lightly sweetened w/lemon	8 fl oz	–	54	–
unsweetened/no lemon	8 fl oz	–	–	–
sweetened	8 fl oz	–	65	–
(Schweppes) iced	8 fl oz	–	90	–
(Snapple)				
cranberry	8 fl oz	–	110	–
just plain tea	8 fl oz	–	80	–
lemon				
decaffeinated	8 fl oz	–	100	–
diet	8 fl oz	–	15	–
regular	8 fl oz	–	110	–
mango	8 fl oz	–	110	–
mint	8 fl oz	–	120	–
orange	8 fl oz	–	110	–
passion fruit	8 fl oz	–	110	–
peach				
diet	8 fl oz	–	–	–
regular	8 fl oz	–	110	–
raspberry				
diet	8 fl oz	–	–	–
regular	8 fl oz	–	120	–
strawberry	8 fl oz	–	100	–
(Southwest) sun tea				
diet	12 fl oz	–	–	–
regular	12 fl oz	–	135	–
(Tropicana) fruit tea				
lemon				
diet	8 fl oz	–	15	–
regular	8 fl oz	–	100	–
peach	10 fl oz	–	140	–
	11.5 fl oz	–	160	–
raspberry				
diet	8 fl oz	–	15	–
regular	8 fl oz	–	120	–
	10 fl oz	–	140	–
	11.5 fl oz	–	160	–
tangerine	10 fl oz	–	140	–
	11.5 fl oz	–	170	–
brewed				
Russian tea	8 fl oz	–	110	–
loose				
(Lipton)	1 tsp	–	–	–

Food and Description	Amount	Fat Grams	Total Calories	% Fat Calories
mix/instant				
(Crystal Light) mix only				
iced tea				
decaffeinated	⅛ tub	–	5	–
regular	⅛ tub	–	5	–
(Lipton) prepared				
citrus	8 fl oz	–	90	–
lemon				
sugar-sweetened	8 fl oz	–	90	–
w/nutrasweet	8 fl oz	–	5	–
plain				
decaffeinated	8 fl oz	–	90	–
sugar-free/decaffeinated or regular	8 fl oz	–	1	–
w/nutrasweet	8 fl oz	–	5	–
(Maxwell House) prepared				
concentrate				
sweetened	8 fl oz	–	80	–
unsweetened	8 fl oz	–	2	–
powder	6 fl oz	–	2	–
(Nestea)				
Ice Teasers				
citrus	8 fl oz	–	5	–
lemon	8 fl oz	–	5	–
orange	8 fl oz	–	5	–
tropical	8 fl oz	–	5	–
wild cherry	8 fl oz	–	5	–
regular				
100%				
decaffeinated	8 fl oz	–	–	–
regular	8 fl oz	–	2	–
lemon & sugar	8 fl oz	–	70	–
sugar-free lemon	8 fl oz	–	2	–
TEFF				
(Arrowhead Mills) seeds	¼ cup	1.0	160	6%
TEMPEH	½ cup	6.0	165	33%
TEMPURA BATTER (See also BAKE & FRY MIX)				
mix				
(Krusteaz)	¼ cup	0.5	110	4%
(SB Sunbird)	1 pkg	0.5	110	4%
TEQUILA (See LIQUOR, DISTILLED)				
TERIYAKI SAUCE (See SAUCE)				
TERRAPIN/baked	¾ cup	4.0	161	22%
THIRST QUENCHER (See SPORTS DRINK; individual flavor listings)				
THURINGER SAUSAGE (See SAUSAGE)				
THYME/ground	1 tsp	–	4	–
TILEFISH				
cooked-dry heat	3 oz	3.0	125	22%
raw	3 oz	2.0	80	23%

Food and Description	Amount	Fat Grams	Total Calories	% Fat Calories
TOASTER PASTRY (*See* PASTRY, TOASTER)				
TOFU (*See also* VEGETARIAN FOODS)				
(Azumaya)				
blue label	3.5 oz	1.0	50	18%
green label	3.5 oz	2.0	70	26%
name age/fried	3.5 oz	4.0	145	25%
red label	3.5 oz	1.0	70	13%
generic				
firm/raw	¼ block	7.0	118	53%
	½ cup	11.0	183	54%
fried	~½ oz	2.6	35	67%
fuyu/salted & fermented	1 block	1.0	13	69%
koyadofu/dried-frozen	~½ oz	5.0	82	55%
Okara	½ cup	1.0	47	19%
regular/raw	¼ block	5.6	88	57%
	½ cup	5.9	94	57%
(Hinoichi)				
Chinese	4 oz	3.0	70	39%
Japanese	4 oz	2.0	60	30%
kinugoshi	4 oz	2.0	50	36%
(Mori-Nu) silken				
firm	5.25 oz	4.0	90	40%
lite	3 oz	1.0	35	26%
soft	5.25 oz	4.0	80	45%
(Nasoya)				
extra firm	3 oz	5.0	90	50%
firm	3 oz	4.0	80	45%
silken	3 oz	2.0	50	36%
soft	3 oz	3.0	60	45%
spicy	3 oz	4.0	70	51%
TOFU DISH (*See* VEGETARIAN FOODS)				
TOFU FROZEN DESSERT				
(Tofutti)				
Better Than Yogurt/low-fat				
chocolate fudge	4 oz	2.0	120	15%
coffee marshmallow	4 oz	1.0	100	9%
passion island fruit	4 oz	1.0	100	9%
peach mango	4 oz	2.0	100	9%
strawberry banana	4 oz	1.0	100	9%
vanilla fudge	4 oz	2.0	120	15%
chocolate fudge treat	1 bar	–	30	–
Cuties sandwiches				
chocolate	1 sandwich	5.0	120	38%
vanilla	1 sandwich	5.0	120	38%
Fruitti				
apricot mango	4 oz	–	100	–
three berry	4 oz	–	100	–
vanilla apple orchard	4 oz	–	100	–

Food and Description	Amount	Fat Grams	Total Calories	% Fat Calories
soft serve				
chocolate				
lite	4 oz	1.0	90	10%
regular	4 oz	4.0	190	19%
peanut butter	4 oz	4.0	190	19%
vanilla				
lite	4 oz	1.0	90	10%
regular	4 oz	4.0	190	19%
wild strawberry/lite	4 oz	1.0	90	10%
sorbet				
chocolate	4 oz	–	90	–
coffee	4 oz	–	80	–
lemon	4 oz	–	90	–
orange peach mango	4 oz	–	90	–
raspberry tea	4 oz	–	80	–
strawberry	4 oz	–	80	–
supreme				
better pecan	4 oz	13.0	220	53%
chocolate	4 oz	11.0	180	55%
chocolate cookies	4 oz	11.0	210	47%
vanilla	4 oz	11.0	190	52%
vanilla almond bark	4 oz	13.0	210	56%
vanilla fudge	4 oz	9.0	190	43%
wildberry	4 oz	9.0	190	43%
Teddy Fudge Bar	1 bar	1.0	70	13%
TOMATO				
canned or jarred				
(Claussen) halves	1 oz	–	5	–
(Contadina)				
crushed	¼ cup	–	20	–
Italian-style/pear	½ cup	–	25	–
pasta-ready	½ cup	2.0	40	45%
primavera	½ cup	1.5	50	27%
w/crushed red pepper	½ cup	3.0	60	45%
w/mushrooms	½ cup	1.5	50	27%
w/olives	½ cup	3.0	60	45%
w/three cheeses	½ cup	4.0	70	51%
recipe-ready	½ cup	–	25	–
(Del Monte)				
diced				
original	½ cup	–	25	–
w/basil, garlic, & oregano	½ cup	–	50	–
w/onion & garlic	½ cup	–	35	–
wedges	½ cup	–	35	–
whole/peeled	½ cup	–	25	–
(Hunt's)				
choice				
cut	½ cup	–	22	–

Food and Description	Amount	Fat Grams	Total Calories	% Fat Calories
cut/diced				
w/green chilies	2 Tbs	–	1	–
w/roasted garlic	½ cup	–	24	–
w/Italian herb	½ cup	–	24	–
crushed				
Angela Mia	½ cup	–	27	–
original	½ cup	<1.0	30	15%
pear-shaped	½ cup	–	20	–
whole				
no salt added	2 tomatoes	<1.0	20	22%
original	2 tomatoes	–	20	–
(Progresso)				
crushed	¼ cup	–	20	–
imported w/basil/peeled	½ cup	–	25	–
whole/peeled	½ cup	–	25	–
w/basil/peeled	½ cup	–	25	–
(Ro*Tel)				
diced/w/chili peppers/extra hot	½ cup	–	20	–
diced/w/green chilies	½ cup	–	20	–
whole/w/green chilies	½ cup	–	20	–
(S&W)				
crushed	½ cup	–	20	–
Italian style/pear	½ cup	–	25	–
no salt	½ cup	–	35	–
ready-cut				
in puree	½ cup	–	30	–
Italian style	½ cup	–	25	–
no salt	½ cup	–	25	–
pasta sauce	¼ cup	–	20	–
peeled	½ cup	–	25	–
salsa				
medium	¼ cup	–	20	–
mild	¼ cup	–	20	–
w/chipotle	¼ cup	–	20	–
w/cilantro	¼ cup	–	20	–
whole				
no salt	½ cup	–	20	–
peeled	½ cup	–	25	–
(Stokely) whole	½ cup	–	25	–
fresh				
green	1 medium	–	30	–
red				
chopped or diced	1 cup	–	35	–
whole	1 medium	–	24	–
sun-dried				
generic				
in oil	1 piece	1.0	6	–
	1 cup	15.0	235	57%

Food and Description	Amount	Fat Grams	Total Calories	% Fat Calories
plain	1 piece	–	5	–
	1 cup	2.0	140	3%
(Sonoma)				
bits	2-3 tsp	–	15	–
halves	2-3 halves	–	15	–
TOMATO ASPIC/canned				
(S&W) supreme	½ cup	–	50	–
TOMATO DISH				
canned or jarred				
(Contadina) stewed				
Italian style	½ cup	–	40	–
Mexican style	½ cup	–	40	–
original	½ cup	–	40	–
(Del Monte) stewed				
Cajun style	½ cup	–	35	–
chunky chili	½ cup	–	30	–
chunky pasta	½ cup	–	45	–
chunky salsa	½ cup	–	35	–
Italian style	½ cup	–	30	–
Mexican style	½ cup	–	35	–
original style				
no salt added	½ cup	–	35	–
regular	½ cup	–	35	–
(Green Giant) stewed				
classic recipe	½ cup	–	35	–
Italian recipe	½ cup	–	30	–
Mexican recipe	½ cup	–	35	–
(Hebrew National) pickled	1 oz	–	4	–
(Hunt's) stewed				
no salt added	½ cup	<1.0	33	8%
original	½ cup	<1.0	33	8%
(Rosoff's) half sour	1 oz	–	5	–
(S&W) stewed				
Italian style	½ cup	–	35	–
regular	½ cup	–	35	–
(Schorr's) pickled	1 oz	–	4	–
(Stokely) stewed	½ cup	–	35	–
homemade/USDA Standard Home Recipe				
stewed	1 cup	2.0	60	30%
TOMATO JUICE/JUICE BLEND				
(Campbell's)	5.5 fl oz	–	30	–
	8 fl oz	–	50	–
	11.5 fl oz	-	70	–
(Del Monte)				
Snap-E-Tom	8 fl oz	–	50	–
Snap-E-Tomato & Chile Cocktail	6 fl oz	–	40	–
generic				
plain	6 fl oz	–	32	–

Food and Description	Amount	Fat Grams	Total Calories	% Fat Calories
tomato & clam	5.5 fl oz	–	77	–
tomato w/beef broth	5.5 fl oz	–	60	–
(Hunt's)				
no salt added	6 fl oz	–	30	–
original	8 fl oz	<1.0	34	9%
(Knudsen)				
organic	8 fl oz	–	60	–
tomato garlic	8 fl oz	–	60	–
(Libby's)	6 fl oz	–	35	–
(Mott's)				
Beefamato	8 fl oz	–	80	–
Clamato	8 fl oz	–	100	–
Clamato Caesar	8 fl oz	–	100	–
(S&W)	5.5 fl oz	–	30	–
	8 fl oz	–	40	–
(Stokely)	4 fl oz	–	20	–
TOMATO PASTE/canned				
(Contadina) stewed				
Italian Style	2 Tbs	1.0	40	23%
original	2 Tbs	–	30	–
(Del Monte)	2 Tbs	–	30	–
generic	½ cup	1.0	110	8%
(Hunt's)				
Italian style	2 Tbs	<1.0	30	15%
no salt added	2 Tbs	<1.0	30	15%
original	2 Tbs	<1.0	27	16%
w/garlic	2 Tbs	<1.0	28	9%
(Progresso)	2 Tbs	–	30	–
(S&W)	6 oz	–	150	–
TOMATO POWDER	4 oz	<1.0	342	1%
TOMATO PURÉE/canned				
(Contadina)	¼ cup	–	20	–
(Hunt's)	4 oz	–	45	–
(Progresso)				
original	¼ cup	–	25	–
thick style	¼ cup	–	30	–
(S&W)				
original	4 oz	–	60	–
w/diced tomatoes	4 oz	–	35	–
TOMATO SAUCE (See also MEXICAN FOOD; SAUCE)				
canned				
(Contadina)				
Italian	¼ cup	–	15	–
original	¼ cup	–	20	–
thick & zesty	¼ cup	–	20	–
(Del Monte)				
original	¼ cup	–	20	–
no salt added	¼ cup	–	20	–

Food and Description	Amount	Fat Grams	Total Calories	% Fat Calories
(Hunt's)				
ready sauce				
chunky chili	¼ cup	<1.0	21	18%
chunky Italian	¼ cup	<1.0	26	14%
chunky Mexican	¼ cup	–	21	–
chunky special	¼ cup	<1.0	21	25%
chunky tomato	¼ cup	–	15	–
country herb	¼ cup	1.0	33	27%
garlic	¼ cup	1.0	29	31%
garlic & herb	¼ cup	<1.0	26	12%
meat loaf fixins	¼ cup	<1.0	23	19%
original Italian	¼ cup	1.0	30	30%
salsa	¼ cup	–	17	–
regular				
Italian	¼ cup	1.0	32	28%
no salt added	¼ cup	–	15	–
original	¼ cup	–	15	–
w/herb	¼ cup	1.0	32	28%
(Progresso)	¼ cup	–	20	–
(S&W)				
garden Italian herb	¼ cup	–	35	–
garden mild Mexican	¼ cup	–	20	–
garden original garden	¼ cup	–	20	–
plain	¼ cup	–	20	–
TOMATO SOUP (See SOUP)				
TONIC WATER (See COCKTAIL MIXER)				
TORTELLINI (See PASTA)				
TORTILLA (See MEXICAN FOOD)				
TORTILLA CHIPS/CORN CHIPS				
(Arizona)				
original	1 oz	6.0	140	39%
restaurant syle	1 oz	7.0	140	45%
(Azteca) Buenitos	1 oz	7.0	140	45%
(Borden)				
corn chips	1 oz	10.0	160	56%
Dipsy Doodles				
mesquite barbecue	1 oz	10.0	160	56%
rippled	1 oz	10.0	160	56%
Doodle Twisters				
nacho cheese	1 oz	10.0	160	56%
nacho chips/thinner crispier	1 oz	8.0	150	48%
white tortilla chips				
crispy rounds	1 oz	8.0	150	48%
quarter rounds/restaurant style	1 oz	8.0	150	48%
yellow tortilla chips				
deli chips/triangles	1 oz	8.0	150	48%
deli rounds	1 oz	8.0	150	48%
(Chi-Chi's)	1 oz	8.0	142	51%

Food and Description	Amount	Fat Grams	Total Calories	% Fat Calories
(Doritos)				
cooler ranch	1 oz	7.0	140	45%
nacho cheesier	1 oz	7.0	140	45%
original thins	1 oz	7.0	140	45%
salsa n cheese thins	1 oz	8.0	150	48%
taco supreme	1 oz	7.0	140	45%
toasted corn	1 oz	6.0	140	39%
zesty salsa	1 oz	7.0	140	45%
(Eagle)				
restaurant style				
white				
nacho/canola oil	1 oz	7.0	140	45%
round				
canola oil	1 oz	6.0	140	39%
El Grande	1 oz	6.0	140	39%
regular	1 oz	6.0	140	39%
salt free/canola oil	1 oz	6.0	140	39%
strips/canola oil	1 oz	6.0	140	39%
yellow				
canola oil	1 oz	6.0	140	39%
regular	1 oz	7.0	140	45%
thins				
nacho	1 oz	7.0	150	42%
ranch	1 oz	7.0	150	42%
(Featherweight) corn chips	1 oz	8.0	150	48%
(Fritos)				
Bar-B-Q	1 oz	10.0	150	60%
cheddar & sour cream	1 oz	10.0	160	56%
choice	1 oz	10.0	160	56%
mesquite grille BBQ	1 oz	10.0	160	56%
original	1 oz	10.0	160	56%
ranch	1 oz	9.0	150	54%
(Garden of Eatin')				
black bean	1 oz	7.0	150	42%
blue corn	1 oz	7.0	150	42%
jalapeño				
no salt added	1 oz	7.0	140	45%
salted	1 oz	7.0	140	45%
mini	1 oz	7.0	150	42%
red hot blues	1 oz	7.0	150	42%
(Guiltless Gourmet) baked				
blue corn	1 oz	1.0	110	8%
chili & lime	1 oz	1.0	110	8%
nacho	1 oz	1.0	110	8%
original style				
no salt	1 oz	1.0	110	8%
regular	1 oz	1.0	110	8%
white corn	1 oz	1.0	110	8%

Food and Description	Amount	Fat Grams	Total Calories	% Fat Calories
(Hain)				
sesame				
no salt	1 oz	7.0	140	45%
regular	1 oz	7.0	140	45%
sesame cheese	1 oz	8.0	160	45%
taco style/no salt	1 oz	11.0	160	62%
(Keebler) Chacho's flour tortilla chips				
cheesy quesadilla	14 chips	5.0	150	30%
cinnamon crispana	13 chips	7.0	150	42%
restaurant style original	15 chips	8.0	150	48%
(Kettle Tias)				
5-grain chips	1 oz	6.0	140	39%
yellow corn	1 oz	6.0	140	39%
(La Famous)				
no salt	1 oz	7.0	140	45%
regular	1 oz	7.0	140	45%
(Lance)				
corn chips				
BBQ	1 oz	11.0	160	62%
hot BBQ	1¼ oz	14.0	210	60%
plain	1 oz	10.0	160	56%
	1¼ oz	11.0	200	50%
	1½ oz	15.0	240	56%
tortilla chips				
fiesta salsa	1 oz	7.0	140	45%
	1¾ oz	12.0	250	43%
nacho chips	1 oz	7.0	140	45%
nacho mini round	1 oz	7.0	140	45%
	1¼ oz	9.0	180	45%
nacho triangles	1¾ oz	12.0	250	43%
(Laura Scudder's)				
nacho				
jalapeño strips	1 oz	7.0	150	42%
triangles	1 oz	7.0	140	45%
restaurant style				
lightly salted	1 oz	7.0	140	45%
picante strips	1 oz	7.0	150	42%
(Louise's) 95% fat-free	1 oz	1.5	120	11%
(Mexi-Snax)				
hot	12 chips	6.0	144	38%
Louisiana cajun/blue	12 chips	6.0	144	38%
sesame	12 chips	5.0	140	32%
tomato & basil	12 chips	6.0	144	38%
vegetable medley	12 chips	5.0	140	32%
(Mi Ranchito) traditional & supreme lights	1 oz	6.0	140	39%
(Michael Season's) organic				
lightly salted	1 oz	5.0	135	33%
salsa	1 oz	5.0	135	33%

Food and Description	Amount	Fat Grams	Total Calories	% Fat Calories
tostados/bite-size	1 oz	5.0	135	34%
white corn/lightly salted	1 oz	6.0	135	43%
(Mission)				
authentic Mexican tortilla chips				
blue corn	1 oz	7.0	140	45%
strips				
regular	1 oz	7.0	140	45%
unsalted	1 oz	7.0	140	45%
tortilla strips				
regular	1 oz	7.0	140	45%
unsalted	1 oz	7.0	140	45%
(Nabisco) Mr. Phipps tortilla crisps				
nacho	28 crisps	7.0	130	48%
original	28 crisps	7.0	130	48%
(Old El Paso)				
Nachips	9 chips	8.0	150	48%
white corn	11 chips	8.0	140	51%
(Old Vienna) deli rounds				
salted	1 oz	7.0	150	42%
white corn	1 oz	6.0	140	39%
(Pepperidge Farm) tortilla crisps				
chili cheese	36 pieces	7.0	130	48%
original	36 pieces	6.0	130	42%
salsa	36 pieces	7.0	130	48%
(Planters)				
king size	1 oz	10.0	160	56%
plain	1 oz	10.0	170	53%
Snacks-To-Go	1.5 oz	14.5	240	54%
(Pringles)				
fresh roasted	1 oz	7.0	140	45%
mild nacho cheese	1 oz	7.0	140	45%
(Rancho California)				
guacamole	1 oz	7.0	155	41%
macho nacho	1 oz	7.0	150	42%
(Santitas) restaurant style				
chips	1 oz	6.0	140	39%
100 % white corn	1 oz	6.0	140	39%
strips	1 oz	6.0	140	39%
(Skinny) natural low-fat corn chips				
barbeque	¾ oz	1.5	90	15%
	2 cups	2.0	120	15%
nacho cheese	¾ oz	1.5	90	15%
	2 cups	2.0	120	15%
original				
lightly salted	¾ oz	1.5	90	15%
	2 cups	2.0	120	15%
no salt	2 cups	2.0	120	15%

Food and Description	Amount	Fat Grams	Total Calories	% Fat Calories
sour cream & onion	1 cup	1.0	60	15%
	2 cups	2.0	130	14%
(Snyder's)				
enchilada	1 oz	7.0	140	45%
nacho cheese	1 oz	7.0	140	45%
original				
no salt	1 oz	7.0	140	45%
regular	1 oz	7.0	140	45%
ranch	1 oz	7.0	140	45%
(Taco Bell) restaurant style	12 chips	6.0	140	39%
(Tostitos)				
baked				
cool ranch	1 oz	3.0	120	23%
original	1 oz	1.0	110	8%
unsalted	1 oz	1.0	110	8%
original				
bite-size	1 oz	8.0	140	51%
lime 'n chile	1 oz	7.0	150	42%
round	1 oz	8.0	150	48%
white corn/restaurant	1 oz	6.0	130	42%
(Tyson)				
nacho cheese	1 oz	7.0	140	45%
ranch flavor	1 oz	7.0	140	45%
traditional	1 oz	7.0	140	45%
unsalted	1 oz	7.0	140	45%
(Weaver's)				
deli rounds				
nacho cheese	1½ oz	14.0	250	50%
salted	1 oz	7.0	150	42%
	1½ oz	15.0	240	56%
white corn	1 oz	6.0	140	39%
Sundance				
BBQ	1½ oz	13.0	230	51%
hot	⅔ cup	8.0	150	48%
plain	1½ oz	15.0	240	56%
(Wise) Bravos				
nacho cheese flavor	1 oz	8.0	150	48%
TRAIL MIX (See CEREAL; FRUIT SNACK; SNACK MIX)				
TREACLE (See MOLASSES)				
TRIPE				
(Armour/Armour Star)				
Banner sausage				
stomachs	2 oz	5.0	90	50%
tripe	2 oz	5.0	90	50%
beef tripe	3 oz	1.5	90	20%
TRITICALE (See also FLOUR)				
whole-grain	1 oz	0.5	95	5%
	1 cup	4.0	645	6%

Food and Description	Amount	Fat Grams	Total Calories	% Fat Calories
TROUT				
mixed species				
cooked-dry heat	3 oz	6.5	165	35%
raw	3 oz	5.0	125	36%
rainbow				
farmed				
cooked-dry heat	3 oz	5.5	145	34%
raw	3 oz	4.0	120	30%
wild				
cooked-dry heat	3 oz	4.5	130	31%
raw	3 oz	2.6	100	23%
smoked	3 oz	3.0	153	18%
sea/mixed species				
cooked-dry heat	3 oz	3.0	115	23%
raw	3 oz	2.0	90	20%
TUNA (*See also* SEAFOOD ENTRÉE/DINNER; TUNA DISH; VEGETARIAN FOODS)				
canned/drained				
(Bumble Bee)				
chunk light				
in oil	2 oz	12.0	160	68%
in water	2 oz	1.0	60	15%
chunk white				
in oil	2 oz	12.0	160	68%
in water	2 oz	2.0	70	26%
solid white				
in oil	2 oz	8.0	130	55%
in water	2 oz	2.0	70	26%
(Carnation) chunk light				
in oil	2 oz	8.0	125	58%
in water	2 oz	2.0	70	26%
(Chicken Of The Sea)				
chunk light				
in canola oil	2 oz	6.0	110	49%
in spring water				
50% less salt	2 oz	0.5	60	8%
low sodium	2 oz	0.5	60	8%
regular	2 oz	0.5	60	8%
chunk white				
albacore/in spring water	2 oz	1.0	60	15%
very low sodium/in spring water	2 oz	0.5	60	15%
solid light Genova tonno/ in olive oil	2 oz	8.0	130	55%
solid white				
in canola oil	2 oz	3.0	90	30%
in spring water	2 oz	1.0	70	13%
(Empress) chunk light/in water	2 oz	1.0	60	15%
(Featherweight) chunk light/in water	¼ cup	0.5	60	8%

Food and Description	Amount	Fat Grams	Total Calories	% Fat Calories
generic				
light				
in oil	3 oz	7.0	169	37%
in water	3 oz	<1.0	111	4%
white				
in oil	2 oz	6.9	158	39%
in water	2 oz	2.0	116	16%
(S&W)				
chunk light				
in oil	2 oz	6.0	110	33%
in water	2 oz	0.5	70	6%
solid white/in oil	2 oz	1.5	80	17%
(StarKist)				
chunk light				
in oil	2 oz	6.0	110	49%
	2.7 oz	8.0	140	51%
in water	2 oz	0.5	60	8%
	2.7 oz	1.0	80	11%
chunk white				
low-salt, low-fat				
in-distilled water	2 oz	0.5	60	8%
	2.7 oz	0.5	80	9%
in spring water	2 oz	0.5	60	8%
	2.7 oz	0.5	70	6%
regular/in water	2 oz	1.0	60	15%
	2.8 oz	1.0	80	11%
solid light				
hickory smoke/in water	2 oz	1.0	60	15%
Prime Catch/in water	2 oz	1.0	60	15%
	2.8 oz	1.0	80	11%
solid white				
hickory smoke/in water	2 oz	1.0	70	13%
regular				
in oil	2 oz	3.0	90	30%
	2.8 oz	5.0	130	35%
in water	2 oz	1.0	70	13%
	2.8 oz	1.0	100	9%
fresh				
bluefin				
cooked-dry heat	3 oz	5.0	157	29%
raw	3 oz	4.0	122	30%
skipjack				
cooked-dry heat	3 oz	1.0	112	8%
raw	3 oz	1.0	88	10%
yellowfin				
cooked-dry heat	3 oz	1.0	118	8%
raw	3 oz	1.0	90	10%

Food and Description	Amount	Fat Grams	Total Calories	% Fat Calories
TUNA DISH (*See also* FROZEN ENTRÉE/DINNER; SEAFOOD ENTRÉE/DINNER)				
canned				
(Libby's) The Spredables tuna salad	⅓ cup	8.0	130	55%
frozen				
(Peter Pan) steaks/skinless-boneless/raw				
white albacore	3.5 oz	5.0	100	45%
yellowfin	3.5 oz	4.0	130	28%
homemade/USDA Standard Home Recipe				
tuna patty	3 oz	3.0	80	34%
tuna salad made w/salad dressing & tuna canned in oil/no egg	1 cup	19.0	375	46%
mix/kit				
(Bumble Bee) Tuna Mix-Ins/mix only				
classic Italian	⅓ pkg	–	25	–
garden & herb	⅓ pkg	–	25	–
lemon herb	⅓ pkg	–	25	–
zesty tomato	⅓ pkg	–	25	–
(Featherweight) tuna combo kit	1 kit	3.5	230	14%
(Betty Crocker) Tuna Helper				
au gratin				
mix only	½ cup	4.0	190	19%
prepared	1 cup	12.0	300	36%
cheesy noodles				
mix only	⅔ cup	4.0	170	21%
prepared	1 cup	12.0	290	37%
creamy broccoli				
mix only	⅔ cup	5.0	190	24%
prepared	1 cup	13.0	310	38%
creamy noodles				
mix only	¾ cup	6.0	190	28%
prepared	1 cup	14.0	310	41%
fettuccine Alfredo				
mix only	1 cup	4.0	180	20%
prepared	1 cup	16.0	340	42%
garden cheddar				
mix only	⅔ cup	4.0	190	19%
prepared	1 cup	12.0	310	35%
pasta salad				
mix only	⅓ cup	0.5	120	4%
prepared				
low-fat recipe	⅓ cup	1.5	230	6%
regular recipe	⅔ cup	27.0	380	64%
tetrazzini				
mix only	½ cup	3.0	180	15%
prepared	1 cup	12.0	310	35%
tuna pot pie				
mix only	½ cup	20.0	340	53%
prepared	⅕ pie	24.0	440	49%

Food and Description	Amount	Fat Grams	Total Calories	% Fat Calories
tuna Romanoff				
mix only	⅔ cup	3.0	210	13%
prepared	1 cup	8.0	280	26%
(StarKist) Charlie's Lunch Kits/prepared w/low-fat mayonnaise				
chunk light tuna	1 serving	9.0	230	35%
chunk white tuna	1 serving	9.0	230	35%
TURBINADO SUGAR (See SUGAR)				
TURBOT				
cooked-dry heat	3 oz	3.0	104	26%
raw	3 oz	2.5	81	28%
TURKEY (See also FRANKFURTER; LUNCHEON MEAT; SAUSAGE)				
■ **TURKEY & TURKEY PARTS/FRESH**				
all classes				
dark meat only/roasted				
w/skin	~2 lb	93.0	1789	47%
w/o skin	~5 oz	10.0	262	34%
chopped/diced	1 cup	9.0	223	36%
giblets & organs/simmered				
giblets	~5 oz	7.0	243	26%
gizzard	~5 oz	5.6	236	21%
heart	~5 oz	8.0	257	28%
liver	~5 oz	8.0	237	30%
light meat only				
w/skin	2¼ lb	87.0	206	38%
w/o skin	~5 oz	4.5	219	19%
chopped/diced	1 cup	4.0	194	19%
meat & skin/dark & light/no giblets or neck	~4 lb	180.6	3857	42%
meat only/dark & light	~5 oz	7.0	238	26%
whole/including meat, skin, giblets, & neck/roasted	~9 lb	380.0	8245	42%
fryer/roaster/roasted				
back				
w/skin	4 oz	11.5	230	45%
w/o skin	4 oz	6.5	195	30%
breast				
w/skin	4 oz	3.6	175	19%
w/o skin	4 oz	1.0	155	6%
dark meat				
w/skin	4 oz	8.0	206	35%
w/o skin	4 oz	5.0	185	24%
chopped/diced	1 cup	6.0	227	24%
leg				
w/skin	4 oz	6.0	193	28%
w/o skin	4 oz	4.3	180	22%
light meat				
w/skin	4 oz	5.0	185	24%

Food and Description	Amount	Fat Grams	Total Calories	% Fat Calories
w/o skin	4 oz	1.3	159	7%
chopped/diced	1 cup	1.7	195	8%
wing				
w/skin	4 oz	11.2	235	43%
w/o skin	4 oz	3.9	185	19%
young hen/roasted				
back w/skin	4 oz	17.7	288	55%
breast w/skin	4 oz	9.0	220	37%
dark meat				
w/skin	4 oz	14.5	265	49%
w/o skin	4 oz	9.0	220	37%
chopped/diced	1 cup	11.0	270	37%
leg w/skin	4 oz	12.0	245	40%
light meat				
w/skin	4 oz	10.7	235	41%
w/o skin	4 oz	4.0	180	20%
chopped/diced	1 cup	5.0	225	20%
wing-w/skin	4 oz	15.3	270	51%
young tom/roasted				
back w/skin	4 oz	15.5	270	52%
breast w/skin	4 oz	8.4	214	35%
dark meat				
w/skin	4 oz	12.3	245	45%
w/o skin	4 oz	8.0	210	34%
chopped/diced	1 cup	10.0	260	35%
leg w/skin	4 oz	11.0	235	42%
light meat				
w/skin	4 oz	8.7	217	36%
w/o skin	4 oz	3.3	175	17%
chopped/diced	1 cup	4.0	215	17%
wing-w/skin	4 oz	13.0	251	47%
■ TURKEY & TURKEY PARTS/FRESH, FROZEN, OR CANNED/BRAND NAME				
(Alpine Lace) breast of turkey/skinless/ oven-roasted	1 oz	–	45	–
(Armour)				
Golden Star	1 oz	4.0	50	72%
Turkey Selects/boneless				
breast				
roast	3 oz	5.0	120	38%
slices	3 oz	1.0	90	10%
tenderloins	3 oz	1.0	90	10%
ground	3 oz	6.0	120	45%
strips	3 oz	4.0	100	36%
(Armour Star)				
broth-basted				
w/sugar	4 oz	10.0	180	50%
w/o sugar	4 oz	10.0	180	50%
butter-basted	4 oz	10.0	190	47%

Food and Description	Amount	Fat Grams	Total Calories	% Fat Calories
(Butterball) fresh premium turkey cuts				
breast				
cutlets	1 cutlet	0.5	80	6%
medallions	4 pieces	1.0	130	7%
roast	4 oz	6.0	160	34%
strips	4 oz	1.0	120	8%
tenderloins/boneless	4 oz	1.0	120	8%
burger patties (turkey)	1 piece	9.0	170	48%
ground				
all white	4 oz	3.0	130	21%
regular	4 oz	10.0	180	50%
(Honeysuckle White)				
breast steaks	4 oz	2.5	120	19%
ground/white meat	4 oz	10.0	190	47%
(Hormel) Jennie-O turkey roast w/gravy				
white & dark meat	4 oz	7.0	150	42%
white meat	4 oz	7.0	150	42%
(Louis Rich)				
ground	4 oz	12.0	190	57%
nuggets/breaded	4 nuggets	16.0	260	55%
patties/breaded	1 patty	13.0	220	53%
sticks/breaded	3 sticks	15.0	230	59%
(Mr. Turkey) cooked				
breast quarter				
BBQ	1 oz	1.0	34	26%
oven roasted	1 oz	1.0	34	26%
patties	3 oz	11.0	195	51%
smoked	1 oz	1.0	35	26%
diced white meat	2 oz	2.0	84	21%
ground	1 oz	4.0	54	67%
(Perdue) fresh roasted/w/ or w/o skin, as packaged				
breast				
Fit 'n Easy	1 oz	<1.0	31	15%
hotel-style	1 oz	2.0	42	43%
regular	1 oz	2.0	42	43%
drumsticks	1 oz	2.0	41	44%
breast cutlets/Fit 'n Easy	1 oz	<1.0	31	15%
breast tenderloins/Fit 'n Easy	1 oz	<1.0	31	15%
ground				
breast meat	1 oz	<1.0	32	14%
lean	1 oz	2.0	38	47%
thigh				
Fit 'n Easy	1 oz	2.0	37	49%
regular	1 oz	3.0	48	56%
whole turkey				
dark meat	1 oz	3.0	47	57%
white meat	1 oz	2.0	42	43%

Food and Description	Amount	Fat Grams	Total Calories	% Fat Calories
wing drummettes	1 oz	2.0	42	43%
wing portions	1 oz	3.0	48	56%
wings	1 oz	2.0	46	39%
(Shady Brook) fresh/raw				
breast				
boneless	3 oz	4.0	120	30%
half	3 oz	4.0	120	30%
whole	3 oz	7.0	140	45%
drumsticks	3 oz	6.0	120	45%
ground				
breast	3 oz	1.0	90	10%
light & dark meat	3 oz	6.0	120	45%
thighs/no skin	3 oz	6.0	120	45%
wings	3 oz	6.0	130	42%
(Shelton's) turkey burger	1 burger	10.0	170	53%
(The Turkey Store) fresh				
breast				
Cajun style/fat-free	2 oz	–	60	–
cutlets	3 oz	1.0	90	10%
hickory smoked/fat-free	2 oz	–	60	–
patties/seasoned	4 oz	3.0	130	21%
roast	3 oz	6.0	130	42%
slices	3 oz	1.0	90	10%
strips	3 oz	1.0	90	10%
tenders	3 oz	1.0	90	10%
burger patties				
plain	4 oz	8.0	160	45%
seasoned	4 oz	8.0	160	45%
ground				
breast	4 oz	1.5	120	11%
lean	4 oz	8.0	160	45%
(Wampler Longacre)				
breast				
skinless				
gourmet high yield	1 oz	–	28	–
premium				
brown & glazed	1 oz	1.0	26	35%
plain	1 oz	–	28	–
skin-on				
gourmet				
brown & glazed	1 oz	2.0	28	64%
plain	1 oz	2.0	31	58%
premium				
brown & glazed	1 oz	2.0	29	62%
plain	1 oz	2.0	29	62%
ground/raw/frozen	4 oz	15.0	210	64%

TURKEY ALTERNATIVE (*See* VEGETARIAN FOODS)
TURKEY BACON (*See* BACON)

Food and Description	Amount	Fat Grams	Total Calories	% Fat Calories
TURKEY ENTRÉE/DINNER (*See also* FROZEN ENTRÉE/DINNER; PASTA ENTRÉE/DINNER)				
can or microwave container				
(Dinty Moore)				
turkey & dressing w/gravy/ American Classics	1 bowl	8.0	290	25%
turkey stew				
canned	1 cup	3.0	150	18%
microwave cup	1 cup	2.5	130	17%
(Libby's) Diner/gravy w/turkey & dressing	7 oz	7.0	180	35%
(Luck's) gravy w/turkey over cornbread dressing/microwave bowl	1 bowl	2.5	190	12%
(Mary Kitchen) roast turkey hash	1 cup	3.0	210	13%
frozen				
generic				
light	2 oz	2.0	42	43%
light & dark	2 oz	2.0	42	43%
turkey roast/light & dark meat	3 oz	5.0	130	35%
	~7 oz	11.0	304	33%
turkey roll				
(Stouffer's) Lean Cuisine				
pot pie	9.5 oz	9.0	300	27%
turkey Dijon	9⅜ oz	6.0	220	25%
(Morton)	7 oz	18.0	300	54%
(Perdue) Perdue Done It!/fully cooked				
breast nuggets	3 oz	9.0	180	45%
fun shapes/turkey-shaped nuggets	3 oz	9.0	180	45%
(Schwan's) turkey breast/partially or fully cooked				
unbreaded	3 oz	–	70	–
w/gravy	5 oz	4.0	130	28%
(Stouffer's)				
pot pie	10 oz	33.0	530	56%
turkey tetrazzini	10 oz	17.0	360	43%
(Swanson) pot pie				
Hungry Man	1 pie	34.0	650	47%
original	1 pie	21.0	390	48%
(Weight Watchers) turkey sandwich				
honey Dijon pretzel	1 sandwich	4.0	230	16%
stuffed breast	8.75 oz	8.0	240	30%
homemade/USDA Standard Home Recipe				
scalloped turkey	~7 oz	5.6	253	20%
turkey loaf	5 oz	15.0	280	48%
turkey sticks/breaded or battered & fried	5 oz	24.0	397	54%
TURKEY HAM (*See* HAM; LUNCHEON MEAT)				
TURKEY SAUSAGE (*See* SAUSAGE)				
TURKEY SOUP (*See* SOUP)				
TURMERIC/ground	1 tsp	–	8	–

Food and Description	Amount	Fat Grams	Total Calories	% Fat Calories
TURNIP				
fresh				
boiled	½ cup	–	14	–
raw	½ cup	–	18	–
frozen	½ cup	–	26	–
TURNIP GREENS				
canned				
(Bush's Best)	½ cup	–	25	–
generic	½ cup	–	17	–
(Glory Foods)	½ cup	0.5	45	10%
(Luck's) w/diced turnips/seasoned w/pork	½ cup	1.5	35	39%
(Stokely)	½ cup	–	20	–
fresh				
boiled-drained	½ cup	–	15	–
raw	½ cup	–	7	–
frozen				
generic				
plain	½ cup	–	24	–
	10 oz	1.0	60	15%
w/diced turnips	10 oz	0.5	60	8%
(Pictsweet) w/diced turnips	3.3 oz	–	20	–
TURTLE/green				
canned	3 oz	0.6	91	6%
raw	3 oz	<1.0	76	6%

V

Food and Description	Amount	Fat Grams	Total Calories	% Fat Calories
VEAL				
(NOTE: All serving sizes are for cooked portions, unless otherwise stated. "Lean" means veal trimmed of separable fat before cooking. "Lean & fat" means untrimmed and cooked or eaten as purchased. In most cases, 4 ounces of raw veal yields approximately 3 ounces cooked.)				
chop				
lean w/bone/raw	6.5 oz	5.0	170	26%
cutlet, steak				
lean/boneless/braised or broiled	3 oz	4.0	170	21%
ground/broiled	3 oz	6.0	146	37%

Food and Description	Amount	Fat Grams	Total Calories	% Fat Calories
loin				
lean				
braised or broiled	3 oz	8.0	195	37%
roasted	3 oz	6.0	150	36%
lean & fat				
braised or broiled	3 oz	15.0	240	56%
roasted	3 oz	11.0	185	54%
organs				
brain				
braised	3 oz	8.0	120	60%
fried	3 oz	14.0	180	70%
heart/braised	3 oz	6.0	160	34%
kidney/braised	3 oz	5.0	140	32%
liver				
braised	3 oz	6.0	140	39%
fried	3 oz	10.0	210	43%
spleen/braised	3 oz	3.0	110	25%
sweetbreads/braised	3 oz	3.0	145	19%
tongue/braised	3 oz	9.0	170	48%
rib roast				
lean				
braised or broiled	3 oz	7.0	185	34%
roasted	3 oz	6.0	150	36%
lean & fat				
braised or broiled	3 oz	11.0	214	46%
roasted	3 oz	12.0	195	55%
round w/rump				
roasts & leg cutlets/lean/braised or broiled	3 oz	4.0	175	20%
sirloin				
lean				
braised or broiled	3 oz	6.0	175	31%
braised or broiled/chopped	1 cup	9.0	290	28%
roasted	3 oz	5.0	145	31%
roasted/chopped	1 cup	9.0	235	34%
lean & fat				
braised or broiled	3 oz	11.0	220	45%
braised or broiled/chopped	1 cup	18.0	355	45%
roasted	3 oz	9.0	175	46%
roasted/chopped	1 cup	15.0	285	47%
top round				
lean				
roasted	4 oz	6.0	230	23%
roasted/chopped	1 cup	5.0	210	21%
lean & fat				
braised or broiled	4 oz	6.0	230	23%
braised or broiled/chopped	1 cup	7.0	285	22%
roasted	4 oz	5.0	180	25%

Food and Description	Amount	Fat Grams	Total Calories	% Fat Calories
roasted/chopped	1 cup	7.0	225	28%

VEAL DISH (See also FROZEN ENTRÉE/DINNER)
homemade/USDA Standard Home Recipe

veal Parmigiana	~6.5 oz	20.0	351	51%
veal scallopini w/sauce	~3.5 oz	19.0	255	67%

VEGETABLE DISH (See FROZEN ENTRÉE/DINNER; VEGETARIAN FOODS; individual vegetable listings)

VEGETABLE JUICE/JUICE COCKTAIL
bottled, boxed, or canned
(Campbell's) V-8

lightly tangy	8 fl oz	–	60	–
low-sodium	8 fl oz	–	60	–
original	5.5 fl oz	–	35	–
	8 fl oz	–	50	–
	10 fl oz	–	60	–
picante	8 fl oz	–	50	–
	11.5 fl oz	–	70	–
plus	5.5 fl oz	–	40	–
	8 fl oz	–	50	–
spicy hot	11.5 oz	–	70	–
generic	6 fl oz	–	34	–
(Knudsen)				
Very Veggie	8 fl oz	1.0	50	18%
Viva Vegetable	8 fl oz	–	60	–
(Mott's)	10 fl oz	–	60	–

VEGETABLE OIL (See COOKING SPRAY; OIL)
VEGETABLE SOUP (See SOUP)
VEGETABLES, MIXED (See also ASIAN FOOD; FROZEN ENTRÉE/DINNER; SUCCOTASH)

■ CANNED OR JARRED

(Bush's Best) mixed greens	½ cup	–	20	–
(Del Monte)				
mixed vegetables	½ cup	–	40	–
peas & carrots	½ cup	–	60	–
(Freshlike)				
no salt	½ cup	–	35	–
no salt or sugar	½ cup	–	35	–
generic				
beets w/onions	½ cup	–	80	–
peas & carrots	½ cup	–	48	–
peas & onions	½ cup	–	30	–
(Green Giant)				
garden medley	½ cup	–	40	–
mixed vegetables	½ cup	–	60	–
peas & carrots	½ cup	–	50	–
sweet peas w/tiny pearl onions	½ cup	–	60	–
(La Choy) vegetables				
Chinese	⅔ cup	–	10	–

Food and Description	Amount	Fat Grams	Total Calories	% Fat Calories
chop suey	½ cup	–	15	–
(LeSueur)				
early peas w/mushrooms & pearl onions	½ cup	–	60	–
(S&W)				
old fashioned harvest time mixed	½ cup	–	35	–
peas & carrots	½ cup	–	50	–
peas & onions	½ cup	–	40	–
(Seneca)				
mixed vegetables	4.4 oz	–	45	–
peas & carrots	4.4 oz	–	60	–
vegetables for stew	4.4 oz	–	40	–
(Stokely)				
no salt or sugar added	½ cup	–	40	–
regular	½ cup	–	40	–
(Veg-All)				
homestyle	½ cup	–	35	–
lite	½ cup	–	35	–
original	½ cup	–	35	–
(Vlasic) hot & spicy garden mix	1 oz	–	4	–
■ FROZEN				
(Birds Eye)				
Combination Vegetables				
baby carrots, peas, & pearl onions	½ cup	–	50	–
broccoli, baby carrots, & water chestnuts	½ cup	–	30	–
broccoli, carrots, & water chestnuts	½ cup	–	30	–
broccoli, cauliflower, & carrots	½ cup	–	25	–
broccoli, corn, & red peppers	⅔ cup	1.0	60	15%
broccoli, green beans, pearl onions, & red peppers	¾ cup	–	35	–
broccoli, red peppers, bamboo shoots, & straw mushrooms	¾ cup	–	30	–
Brussels sprouts, cauliflower, & carrots	¾ cup	–	40	–
carrots, peas, & pearl onions	½ cup	–	48	–
cauliflower, baby carrots, & snow peas	⅔ cup	–	35	–
corn, green beans, & pasta curls	½ cup	5.0	110	41%
green peas & pearl onions	½ cup	–	70	–
peas & carrots	½ cup	–	40	–
peas & onions	½ cup	–	40	–
rice, green peas, & mushrooms	½ cup	–	110	–
International Recipe				
Austrian	½ cup	3.0	70	39%
Bavarian	½ cup	5.0	90	50%
California	½ cup	4.0	90	36%
Chinese	½ cup	4.0	70	51%

Food and Description	Amount	Fat Grams	Total Calories	% Fat Calories
chow mein	½ cup	4.0	90	40%
country	½ cup	–	90	–
French country	½ cup	4.0	70	51%
Italian	½ cup	5.0	100	45%
Japanese	½ cup	–	30	–
Mandarin	½ cup	4.0	90	40%
New England	½ cup	6.0	125	43%
Oriental	½ cup	4.0	70	51%
San Francisco	½ cup	5.0	100	45%
Spanish	½ cup	–	110	–
Stir-Fry Vegetables				
broccoli	1 cup	–	30	–
Chinese	½ cup	–	35	–
Japanese	½ cup	–	30	–
Oriental	2¼ cups	4.0	210	17%
pepper	3 oz	–	25	–
teriyaki	2 cups	2.5	210	11%
(C&W)				
regular				
corn & black bean salad	⅔ cup	–	80	–
early harvest petite peas & baby carrots	⅔ cup	–	60	–
fancy mixed vegetables	¾ cup	–	60	–
petite peas w/pearl onions	⅔ cup	–	70	–
rancho fiesta blend	⅔ cup	–	60	–
vegetable stand combinations				
broccoli florets, julienne red peppers, sugar snap peas, & water chestnuts	1 cup	–	40	–
early harvest corn, broccoli florets, & julienne red peppers	⅔ cup	0.5	60	8%
petite peas, early harvest corn, baby carrots, & sugar snap peas	⅔ cup	0.5	60	8%
sugar snap peas, baby carrots, cauliflower, & broccoli florets	1 cup	–	30	–
(Freshlike)				
California blend	3.3 oz	–	30	–
chuckwagon blend	3.3 oz	–	70	–
Italian blend	3.3 oz	–	30	–
Midwestern blend	3.3 oz	–	40	–
mixed vegetables	3.3 oz	–	70	–
Oriental blend	3.3 oz	–	25	–
Scandinavian blend	3.3 oz	–	45	–
vegetables for soup	3.3 oz	–	50	–
vegetables for stew	3.3 oz	–	50	–
winter blend	3.3 oz	–	95	–
Wisconsin blend	3.3 oz	–	50	–

Food and Description	Amount	Fat Grams	Total Calories	% Fat Calories
(Green Giant)				
American Mixtures				
California style	¾ cup	–	25	–
Heartland style	1 cup	–	30	–
Manhattan style	1 cup	–	25	–
New England style	⅔ cup	1.5	70	19%
San Francisco style	¾ cup	–	30	–
Santa Fe	¾ cup	–	60	–
Seattle style	¾ cup	–	25	–
Western style	¾ cup	1.5	50	27%
Butter Sauce Vegetables				
broccoli, cauliflower, carrots, corn, & sweet peas	¾ cup	2.0	60	30%
broccoli, pasta, sweet peas, corn, & red peppers	¾ cup	2.0	70	26%
mixed vegetables	¾ cup	2.0	70	26%
cheese & cream sauce vegetables				
broccoli, cauliflower & carrots	⅔ cup	2.5	80	28%
Create a Meal! vegetables				
broccoli stir-fry	2⅓ cups	3.5	120	26%
lo mein stir-fry	2⅓ cups	0.5	160	3%
sweet & sour stir-fry	1¾ cups	–	130	–
Szechuan stir-fry	1¾ cups	5.0	150	30%
teriyaki stir-fry	1¾ cups	–	100	–
vegetable almond stir-fry	1¾ cups	4.5	150	27%
Harvest Fresh				
broccoli, cauliflower, & carrots	1 cup	–	30	–
mixed vegetables	⅔ cup	–	50	–
sweet peas & pearl onions	½ cup	–	50	–
International Mixtures				
English style cheddar	4 oz	5.0	120	38%
French style garlic Dijon	4 oz	3.0	60	45%
Italian style Parmesan	4 oz	2.5	70	32%
Japanese style teriyaki	4 oz	–	50	–
Normandy style mushroom	4 oz	3.0	80	34%
Oriental style rice	8 oz	0.5	180	3%
regular/mixed vegetables	¾ cup	–	50	–
Select/sweet peas & pearl onions	⅔ cup	–	60	–
(Hanover)				
mixed vegetables	½ cup	–	50	–
Oriental blend	½ cup	–	25	–
soup vegetables	½ cup	–	60	–
stew mix	½ cup	–	50	–
summer vegetables	½ cup	–	35	–
(LeSueur) early June peas w/mushrooms	¾ cup	–	60	–
(Ore Ida) stew vegetables	⅔ cup	–	50	–

Food and Description	Amount	Fat Grams	Total Calories	% Fat Calories
(Pictsweet)				
Express/microwave				
broccoli, carrots, & cauliflower	2.5 oz	–	20	–
broccoli, carrots, & water chestnuts	2.5 oz	–	25	–
broccoli, corn, & red peppers	2.5 oz	–	25	–
broccoli, French Beans, onions, & red peppers	2.5 oz	–	20	–
broccoli & cauliflower	2.5 oz	–	20	–
peas, pearl onions, & mushrooms	2.5 oz	–	45	–
squash, onion, & peppers	2.5 oz	–	18	–
mixed vegetables				
Belgian	3.2 oz	–	30	–
California	¾ cup	–	20	–
Cantonese	1 cup	–	35	–
del sol	1 cup	–	30	–
for stir-fry				
prepared as directed	3.5 oz	4.0	75	48%
vegetables only	¾ cup	–	35	–
grande	¾ cup	0.5	45	10
Italian	3.2 oz	–	20	–
Japanese	3.2 oz	–	25	–
Milano	3.2 oz	–	40	–
New England	3.2 oz	–	40	–
Oriental	3.2 oz	–	25	–
Parisian	3.2 oz	–	30	–
regular	3.2 oz	–	60	–
Romano	3.2 oz	–	50	–
Swiss	3.2 oz	–	25	–
Western	3.2 oz	–	50	–
(Seneca)				
broccoli				
Italian blend	¾ cup	–	30	–
Normandy	1 cup	–	30	–
stir-fry blend	1 cup	–	30	–
mixed vegetables	⅔ cup	–	60	–
Oriental				
blend	¾ cup	–	25	–
stir-fry blend	¾ cup	–	25	–
peas & carrots	⅔ cup	–	50	–
peas & onions	⅔ cup	–	70	–
Scandinavian blend	¾ cup	–	40	–
soup mix	¾ cup	–	40	–
winter blend	1 cup	–	25	–
(Stokely) Singles				
broccoli, carrots, & water chestnuts	3 oz	1.0	30	30%
broccoli & cauliflower	3 oz	1.0	20	45%
broccoli, cauliflower, & carrots	3 oz	1.0	25	36%

Food and Description	Amount	Fat Grams	Total Calories	% Fat Calories
(Veg-All)				
mixed vegetables	3.3 oz	–	70	–
soup vegetables	3.3 oz	–	50	–
stew vegetables				
5-ways	3.3 oz	–	50	–
4-ways	3.3 oz	–	50	–
vegetable blends				
California	3.3 oz	–	30	–
chuckwagon	3.3 oz	1.0	70	13%
country	3.3 oz	–	50	–
Italian	3.3 oz	–	30	–
Midwestern	3.3 oz	–	40	–
Oriental	3.3 oz	–	25	–
Scandinavian	3.3 oz	–	45	–
winter	3.3 oz	–	25	–

VEGETARIAN FOODS

(NOTE: Some of the foods listed in this category were designed to be substitutes for meat and foods traditionally made with meat, and their names may therefore reflect the items they are intended to replace. However, all products listed here are meatless.)

■ (Amy's)

Food and Description	Amount	Fat Grams	Total Calories	% Fat Calories
frozen				
bean & rice burrito	6 oz	5.0	250	18%
bean, rice, & cheese burrito	6 oz	8.0	280	26%
black bean burrito	6 oz	8.0	320	23%
black bean & vegetable enchilada	4.75 oz	4.0	130	28%
breakfast burrito	6 oz	5.0	230	20%
California veggie burger	2.5 oz	3.0	100	27%
cannelloni dinner	9 oz	11.0	260	38%
cheese enchilada	4.75 oz	9.0	210	39%
cheese ravioli	8 oz	12.0	340	32%
Chicago Veggie Burger	2.5 oz	5.0	160	28%
country dinner	11 oz	21.0	480	39%
enchilada dinner	10 oz	8.0	250	29%
macaroni & cheese	1 serving	19.0	450	38%
macaroni & soy cheese	1 serving	14.0	360	35%
Mexican tamale pie	1 pie	3.0	220	12%
pizza pocket	4.5 oz	9.0	290	28%
pot pies				
broccoli	1 pie	22.0	430	46%
vegetable tofu	1 pie	18.0	360	45%
shepherd's pie	1 pie	4.0	160	23%
tofu-vegetable lasagna	9.5 oz	10.0	300	30%
vegetable lasagna w/cheese	9.5 oz	10.0	300	30%
veggie loaf dinner	10 oz	5.0	260	17%

■ (Fantastic Foods)

Food and Description	Amount	Fat Grams	Total Calories	% Fat Calories
mix				
quick pilaf/three grain w/herbs				
mix only	⅓ cup	2.0	240	8%

Food and Description	Amount	Fat Grams	Total Calories	% Fat Calories
prepared	1 cup	2.0	240	8%
tofu classics				
creamy stroganoff				
mix only	½ cup	5.0	190	24%
w/tofu	1 cup	12.0	430	25%
Mandarin chow mein				
mix only	⅝ cup	1.5	170	8%
w/tofu	1 cup	5.0	330	14%
shells 'n curry				
mix only	½ cup	1.5	200	7%
w/tofu	1 cup	6.0	440	12%
tofu burger	⅛ cup	1.5	70	19%
tofu scrambler	2½ Tbs	0.5	60	8%
vegetarian entrees				
Nature's Burger				
BBQ				
mix only	⅓ cup	1.5	170	8%
prepared	1 patty	1.5	170	8%
original				
mix only	¼ cup	3.0	170	16%
prepared	1 patty	3.0	170	16%
Nature's Sausage/mix only	2 Tbs	1.5	65	21%
vegetarian chili				
mix only	~⅛ cup	–	50	–
prepared	½ cup	–	50	–
■ (Green Giant)				
frozen				
breakfast patties	2 patties	4.0	100	36%
breakfast links	3 links	5.0	110	41%
Harvest Burgers				
Italian style	1 burger	4.5	140	29%
original	1 burger	4.0	140	26%
Southwestern style	1 burger	4.0	140	26%
■ (Hain)				
Vegetarian Classics				
Hawaiian nuggets	10 oz	5.0	310	15%
Mexican style taco	10 oz	9.0	420	19%
pepper steak	10 oz	6.0	210	17%
radiatore Bolognese	10 oz	2.5	290	8%
■ (Ken & Robert's)				
frozen				
Veggi Burger	1 burger	1.0	130	7%
Veggi Pockets				
Greek	1 pocket	8.0	250	29%
Italian	1 pocket	8.0	260	28%
Oriental	1 pocket	8.0	250	29%
pizza	1 pocket	8.0	270	27%
potato & cheddar	1 pocket	8.0	260	28%

Food and Description	Amount	Fat Grams	Total Calories	% Fat Calories
Tex-Mex	1 pocket	8.0	280	26%
■ **(Lightlife)**				
frozen				
vegetarian hot dogs				
Smart Dogs	1 link	–	45	–
Tofu Pups	1 link	2.5	60	38%
Wonderdogs	1 link	1.0	55	16%
Vegetarian Request dinners				
traditional "meat loaf"	13 oz	5.0	300	15%
vegetable croquette	13 oz	5.0	270	17%
penne pasta Bolognese	12 oz	3.0	410	7%
stew				
French country	12 oz	3.0	340	8%
Moroccan lentil	12 oz	2.0	400	5%
Tuscan white bean	12 oz	3.0	340	8%
■ **(Loma Linda)**				
canned or dry-packed				
Big Franks	1.8 oz	7.0	110	57%
chicken supreme/mix only	⅓ cup	1.0	90	10%
dinner cuts	1 slice	1.5	80	17%
fried chik'n/gravy	2 pieces	31.0	390	72%
gravy/quik/mix only				
brown	1 Tbs	–	20	–
chicken style	1 Tbs	–	20	–
country style	1 Tbs	0.5	25	18%
mushroom	1 Tbs	–	15	–
onion	1 Tbs	–	20	–
Linketts	1 link	4.5	70	58%
Little Links	2 links	6.0	90	60%
Nuteena luncheon loaf	⅜" slice	13.0	160	73%
ocean platter mix/mix only	⅓ cup	1.0	90	10%
patty mix/mix only	⅓ cup	1.0	90	10%
Redi-Burger	⅝" slice	10.0	170	53%
sandwich spread	¼ cup	4.5	80	51%
savory dinner loaf/mix only	⅓ cup	1.5	90	15%
Swiss Stake	1 piece	6.0	120	45%
Tender Bits	6 pieces	4.5	110	37%
Tender Rounds	8 pieces	5.0	120	38%
Vege-Burger	¼ cup	1.5	70	19%
Vitaburger/mix only				
chunks	¼ cup	1.0	70	13%
granules	3 Tbs	1.0	70	13%
frozen				
Chik Nuggets	5 pieces	16.0	240	60%
corn dog	1 piece	9.0	200	41%
fried chicken	1 piece	15.0	180	75%
griddle steak	1 piece	7.0	130	48%
sizzle burger	1 patty	12.0	200	54%

Food and Description	Amount	Fat Grams	Total Calories	% Fat Calories
mix				
Soyagen/mix only				
all-purpose	¼ cup	6.0	130	42%
carob	¼ cup	6.0	130	42%
no sucrose	¼ cup	6.0	130	42%
■ (Morningstar Farms)				
frozen				
Better 'n Burgers	1 patty	–	70	–
Better 'n Eggs	¼ cup	–	20	–
breakfast links	2 links	2.5	60	38%
breakfast patties	1 patty	3.0	70	39%
breakfast strips	2 strips	4.5	60	68%
Chik Patties	1 patty	10.0	170	53%
deli franks	1 link	7.0	110	57%
garden grain patty	1 patty	2.5	120	19%
Grillers	1 patty	7.0	140	45%
ground meatless	½ cup	–	60	–
homestyle noodles	½ cup	–	160	–
Prime Patties	1 patty	5.0	130	35%
Scramblers	¼ cup	–	35	–
spicy black bean burger	1 patty	1.0	100	9%
vege patties	1 patty	2.5	100	23%
■ (Mudpie)				
frozen/veggi burger	1 burger	4.5	180	23%
■ (Natural Touch)				
canned/vegetarian chili	1 cup	12.0	270	40%
mix/mix only				
loaf	4 Tbs	0.5	100	5%
stroganoff	4 Tbs	3.5	90	35%
taco	3 Tbs	1.0	60	15%
frozen				
dinner entrée	1 patty	15.0	220	61%
garden vege patty	1 patty	4.0	110	33%
lentil rice loaf	1" slice	9.0	170	48%
nine bean loaf	1" slice	8.0	160	45%
okra patty	1 patty	5.0	110	41%
vegan burger	1 patty	–	70	–
vege burger	1 patty	6.0	140	39%
vege-frank	1 link	6.0	100	54%
■ (Near East)				
vegetable burger mix				
broiled	1½ patties	1.5	110	12%
fried	2½ patties	15.0	230	59%
■ (NewMenu)				
refrigerated				
Vegi-Burger	1 patty	1.0	110	8%
Vegidogs	1 link	–	45	–

ood and Description	Amount	Fat Grams	Total Calories	% Fat Calories
(Van's)				
ozen/eggless/dairy-free				
pancakes/multigrain	2 pancakes	1.5	180	9%
waffles				
Belgian				
original	2 waffles	4.0	160	23%
7 grain	2 waffles	3.5	150	21%
blueberry	2 waffles	4.5	195	21%
toaster	2 waffles	3.5	145	22%
(Wholesome & Hearty)				
ozen				
Gardenburger				
Mexi				
2.5-oz patty	1 patty	2.5	215	10%
3.4-oz patty	1 patty	3.0	290	9%
plain				
2.5-oz patty	1 patty	2.5	140	16%
3.4-oz patty	1 patty	3.0	190	14%
sub/3.1-oz patty	1 patty	3.0	170	16%
veggie				
2.5-oz patty	1 patty	–	190	–
3.4-oz patty	1 patty	–	260	–
Gardendog	2 oz	2.5	120	19%
	2.67 oz	3.0	140	19%
Gardensausage				
1.2 oz patty	1 patty	1.0	120	8%
2.5 oz patty	1 patty	2.5	240	9%
(Worthington)				
anned or dry-packed				
Chik				
diced/drained	¼ cup	3.5	60	53%
sliced/drained	3 slices	6.0	90	60%
chili	1 cup	15.0	290	47%
choplets	2 slices	1.5	90	15%
country stew	1 cup	9.0	210	34%
cutlets	1 slice	1.0	70	13%
Fri Chik	2 pieces	8.0	120	60%
Granburger	3 Tbs	0.5	60	8%
Numete	⅜" slice	10.0	130	69%
Prime Stakes	1 piece	9.0	140	58%
Protose	⅜" slice	7.0	130	48%
Saucettes	1 link	6.0	90	60%
savory slices	3 slices	9.0	150	54%
turkee slices	3 slices	14.0	190	66%
vegetable skallops	½ cup	1.5	90	15%
vegetable steaks	2 pieces	1.5	80	17%
vegetarian burger	¼ cup	2.0	60	30%
Veja-Links	1 link	3.0	50	54%

Food and Description	Amount	Fat Grams	Total Calories	% Fat Calories
frozen				
beef pie	1 pie	24.0	410	53%
beef style	3⁄8" slice	7.0	110	57%
Bolono	3 slices	3.5	80	39%
chicken pie	1 pie	27.0	450	54%
chicken slices	2 slices	4.5	80	23%
Chic-ketts roll	2 3⁄8" slice	7.0	120	53%
Chik Stiks	1 piece	7.0	110	57%
corned beef	4 slices	9.0	140	58%
Crispy Chik	1 patty	9.0	170	48%
Diced Chik	1⁄4 cup	4.5	80	51%
dinner roast	3⁄4" slice	12.0	180	60%
egg roll	1 piece	8.0	180	40%
fillet	2 fillets	10.0	180	50%
Fripats	1 patty	6.0	130	42%
golden croquettes	4 pieces	10.0	210	43%
ground beef	1⁄2 cup	2.5	80	28%
Leanies	1 link	8.0	110	65%
multigrain cutlets	2 slices	2.0	100	18%
Prosage				
links	2 links	2.5	60	38%
patties	2 patties	7.0	100	63%
roll	5⁄8" slice	10.0	140	64%
salami	3 slices	8.0	130	55%
sausage	1⁄2 cup	6.0	110	49%
smoked beef	6 slices	6.0	120	45%
smoked turkey	3 slices	10.0	140	64%
Stakelets	1 piece	8.0	140	51%
Stripples	2 strips	4.5	60	68%
Tuno/drained	1⁄2 cup	6.0	80	68%
Veelets	1 patty	9.0	180	45%
Wham	2 slices	5.0	80	56%
■ (Yves)				
Veggie Cuisine				
burger burgers	1 burger	–	92	–
chili dogs	1 link	–	70	–
deli slices	3½ slices	–	70	–
garden vegetable patties	1 patty	2.0	123	15%
tofu wieners	1 link	0.5	57	8%
veggi pepperoni	3½ slices	–	79	–
veggi wieners	1 link	–	60	–
VENISON/boneless				
cured	3 oz	5.0	151	30%
raw				
lean meat	3 oz	3.0	107	25%
steak	3 oz	5.0	153	29%
roasted	3 oz	3.0	135	20%
stewed	3 oz	5.0	153	29%

Food and Description	Amount	Fat Grams	Total Calories	% Fat Calories
VICHYSSOISE (*See* SOUP)				
VIENNA SAUSAGE (*See* SAUSAGE)				
VINE SPINACH				
fresh/raw	4 oz	–	22	–
VINEGAR				
(China Bowl) white rice	1 Tbs	–	–	–
generic				
cider	1 oz	–	–	–
	½ cup	–	15	–
distilled	1 Tbs	–	2	–
	1 cup	–	29	–
(Great Impressions)				
apple cider	1 Tbs	–	7	–
basil	1 Tbs	–	7	–
hot paprika	1 Tbs	–	6	–
raspberry	1 Tbs	–	7	–
(Grey Poupon)				
balsamic	1 Tbs	–	–	–
garden herb	1 Tbs	–	10	–
raspberry	1 Tbs	–	10	–
(Hain)				
apple cider/raw-unpasteurized	1 Tbs	–	2	–
cider	1 Tbs	–	2	–
(Heinz)				
apple cider	1 Tbs	–	2	–
white	1 Tbs	–	2	–
wine				
regular/gourmet decanter	1 Tbs	–	4	–
tarragon	1 Tbs	–	2	–
(Indian Summer)				
apple cider	1 Tbs	–	3	–
	1 cup	–	40	–
white	1 Tbs	–	2	–
	1 cup	–	30	–
(LuvYu)				
pineapple salad	1 Tbs	–	10	–
rice	1 Tbs	–	11	–
(Musselman's)				
apple cider	2 Tbs	–	4	–
red wine	2 Tbs	–	–	–
white	2 Tbs	–	4	–
(Nakano)	1 Tbs	--	--	--
(Progresso)				
garlic	1 Tbs	--	2	--
red wine	1 Tbs	--	2	--
red wine flavored	1 Tbs	--	2	--
(Regina) wine				
red/garlic or regular	1 oz	--	4	--

Food and Description	Amount	Fat Grams	Total Calories	% Fat Calories
white	1 oz	--	4	--
(S&W)				
cider	1 Tbs	–	–	–
international				
garlic wine	1 Tbs	–	–	–
Italian herb	1 Tbs	–	–	–
malt ale	1 Tbs	–	–	–
red wine	1 Tbs	–	–	–
tarragon	1 Tbs	–	–	–
white distilled	1 Tbs	–	–	–
(Spectrum Naturals) organic				
brown rice	1 Tbs	–	–	–
wine				
garlic	1 Tbs	–	–	–
Italian herb	1 Tbs	–	–	–
raspberry	1 Tbs	–	10	–
red	1 Tbs	–	–	–
white	1 Tbs	–	–	–
(White House)				
apple cider	2 Tbs	--	2	--
red wine	2 Tbs	--	4	--

VODKA (See LIQUOR, DISTILLED)

W

Food and Description	Amount	Fat Grams	Total Calories	% Fat Calories
WAFFLE (See also PANCAKE/WAFFLE MIX)				
(Aunt Jemima) frozen				
blueberry	2 waffles	7.0	190	33%
buttermilk	2 waffles	6.0	170	32%
cinnamon	2 waffles	6.0	180	30%
low-fat	2 waffles	1.5	160	8%
oatmeal	2 waffles	7.0	170	37%
whole-grain	2 waffles	7.0	170	37%
(Belgian Chef) frozen	2 waffles	2.5	140	16%
(Downyflake) frozen				
blueberry	2 waffles	4.0	180	20%
butter & syrup	2 waffles	4.0	150	24%
buttermilk	2 waffles	4.0	160	23%

Food and Description	Amount	Fat Grams	Total Calories	% Fat Calories
crisp & healthy				
apple & cinnamon	2 waffles	2.0	170	11%
original	2 waffles	2.0	180	10%
homestyle				
jumbo	2 waffles	4.0	170	22%
regular	4 waffles	5.0	230	20%
hot-n-buttery	2 waffles	4.0	170	22%
(Kellogg's) frozen				
Common Sense				
oat bran	2 waffles	7.0	200	32%
oat bran w/fruit & nut	2 waffles	8.0	220	33%
Eggo				
apple cinnamon	2 waffles	8.0	220	33%
blueberry				
mini	12 waffles	8.0	240	45%
original	2 waffles	8.0	220	33%
buttermilk	2 waffles	8.0	220	33%
cinnamon toast	2 waffles	9.0	280	29%
homestyle				
original	2 waffles	8.0	220	33%
mini	12 waffles	8.0	240	30%
nut & honey	2 waffles	10.0	240	38%
strawberry	2 waffles	8.0	220	33%
Nutri-Grain				
multi-bran	2 waffles	6.0	180	30%
plain	2 waffles	6.0	190	28%
raisin & bran	2 waffles	6.0	210	26%
Special K	2 waffles	–	140	–
(Krusteaz)				
frozen				
blueberry	2 waffles	8.0	230	31%
buttermilk	2 waffles	8.0	220	33%
homestyle	2 waffles	8.0	220	33%
mix/Belgian				
mix only	½ cup	2.0	280	6%
prepared/7"-dia waffle	1 waffle	19.0	440	39%
(Schwan's) frozen	4 pieces	18.0	320	51%
(Swanson) Kid's Breakfast Blast				
waffle stix w/syrup	1 meal	17.0	330	46%
(Van's) frozen/vegetarian-eggless & dairy-free				
Belgian				
original	2 waffles	4.0	160	23%
7 grain	2 waffles	3.5	150	21%
blueberry	2 waffles	4.5	195	21%
toaster	2 waffles	3.5	145	22%

WAFFLE SYRUP (*See* MAPLE SYRUP; PANCAKE/WAFFLE SYRUP)
WAKAME (*See* SEAWEED)

Food and Description	Amount	Fat Grams	Total Calories	% Fat Calories
WALNUT				
(Ann's House of Nuts) English	1 oz	18.0	180	90%
(Azar) English/pieces	1 oz	19.0	190	90%
(Diamond) English				
pieces	¼ cup	19.0	190	90%
shelled	¼ cup	19.0	190	90%
generic				
dried				
black/shelled	1 oz	16.0	172	84%
ground	1 cup	45.0	490	83%
pieces	1 cup	71.0	760	84%
English or Persian				
pieces	1 cup	74.0	770	87%
shelled	1 oz	18.0	190	85%
(Planters)				
black	2 oz	31.0	340	82%
English or Persian				
halves				
Gold Measure	2 oz	38.0	380	90%
regular	⅓ cup	22.0	220	90%
pieces	¼ cup	20.0	190	95%
WATER (See also SOFT DRINK; COCKTAIL MIXER)				
bottled				
(Arrowhead)				
distilled	1 liter	–	–	–
drinking	1 liter	–	–	–
fluoridated	1 liter	–	–	–
spring	1 liter	–	–	–
(Canada Dry) seltzer/sparkling water	8 fl oz	–	–	–
cherry	8 fl oz	–	–	–
cranberry	8 fl oz	–	–	–
grapefruit	8 fl oz	–	–	–
lemon lime	8 fl oz	–	–	–
Mandarin orange	8 fl oz	–	–	–
peach	8 fl oz	–	–	–
raspberry	8 fl oz	–	–	–
strawberry	8 fl oz	–	–	–
tropical	8 fl oz	–	–	–
(Cascadia) sparkling water w/juice				
cherry-blackberry	6 fl oz	–	2	–
grapefruit	6 fl oz	–	2	–
guava-berry	6 fl oz	–	2	–
lemonaid	6 fl oz	–	2	–
(Clearly Canadian) sparkling water				
blackberry	8 fl oz	–	100	–
cherry	8 fl oz	–	90	–
cranberry	8 fl oz	–	90	–
peach	8 fl oz	–	90	–

Food and Description	Amount	Fat Grams	Total Calories	% Fat Calories
raspberry	8 fl oz	–	80	–
(Coor's) Rocky Mountain sparkling water				
cherry	8 fl oz	–	–	–
lemon lime	8 fl oz	–	–	–
original	8 fl oz	–	–	–
(Crystal Geyser) seltzer water/light				
black cherry cider	6 fl oz	–	60	–
cranberry-raspberry	6 fl oz	–	60	–
kiwi lemonade	6 fl oz	–	60	–
natural peach	6 fl oz	–	60	–
vanilla creme	6 fl oz	–	60	–
(Evian) spring water	8 fl oz	–	–	–
generic				
pain/all types	any amount	–	–	–
seltzer water/flavored				
lemon	12 fl oz	–	–	–
lime	12 fl oz	–	–	–
orange	12 fl oz	–	–	–
strawberry	12 fl oz	–	–	–
(Perrier) mineral water with-a-twist				
lemon	12 fl oz	–	–	–
lime	12 fl oz	–	–	–
(Poland Spring) spring water	8 fl oz	–	–	–
(Polar) spring water	8 fl oz	–	–	–
(Quest) sparkling water				
black cherry	8 fl oz	–	–	–
peach	8 fl oz	–	–	–
raspberry	8 fl oz	–	–	–
red raspberry	8 fl oz	–	–	–
strawberry-kiwi	8 fl oz	–	–	–
tangerine-lemon	8 fl oz	–	–	–
tangerine-lime	8 fl oz	–	–	–
(San Francisco) sweetened seltzer				
almond cream	8 fl oz	–	100	–
black cherry	8 fl oz	–	110	–
peach	8 fl oz	–	100	–
raspberry	8 fl oz	–	110	–
(Savoir Faire) natural spring water	8 fl oz	–	–	–
(Schweppes) seltzer/sparkling water				
black cherry	8 fl oz	–	–	–
lemon	8 fl oz	–	–	–
lemon lime	8 fl oz	–	–	–
lime	8 fl oz	–	–	–
orange	8 fl oz	–	–	–
peaches & cream	8 fl oz	–	–	–
raspberry	8 fl oz	–	–	–
(Water Joe) caffeine-enhanced natural artesian water	8 fl oz	–	–	–

Food and Description	Amount	Fat Grams	Total Calories	% Fat Calories
WATER CHESTNUT (*See also* ASIAN FOOD)				
canned/sliced	½ cup	–	35	–
fresh/raw/sliced	½ cup	–	66	–
WATERCRESS/fresh/raw				
chopped	½ cup	–	2	–
whole	1 sprig	–	–	–
WATERCRESS SOUP (*See* SOUP)				
WATERMELON (*See also* WATERMELON RIND)				
fresh				
wedges/10" dia	1/16 wedge	2.0	152	12%
cubed	1 cup	0.7	50	12%
WATERMELON DRINK (*See also* FRUIT PUNCH; SOFT DRINK; SOFT DRINK MIX; TEA)				
bottled, boxed, or canned				
(Betty Crocker) Squeezit	6.76 fl oz	–	110	–
WATERMELON RIND				
(Old South)	2 cubes	–	70	–
WATERMELON SEEDS/KERNELS				
dried	1 oz	13.0	158	74%
	1 cup	51.0	602	76%
WAX BEAN				
canned				
(Del Monte) golden-cut	½ cup	–	20	–
generic	½ cup	–	25	–
(S&W) premium golden-cut	½ cup	–	20	–
(Seneca) cuts	½ cup	–	25	–
(Stokely)				
no salt or sugar	½ cup	–	20	–
regular	½ cup	–	20	–
frozen				
(Seabrook) cut	½ cup	–	25	–
WAX GOURD/fresh				
boiled	1 cup	–	23	–
raw	1 cup	–	17	–
WEAKFISH				
broiled w/butter or margarine	3 oz	9.6	177	49%
WELSH RAREBIT (*See also* FROZEN ENTRÉE/DINNER; SAUCE)				
homemade/USDA Standard Home Recipe	1 cup	32.0	415	69%
WHALE/raw	3 oz	6.0	130	42%
WHEAT (*See* BULGUR; FLOUR; WHEAT GERM)				
WHEAT GERM (*See also* CEREAL)				
(Bob's Red Mill) natural raw	⅛ cup	1.0	52	17%
generic				
crude	¼ cup	3.0	105	26%
toasted	¼ cup	3.0	110	25%
(Hodgson Mill)	2 Tbs	1.0	55	16%
(Kretschmer)				
honey crunch	2 Tbs	1.0	50	18%

Food and Description	Amount	Fat Grams	Total Calories	% Fat Calories
plain	1⅔ Tbs	1.0	50	18%
(Mother's) toasted	2 Tbs	1.0	50	18%
WHELK (*See* SNAIL)				
WHEY				
dried				
acid	1 Tbs	–	10	–
	1 cup	–	193	–
sweet	1 Tbs	–	26	–
	1 cup	–	512	–
fluid				
acid	1 Tbs	–	4	–
	1 cup	<1.0	60	8%
sweet	1 Tbs	–	4	–
	1 cup	0.7	65	10%
WHIPPED TOPPING (*See also* CREAM)				
(NOTE: Unless specified otherwise, 1 serving of mix = the amount in 2 Tbs prepared)				
(Birds Eye) Cool Whip				
extra creamy	2 Tbs	2.0	30	60%
lite	2 Tbs	1.0	20	45%
nondairy	2 Tbs	1.5	25	54%
(Dream Whip)				
mix only	1 serving	0.5	15	30%
prepared w/2% milk	2 Tbs	1.0	20	45%
(D-Zerta) mix only	1 serving	1.0	10	100%
(Estee)				
mix/mix only	¾ tsp	0.5	10	45%
ready to use	1 Tbs	<1.0	8	70%
generic				
frozen				
nondairy	1 Tbs	0.8	11	66%
regular	1 Tbs	1.0	15	60%
powdered				
low calorie	1 Tbs	1.0	8	100%
w/whole milk	1 Tbs	–	10	–
	1 cup	10.0	150	60%
pressurized				
cream	1 Tbs	1.0	8	100%
	½ cup	7.0	75	84%
nondairy	1 Tbs	1.0	10	81%
	1 cup	16.0	185	78%
(Kraft)				
real whipped cream	2 Tbs	1.5	20	68%
whipped nondairy	2 Tbs	1.5	20	68%
(LaCreme) lite	2 Tbs	1.0	15	60%
(Pet) whip	2 Tbs	2.0	30	60%
(Rich's)				
nondairy				
aerosol	2 Tbs	2.0	25	72%

Food and Description	Amount	Fat Grams	Total Calories	% Fat Calories
bowl	2 Tbs	1.5	25	54%
Richwhip				
liquid	2 Tbs	2.0	25	72%
whipped	2 Tbs	2.0	25	72%
WHISKEY (See LIQUOR, DISTILLED)				
WHITE BEAN				
canned				
generic	½ cup	–	153	–
(Goya) Spanish style	½ cup	0.5	125	4%
dried				
boiled				
regular	½ cup	–	125	–
small	½ cup	0.5	127	4%
raw				
regular	½ cup	1.0	340	3%
small	½ cup	1.5	365	4%
WHITE PERCH/raw	3 oz	3.0	100	27%
WHITE SAUCE (See SAUCE)				
WHITEFISH/mixed species				
fresh				
cooked-dry heat	3 oz	5.5	145	34%
raw	1 oz	1.7	38	39%
	3 oz	5.0	115	39%
jarred				
(Mother's)				
jellied	1 fishball	1.0	46	20%
jellied in broth	1 fishball	1.0	70	13%
smoked	1 oz	<1.0	30	6%
	3 oz	<1.0	92	7%
WHITEFISH & PIKE				
jarred				
(Manischewitz)				
regular	3.5 oz	3.6	99	33%
sweet	3.5 oz	4.0	129	28%
(Mother's) jellied in broth	1 fishball	2.0	60	15%
(Rokeach) jellied	1 fishball	1.0	60	15%
WHITING (See also SEAFOOD ENTREE/DINNER)				
breaded & fried	3 oz	9.7	171	51%
cooked-dry heat	3 oz	1.0	98	9%
raw	3 oz	1.0	77	12%
WIENER (See FRANKFURTER; FRANKFURTER, VEGETARIAN; SAUSAGE; VEGETARIAN FOODS)				
WILD CELERY (See CELERIAC)				
WINE				
(Andre) champagne				
blush	1 fl oz	–	22	–
brut	1 fl oz	–	25	–

Food and Description	Amount	Fat Grams	Total Calories	% Fat Calories
cold duck	1 fl oz	–	25	–
extra dry	1 fl oz	–	24	–
(Carl Jung) white/alcohol removed	3 fl oz	–	20	–
(Carlo Rossi)				
blush	1 fl oz	–	21	–
burgundy	1 fl oz	–	22	–
chablis	1 fl oz	–	21	–
paisano	1 fl oz	–	23	–
red sangria	1 fl oz	–	24	–
rhine	1 fl oz	–	21	–
vin rose	1 fl oz	–	21	–
white grenache	1 fl oz	–	20	–
(Eden Roc)				
brut	1 fl oz	–	21	–
brut rose	1 fl oz	–	22	–
extra dry	1 fl oz	–	21	–
(Gallo)				
Gallo label				
vermouth				
extra dry	1 fl oz	–	28	–
sweet	1 fl oz	–	43	–
Fairbanks label				
sherry				
cocktail/pale dry	1 fl oz	–	31	–
cream	1 fl oz	–	42	–
regular	1 fl oz	–	34	–
port				
regular	1 fl oz	–	44	–
white	1 fl oz	–	44	–
Ernest & Julio Gallo label				
cabernet sauvignon	1 fl oz	–	22	–
chardonnay	1 fl oz	–	22	–
classic Burgundy	1 fl oz	–	22	–
Johannisberg riesling	1 fl oz	–	20	–
sauvignon blanc	1 fl oz	–	20	–
white grenache	1 fl oz	–	20	–
zinfandel	1 fl oz	–	23	–
Gallo Livingston label				
blush chablis	1 fl oz	–	22	–
Burgundy	1 fl oz	–	22	–
chablis blanc	1 fl oz	–	20	–
chenin blanc	1 fl oz	–	20	–
French colombard	1 fl oz	–	21	–
pink chablis	1 fl oz	–	20	–
red rosé	1 fl oz	–	23	–
Rhine	1 fl oz	–	22	–
white grenache	1 fl oz	–	20	–

Food and Description	Amount	Fat Grams	Total Calories	% Fat Calories
white zinfindel	1 fl oz	–	20	–
Sheffield label				
sherry				
cream	1 fl oz	–	44	–
very dry	1 fl oz	–	32	–
tawny port	1 fl oz	–	45	–
general				
barbera/white	4 fl oz	–	91	–
Beaujolais-12% alcohol	4 fl oz	–	96	–
Bordeaux/red-12% alcohol	4 fl oz	–	96	–
Burgundy				
cooking	¼ cup	–	2	–
red-12% alcohol	4 fl oz	–	96	–
sparkling-12% alcohol	4 fl oz	–	116	–
white-12% alcohol	4 fl oz	–	90	–
cabernet sauvignon	4 fl oz	–	88	–
chablis	4 fl oz	–	84	–
emerald	4 fl oz	–	102	–
gold	4 fl oz	–	97	–
pink	4 fl oz	–	98	–
ruby	4 fl oz	–	104	–
champagne				
brut	4 fl oz	–	100	–
domestic	4 fl oz	–	84	–
extra dry	4 fl oz	–	105	–
pink	4 fl oz	–	98	–
chardonnay	4 fl oz	–	88	–
Chenin Blanc	4 fl oz	–	86	–
chianti	4 fl oz	–	100	–
cold duck	4 fl oz	–	108	–
dessert	4 fl oz	–	180	–
Dubonnet	4 fl oz	–	160	–
French colombard	4 fl oz	–	88	–
Liebfraumilch-10% alcohol	4 fl oz	–	84	–
Madeira-19% alcohol	4 fl oz	–	160	–
muscatel	3.5 fl oz	–	158	–
port				
ruby-20% alcohol	4 fl oz	–	184	–
tawny-20% alcohol	4 fl oz	–	184	–
white	4 fl oz	–	172	–
Reisling-12% alcohol	4 fl oz	–	90	–
Rhine-11% alcohol	4 fl oz	–	96	–
Rhone-12% alcohol	4 fl oz	–	96	–
rosé	4 fl oz	–	90	–
sake/saki	1.5 fl oz	–	36	–
sauternes				
cooking	¼ cup	–	2	–
dry-12% alcohol	4 fl oz	–	108	–

Food and Description	Amount	Fat Grams	Total Calories	% Fat Calories
12% alcohol	4 fl oz	–	116	–
sauvignon blanc	4 fl oz	–	80	–
sherry				
cooking	¼ cup	–	20	–
cream-19.5% alcohol	4 fl oz	–	200	–
dry-19% alcohol	4 fl oz	–	162	–
sweet	4 fl oz	–	165	–
sylvaner-12% alcohol	4 fl oz	–	90	–
table				
red	3.5 fl oz	–	74	–
rose	3.5 fl oz	–	73	–
white	3.5 fl oz	–	70	–
Tokay	4 fl oz	–	164	–
vermouth				
dry-17% alcohol	4 fl oz	–	136	–
sweet-17% alcohol	4 fl oz	–	180	–
wine spritzer	5 fl oz	–	61	–
zinfandel				
red	4 fl oz	–	92	–
white	4 fl oz	–	82	–
(Grey Poupon) cooking wine				
Burgundy	1 fl oz	–	20	–
sherry	1 fl oz	–	35	–
white	1 fl oz	–	20	–
(Holland House) cooking wine				
Marsala	1 fl oz	–	9	–
red	1 fl oz	–	6	–
sherry	1 fl oz	–	5	–
vermouth	1 fl oz	–	2	–
white	1 fl oz	–	2	–
(Regina) cooking wine				
Burgundy	¼ cup	–	2	–
sauternes	¼ cup	–	2	–
sherry	¼ cup	–	20	–
WINE COOLER				
(Bartles & Jaymes)				
berry	12 fl oz	–	210	–
margarita	12 fl oz	–	260	–
original	12 fl oz	–	190	–
peach	12 fl oz	–	210	–
piña colada	12 fl oz	–	280	–
planter's punch	12 fl oz	–	230	–
strawberry	12 fl oz	–	210	–
strawberry daiquiri	12 fl oz	–	230	–
tropical	12 fl oz	–	230	–
(Boone's)				
country kwencher	1 fl oz	–	24	–
delicious apple	1 fl oz	–	21	–

Food and Description	Amount	Fat Grams	Total Calories	% Fat Calories
sangria	1 fl oz	–	22	-
snow creek berry	1 fl oz	–	18	–
strawberry hill	1 fl oz	–	22	–
sun peak peach	1 fl oz	–	18	–
wild island	1 fl oz	–	18	–
generic	7 fl oz	–	100	–
	12 fl oz	–	192	–
WINGED BEAN				
cooked	½ cup	5.0	126	36%
raw	½ cup	15.0	375	36%
WOLFFISH				
Atlantic/fresh				
cooked-dry heat	3 oz	2.0	105	17%
raw	3 oz	2.0	80	23%

WON TON (See ASIAN FOOD)
WON TON SOUP (See SOUP)
WON TON WRAPPER (See ASIAN FOOD)
WORCESTERSHIRE SAUCE (See SAUCE)

Y

Food and Description	Amount	Fat Grams	Total Calories	% Fat Calories
YAM (See also SWEET POTATO)				
canned				
(Bruce's)				
candied	½ cup	–	170	–
cut or whole	½ cup	1.0	140	6%
mashed	½ cup	1.0	130	7%
(Bush's Best)	½ cup	–	120	–
generic				
in heavy syrup	½ cup	–	120	–
in light syrup	½ cup	–	110	–
mashed	½ cup	–	90	–
w/pineapple-orange sauce	½ cup	–	190	–
(S&W) candied/old-fashioned	½ cup	–	170	–
(Trappey's) golden/whole in heavy syrup	½ cup	–	130	–
fresh				
Hawaii/mountain				
cooked/cubed	½ cup	–	59	–

Food and Description	Amount	Fat Grams	Total Calories	% Fat Calories
raw				
cubed	½ cup	–	46	–
whole/8¼" long/2½" dia	1 yam	0.5	280	2%
regular				
boiled or baked/cubed	1 cup	–	158	–
raw/cubed	1 cup	–	177	–
YAM BEAN-TUBER (*See* JICAMA)				
YARDLONG BEAN				
dried				
boiled	½ cup	<1.0	100	4%
raw	½ cup	1.0	290	3%
fresh				
boiled/drained/sliced	½ cup	–	25	–
raw/sliced	½ cup	–	22	–
YEAST				
baker's				
(Fleischmann's)				
active dry & rapid rise/packet or jar	¼ oz	–	20	–
fresh active	0.6 oz	–	15	–
household	0.5 oz	–	15	–
generic/active dry				
compressed	1 oz	1.0	24	38%
powdered	1 oz	0.5	80	6%
(Red Star) active dry	¼ oz	–	15	–
brewer's				
generic	1 Tbs	–	25	–
	1 oz	–	80	–
(Louis Laboratories)	2 Tbs	1.0	114	8%
torula	1 oz	–	79	–
YELLOWEYE BEAN				
canned				
(B&M) baked	½ cup	2.0	170	11%
dried				
(Bean Cuisine)	½ cup	1.0	115	8%
YELLOWTAIL				
mixed species/fresh				
cooked-dry heat	3 oz	5.5	160	31%
raw	3 oz	4.5	125	32%
YOGURT, DAIRY				
(Alta Dena)				
black cherry	1 cup	–	200	–
mixed berries	1 cup	–	190	–
peach	1 cup	–	210	–
piña colada	1 cup	–	220	–
raspberry	1 cup	–	190	–
vanilla	1 cup	–	180	–
(Breyers)				
light/fat-free/all flavors	8 oz	–	130	–

Food and Description	Amount	Fat Grams	Total Calories	% Fat Calories
low-fat/1% milkfat				
black cherry	8 oz	2.5	260	9%
blueberry	8 oz	2.5	250	9%
mixed berry	8 oz	2.5	250	9%
peach	8 oz	2.5	250	9%
pineapple	8 oz	2.5	250	9%
red raspberry	8 oz	2.5	250	9%
strawberry	8 oz	2.5	250	9%
strawberry-banana	8 oz	2.5	250	9%
low-fat/1.5% milkfat				
coffee	8 oz	3.0	220	12%
creamy lemon	8 oz	3.0	220	12%
plain	8 oz	3.0	130	21%
vanilla	8 oz	3.0	220	12%
(Colombo)				
fat-free				
apples 'n spice	8 oz	–	190	–
apricot	8 oz	–	190	–
banana-strawberry	8 oz	–	200	–
blueberry	8 oz	–	190	–
cappuccino	8 oz	–	180	–
cherry	8 oz	–	190	–
cranberry strawberry	8 oz	–	200	–
French roast	8 oz	–	180	–
fruit cocktail	8 oz	–	190	–
lemon	8 oz	–	170	–
peach	8 oz	–	190	–
plain	8 oz	–	110	–
raspberry	8 oz	–	190	–
strawberry	8 oz	–	190	–
strawberry pineapple orange	8 oz	–	190	–
vanilla	8 oz	–	170	–
Light 100/all flavors	8 oz	–	100	–
low-fat				
banana-strawberry	8 oz	4.0	210	17%
black cherry	8 oz	4.0	200	18%
blueberry	8 oz	4.0	200	18%
French vanilla	8 oz	4.0	180	20%
peach melba	8 oz	4.0	200	18%
plain	8 oz	5.0	120	38%
raspberry	8 oz	4.0	200	18%
(Dannon)				
blended				
blueberry	6 oz	–	160	–
French vanilla	6 oz	–	160	–
lemon chiffon	6 oz	–	150	–
peach	6 oz	–	150	–
raspberry	6 oz	–	160	–

Food and Description	Amount	Fat Grams	Total Calories	% Fat Calories
strawberry	6 oz	–	150	–
strawberry-banana	6 oz	–	150	–
Danimals/low-fat				
blueberry	4.4 oz	2.0	140	13%
grape lemonade	4.4 oz	2.0	130	14%
lemon ice	4.4 oz	2.0	130	14%
orange-banana	4.4 oz	2.0	140	13%
strawberry	4.4 oz	2.0	140	13%
tropical punch	4.4 oz	2.0	140	13%
wild raspberry	4.4 oz	2.0	130	14%
vanilla	4.4 oz	2.0	140	13%
Double Delights/lowfat w/fruit toppings				
banana creme w/strawberry	6 oz	2.5	170	13%
Bavarian creme w/raspberry	6 oz	2.5	170	13%
cheesecake				
w/cherry	6 oz	2.5	170	13%
w/strawberry	6 oz	2.5	170	13%
vanilla				
w/peach & apricot	6 oz	2.5	170	13%
w/strawberry	6 oz	2.5	170	13%
fruit on the bottom/low-fat				
apple cinnamon	8 oz	3.0	240	11%
banana	8 oz	3.0	240	11%
blueberry	8 oz	3.0	240	11%
boysenberry	8 oz	3.0	240	11%
cherry	8 oz	3.0	240	11%
mixed berry	8 oz	3.0	240	11%
nonfat	8 oz	–	110	–
orange	8 oz	3.0	240	11%
peach	8 oz	3.0	240	11%
pear	8 oz	3.0	240	11%
plum	8 oz	3.0	240	11%
raspberry	8 oz	3.0	240	11%
strawberry	8 oz	3.0	240	11%
strawberry-banana	8 oz	3.0	240	11%
light/nonfat				
banana cream pie				
8-oz container	8 oz	–	100	–
mini-pack	4.4 oz	–	60	–
blueberry	8 oz	–	100	–
cappuccino	8 oz	–	100	–
cherry vanilla				
8-oz container	8 oz	–	100	–
quart container	1 cup	–	110	–
creme caramel	8 oz	–	100	–
lemon	8 oz	–	100	–
lemon chiffon/mini-pack	4.4 oz	–	60	–
mint chocolate cream pie	8 oz	–	100	–

Food and Description	Amount	Fat Grams	Total Calories	% Fat Calories
peach				
8-oz container	8 oz	–	100	–
mini-pack	4.4 oz	–	50	–
plain				
8-oz container	1 container	–	110	–
16- or 32-oz container	1 cup	–	120	–
raspberry	8 oz	–	100	–
strawberry				
8-oz container	8 oz	–	100	–
mini-pack	4.4 oz	–	50	–
quart container	1 cup	–	110	–
strawberry-banana	8 oz	–	100	–
strawberry-kiwi	8 oz	–	100	–
tangerine chiffon	8 oz	–	100	–
tropical fruit	8 oz	–	100	–
vanilla				
8-oz container	8 oz	–	100	–
quart container	1 cup	–	110	–
Llight 'n Ccrunchy				
cappuccino w/chocolate	8 oz	–	150	–
caramel apple crunch	8 oz	–	150	–
lemon chiffon w/blueberry	8 oz	–	140	–
raspberry w/granola	8 oz	–	150	–
vanilla w/chocolate	8 oz	–	150	–
lowfat				
coffee				
8-oz container	1 container	3.0	210	13%
16-oz container	1 cup	3.5	230	14%
cranberry-raspberry	8 oz	3.0	210	13%
lemon				
8-oz container	1 container	3.0	210	13%
16-oz container	1 cup	3.5	230	14%
plain				
8-oz container	1 container	4.0	140	26%
16-oz container	1 cup	4.0	150	24%
32-oz container	1 cup	4.0	150	24%
vanilla				
8-oz container	1 container	3.0	210	13%
16-oz container	1 cup	3.5	230	14%
Sprinkl'ins				
crazy crunch				
cherry w/honey grahams	4.4 oz	3.0	170	16%
grape w/chocolate grahams	4.4 oz	2.5	160	14%
vanilla				
w/chocolate grahams	4.4 oz	2.5	160	14%
w/honey grahams	4.4 oz	3.0	170	16%
regular				
banana	4.1 oz	2.5	140	16%

Food and Description	Amount	Fat Grams	Total Calories	% Fat Calories
cherry vanilla	4.1 oz	2.5	140	16%
strawberry	4.1 oz	2.5	140	16%
strawberry-banana	4.1 oz	2.5	140	16%
Tropifruit/nonfat				
banana	6 oz	–	150	–
guava	6 oz	–	150	–
mango	6 oz	–	150	–
papaya-pineapple	6 oz	–	150	–
piña colada	6 oz	–	150	–
strawberry	6 oz	–	150	–
strawberry-banana	6 oz	–	150	–
strawberry-kiwi	6 oz	–	150	–
generic				
lowfat				
coffee or vanilla	4 oz	1.0	100	9%
fruit flavors	4 oz	1.0	115	8%
plain	4 oz	2.0	75	24%
nonfat	4 oz	–	65	–
whole-milk	4 oz	4.0	70	51%
(Jell-O) Jigglers Bits & Yyogurt				
berry blue	6 oz	1.5	230	6%
cherry	6 oz	1.5	220	6%
orange	6 oz	1.5	220	6%
strawberry	6 oz	1.5	220	6%
(Kemps)				
classic yogurt/strawberry	6 oz	2.0	150	12%
vanilla & fruit/strawberry	6 oz	2.0	160	11%
Yogurt Jr.'s/strawberry	4 oz	1.0	130	7%
(Knudsen) Cal 70/nonfat				
black cherry	6 oz	–	70	–
blueberry	6 oz	–	70	–
lemon	6 oz	–	70	–
peach	6 oz	–	70	–
pineapple	6 oz	–	70	–
red raspberry	6 oz	–	70	–
strawberry	6 oz	–	70	–
strawberry fruit basket	6 oz	–	70	–
strawberry-banana	6 oz	–	70	–
vanilla	6 oz	–	70	–
(La Carona)				
low-fat				
blackberry	8 oz	3.0	210	13%
blueberry	8 oz	3.0	210	13%
cherry	8 oz	3.0	210	13%
cherry vanilla	8 oz	3.0	210	13%
French vanilla	8 oz	3.0	200	14%
lemon	8 oz	3.0	210	13%
peach	8 oz	3.0	210	13%

Food and Description	Amount	Fat Grams	Total Calories	% Fat Calories
raspberry	8 oz	3.0	210	13%
strawberry	8 oz	3.0	210	13%
strawberry cheesecake	8 oz	3.0	210	13%
strawberry-banana	8 oz	3.0	210	13%
nonfat/plain	8 oz	–	110	–
(La Yogurt)				
regular				
blueberry	6 oz	4.0	190	19%
cherry	6 oz	4.0	190	19%
cherry vanilla	6 oz	4.0	190	19%
key lime	6 oz	4.0	190	19%
peach	6 oz	4.0	190	19%
piña colada	6 oz	4.0	190	19%
plain	6 oz	6.0	140	39%
strawberry	6 oz	4.0	190	19%
strawberry fruit cup	6 oz	4.0	190	19%
strawberry-banana	6 oz	4.0	290	19%
tropical orange	6 oz	4.0	190	19%
vanilla	6 oz	4.0	160	23%
Yogurt-25/fat-free				
blueberry	8 oz	–	200	–
cherry	8 oz	–	200	–
raspberry	8 oz	–	200	–
strawberry	8 oz	–	200	–
strawberry-banana	8 oz	–	200	–
(Light n' Lively)				
Free				
50 calories				
blueberry	4.4 oz	–	50	–
peach	4.4 oz	–	50	–
red raspberry	4.4 oz	–	50	–
strawberry	4.4 oz	–	50	–
strawberry fruit cup	4.4 oz	–	50	–
strawberry-banana	4.4 oz	–	50	–
nonfat				
blueberry	6 oz	–	190	–
lemon	6 oz	–	170	–
mixed berry	6 oz	–	170	–
peach	6 oz	–	170	–
red raspberry	6 oz	–	180	–
strawberry	6 oz	–	180	–
strawberry fruit cup	6 oz	–	170	–
vanilla	6 oz	–	160	–
70 calories				
black cherry	6 oz	–	70	–
blueberry	6 oz	–	70	–
lemon	6 oz	–	70	–
peach	6 oz	–	70	–

Food and Description	Amount	Fat Grams	Total Calories	% Fat Calories
red raspberry	6 oz	–	70	–
strawberry	6 oz	–	70	–
strawberry fruit cup	6 oz	–	70	–
strawberry-banana	6 oz	–	70	–
low-fat/1% milk fat				
kid pack				
banana berry	4.4 oz	1.0	130	7%
berry blue	4.4 oz	1.0	150	6%
cherry	4.4 oz	1.0	140	6%
grape	4.4 oz	1.0	130	7%
outrageous orange	4.4 oz	1.0	150	6%
tropical punch	4.4 oz	1.0	140	6%
wild berry	4.4 oz	1.0	140	6%
wild strawberry	4.4 oz	1.0	140	6%
multi-pack				
blueberry	4.4 oz	1.0	140	6%
peach	4.4 oz	1.0	140	6%
pineapple	4.4 oz	1.0	140	6%
red raspberry	4.4 oz	1.0	140	6%
strawberry	4.4 oz	1.0	140	6%
strawberry banana	4.4 oz	1.0	140	6%
strawberry fruit cup	4.4 oz	1.0	140	6%
(Lite-Line) low-fat				
plain	8 oz	2.0	140	13%
Swiss style/natural				
cherry vanilla	8 oz	2.0	240	8%
peach	8 oz	2.0	240	8%
strawberry	8 oz	2.0	240	8%
(Lucerne) nonfat				
blueberry	8 oz	–	180	–
cherry	8 oz	–	180	–
peach	8 oz	–	180	–
plain	8 oz	–	130	–
strawberry	8 oz	–	180	–
(Meadow Gold)				
low-fat/plain/2% milkfat	8 oz	5.0	160	28%
sundae style/raspberry/1.5% milkfat	8 oz	4.0	250	14%
(Mountain High)				
fat-free				
black cherry	6 oz	–	120	–
blueberry	6 oz	–	120	–
cherry	6 oz	–	120	–
key lime	6 oz	–	120	–
plain	6 oz	–	120	–
raspberry	6 oz	–	120	–
strawberry	6 oz	–	120	–
strawberry-banana	6 oz	–	120	–
honey light/all flavors	8 oz	<1.0	190	2%

Food and Description	Amount	Fat Grams	Total Calories	% Fat Calories
(Nabisco) SnackWell's/nonfat				
almond	6 oz	–	190	–
banana	6 oz	–	190	–
cappuccino	6 oz	–	190	–
cherry	6 oz	–	190	–
double chocolate	6 oz	–	190	–
raspberry	6 oz	–	190	–
(New Country) low-fat				
apple crisp	6 oz	2.0	150	12%
blueberry supreme	6 oz	2.0	150	12%
cherry supreme	6 oz	2.0	150	12%
French vanilla	6 oz	2.0	150	12%
fruit crunch	6 oz	2.0	150	12%
Hawaiian salad	6 oz	2.0	150	12%
lemon supreme	6 oz	2.0	150	12%
mixed berries	6 oz	2.0	150	12%
orange supreme	6 oz	2.0	150	12%
peaches 'n cream	6 oz	2.0	150	12%
raspberry supreme	6 oz	2.0	150	12%
strawberry fruit cup	6 oz	2.0	150	12%
strawberry supreme	6 oz	2.0	150	12%
strawberry-banana supreme	6 oz	2.0	150	12%
(TCBY)				
light				
black cherry	8 oz	–	100	–
blueberry	8 oz	–	100	–
strawberry	8 oz	–	100	–
strawberry-banana	8 oz	–	100	–
low-fat				
blueberry	8 oz	2.0	220	8%
cherry-vanilla	8 oz	2.0	220	8%
peach	8 oz	2.0	220	8%
raspberry	8 oz	2.0	220	8%
strawberry	8 oz	2.0	220	8%
strawberry-banana	8 oz	2.0	220	8%
(Weight Watchers) Ultimate 90				
blueberries 'n creme	1 cup	–	90	–
cappuccino	1 cup	–	90	–
cherries jubilee	1 cup	–	90	–
cranberry raspberry	1 cup	–	90	–
lemon chiffon	1 cup	–	90	–
peach	1 cup	–	90	–
plain	1 cup	–	90	–
raspberries 'n creme	1 cup	–	90	–
strawberry	1 cup	–	90	–
strawberry-banana	1 cup	–	90	–
vanilla	1 cup	–	90	–

Food and Description	Amount	Fat Grams	Total Calories	% Fat Calories
(Whitney's)				
light/all flavors	6 oz	–	130	–
original				
apples & raisins	6 oz	5.0	190	24%
blueberry	6 oz	5.0	190	24%
boysenberry	6 oz	5.0	190	24%
cherry	6 oz	5.0	190	24%
coffee	6 oz	6.0	200	27%
lemon	6 oz	6.0	200	27%
peach	6 oz	5.0	190	24%
piña colada	6 oz	7.0	210	30%
plain	6 oz	7.0	150	42%
raspberry	6 oz	5.0	190	24%
strawberry	6 oz	5.0	190	24%
strawberry-banana	6 oz	5.0	190	24%
tropical fruits	6 oz	6.0	200	27%
vanilla	6 oz	6.0	200	27%
wild berries	6 oz	5.0	190	24%
(Yoplait)				
breakfast/low-fat				
mixed berry	6 oz	2.0	200	9%
strawberry-banana	6 oz	2.0	200	9%
tropical fruit	6 oz	2.5	210	11%
Crunch 'n Yogurt				
light				
cappuccino w/chocolate nuggets	7 oz	1.5	130	10%
cherry cheesecake w/graham crunch	7 oz	1.0	130	7%
raspberry w/granola	7 oz	1.0	130	7%
strawberry w/granola	7 oz	1.0	130	7%
regular				
peach w/granola	7 oz	1.5	220	6%
strawberry				
w/cereal nuggets	7 oz	0.5	200	2%
w/granola	7 oz	1.5	220	6%
vanilla				
w/chocolate crunchies	7 oz	1.5	220	6%
w/granola	7 oz	1.5	220	6%
custard style				
fruit flavors				
multi-pack	4 oz	2.0	110	16%
regular size	6 oz	2.5	170	13%
vanilla				
multi-pack	4 oz	2.0	110	16%
regular size	6 oz	2.5	170	13%
extra creamy/nonfat				
plain	1 cup	–	140	–
vanilla	1 cup	–	210	–

Food and Description	Amount	Fat Grams	Total Calories	% Fat Calories
fruit-on-the-bottom/fat-free				
all fruit flavors	6 oz	–	160	–
light				
all fruit flavors	6 oz	–	90	–
custard style	6 oz	–	90	–
original/99% fat free				
all fruit flavors	4 oz	1.0	110	8%
	6 oz	1.5	180	8%
nonfat plain	6 oz	–	100	–
vanilla	6 oz	1.0	170	5%
Trix				
all fruit flavors				
multi-pack	4 oz	2.0	120	15%
regular size	6 oz	3.0	180	15%
YOGURT, FROZEN				
■ BARS & NOVELTIES				
(Ben & Jerry's) Cherry Garcia pop	1 pop	16.0	290	50%
(Breyer's) chocolate chip cup	1 cup	5.0	220	20%
(Haagen-Dazs) bar				
cherry chocolate fudge	1 bar	13.0	240	49%
peach	1 bar	1.0	90	10%
piña colada	1 bar	1.0	100	9%
raspberry & vanilla	1 bar	1.0	90	10%
strawberry daiquiri	1 bar	1.0	90	10%
tropical orange passion	1 bar	1.0	100	9%
(Popsicle) Creamsicle frozen yogurt bar	1 bar	1.0	100	9%
(Schwan's) Push-Em				
raspberry	1 pop	2.5	100	23%
strawberry	1 pop	2.5	100	23%
(Yoplait) bar				
low-fat				
vanilla-orange cream	1 bar	0.5	30	15%
nonfat				
chocolate mousse	1 bar	–	30	–
cherry	1 bar	–	45	–
double fruit	1 bar	–	45	–
peach	1 bar	–	45	–
strawberry	1 bar	–	45	–
triple-dipped				
chocolate	1 bar	6.0	110	49%
vanilla	1 bar	6.0	110	49%
strawberry	1 bar	6.0	110	49%
■ REGULAR & SOFT-SERVE/CARTON OR PACKAGE				
(Baskin-Robbins)				
Gone Crazy hard-packed				
low-fat				
Major Brownie Madness	½ cup	3.0	140	19%
Perils of Praline	½ cup	3.0	130	21%

Food and Description	Amount	Fat Grams	Total Calories	% Fat Calories
Raspberry Cheese Louise	½ cup	3.0	130	21%
regular				
Boom Choco Laka	½ cup	5.0	160	28%
For Heaven's Cake	½ cup	2.0	120	15%
soft serve				
low-fat				
blueberry	½ cup	1.5	120	11%
cheesecake	½ cup	1.5	120	11%
chocolate	½ cup	1.5	120	11%
vanilla	½ cup	2.0	120	15%
nonfat				
black cherry	½ cup	–	110	–
chocolate mint	½ cup	–	100	–
Dutch chocolate	½ cup	–	100	–
Kahlua	½ cup	–	100	–
key lime	½ cup	–	100	–
maple walnut	½ cup	–	100	–
peach	½ cup	–	100	–
peppermint twist	½ cup	–	100	–
piña colada	½ cup	–	110	–
raspberry	½ cup	–	100	–
strawberry	½ cup	–	100	–
vanilla	½ cup	–	110	–
Truly Free				
apple pie	½ cup	–	80	–
cafe moca	½ cup	–	80	–
chocolate	½ cup	–	80	–
triple berry delight	½ cup	–	90	–
vanilla	½ cup	–	80	–
Whata Banana	½ cup	–	80	–
(Ben & Jerry's)				
nonfat				
cappuccino	½ cup	–	140	–
strawberry	½ cup	–	140	–
vanilla fudge	½ cup	–	150	–
original				
Cherry Garcia	½ cup	3.0	170	16%
chocolate fudge brownie	½ cup	2.0	180	10%
coffee almond fudge	½ cup	7.0	200	32%
English Toffee crunch	½ cup	6.0	190	28%
(Breyers)				
fat-free				
cookies in cream	½ cup	–	110	–
fudge twirl	½ cup	–	105	–
strawberry	½ cup	–	95	–
vanilla	½ cup	–	100	–
vanilla/chocolate	½ cup	–	100	–

Food and Description	Amount	Fat Grams	Total Calories	% Fat Calories
low-fat				
black cherry	½ cup	3.0	140	19%
chocolate	½ cup	3.0	160	17%
chocolate chip cookie dough	½ cup	3.0	160	17%
chocolate fudge brownie	½ cup	3.0	160	17%
mint chocolate chip	½ cup	3.0	160	17%
peach	½ cup	3.0	140	19%
strawberry	½ cup	3.0	130	21%
strawberry cheesecake	½ cup	3.0	140	19%
toffee bar crunch	½ cup	3.0	160	17%
vanilla	½ cup	3.0	140	19%
vanilla fudge twirl	½ cup	3.0	140	19%
vanilla raspberry twirl	½ cup	3.0	130	21%
vanilla/chocolate/strawberry	½ cup	3.0	140	19%
no sugar added/vanilla	½ cup	5.0	100	45%
regular/butter pecan	½ cup	7.0	170	38%
Viennetta/strawberry				
mini	1 piece	10.0	185	49%
regular	1 slice	8.0	170	42%
(Colombo)				
gourmet				
Bavarian chocolate chunk	½ cup	4.0	120	30%
caramel-pecan chunk	½ cup	3.0	120	23%
dream	½ cup	2.0	90	20%
Heath Bar crunch	½ cup	5.0	130	35%
mocha Swiss almond	½ cup	5.0	120	38%
peanut butter cup	½ cup	7.0	140	45%
strawberry passion	½ cup	2.0	100	18%
wild raspberry cheesecake	½ cup	2.0	100	18%
sundae style				
banana split	½ cup	1.0	100	9%
caramel fudge sundae	½ cup	1.0	100	9%
chocolate peanut butter	½ cup	3.0	110	25%
(Dannon)				
light				
cappuccino	½ cup	–	80	–
cherry vanilla	½ cup	–	90	–
chocolate	½ cup	–	80	–
lemon chiffon	½ cup	–	90	–
peach raspberry melba	½ cup	–	90	–
strawberry cheesecake	½ cup	–	90	–
vanilla	½ cup	–	80	–
Light 'n Crunchy				
banana cream pie	½ cup	1.0	110	8%
mocha chocolate chunk	½ cup	1.0	110	8%
peanut chocolate crunch	½ cup	–	110	–
triple chocolate	½ cup	–	110	–
vanilla blueberry swirl	½ cup	1.0	110	8%

Food and Description	Amount	Fat Grams	Total Calories	% Fat Calories
Pure Indulgence				
cherry chocolate cherry	½ cup	3.0	150	18%
chunky chocolate nut	½ cup	3.0	150	18%
coco-nut fudge	½ cup	3.0	160	17%
cookies 'n cream	½ cup	3.0	150	18%
crunchy espresso	½ cup	3.0	150	18%
Heath toffee crunch	½ cup	3.0	150	18%
vanilla raspberry truffle	½ cup	3.0	150	18%
(Dreyer's)				
fat-free				
black cherry vanilla swirl	½ cup	–	90	–
caramel praline crunch	½ cup	–	100	–
chocolate	½ cup	–	90	–
chocolate fudge	½ cup	–	100	–
coffee fudge sundae	½ cup	–	100	–
marble fudge	½ cup	–	100	–
pine-orange paradise	½ cup	–	90	–
raspberry	½ cup	–	90	–
strawberry	½ cup	–	90	–
vanilla	½ cup	–	90	–
vanilla chocolate swirl	½ cup	–	90	–
regular				
boysenberry vanilla swirl	½ cup	2.5	100	23%
chocolate	½ cup	3.0	100	27%
chocolate brownie chunk	½ cup	4.0	110	33%
citrus heights	½ cup	2.5	80	28%
cookies 'n cream	½ cup	4.0	120	30%
espresso chip	½ cup	4.0	110	33%
Heath Bar Crunch	½ cup	4.0	120	30%
orange vanilla swirl	½ cup	2.5	100	23%
perfectly peach	½ cup	2.5	100	23%
raspberry	½ cup	2.5	100	23%
raspberry vanilla	½ cup	2.5	100	23%
strawberry chocolate chip	½ cup	4.0	120	30%
vanilla	½ cup	2.5	100	23%
(Edy's)				
fat-free				
black cherry vanilla swirl	½ cup	–	90	–
caramel praline crunch	½ cup	–	100	–
chocolate	½ cup	–	90	–
chocolate fudge	½ cup	–	100	–
coffee fudge sundae	½ cup	–	100	–
marble fudge	½ cup	–	100	–
pine-orange paradise	½ cup	–	90	–
raspberry	½ cup	–	90	–
strawberry	½ cup	–	90	–
vanilla	½ cup	–	90	–
vanilla chocolate swirl	½ cup	–	90	–

Food and Description	Amount	Fat Grams	Total Calories	% Fat Calories
regular				
chocolate	½ cup	2.5	100	23%
chocolate brownie chunk	½ cup	4.0	110	33%
citrus heights	½ cup	2.5	80	28%
cookies 'n cream	½ cup	4.0	120	30%
Heath Bar crunch	½ cup	4.0	120	30%
marble fudge	½ cup	3.0	110	25%
orange vanilla swirl	½ cup	2.5	100	23%
perfectly peach	½ cup	2.5	100	23%
raspberry	½ cup	2.5	100	23%
raspberry vanilla swirl	½ cup	2.5	100	23%
strawberry	½ cup	2.5	100	23%
strawberry chocolate chip	½ cup	4.0	120	30%
vanilla	½ cup	2.5	100	23%
(Elan)				
caramel almond praline	½ cup	4.0	150	24%
chocolate	½ cup	3.0	130	21%
chocolate almond	½ cup	6.0	160	34%
coffee	½ cup	3.0	130	21%
peach	½ cup	3.0	130	21%
rum raisin	½ cup	3.0	135	20%
strawberry	½ cup	3.0	125	22%
vanilla	½ cup	3.0	130	21%
(Haagen-Dazs)				
Extraas				
brownie nut blast	½ cup	8.0	220	33%
strawberry cheesecake craze	½ cup	8.0	220	33%
regular				
chocolate	½ cup	2.5	160	14%
coffee	½ cup	2.5	160	14%
orange tango	½ cup	1.0	130	7%
piña colada	½ cup	1.5	130	10%
raspberry rendezvous	½ cup	1.5	130	10%
strawberry duet	½ cup	2.0	130	14%
vanilla	½ cup	2.5	160	14%
(Honey Hill)				
chocolate thunder	½ cup	3.0	110	25%
cookie jar	½ cup	5.0	130	35%
peach	½ cup	3.0	110	25%
vanilla velvet	½ cup	4.0	110	33%
white almond chocolate	½ cup	5.0	120	38%
(Kemp's)				
nonfat				
chocolate	½ cup	–	110	–
cookies 'n cream	½ cup	–	120	–
fudge marble	½ cup	–	110	–
mint fudge	½ cup	–	110	–
peach	½ cup	–	90	–

Food and Description	Amount	Fat Grams	Total Calories	% Fat Calories
rocky road	½ cup	–	130	–
strawberry	½ cup	–	90	–
strawberry shortcake	½ cup	–	100	–
vanilla	½ cup	–	110	–
regular/praline caramel	½ cup	4.0	150	24%
sundae topper				
chocolate chip cookie dough	½ cup	4.0	140	50%
Heath Bar Crunch	½ cup	4.0	140	50%
(La Corona)				
blueberry	½ cup	1.0	80	11%
chocolate	½ cup	2.0	90	20%
strawberry	½ cup	1.0	80	11%
strawberry-banana	½ cup	1.0	90	10%
(Miss Karen's) gourmet				
low-fat				
chocolate	½ cup	3.0	140	19%
premium	½ cup	1.5	100	14%
original	½ cup	1.5	80	17%
nonfat				
chocolate temptation	½ cup	–	90	–
original	½ cup	–	70	–
vanilla bean	½ cup	–	90	–
select	½ cup	–	70	–
(Rhapsody Farms)				
nonfat				
chocolate peanut butter	½ cup	–	85	–
Dutch chocolate	½ cup	–	85	–
mocha madness	½ cup	–	85	–
peach	½ cup	–	85	–
strawberry extravaganza	½ cup	–	85	–
regular				
mocha almond	½ cup	2.0	89	20%
red raspberry	½ cup	2.0	89	20%
vanilla	½ cup	2.0	89	20%
(Schwan's) premium lowfat				
black cherry	½ cup	2.5	120	19%
chocolate	½ cup	3.0	120	23%
peach	½ cup	2.0	110	16%
strawberry	½ cup	2.5	110	20%
vanilla	½ cup	3.0	110	25%
(Sealtest)				
low-fat				
cherry chocolate cordial	½ cup	2.5	140	16%
chocolate	½ cup	1.5	120	11%
mint cookies & cream	½ cup	2.0	140	13%
mocha fudge	½ cup	2.0	130	14%
vanilla	½ cup	1.5	120	11%
nonfat				

Food and Description	Amount	Fat Grams	Total Calories	% Fat Calories
black cherry	½ cup	–	110	–
peach	½ cup	–	100	–
red raspberry	½ cup	–	100	–
strawberry	½ cup	–	100	–
(TCBY)				
banana pudding	½ cup	2.0	120	15%
classic vanilla	½ cup	1.5	110	12%
Dutch chocolate	½ cup	1.5	100	14%
peach	½ cup	1.0	110	8%
peanut butter fudge sundae	½ cup	1.5	110	12%
summertime strawberry	½ cup	1.0	100	9%
YOGURT BAR (See CANDY; YOGURT, FROZEN)				
YOGURT DRINK				
(Dannon) all flavors	8 fl oz	4.0	190	19%
(Glen Oaks) all flavors	8 fl oz	4.0	212	17%
(Kemp's) Yo-G yogurt-juice blend/all flavors	1 cup	–	150	–
(Yogloo) all flavors	10 oz	–	170	–
(Yonique) low-fat				
banana	7 oz	2.0	190	9%
blackberry	7 oz	2.0	190	9%
guanabana	7 oz	2.0	190	9%
guava	7 oz	2.0	190	9%
mango	7 oz	2.0	210	9%
peach	7 oz	2.0	190	9%
strawberry	7 oz	2.0	210	9%

Z

Food and Description	Amount	Fat Grams	Total Calories	% Fat Calories
ZABAGLIONE (See CUSTARD)				
ZUCCHINI (See SQUASH)				
ZWIEBACK (See BABY FOOD; COOKIE)				

Fast Food

Food and Description	Amount	Fat Grams	Total Calories	% Fat Calories
GENERAL (USDA averages derived from several restaurant chains)				
■ **BREAKFAST**				
biscuit/plain	1 biscuit	13.0	276	42%
croissant				
w/egg, cheese, & bacon	1 croissant	28.0	413	61%
w/egg, cheese, & ham	1 croissant	33.6	475	64%
w/egg, cheese, & sausage	1 croissant	38.0	524	65%
w/egg & cheese	1 croissant	24.7	369	60%
Danish				
cheese	1 Danish	24.6	353	63%
cinnamon	1 Danish	16.7	349	43%
fruit	1 Danish	15.9	335	43%
egg/scrambled	2 eggs	15.0	200	68%
English muffin				
w/butter	1 muffin	5.8	189	27%
w/cheese & sausage	1 muffin	24.0	394	55%
w/egg, cheese, & Canadian bacon	1 muffin	19.8	383	46%
w/egg, cheese, & sausage	1 muffin	30.9	487	57%
French toast w/butter	2 slices	18.8	356	47%
French toast stick	5 sticks	29.0	479	55%
omelet/ham & cheese	2 egg	17.7	255	62%
pancakes w/syrup & butter	3 pancakes	14.0	519	24%
potatoes/hash brown	½ cup	9.0	151	54%
sausage	1 patty	8.0	100	72%
■ **BURGERS, HOT DOGS, & BEEF**				
(NOTE: A regular meat patty = 2 oz; large = 4 oz [1/4 lb]. Single burgers contain 1 patty; double burgers contain 2 patties; triple burgers contain 3 patties. All burgers and hot dogs are served on appropriate size buns. Items marked with an asterisk [*] do not not include condiments or garnishes such as pickle, catsup, lettuce, onions, tomato, mustard, or mayonnaise-type dressing.)				
cheeseburger				
large patty/w/bacon				
double	1 burger	43.7	706	56%
single	1 burger	36.8	609	60%
regular patty/double	1 burger	28.0	457	55%
cheeseburger*				
large patty				
single	1 burger	33.0	608	49%
triple	1 burger	51.0	796	57%

Food and Description	Amount	Fat Grams	Total Calories	% Fat Calories
regular patty				
single	1 burger	15.0	320	42%
double/double bun	1 burger	21.6	461	42%
corn dog*	1 corn dog	18.9	460	37%
hamburger				
large patty				
single	1 burger	27.0	511	48%
triple	1 burger	41.0	693	53%
regular patty				
single	1 burger	13.0	279	42%
double	1 burger	32.0	576	50%
hamburger*				
large patty/single	1 burger	22.9	400	52%
regular patty				
double	1 burger	27.9	544	46%
single	1 burger	11.8	275	39%
hot dog*				
plain	1 hot dog	14.5	242	54%
w/chili	1 hot dog	17.5	324	49%
roast beef on bun*				
plain				
regular	1 sandwich	13.8	346	36%
super	1 sandwich	28.0	620	41%
w/cheese*	1 sandwich	18.0	402	40%

■ CHICKEN, EGG, HAM, & SEAFOOD

(NOTE: Items marked with an asterisk [*] do not not include condiments or garnishes such as pickle, catsup, lettuce, onions, tomato, mustard, or mayonnaise-type dressing.)

Food and Description	Amount	Fat Grams	Total Calories	% Fat Calories
chicken/breaded & fried				
dark meat	2 pieces	26.7	430	56%
wing & breast	2 pieces	29.5	494	54%
chicken fillet sandwich*				
plain	1 sandwich	29.0	515	51%
w/cheese	1 sandwich	38.8	632	55%
chicken nuggets				
plain	1 piece	3.0	48	55%
	6 pieces	17.7	290	55%
w/barbecue sauce	6 pieces	18.0	330	49%
w/honey	6 pieces	17.5	329	48%
w/mustard sauce	6 pieces	18.9	323	53%
w/sweet & sour sauce	6 pieces	18.0	346	47%
clams/breaded & fried	¾ cup	26.0	451	52%
crab/soft shell/fried	1 serving	17.9	334	48%
crab cake				
baked	1 cake	1.0	88	10%
fried	1 cake	18.8	290	58%
fish fillet/battered or breaded & fried	1 fillet	11.0	211	47%
fish fillet sandwich*				
plain	1 sandwich	22.8	431	48%

Food and Description	Amount	Fat Grams	Total Calories	% Fat Calories
w/tartar sauce & cheese	1 sandwich	28.6	524	49%
ham, egg, & cheese on bun*	1 sandwich	16.0	348	41%
ham & cheese on bun*	1 sandwich	15.0	353	38%
oysters/battered or breaded & fried	6 pieces	17.9	368	44%
scallops/breaded & fried	6 pieces	19.0	386	44%
shrimp/breaded & fried	6-8 pieces	24.9	454	49%
■ CONDIMENTS (*See also* Salad & Salad Bar Items in this section)				
butter/½-oz pkt	1 pkt	11.0	100	100%
catsup/¼-oz pkt	1 pkt	–	3	–
half & half/½-oz pkt	1 pkt	1.6	18	80%
honey/½-oz pkt	1 pkt	–	43	–
jelly/¾-oz pkt	1 pkt	–	58	–
lemon/½-oz pkt	1 pkt	–	3	–
lettuce	2 leaves	–	2	–
mayonnaise/²⁄₅-oz pkt	1 pkt	9.0	81	100%
mustard/⅕-oz pkt	1 pkt	–	4	–
nondairy creamer/²⁄₅-oz pkt	1 pkt	3.5	55	57%
onion	2 slices	–	7	–
pickle	2 slices	–	2	–
sugar	1 pkt	–	25	–
sugar substitute	1 pkt	–	4	–
syrup/1½-oz pkt	1 pkt	–	122	–
tartar sauce/½-oz pkt	1 pkt	8.0	74	97%
tomato	1 slice	–	5	–
■ DESSERT				
brownie	1 brownie	10.0	243	37%
fried pie	1 pie	14.0	266	47%
ice cream cone				
chocolate-dipped	1 small	7.0	150	42%
	1 medium	13.0	300	39%
	1 large	20.0	450	40%
plain	1 small	3.0	110	25%
	1 medium	7.0	230	27%
	1 large	10.0	340	27%
ice cream sandwich	1 sandwich	4.0	140	26%
ice milk/soft serve w/cone	1 oz	6.0	164	33%
sundae				
caramel	1 sundae	9.0	303	27%
hot fudge	1 sundae	8.6	284	27%
strawberry	1 sundae	7.9	269	26%
■ MEXICAN FOOD				
burrito				
bean	2 burritos	13.5	448	27%
bean & cheese	2 burritos	11.7	377	28%
bean & chili peppers	2 burritos	14.7	413	32%
bean & meat	2 burritos	17.8	508	32%
bean, cheese, & beef	2 burritos	13.0	331	35%
beef	2 burritos	20.8	523	36%

Food and Description	Amount	Fat Grams	Total Calories	% Fat Calories
beef & chili peppers	2 burritos	16.5	426	35%
beef, cheese, & chili peppers	2 burritos	24.8	634	35%
chili con carne	1 cup	8.0	254	28%
chimichanga				
beef	1 piece	19.7	425	42%
beef & cheese	1 piece	23.5	443	48%
beef & red chili peppers	1 piece	19.0	424	40%
beef, cheese, & red chili peppers	1 piece	17.6	364	43%
enchilada				
cheese, beef, & beans	1 enchilada	16.0	344	42%
cheese & beef	1 enchilada	17.6	324	49%
cheese & sour cream	1 enchilada	18.9	320	53%
frijoles/cheese	1 cup	7.8	226	31%
nachos				
cheese	6-8 pieces	19.0	345	49%
cheese & jalapeño pepper	6-8 pieces	34.0	607	50%
cheese, ground beef, beans & jalapeño pepper	6-8 pieces	30.7	568	49%
cinnamon & sugar	6-8 pieces	36.0	592	55%
taco	1 small	20.6	370	50%
	1 large	31.6	569	50%
taco salad/lettuce, tomato, chili sauce, ground beef, cheese, & taco shell	1½ cups	14.8	279	47%
w/chili con carne	1½ cups	13.0	288	41%
tostada				
bean, beef, & cheese	1 tostada	16.9	334	46%
bean & cheese	1 tostada	9.9	223	40%
beef, cheese, & guacomole	2 tostadas	23.0	360	58%
beef & cheese	1 tostada	16.0	315	46%
■ SALAD & SALAD BAR ITEMS				
alfalfa sprouts	1 oz	–	10	–
bacon bits	2 Tbs	3.0	54	50%
broccoli	~2 oz	–	6	–
carrots	~2 oz	–	12	–
cauliflower	~2 oz	–	14	–
cheese				
cheddar/shredded	3 Tbs	7.0	84	75%
cottage	½ cup	5.0	117	39%
mozzarella	1 oz	7.0	90	70%
Parmesan	3 Tbs	4.5	70	58%
chef's salad w/cheese, turkey, ham, & egg	1½ cups	16.0	267	54%
coleslaw	½ cup	8.0	90	80%
croutons	18 pieces	1.0	35	26%
cucumber/sliced	3 slices	–	2	–
egg/hard-cooked/chopped	2 Tbs	2.0	30	60%
garbanzo beans	1 Tbs	–	11	–
green peas	½ cup	–	60	–
lettuce	½ cup	–	5	–

Food and Description	Amount	Fat Grams	Total Calories	% Fat Calories
mushroom/pieces	¼ cup	–	6	–
onion	2 Tbs	–	4	–
green pepper	2 Tbs	–	4	–
salad dressing (Note: 2 oz of dressing = 4 level Tbs)				
blue cheese/2½-oz pkt	1 pkt	34.0	342	90%
French/2-oz pkt	1 pkt	20.6	228	81%
Italian/2-oz pkt	1 pkt	34.0	326	94%
low-calorie/2-oz pkt	1 pkt	2.0	50	36%
Oriental/2-oz pkt	1 pkt	1.0	102	9%
Thousand Island/2½-oz pkt	1 pkt	39.0	396	89%
wine vinegar	1 Tbs	–	2	–
tossed salad w/lettuce, tomato, radishes, carrots, cabbage, cucumber, & green pepper				
plain/no dressing	1½ cups	–	32	–
w/cheese & egg	1½ cups	5.8	102	51%
w/chicken	1½ cups	2.0	105	17%
w/pasta & seafood	1½ cups	20.9	380	49%
w/shrimp	1½ cups	2.0	107	17%
tomato	1 oz	–	6	–

■ SANDWICHES

(NOTE: Unless otherwise stated, regular sandwiches are on sliced whole wheat bread w/average portions. Subs are on rolls, 6 to 8 inches long [8 to 12 ounces].)

Food and Description	Amount	Fat Grams	Total Calories	% Fat Calories
regular				
bacon, lettuce, & tomato	1 sandwich	16.0	290	50%
bologna/plain	1 sandwich	16.0	305	47%
chicken/sliced w/lettuce	1 sandwich	15.0	310	44%
chicken salad	1 sandwich	20.0	255	71%
club/chicken, bacon, & tomato	1 sandwich	26.0	570	41%
corned beef/plain	1 sandwich	10.0	296	30%
cream cheese & jelly	1 sandwich	16.0	370	39%
egg salad	1 sandwich	13.0	285	41%
ham/plain	1 sandwich	16.0	285	51%
ham & Swiss	1 sandwich	24.0	390	55%
ham salad	1 sandwich	17.0	321	48%
liverwurst/plain	1 sandwich	12.0	260	42%
peanut butter	1 sandwich	20.0	350	51%
peanut butter & jelly	1 sandwich	15.0	385	35%
roast beef/hot w/gravy	1 sandwich	25.0	421	53%
roast pork/hot w/gravy	1 sandwich	31.0	503	56%
steak/sirloin/lean & fat/3 oz	1 sandwich	12.0	325	33%
tuna salad	1 sandwich	14.0	275	46%
turkey/plain	1 sandwich	19.0	400	43%
subs/heroes				
roast beef, lettuce, tomato, & mayonnaise	1 sandwich	13.0	411	28%
salami, ham, cheese, lettuce, tomato, & onion	1 sandwich	18.6	456	37%

Food and Description	Amount	Fat Grams	Total Calories	% Fat Calories
tuna salad	1 sandwich	28.0	584	43%

■ SIDE ORDERS (*See also* Salad & Salad Bar Items in this section)

Food and Description	Amount	Fat Grams	Total Calories	% Fat Calories
baked potato				
w/cheese	1 potato	28.7	475	54%
w/cheese & bacon	1 potato	25.9	451	52%
w/cheese sauce & broccoli	1 potato	21.0	402	47%
w/cheese sauce & chili	1 potato	21.9	481	41%
w/sour cream & chives	1 potato	22.0	394	50%
chili	1 cup	9.0	268	30%
coleslaw	¾ cup	11.0	147	67%
corn on the cob				
plain	1 ear	1.0	125	7%
w/butter	1 ear	3.0	155	17%
French fries				
fried in beef tallow	regular	12.0	237	46%
	large	18.5	358	47%
fried in beef tallow & vegetable oil	regular	12.0	237	46%
	large	18.5	358	47%
fried in vegetable oil	regular	12.0	235	46%
	large	18.5	355	47%
hushpuppies	5 pieces	12.0	256	41%
macaroni salad w/mayonnaise	½ cup	6.0	168	32%
mashed potatoes w/whole milk & margarine	⅓ cup	1.0	66	13%
onion rings	8-9 pieces	15.5	175	80%
potato chips	10 chips	7.0	105	60%
	1 oz	10.0	148	61%
potato salad	⅓ cup	5.7	108	48%
Waldorf salad	½ cup	5.0	90	50%

ARBY'S
■ BEVERAGES

Food and Description	Amount	Fat Grams	Total Calories	% Fat Calories
chocolate shake	12 fl oz	12.0	451	24%
Coca-Cola				
classic	12 fl oz	–	140	–
Diet Coke	12 fl oz	–	1	–
coffee	8 fl oz	–	3	–
Diet Rite cola	12 fl oz	–	1	–
Dr. Pepper	12 fl oz	–	160	–
hot chocolate	8 fl oz	1.0	110	8%
iced tea	16 fl oz	–	6	–
jamocha shake	11.5 fl oz	10.0	384	23%
milk/2% reduced fat	8 fl oz	4.4	121	33%
Nehi Orange	12 fl oz	–	195	–
orange juice	6 fl oz	–	82	–
Pepsi				
diet	12 fl oz	–	–	–
regular	12 fl oz	–	150	–

Food and Description	Amount	Fat Grams	Total Calories	% Fat Calories
R.C. cola	12 fl oz	–	165	–
7-Up				
diet	12 fl oz	–	4	–
regular	12 fl oz	–	144	–
Upper Ten	12 fl oz	–	169	–
vanilla shake	11 fl oz	12.0	360	30%
■ BREAKFAST				
bacon	2 strips	7.0	90	70%
biscuit/plain	1 biscuit	15.0	280	48%
blueberry muffin	1 muffin	9.0	230	35%
cinnamon nut Danish	1 Danish	11.0	360	28%
croissant/plain	1 croissant	12.0	220	49%
egg	1 egg	8.0	95	76%
ham	1.5 oz	1.0	45	20%
maple syrup	1 oz	–	120	–
sausage	1.3 oz	15.0	163	83%
Swiss cheese	0.5 oz	3.0	45	60%
toastix	6 pieces	21.1	430	44%
■ CONDIMENTS (*See also* Salads & Related Items in this section)				
Arby's sauce	½ oz	0.2	15	12%
au jus sauce	4 oz	–	10	–
BBQ sauce	½ oz	–	30	–
catsup	½ oz	–	16	–
cheddar cheese sauce	¾ oz	3.0	35	77%
horsey sauce	½ oz	5.0	60	82%
Italian sub sauce	½ oz	7.0	70	90%
mayonnaise				
light	¼ oz	1.0	12	75%
reduced calorie honey	½ oz	7.0	70	90%
regular	½ oz	12.0	110	98%
mustard	1 pkt	–	5	–
Parmesan cheese sauce	½ oz	7.0	70	90%
sugar substitute	1 pkt	–	4	–
tartar sauce	1 oz	15.0	140	96%
■ DESSERT				
cheesecake	3 oz	23.0	320	65%
chocolate chip cookie	1 oz	6.0	125	43%
Polar Swirl				
Butterfinger	11.6 oz	18.0	457	35%
Heath	11.6 oz	22.0	543	36%
Oreo	11.6 oz	22.0	482	41%
peanut butter cup	11.6 oz	24.0	517	42%
Snickers	11.6 oz	19.0	511	33%
turnover				
apple	1 turnover	14.0	330	38%
cherry	1 turnover	13.0	320	37%
■ SALADS & RELATED ITEMS				
croutons	½ oz	2.2	59	34%

Food and Description	Amount	Fat Grams	Total Calories	% Fat Calories
garden salad	1 serving	<1.0	61	7%
roast chicken salad	1 serving	2.0	149	12%
salad dressing				
blue cheese	2 oz	31.0	290	96%
buttermilk ranch/light	2 oz	–	50	–
honey French	2 oz	23.0	280	74%
Italian/light	2 oz	1.0	20	45%
red ranch	½ oz	6.0	75	72%
Thousand Island	2 oz	26.0	260	90%
side salad	1 serving	–	23	–
■ SANDWICHES				
chicken				
breast fillet	1 sandwich	28.0	536	47%
cordon bleu	1 sandwich	33.0	623	48%
grilled barbeque	1 sandwich	13.0	388	30%
grilled deluxe	1 sandwich	20.0	430	42%
roast club	1 sandwich	31.0	546	51%
roast deluxe				
light	1 sandwich	6.0	276	20%
regular	1 sandwich	22.0	433	46%
roast Santa Fe	1 sandwich	22.0	436	45%
fish fillet	1 sandwich	27.0	529	46%
ham 'n cheese melt	1 sandwich	13.0	329	36%
roast beef				
Arby Q	1 sandwich	18.0	431	38%
Arby's melt w/cheddar	1 sandwich	18.0	368	44%
bac'n cheddar deluxe	1 sandwich	34.0	539	57%
beef & cheddar	1 sandwich	28.0	487	52%
deluxe/light	1 sandwich	10.0	296	30%
original				
giant	1 sandwich	28.0	555	45%
junior	1 sandwich	14.0	324	39%
regular	1 sandwich	19.0	388	44%
super	1 sandwich	27.0	523	46%
roast turkey deluxe/light	1 sandwich	7.0	260	24%
Sub Shop				
French dip	1 sandwich	22.0	475	42%
hot ham & Swiss	1 sandwich	23.0	500	41%
Italian	1 sandwich	36.0	675	48%
Philly beef & Swiss	1 sandwich	47.0	755	56%
roast beef	1 sandwich	42.0	700	54%
triple cheese melt	1 sandwich	45.0	720	56%
turkey	1 sandwich	27.0	550	44%
■ SIDE ORDERS				
baked potato				
broccoli & cheddar	1 potato	20.0	571	32%
deluxe	1 potato	36.0	736	44%
plain	1 potato	<1.0	355	<1%

Food and Description	Amount	Fat Grams	Total Calories	% Fat Calories
w/butter or margarine & sour cream	1 potato	24.0	578	37%
curly fries				
cheddar	4.25 oz	18.0	333	49%
regular	3.5 oz	15.0	300	45%
French fries	2.5 oz	13.0	246	48%
potato cakes	3 oz	12.0	204	53%
■ SOUP				
Boston clam chowder	8 oz	9.0	190	43%
cream of broccoli	8 oz	8.0	160	45%
lumberjack mixed vegetable	8 oz	4.0	90	40%
old-fashioned chicken noodle	8 oz	2.0	80	23%
potato w/bacon	8 oz	7.0	170	37%
timberline chili	8 oz	10.0	220	41%
Wisconsin cheese	8 oz	18.0	280	58%
ARTHUR TREACHER'S				
chicken patty	2 patties	21.6	369	53%
chicken sandwich	1 sandwich	19.2	413	42%
chips	4 oz	13.2	276	43%
cod/tail shape/bake 'n broil	5 oz	14.2	245	52%
coleslaw	3 oz	8.2	123	60%
fish	2 pieces	19.8	355	50%
fish sandwich	1 sandwich	24.0	440	49%
Krunch Pup	1-2 oz	14.8	203	66%
Lemon Luv	1-3 oz	13.9	276	45%
shrimp	7 pieces	24.4	381	58%
AU BON PAIN				
■ ACCOMPANIMENTS				
cream cheese/lite	1.8 oz	9.0	110	74%
whipped cream	1.2 oz	11.0	160	62%
■ BAGELS				
cinnamon raisin	1 bagel	1.5	360	4%
onion	1 bagel	1.5	370	4%
plain	1 bagel	1.5	350	4%
poppy seed	1 bagel	3.5	380	8%
sesame	1 bagel	5.0	390	12%
■ BEVERAGES				
caffe latte				
hot	1 small	4.0	110	33%
	1 medium	6.0	150	36%
	1 large	8.0	200	36%
iced	1 small	5.0	130	35%
	1 medium	6.0	150	36%
	1 large	10.0	270	33%
cappuccino				
hot	1 small	4.0	110	33%
	1 medium	6.0	150	36%
	1 large	8.0	200	36%

Food and Description	Amount	Fat Grams	Total Calories	% Fat Calories
iced	1 small	4.0	110	33%
	1 medium	6.0	150	36%
	1 large	10.0	270	33%
cocoa				
hot	1 small	6.0	220	10%
	1 medium	8.0	320	23%
	1 large	11.0	420	24%
iced	1 small	6.0	200	27%
	1 medium	6.0	280	19%
	1 large	11.0	440	23%
mocha blast				
hot	1 small	4.0	160	23%
	1 medium	6.0	260	21%
	1 large	8.0	310	23%
iced	1 small	4.5	180	23%
	1 medium	6.0	260	21%
	1 large	10.0	360	25%
raspberry breeze/iced	1 small	–	130	–
	1 medium	–	190	–
	1 large	–	260	–
raspberry mocha blast				
hot	1 small	4.0	180	20%
	1 medium	6.0	300	18%
	1 large	8.0	350	21%
iced	1 small	3.5	160	20%
	1 medium	5.0	210	21%
	1 large	7.0	330	19%
■ BREAD				
baguette	1 slice	0.5	140	3%
bread bowl for soup (*See* Soup in this section)	1 bowl	3.5	640	5%
cheese loaf	1 slice	3.0	40	68%
four grain	1 slice	1.0	130	7%
multigrain loaf	1 slice	1.0	130	7%
Parisienne	1 slice	0.5	120	4%
rye loaf	1 slice	1.5	110	12%
■ COOKIES				
biscotti				
chocolate	1 cookie	13.0	240	49%
plain	1 cookie	10.0	200	45%
chocolate chip	1 cookie	13.0	280	42%
holiday brownie nut fudge	1 cookie	14.0	260	48%
oatmeal raisin	1 cookie	10.0	250	36%
peanut butter	1 cookie	15.0	280	48%
shortbread	1 cookie	25.0	390	58%
■ CROISSANTS				
dessert				
almond	1 croissant	37.0	560	59%

Food and Description	Amount	Fat Grams	Total Calories	% Fat Calories
apple	1 croissant	10.0	260	35%
chocolate	1 croissant	20.0	390	46%
cinnamon raisin	1 croissant	13.0	380	31%
raspberry cheese	1 croissant	19.0	380	45%
strawberry cheese	1 croissant	19.0	370	46%
sweet cheese	1 croissant	22.0	390	51%
filled/hot				
ham & cheese	1 croissant	20.0	380	47%
spinach & cheese	1 croissant	16.0	270	53%
turkey & cheddar	1 croissant	21.0	390	48%
plain				
regular	1 croissant	15.0	270	50%
sandwich	1 croissant	16.0	310	46%
■ MUFFINS				
gourmet				
blueberry	1 muffin	15.0	410	33%
carrot	1 muffin	23.0	480	43%
chocolate chip	1 muffin	20.0	490	37%
corn	1 muffin	18.0	470	34%
pumpkin w/streusel topping	1 muffin	18.0	470	34%
raisin bran	1 muffin	11.0	390	25%
low-fat				
chocolate cake	1 muffin	3.0	290	9%
cinnamon cranapple	1 muffin	3.0	310	9%
peach cobbler	1 muffin	3.0	310	9%
triple berry	1 muffin	3.0	270	10%
■ PASTRY				
Danish				
raspberry	1 Danish	21.0	370	51%
sweet cheese	1 Danish	26.0	420	56%
pecan roll	1 roll	48.0	900	48%
■ ROLLS				
regular				
country seed	1 roll	3.5	220	14%
hearth	1 roll	1.5	220	6%
petit pain	1 roll	1.0	200	9%
sandwich				
braided	1 roll	5.0	170	26%
French	1 roll	0.5	120	4%
hearth	1 roll	1.5	140	10%
■ SALADS & RELATED ITEMS				
antipasto	1 serving	28.0	410	61%
Caesar salad	1 serving	10.0	270	33%
chicken Caesar salad	1 serving	11.0	360	28%
chicken tarragon salad	1 serving	23.0	470	44%
garden salad	1 small	1.0	100	9%
	1 large	1.5	160	8%
Greek salad	1 serving	22.0	300	66%

Food and Description	Amount	Fat Grams	Total Calories	% Fat Calories
Oriental chicken salad	1 serving	5.0	230	20%
salad dressing				
bleu cheese	3 oz	41.0	410	90%
buttermilk ranch	3 oz	32.0	310	93%
Caesar	3 oz	39.0	380	92%
Greek	3 oz	50.0	440	100%
honey mustard	3 oz	33.0	380	78%
Italian/Lite	3 oz	20.0	230	78%
lemon basil vinaigrette	3 oz	32.0	330	87%
mandarin orange	3 oz	33.0	380	78%
sesame French	3 oz	30.0	370	73%
tomato basil/fat-free	3 oz	–	70	–
tuna salad	1 serving	27.0	490	50%

■ SANDWICH FILLINGS
(Note: Data are for fillings only; bread is not included)

Food and Description	Amount	Fat Grams	Total Calories	% Fat Calories
cheese				
Brie	½ portion	12.0	140	77%
cheddar	½ portion	14.0	170	74%
herb	½ portion	15.0	150	90%
provolone	½ portion	11.0	150	66%
Swiss	½ portion	12.0	160	68%
chicken				
cracked pepper	1 portion	1.6	140	10%
grilled	1 portion	1.6	140	10%
tarragon	1 portion	17.0	240	64%
country ham	1 portion	7.0	150	42%
roast beef	1 portion	4.5	140	29%
tuna salad	1 portion	29.0	360	73%
turkey breast	1 portion	1.0	120	8%

■ SANDWICHES

Food and Description	Amount	Fat Grams	Total Calories	% Fat Calories
Chef's Creation				
Arizona chicken	1 sandwich	33.0	720	41%
California chicken	1 sandwich	44.0	820	48%
fresh mozzarella, tomato, & pesto	1 sandwich	30.0	650	42%
Parmesan chicken	1 sandwich	24.0	740	29%
steak & cheese melt	1 sandwich	32.0	750	38%
Thanksgiving sub	1 sandwich	5.0	520	9%

■ SCONES

Food and Description	Amount	Fat Grams	Total Calories	% Fat Calories
blueberry	1 scone	23.0	430	48%
cinnamon	1 scone	28.0	520	48%
orange	1 scone	23.0	440	47%

■ SOUP

Food and Description	Amount	Fat Grams	Total Calories	% Fat Calories
beef barley				
regular bowl	8 oz	2.0	75	24%
	12 oz	3.0	112	24%
	16 oz	4.0	150	24%
served in a bread bowl	1 serving	7.0	760	8%

Food and Description	Amount	Fat Grams	Total Calories	% Fat Calories
beef stew				
regular bowl	8 oz	7.0	140	45%
	12 oz	10.5	210	45%
	16 oz	14.0	280	45%
served in a bread bowl	1 serving	14.0	850	15%
broccoli, cream of				
regular bowl	8 oz	18.5	220	76%
	12 oz	28.0	330	76%
	16 oz	37.0	440	76%
served in a bread bowl	1 serving	31.0	970	29%
broccoli & cheddar/regular bowl	8 oz	22.0	260	76%
	12 oz	33.0	390	76%
	16 oz	44.0	520	76%
Caribbean black bean				
regular bowl	8 oz	1.0	120	8%
	12 oz	1.5	180	8%
	16 oz	2.0	240	8%
served in a bread bowl	1 serving	5.0	830	5%
chicken, cream of, w/wild rice/regular bowl	8 oz	9.5	165	52%
	12 oz	14.3	250	52%
	16 oz	19.0	330	52%
chicken noodle				
regular bowl	8 oz	1.3	85	13%
	12 oz	1.9	130	13%
	16 oz	2.5	170	13%
served in a bread bowl	1 serving	6.0	760	7%
chicken sausage gumbo				
regular bowl	8 oz	8.5	155	49%
	12 oz	13.0	235	49%
	16 oz	17.0	310	49%
served in a bread bowl	1 serving	17.0	880	17%
chicken wild rice				
regular bowl	8 oz	1.3	90	13%
	12 oz	1.9	135	13%
	16 oz	2.5	180	13%
served in a bread bowl	1 serving	6.0	780	7%
chili				
vegetarian				
regular bowl	8 oz	2.5	140	16%
	12 oz	4.0	210	16%
	16 oz	5.0	280	16%
served in a bread bowl	1 serving	7.0	870	7%
w/meat				
regular bowl	8 oz	9.5	230	37%
	12 oz	14.0	345	37%
	16 oz	19.0	460	37%
served in a bread bowl	1 serving	19.0	990	17%

Food and Description	Amount	Fat Grams	Total Calories	% Fat Calories
clam chowder				
regular bowl	8 oz	19.5	270	65%
	12 oz	29.0	405	65%
	16 oz	39.0	540	65%
served in a bread bowl	1 serving	32.0	1050	27%
corn chowder				
regular bowl	8 oz	16.5	265	56%
	12 oz	25.0	400	56%
	16 oz	33.0	530	56%
served in a bread bowl	1 serving	28.0	1030	24%
garden vegetable				
regular bowl	8 oz	–	30	–
	12 oz	–	45	–
	16 oz	–	60	–
served in a bread bowl	1 serving	3.5	700	5%
northeastern potato & cheese w/ham				
regular bowl	8 oz	7.5	145	47%
	12 oz	11.3	220	47%
	16 oz	15.0	290	47%
served in a bread bowl	1 serving	15.0	860	16%
seafood gumbo	8 oz	6.0	130	42%
	12 oz	9.0	195	42%
	16 oz	12.0	260	42%
split pea				
regular bowl	8 oz	1.5	175	8%
	12 oz	2.3	265	8%
	16 oz	3.0	350	8%
served in a bread bowl	1 serving	6.0	940	6%
tomato Florentine				
regular bowl	8 oz	1.0	60	15%
	12 oz	1.5	90	15%
	16 oz	2.0	120	15%
served in a bread bowl	1 serving	5.0	760	6%
tomato tortellini				
regular bowl	8 oz	1.0	55	16%
	12 oz	1.5	83	16%
	16 oz	2.0	110	16%
served in a bread bowl	1 serving	5.0	730	6%
vegetable stew	8 oz	1.0	65	14%
	12 oz	1.5	100	14%
	16 oz	2.0	130	14%
vegetarian lentil				
regular bowl	8 oz	0.5	135	3%
	12 oz	0.8	205	3%
	16 oz	1.0	270	3%
served in a bread bowl	1 serving	3.5	840	4%

Food and Description	Amount	Fat Grams	Total Calories	% Fat Calories
BLIMPIE				
■ **SANDWICHES**				
Blimpie best	1 sandwich	13.0	410	29%
cheese trio	1 sandwich	23.0	510	41%
club	1 sandwich	13.0	450	26%
5 meatball	1 sandwich	22.0	500	40%
grilled chicken	1 sandwich	9.0	400	20%
grilled chicken salad	1 sandwich	12.0	350	31%
ham & Swiss	1 sandwich	13.0	400	29%
ham, salami, & provolone	1 sandwich	28.0	590	43%
roast beef	1 sandwich	4.0	340	11%
steak & cheese	1 sandwich	26.0	550	43%
tuna	1 sandwich	32.0	570	51%
turkey	1 sandwich	4.5	320	13%
BOSTON MARKET				
■ **DESSERT**				
brownie	1 piece	27.0	450	54%
chocolate chip cookie	1 cookie	17.0	340	45%
oatmeal raisin cookie	1 cookie	13.0	320	37%
■ **ENTRÉES**				
Caesar salad	10 oz	43.0	520	74%
w/o dressing	8 oz	13.0	240	49%
chicken Caesar salad	13 oz	47.0	670	63%
chicken pot pie	1 pie	34.0	750	41%
chunky chicken salad	¾ cup	30.0	390	69%
ham w/cinnamon apples	8 oz	13.0	350	33%
meat loaf				
w/chunky tomato sauce	8 oz	18.0	370	44%
w/brown gravy	7 oz	22.0	390	51%
roast chicken				
¼ chicken				
dark meat				
skinless	1 serving	10.0	210	43%
w/skin	1 serving	22.0	330	60%
white meat				
skinless, w/o wing	1 serving	3.5	160	20%
w/skin	1 serving	17.0	330	46%
½ chicken w/skin	1 serving	37.0	630	53%
turkey breast rotisserie/skinless	5 oz	1.0	170	5%
■ **SANDWICHES**				
chicken				
plain	1 sandwich	3.5	430	7%
w/cheese & sauce	1 sandwich	32.0	760	38%
chicken salad	1 sandwich	33.0	680	44%
ham				
plain	1 sandwich	9.0	450	18%
w/cheese & sauce	1 sandwich	35.0	760	41%

Food and Description	Amount	Fat Grams	Total Calories	% Fat Calories
ham & turkey club				
plain	1 sandwich	6.0	430	13%
w/cheese & sauce	1 sandwich	43.0	890	43%
meat loaf				
plain	1 sandwich	21.0	690	27%
w/cheese	1 sandwich	33.0	860	35%
turkey				
plain	1 sandwich	3.5	400	8%
w/cheese & sauce	1 sandwich	28.0	710	35%
■ SIDE DISHES				
BBQ baked beans	¾ cup	9.0	330	25%
buttered corn	¾ cup	4.0	190	19%
butternut squash	¾ cup	6.0	160	34%
Caesar side salad	4 oz	17.0	210	73%
chicken gravy	1 oz	1.0	15	60%
coleslaw	¾ cup	16.0	280	51%
cornbread	1 loaf	6.0	200	27%
cranberry relish	¾ cup	5.0	370	12%
creamed spinach	¾ cup	24.0	300	72%
fruit salad	¾ cup	0.5	70	6%
hot cinnamon apples	¾ cup	4.5	250	16%
macaroni & cheese	¾ cup	10.0	280	32%
mashed potatoes				
homestyle w/gravy	¾ cup	9.0	200	41%
plain	⅔ cup	8.0	180	40%
Mediterranean pasta salad	¾ cup	10.0	170	53%
new potatoes	¾ cup	3.0	140	19%
rice pilaf	⅔ cup	5.0	180	25%
steamed vegetables	⅔ cup	0.5	35	13%
stuffing	¾ cup	12.0	310	35%
tortellini salad	¾ cup	24.0	380	57%
zucchini marinara	¾ cup	4.0	80	45%
■ SOUP				
chicken	¾ cup	3.0	80	34%
chicken tortilla	1 cup	11.0	220	45%
BURGER KING				
■ BEVERAGES				
chocolate shake				
regular	1 medium	7.0	320	19%
syrup added	1 medium	7.0	440	14%
Coca-Cola				
classic	1 medium	–	280	–
Diet Coke	1 medium	–	1	–
coffee	1 serving	–	5	–
milk/2% reduced fat	1 serving	5.0	130	42%
orange juice	1 serving	–	140	–
Sprite	1 medium	–	260	–

Food and Description	Amount	Fat Grams	Total Calories	% Fat Calories
strawberry shake				
regular	1 medium	7.0	430	15%
syrup added	1 medium	6.0	420	13%
vanilla shake	1 medium	6.0	300	18%
■ **BREAKFAST**				
biscuit				
bacon, egg, & cheese	1 biscuit	31.0	510	55%
sausage	1 biscuit	40.0	590	61%
Croissan'wich/sausage, egg, & cheese	1 sandwich	46.0	600	69%
French toast sticks	1 serving	27.0	500	49%
hash browns	1 serving	12.0	220	49%
■ **BURGERS**				
cheeseburger				
double				
plain	1 burger	36.0	600	54%
w/bacon	1 burger	39.0	640	55%
regular	1 burger	19.0	380	45%
hamburger/regular	1 burger	15.0	330	41%
Whopper				
double				
plain	1 burger	56.0	870	58%
w/cheese	1 burger	63.0	960	59%
original				
plain	1 burger	39.0	640	55%
w/cheese	1 burger	46.0	730	57%
Whopper Jr.				
plain	1 burger	24.0	420	51%
w/cheese	1 burger	28.0	460	55%
■ **CHICKEN & FISH**				
chicken sandwich				
BK Broiler	1 sandwich	29.0	550	47%
regular	1 sandwich	43.0	710	55%
chicken tenders	6 pieces	12.0	230	47%
fish sandwich/BK Big Fish	1 sandwich	41.0	700	53%
■ **CONDIMENTS** (*See also* Salads & Related Items in this section)				
A.M. Express				
grape jam	1 serving	–	30	–
strawberry jam	1 serving	–	30	–
Bull's Eye barbecue sauce	1 Tbs	–	20	–
butter blend/Land O'Lakes Whipped Classic Blend	1 serving	7.0	65	100%
catsup	1 Tbs	–	15	–
cheese/processed American	¾ oz	8.0	90	80%
dipping sauce/1-oz serving				
barbecue	1 serving	–	35	–
Burger King A.M. Express dip	1 serving	–	80	–
honey	1 serving	–	90	–
ranch	1 serving	17.0	170	90%

Food and Description	Amount	Fat Grams	Total Calories	% Fat Calories
sweet & sour	1 serving	–	45	–
lettuce	1 piece	–	–	–
mayonnaise	2 Tbs	23.0	210	99%
mustard	1 serving	–	–	–
pickle	1 serving	–	–	–
tartar sauce	2 Tbs	19.0	180	95%
tomato	1 oz	–	5	–
■ DESSERT				
Dutch apple pie	1 pie	15.0	300	45%
■ SALADS & RELATED ITEMS				
bacon bits	1 serving	1.0	15	60%
broiled chicken salad/no dressing	1 serving	10.0	200	45%
croutons	1 serving	1.0	30	30%
garden salad/no dressing	1 serving	5.0	100	45%
salad dressing				
blue cheese	1 serving	16.0	160	90%
French	1 serving	10.0	140	64%
Italian/light	1 serving	0.5	15	30%
ranch	1 serving	19.0	180	95%
Thousand Island	1 serving	12.0	140	77%
side salad/no dressing	1 serving	3.0	60	45%
■ SIDE ORDERS (See also Salads & Related Items in this section)				
French fries	medium	20.0	370	49%
onion rings	1 serving	14.0	310	41%
CAPTAIN D'S				
■ CAPTAIN'S BROILER				
meals				
chicken lunch	1 meal	9.0	503	16%
chicken platter	1 meal	10.0	802	11%
fish & chicken lunch	1 meal	8.0	478	15%
fish & chicken platter	1 meal	10.0	777	12%
fish lunch	1 meal	7.0	435	14%
fish platter	1 meal	7.0	734	9%
shrimp lunch	1 meal	7.0	421	15%
shrimp platter	1 meal	8.0	720	10%
side dishes				
baked potato	1 potato	–	278	–
breadstick	1 breadstick	4.0	113	32%
rice	1 serving	–	184	–
salad	1 serving	–	20	–
vegetable medley	1 serving	1.0	36	25%
■ CONDIMENTS				
cocktail sauce	side portion	–	34	–
	bulk portion	<1.0	135	3%
creamer/nondairy	1 serving	1.0	14	64%
margarine	1 serving	12.0	102	100%

Food and Description	Amount	Fat Grams	Total Calories	% Fat Calories
salad dressing				
blue cheese	1 packet	11.7	105	100%
French	1 packet	10.7	111	90%
Italian/light	1 serving	0.5	16	28%
ranch	1 packet	10.0	92	98%
sour cream/imitation	1 serving	3.0	29	93%
sugar	1 packet	–	13	–
sweet & sour sauce	side portion	–	52	–
	bulk portion	–	206	–
tartar sauce	side portion	6.9	75	83%
	bulk portion	27.4	298	83%
■ CRAB				
stuffed	1 serving	6.5	91	64%
■ DESSERT				
carrot cake	1 piece	22.8	434	47%
cheesecake	1 piece	31.0	420	66%
chocolate cake	1 piece	10.2	303	30%
lemon pie	1 piece	10.0	351	26%
pecan pie	1 piece	19.8	458	39%
■ SANDWICH				
broiled chicken	1 serving	18.5	451	37%
■ SIDE ORDERS				
coleslaw	1 serving	11.8	158	67%
	1 pint	47.0	635	67%
corn on the cob	1 serving	2.0	250	7%
crackers	4 pieces	1.0	50	18%
Cracklins/w/dinner	1 serving	16.8	218	69%
French fries	1 serving	9.9	302	30%
fried okra	1 serving	15.6	300	47%
green beans	1 serving	2.3	46	45%
hushpuppies	1 piece	4.0	125	29%
	6 pieces	24.5	756	29%
rice	1 serving	–	124	–
white beans	1 serving	0.5	126	4%
CARL'S JR.				
■ BEVERAGES				
chocolate shake	13.5 fl oz	7.0	390	16%
Coca-Cola				
classic	16 fl oz	–	190	–
Diet Coke	16 fl oz	–	1	–
coffee	12 fl oz	–	10	–
Dr. Pepper	16 fl oz	–	200	–
hot chocolate	12 fl oz	1.0	110	8%
iced tea	1 regular	–	5	–
milk/1% low-fat	10 fl oz	3.0	150	18%
Minute Maid Orange	16 fl oz	–	230	–
orange juice	6 fl oz	–	90	–

Food and Description	Amount	Fat Grams	Total Calories	% Fat Calories
Ramblin' Root Beer	16 fl oz	–	230	–
7-Up/diet	16 fl oz	–	–	–
Sprite	16 fl oz	–	190	–
strawberry shake	13.5 fl oz	7.0	400	16%
vanilla shake	13.5 fl oz	8.0	330	22%
■ BREAKFAST				
bacon	2 strips	3.5	40	79%
blueberry muffin	1 muffin	14.0	340	37%
bran muffin	1 muffin	13.0	370	32%
breakfast burrito	1 burrito	26.0	430	54%
breakfast quesadilla	1 quesadilla	14.0	300	42%
cinnamon roll	1 roll	13.0	420	28%
Danish/cheese	1 Danish	22.0	400	50%
eggs/scrambled	1 serving	11.0	160	62%
English muffin w/margarine	1 muffin	10.0	230	39%
French toast dips	1 serving	25.0	410	55%
sausage	1 patty	18.0	200	81%
sunrise sandwich/no bacon or sausage	1 sandwich	21.0	370	51%
■ BURGERS				
cheeseburger/Western bacon				
double	1 burger	57.0	970	53%
regular	1 burger	35.0	870	36%
hamburger				
Big Burger	1 burger	20.0	470	38%
Famous Star	1 burger	38.0	610	56%
regular	1 burger	8.0	200	36%
Super Star	1 burger	53.0	820	58%
■ CHICKEN & FISH				
chicken sandwich				
hot & crispy	1 sandwich	22.0	400	50%
Santa Fe	1 sandwich	29.0	550	47%
fish sandwich/Carl's Catch	1 sandwich	30.0	560	48%
■ CONDIMENTS (See also Salads & Related Items in this section)				
BBQ sauce	1 oz	–	50	–
cheese				
American	1 slice	5.0	60	75%
Swiss	1 slice	3.5	45	70%
grape jelly	1 Tbs	–	35	–
honey sauce	1 oz	–	90	–
mustard sauce	1 oz	0.5	45	10%
salsa	1 oz	–	10	–
strawberry jam	1 Tbs	–	35	–
sweet n' sour sauce	1 oz	–	50	–
table syrup	1 oz	–	90	–
■ DESSERT				
cheesecake/strawberry swirl	1 piece	17.0	300	51%
chocolate cake	1 piece	10.0	300	30%
chocolate chip cookie	1 serving	13.0	330	36%

Food and Description	Amount	Fat Grams	Total Calories	% Fat Calories
▨ POTATOES				
bacon & cheese	1 serving	29.0	630	41%
broccoli & cheese	1 serving	22.0	530	37%
plain	1 serving	–	290	–
sour cream & chive	1 serving	14.0	430	29%
▨ SALADS & RELATED ITEMS				
breadsticks	1 serving	0.5	35	13%
charbroled chicken salad	1 serving	9.0	260	31%
croutons	1 serving	1.0	35	26%
garden salad	1 serving	3.0	50	54%
salad dressing				
blue cheese	2 oz	34.0	310	99%
house	2 oz	22.0	220	90%
Thousand Island	2 oz	24.0	250	86%
▨ SIDE ORDERS (*See also* Salads & Related Items in this section)				
chicken stars	6 pieces	14.0	230	55%
criscut fries	large	34.0	550	56%
French fries	regular	20.0	370	49%
hash brown nuggets	1 serving	17.0	270	57%
onion rings	1 serving	26.0	520	45%
zucchini	1 serving	23.0	380	54%
CHICK-FIL-A				
▨ BEVERAGES				
Coca-Cola				
classic	9 fl oz	–	110	–
Diet Coke	9 fl oz	–	1	–
iced tea				
sweetened	9 fl oz	–	150	–
unsweetened	9 fl oz	–	–	–
lemonade				
diet	9 fl oz	–	5	–
regular	9 fl oz	–	90	–
▨ CHICKEN				
chicken salad sandwich on wheat bread	1 sandwich	5.0	320	14%
Chik-fil-A				
chargrilled				
no bun/no pickles	1 piece	3.0	130	21%
sandwich				
club/no dressing	1 sandwich	12.0	390	28%
deluxe w/lettuce & tomato	1 sandwich	3.0	290	9%
regular	1 sandwich	3.0	280	10%
Grilled 'n Lites	2 skewers	2.0	100	18%
original				
Chick-n Strips	4 pieces	8.0	230	31%
no bun	1 piece	8.0	160	45%
sandwich				
deluxe	1 sandwich	9.0	300	27%

Food and Description	Amount	Fat Grams	Total Calories	% Fat Calories
regular	1 sandwich	9.0	290	28%
nuggets	8 pieces	14.0	290	43%
Chick-n-Q sandwich	1 sandwich	13.0	370	32%
■ DESSERT				
cheesecake				
plain	1 slice	21.0	270	70%
w/blueberry topping	1 slice	23.0	290	71%
w/strawberry topping	1 slice	23.0	290	71%
fudge brownie w/nuts	1 brownie	16.0	350	41%
ice cream				
cone	1 small	4.0	140	26%
cup	1 small	10.0	350	26%
lemon pie	1 slice	22.0	280	71%
■ SALADS				
chargrilled chicken garden salad	1 serving	3.0	170	16%
chicken salad plate	1 serving	5.0	290	16%
Chick-fil-A Chick-n Strips salad	1 serving	9.0	290	28%
tossed salad/plain	1 serving	–	70	–
■ SIDE ORDERS (See also Salads in this section)				
carrot & raisin salad	1 serving	2.0	150	12%
coleslaw	1 serving	6.0	130	42%
waffle potato fries				
salted	small	10.0	290	31%
unsalted	small	10.0	290	31%
■ SOUP				
hearty breast of chicken	1 cup	1.0	110	8%
CHURCH'S CHICKEN				
■ CHICKEN				
breast	2.8 oz	12.4	200	56%
leg	2 oz	9.0	140	58%
tender strip	1.1 oz	4.0	80	45%
thigh	2.8 oz	16.0	230	63%
wing	3.1 oz	16.0	250	58%
■ DESSERT				
apple pie	1 piece	12.3	280	39%
■ SIDE ORDERS				
biscuit	1 biscuit	16.4	250	59%
Cajun rice	1 serving	7.0	130	48%
coleslaw	1 serving	5.5	92	54%
corn on the cob	1 piece	3.2	139	21%
French fries	1 serving	10.5	210	45%
okra	1 serving	16.0	210	69%
potatoes & gravy	1 serving	3.3	90	33%
DAIRY QUEEN				
■ BEVERAGES				
chocolate malt	1 small	18.0	760	21%
	1 regular	25.0	1060	21%

Food and Description	Amount	Fat Grams	Total Calories	% Fat Calories
chocolate shake	1 small	14.0	540	23%
	1 regular	26.0	990	24%
vanilla malt	1 small	14.0	610	21%
vanilla shake	1 small	14.0	520	24%
	1 regular	16.0	600	24%
■ BURGERS & HOT DOGS				
hamburger/DQ homestyle				
double				
deluxe				
plain	1 burger	22.0	440	45%
w/cheese	1 burger	31.0	540	52%
regular				
w/bacon & cheese	1 burger	36.0	610	53%
w/cheese	1 burger	31.0	540	52%
single				
plain	1 burger	12.0	290	37%
w/cheese	1 burger	17.0	340	45%
hot dog				
cheese	1 hot dog	18.0	290	56%
chili	1 hot dog	16.0	280	51%
chili n' cheese	1 hot dog	21.0	330	57%
plain	1 hot dog	14.0	240	53%
■ CHICKEN & FISH				
chicken fillet sandwich				
breaded				
plain	1 sandwich	20.0	430	42%
w/cheese	1 sandwich	25.0	480	47%
grilled	1 sandwich	10.0	310	24%
chicken strip basket				
w/BBQ sauce	1 basket	37.0	810	41%
w/gravy	1 basket	42.0	860	44%
fish fillet sandwich				
plain	1 sandwich	16.0	370	39%
w/cheese	1 sandwich	21.0	420	45%
■ FROZEN DESSERT SPECIALTIES				
banana split	1 serving	11.0	510	19%
Blizzard				
Heath	1 small	23.0	560	37%
	1 regular	36.0	820	40%
strawberry	1 small	12.0	400	22%
	1 regular	16.0	570	19%
Breeze				
Heath	1 small	12.0	450	24%
	1 regular	21.0	680	28%
strawberry	1 small	<1.0	290	2%
	1 regular	1.0	420	2%
Buster Bar	1 bar	29.0	450	58%

Food and Description	Amount	Fat Grams	Total Calories	% Fat Calories
cone				
chocolate	1 small	7.0	230	27%
	1 regular	11.0	350	28%
chocolate-dipped	1 small	16.0	330	44%
vanilla	1 child's	4.0	140	26%
	1 small	7.0	230	27%
	1 regular	10.0	340	26%
Dilly Bar	1 bar	13.0	210	56%
DQ frozen cake slice/undecorated	1 slice	18.0	380	43%
DQ sandwich	1 sandwich	4.0	140	26%
frozen yogurt				
cone	1 small	<1.0	180	3%
	1 regular	<1.0	260	2%
cup	1 small	<1.0	170	3%
	1 regular	<1.0	230	3%
strawberry sundae	1 regular	<1.0	200	2%
Mr. Misty	1 small	–	250	–
Mr. Misty float	1 serving	7.0	390	16%
Mr. Misty freeze	1 serving	12.0	500	22%
nutty double fudge	1 serving	22.0	580	34%
Peanut Buster parfait	1 serving	32.0	710	41%
Queen's Choice Big Scoop				
chocolate	1 serving	14.0	310	41%
vanilla	1 serving	14.0	300	42%
sundae				
chocolate sundae	1 small	7.0	300	21%
hot fudge brownie delight	1 sundae	29.0	710	37%
strawberry waffle cone	1 sundae	12.0	350	31%
■ SALADS & DRESSING				
garden salad/no dressing	1 serving	13.0	200	59%
salad dressing				
French/reduced calorie	1 serving	5.0	90	50%
Thousand Island	1 serving	21.0	225	84%
side salad/no dressing	1 serving	–	25	–
■ SIDE ORDERS (*See also* Salads & Dressing in this section)				
French fries	1 small	10.0	210	43%
	1 regular	14.0	300	42%
	1 large	18.0	390	42%
lettuce	1 piece	–	2	–
onion rings	1 serving	12.0	240	45%
tomato	1 slice	–	3	–

Food and Description	Amount	Fat Grams	Total Calories	% Fat Calories
DEL TACO				
■ **BEVERAGES**				
chocolate shake	1 small	16.0	549	26%
	1 medium	22.0	755	26%
Coca-Cola				
classic	1 small	–	144	–
	1 medium	–	198	–
	1 large	–	267	–
Diet Coke	1 small	–	1	–
	1 medium	–	1	–
	1 large	–	2	–
	1 best value	–	2	–
coffee	1 regular	–	6	–
iced tea	1 small	–	3	–
	1 medium	–	4	–
	1 large	–	6	–
	1 best value	–	8	–
milk	1 regular	3.0	126	21%
Mr. Pibb	1 small	–	142	–
	1 medium	–	195	–
	1 large	–	283	–
	1 best value	–	390	–
orange juice	1 regular	<1.0	83	3%
orange shake	1 small	16.0	609	24%
	1 medium	22.0	837	24%
Sprite	1 small	–	144	–
	1 medium	–	198	–
	1 large	–	287	–
	1 best value	–	395	–
strawberry shake	1 small	16.0	486	30%
	1 medium	22.0	668	30%
vanilla shake	1 small	18.0	514	32%
	1 medium	25.0	707	32%
■ **BURGERS**				
cheeseburger				
Del cheeseburger				
single	1 burger	25.0	439	51%
double	1 burger	39.0	618	57%
regular	1 burger	13.0	284	41%
hamburger				
Del burger	1 burger	20.0	385	47%
regular	1 burger	8.0	231	31%
■ **BURRITOS**				
breakfast				
beef & egg	1 burrito	27.0	529	46%
egg & bean	1 burrito	22.0	470	42%
egg & cheese	1 burrito	22.0	443	45%
regular	1 burrito	11.0	256	39%

Food and Description	Amount	Fat Grams	Total Calories	% Fat Calories
steak & egg	1 burrito	25.0	500	45%
regular				
beef				
Del Beef				
regular	1 burrito	20.0	440	41%
deluxe	1 burrito	23.0	479	43%
nacho	1 burrito	41.0	891	41%
chicken	1 burrito	10.0	264	34%
deluxe	1 burrito	34.0	549	56%
spicy	1 burrito	11.0	392	25%
combination	1 burrito	17.0	413	37%
deluxe	1 burrito	20.0	453	40%
nacho	1 burrito	31.0	774	36%
green	1 burrito	8.0	229	31%
regular	1 burrito	11.0	330	30%
red	1 burrito	8.0	235	31%
regular	1 burrito	12.0	342	32%
The Works	1 burrito	18.0	448	36%
■ CONDIMENTS (*See also* Salads & Dressing in this section)				
American cheese	1 slice	4.0	53	68%
guacamole	1 oz	6.0	60	90%
hot sauce	1 pouch	–	<1	–
nacho cheese sauce	1 serving	8.0	100	72%
salsa	2 oz	<1.0	14	19%
sour dream	1 oz	6.0	60	90%
■ DESSERT				
toppers				
M&M's	1 serving	8.0	256	28%
Oreos	1 serving	10.0	257	35%
Snickers	1 serving	10.0	254	35%
■ KIDS' MEALS				
hamburger	1 meal	20.0	617	29%
taco	1 meal	17.0	532	29%
■ QUESADILLAS				
chicken/regular	1 quesadilla	31.0	544	51%
plain	1 quesadilla	12.0	257	42%
regular	1 quesadilla	27.0	483	50%
Spicy Jack	1 quesadilla	12.0	254	43%
chicken	1 quesadilla	30.0	537	50%
regular	1 quesadilla	27.0	476	51%
■ SALADS & DRESSING				
chicken salad				
regular	1 serving	19.0	254	67%
deluxe	1 serving	47.0	716	59%
salsa dressing	1 oz	3.0	33	82%
taco salad				
regular	1 serving	19.0	235	73%
deluxe	1 serving	49.0	741	60%

Food and Description	Amount	Fat Grams	Total Calories	% Fat Calories
■ **SIDE ORDERS** (*See also* Salads & Dressing in this section)				
beans & cheese	1 serving	3.0	122	22%
fries				
regular	small	11.0	242	41%
	medium	19.0	404	42%
	large	26.0	566	41%
chili cheese				
deluxe	1 serving	33.0	600	50%
nacho	1 serving	34.0	669	46%
regular	1 serving	30.0	562	48%
nachos				
Nacho Nachos	1 serving	61.0	1089	50%
regular	1 serving	23.0	390	53%
■ **TACOS**				
chicken				
regular	1 taco	13.0	186	63%
soft	1 taco	11.0	197	50%
double beef				
deluxe	1 taco	13.0	205	57%
regular	1 taco	10.0	172	52%
soft	1 taco	6.0	178	30%
soft deluxe	1 taco	11.0	211	47%
regular	1 taco	8.0	140	51%
soft	1 taco	6.0	146	37%
■ **TOSTADA**				
regular	1 tostada	8.0	140	51%
DENNY'S				
■ **BREAKFAST**				
All-American Slam/w/o bread	1 serving	84.0	980	77%
applesauce	2 oz	–	40	–
bacon	4 strips	12.0	145	74%
bagel	1 bagel	1.0	230	4%
banana	1 banana	1.0	105	9%
banana strawberry medley	1 serving	–	95	–
Belgian waffle				
plain	1 serving	22.0	320	62%
w/3 oz blueberry topping	1 serving	22.0	430	46%
w/3 oz strawberry topping	1 serving	22.0	400	50%
w/2 oz whipped topping	1 serving	24.0	343	63%
Belgian Waffle Slam/senior	1 serving	46.0	540	74%
biscuit				
plain	1 serving	9.0	215	38%
w/sausage gravy	1 serving	30.0	465	58%
blueberry muffin	1 muffin	14.0	310	41%
buttermilk pancakes				
plain	3 pancakes	6.0	410	13%
w/2 oz syrup	3 pancakes	6.0	570	9%

Food and Description	Amount	Fat Grams	Total Calories	% Fat Calories
w/1 Tbs whipped butter	3 pancakes	13.0	475	25%
w/2 oz syrup & 1 Tbs whipped butter	3 pancakes	13.0	635	18%
canteloupe	¼ melon	–	100	–
chicken fried steak & eggs/w/o bread	1 serving	49.0	650	68%
cinnamon roll	1 roll	30.0	670	40%
cream cheese	1 oz	10.0	100	90%
egg	1 egg	10.0	120	75%
English muffin	1 muffin	1.0	150	6%
French Slam	1 serving	60.0	915	59%
French toast	1 serving	19.0	325	53%
Grand Slam				
regular	1 serving	45.0	860	47%
senior	1 serving	24.0	535	40%
grapefruit	½ fruit	–	40	–
grapes	1 serving	–	55	–
grits	1 serving	<1.0	160	3%
ham	1 serving	8.0	170	42%
Harvest Slam	1 serving	56.0	1055	48%
hash browns	1 serving	13.0	210	56%
honeydew	¼ melon	–	125	–
International Slam	1 serving	68.0	975	63%
Moons Over My Hammy	1 serving	66.0	980	61%
omelette				
chili-cheese	1 serving	33.0	445	67%
Denver	1 serving	63.0	735	77%
ham 'n cheddar	1 serving	34.0	490	62%
Mexican	1 serving	41.0	550	67%
senior	1 serving	58.0	650	80%
ultimate	1 serving	64.0	745	77%
vegetable	1 serving	48.0	585	74%
orange juice	10 fl oz	–	130	–
sausage	4 links	22.0	225	88%
Scram Slam/w/o bread	1 serving	91.0	1080	76%
Senior Starter	1 serving	45.0	550	74%
Southern Slam	1 serving	71.0	895	71%
steak & eggs	1 serving	51.0	800	57%
syrup	2 oz	–	160	–
toast/no butter	2 pieces	2.0	140	13%
■ BURGERS				
bacon-Swiss	1 burger	45.0	745	54%
Denny burger	1 burger	25.0	485	46%
patty melt	1 burger	58.0	780	67%
Works Burger	1 burger	66.0	950	63%
■ DESSERT				
apple pie				
regular	1 slice	30.0	520	52%
sweetened w/Equal	1 slice	30.0	460	59%
blueberry cream cheese pie	1 slice	37.0	700	48%

Food and Description	Amount	Fat Grams	Total Calories	% Fat Calories
cherry pie				
regular	1 slice	30.0	635	43%
sweetened w/Equal	1 slice	30.0	510	53%
cherry cream cheese pie	1 slice	37.0	685	49%
coconut cream pie	1 slice	27.0	480	51%
French silk pie	1 slice	30.0	510	53%
Key lime pie	1 slice	27.0	590	41%
■ ENTRÉES				
beef				
prime rib	8 oz	46.0	570	73%
roast beef				
senior selection/w/o vegetable	1 meal	9.0	280	29%
w/bread, gravy, & potatoes	1 serving	19.0	600	29%
sirloin tips/senior selection/w/o vegetable	1 meal	5.0	220	20%
catfish				
dinner/senior selection/w/o vegetable	1 meal	32.0	450	64%
grilled	1 serving	43.0	475	81%
chicken				
breast/grilled	4 oz	3.0	125	22%
	6 oz	5.0	190	24%
fried				
regular	1 serving	27.0	460	53%
senior selection/w/o vegetable	1 meal	23.0	480	43%
grilled chicken dinner/senior selection/ w/o vegetable	1 meal	7.0	245	26%
stir-fry w/vegetables & rice pilaf	1 serving	21.0	435	43%
strips	1 serving	25.0	580	39%
chicken-fried steak				
regular	1 serving	38.0	465	74%
senior selection	1 meal	23.0	425	49%
liver w/bacon & onions				
regular	1 serving	41.0	585	63%
senior selection/w/o vegetable	1 meal	27.0	435	56%
rainbow trout/grilled	1 serving	34.0	490	62%
roast turkey w/stuffing & gravy				
regular	1 serving	26.0	490	48%
senior selection/w/o vegetable	1 meal	16.0	440	33%
spaghetti				
w/meatballs				
regular	1 serving	38.0	1000	34%
senior selection/w/o vegetable	1 meal	25.0	580	39%
w/sauce	1 serving	9.0	605	13%
■ SALADS & DRESSING				
Caesar salad	1 serving	23.0	325	64%
California grilled chicken salad	1 serving	12.0	290	37%
Chef's salad	1 serving	26.0	370	63%
crispy chicken salad				
regular	1 serving	55.0	905	55%

Food and Description	Amount	Fat Grams	Total Calories	% Fat Calories
w/o tortilla shell	1 serving	25.0	465	48%
garden salad	1 serving	4.0	115	31%
grilled chicken Caesar salad	1 serving	41.0	655	56%
salad dressing				
blue cheese	2 Tbs	14.0	120	100%
French				
regular	2 Tbs	12.0	100	100%
reduced calorie	2 Tbs	4.0	70	51%
Italian				
creamy	2 Tbs	10.0	100	90%
reduced calorie	2 Tbs	1.0	16	56%
honey mustard	2 Tbs	6.0	100	54%
ranch	2 Tbs	11.0	110	90%
Thousand Island	2 Tbs	11.0	120	83%
taco salad				
regular	1 serving	55.0	905	55%
w/o tortilla shell	1 serving	25.0	470	48%
■ SANDWICHES				
bacon, lettuce, & tomato	1 sandwich	37.0	490	68%
chicken melt	1 sandwich	41.0	700	53%
club	1 sandwich	35.0	485	65%
French dip	1 sandwich	40.0	575	63%
grilled cheese				
regular	1 sandwich	49.0	715	62%
senior selection	1 sandwich	25.0	360	63%
grilled chicken	1 sandwich	34.0	665	46%
Mega Melt	1 sandwich	63.0	945	60%
Prime Time	1 sandwich	70.0	930	86%
roast beef deluxe	1 sandwich	56.0	850	59%
Super Bird	1 sandwich	35.0	585	54%
tuna melt supreme	1 sandwich	58.0	805	65%
tuna salad/senior selection	1 sandwich	17.0	260	59%
turkey/senior selection	1 sandwich	27.0	340	71%
veggie cheese melt	1 sandwich	40.0	565	64%
■ SIDE ORDERS & APPETIZERS (See also Salads & Dressing in this section)				
Buffalo wings/w/o dressing	1 serving	22.0	350	57%
chicken strips/w/o dressing	1 serving	25.0	580	39%
chili fries	1 serving	25.0	585	38%
coleslaw	1 serving	9.0	105	77%
French fries	1 serving	12.0	285	38%
mozzarella sticks	4 sticks	20.0	350	51%
Nacho Supreme	1 serving	45.0	770	53%
quesadilla				
chicken	1 quesadilla	31.0	580	48%
regular	1 quesadilla	28.0	460	55%
■ SOUP				
broccoli, cream of	1 serving	12.0	200	54%
cheese	1 serving	23.0	315	76%

Food and Description	Amount	Fat Grams	Total Calories	% Fat Calories
chicken noodle	1 serving	2.0	60	30%
chili w/beans	1 serving	6.0	160	34%
clam chowder	1 serving	12.0	220	49%
potato, cream of	1 serving	12.0	230	47%
vegetable beef	1 serving	1.0	80	11%

DOMINO'S PIZZA
■ 12" DEEP-DISH PIZZA

cheese	¼ pizza	24.0	560	39%
extra cheese & pepperoni	¼ pizza	33.0	670	44%
ham	¼ pizza	24.5	577	38%
Italian sausage & mushroom	¼ pizza	28.0	618	41%
pepperoni	¼ pizza	29.5	622	43%
veggie	¼ pizza	25.0	575	39%

■ 12" HAND-TOSSED PIZZA

cheese	¼ pizza	9.5	344	25%
extra cheese & pepperoni	¼ pizza	19.0	455	38%
ham	¼ pizza	10.0	361	25%
Italian sausage & mushroom	¼ pizza	14.0	402	31%
pepperoni	¼ pizza	15.0	406	33%
veggie	¼ pizza	10.5	360	26%

■ 12" THIN-CRUST PIZZA

cheese	⅓ pizza	15.5	365	38%
extra cheese & pepperoni	⅓ pizza	28.0	512	49%
ham	⅓ pizza	16.5	390	38%
Italian sausage & mushroom	⅓ pizza	21.5	445	43%
pepperoni	⅓ pizza	23.0	447	46%
veggie	⅓ pizza	17.0	385	40%

DRUTHER'S
■ BREAKFAST

bacon & egg plate				
fried	1 serving	41.9	721	52%
scrambled	1 serving	43.0	742	52%
bacon & egg w/biscuit	1 serving	16.3	258	57%
biscuits & gravy	1 serving	14.7	331	40%
ham & egg plate				
fried	1 serving	35.3	681	47%
scrambled	1 serving	44.6	762	53%
ham & egg w/biscuit	1 serving	11.2	217	46%
sausage & egg plate				
fried	1 serving	43.4	741	53%
scrambled	1 serving	44.6	762	53%
sausage & egg w/biscuit	1 serving	15.0	246	55%
sausage & biscuit	1 of each	11.1	179	56%
	2 of each	22.3	358	56%

■ BURGERS

cheeseburger				
deluxe quarter	1 burger	37.6	660	51%

Food and Description	Amount	Fat Grams	Total Calories	% Fat Calories
double	1 burger	26.1	500	47%
regular	1 burger	17.8	380	42%
hamburger	1 burger	13.4	327	37%
■ CHICKEN & FISH				
chicken				
2 pieces				
breast & wing	1 serving	30.7	595	46%
w/potatoes & cole slaw	1 serving	49.9	970	46%
leg & thigh	1 serving	29.8	549	49%
w/potatoes & cole slaw	1 serving	49.0	925	48%
3 pieces				
breast, thigh, & leg	1 serving	66.9	1281	47%
breast, thigh, & wing	1 serving	70.3	1309	48%
8 pieces	1 serving	114.0	3664	28%
12 pieces	1 serving	171.0	5496	28%
fish & chips	1 serving	29.8	729	37%
fish dinner	1 serving	31.3	770	37%
fish sandwich	1 sandwich	14.4	349	37%

DUNKIN' DONUTS (See also COOKIE; CROISSANT; DONUT; MUFFIN; PASTRY)

	Amount	Fat Grams	Total Calories	% Fat Calories
■ BAGELS				
cinnamon raisin	1 bagel	1.0	340	3%
egg	1 bagel	2.0	340	5%
everything	1 bagel	2.0	340	5%
garlic	1 bagel	1.0	330	3%
onion	1 bagel	1.0	320	3%
plain	1 bagel	1.0	330	3%
poppy	1 bagel	2.5	340	7%
pumpernickel	1 bagel	1.5	340	4%
salt	1 bagel	1.0	320	3%
sesame	1 bagel	4.0	350	10%
whole wheat	1 bagel	1.5	320	4%
■ CROISSANT SANDWICHES				
broccoli & cheese	1 sandwich	21.0	370	51%
chicken salad	1 sandwich	31.0	540	52%
ham & cheese	1 sandwich	32.0	710	41%
roast beef & cheese	1 sandwich	27.0	490	49%
seafood salad	1 sandwich	26.0	480	49%
tuna salad	1 sandwich	30.0	540	50%
■ SOUP				
beef barley	1 serving	0.5	90	5%
beef noodle	1 serving	1.0	90	10%
chicken noodle	1 serving	1.5	80	17%
chili	1 serving	6.0	170	32%
chili con carne w/beans	1 serving	15.0	300	45%
cream of broccoli	1 serving	11.0	200	50%
cream of potato	1 serving	10.0	190	47%
harvest vegetable	1 serving	2.0	80	23%

Food and Description	Amount	Fat Grams	Total Calories	% Fat Calories
Manhattan clam chowder	1 serving	0.5	70	6%
minestrone	1 serving	1.0	100	9%
New England clam chowder	1 serving	10.0	200	45%
split pea w/ham	1 serving	9.0	190	43%
EL POLLO LOCO				
■ **BURRITOS**				
bean, rice, & cheese	1 burrito	13.0	530	22%
chicken				
classic	1 burrito	20.0	560	32%
loco grande	1 burrito	30.0	680	40%
regular	1 burrito	11.0	310	32%
spicy hot	1 burrito	20.0	570	32%
whole wheat	1 burrito	16.0	510	28%
steak				
grilled	1 burrito	29.0	740	35%
regular	1 burrito	22.0	450	44%
vegetarian	1 burrito	7.0	340	19%
■ **CHICKEN**				
breast	1 piece	6.0	160	34%
leg	1 piece	5.0	90	50%
thigh	1 piece	12.0	180	60%
wing	1 piece	6.0	110	49%
■ **CONDIMENTS** (*See also* Salads & Dressing in this section)				
cheddar cheese	1 oz	5.0	90	50%
guacamole	1 oz	6.0	60	90%
honey Dijon mustard	1 oz	0.5	50	9%
salsa	2 oz	–	10	–
sour cream	1 oz	6.0	60	90%
■ **DESSERT**				
cheesecake	1 slice	18.0	310	52%
churro	1 piece	8.0	130	55%
■ **FAJITAS**				
chicken fajita meal	1 meal	18.0	780	21%
steak fajita meal	1 meal	38.0	1040	33%
■ **SALADS & DRESSING**				
chicken salad	1 serving	4.0	160	23%
salad dressing				
blue cheese	2 oz	6.0	80	68%
French/deluxe	2 Tbs	4.0	60	60%
Italian/reduced calorie	2 Tbs	2.0	25	72%
ranch	2 Tbs	6.0	75	72%
Thousand Island	2 Tbs	10.0	110	82%
side salad	1 serving	1.0	50	18%
■ **SIDE ORDERS** (*See also* Salads & Dressing in this section)				
beans	1 serving	2.5	100	23%
coleslaw	1 serving	8.0	100	72%
corn	1 serving	2.0	110	16%

Food and Description	Amount	Fat Grams	Total Calories	% Fat Calories
potato salad	1 serving	10.0	180	50%
rice	1 serving	1.5	110	12%
■ TACOS				
chicken	1 taco	7.0	180	35%
steak	1 taco	12.0	250	43%
■ TORTILLAS				
corn	1 tortilla	0.5	60	8%
flour	1 tortilla	2.5	90	25%

FAZOLI'S
■ DESSERT

Food and Description	Amount	Fat Grams	Total Calories	% Fat Calories
cheesecake				
plain	1 serving	20.8	270	69%
w/strawberry topping	1 serving	20.8	310	60%
chocolate chocolate chip cheesecake	1 serving	21.8	298	66%
lemon ice	12 oz	–	142	–
■ ENTRÉES				
baked ziti	1 serving	12.7	331	35%
broccoli fettucine				
large	1 serving	19.8	619	29%
regular	1 serving	13.4	424	28%
chicken Parmesan	1 serving	13.7	481	26%
fettucine Alfredo				
large	1 serving	19.7	596	30%
regular	1 serving	13.3	400	30%
lasagna				
broccoli	1 serving	27.1	571	43%
regular	1 serving	24.3	533	41%
meatball sub	1 serving	30.2	650	42%
ravioli				
w/meat sauce	1 serving	16.4	361	41%
w/tomato sauce	1 serving	15.2	332	41%
sampler platter	1 serving	19.8	607	29%
shrimp pasta	1 serving	19.0	552	31%
spaghetti				
w/meat sauce				
large	1 serving	11.7	553	19%
regular	1 serving	8.0	372	19%
w/meatballs				
large	1 serving	33.8	829	37%
regular	1 serving	24.7	582	38%
w/tomato sauce				
large	1 serving	9.9	509	18%
regular	1 serving	6.8	343	18%
■ PIZZA				
cheese	double slice	10.7	360	27%
combination	double slice	20.8	484	39%
pepperoni	double slice	17.0	430	36%

Food and Description	Amount	Fat Grams	Total Calories	% Fat Calories
■ **SALADS & RELATED ITEMS**				
breadstick				
regular	1 breadstick	4.3	131	30%
dry	1 breadstick	0.8	99	7%
garden salad	1 serving	0.3	28	10%
Italian chef salad	1 serving	7.2	174	37%
pasta salad	1 serving	19.7	397	45%
salad dressing				
honey French	1 oz	14.0	160	79%
house Italian				
reduced calorie	1 oz	3.5	69	46%
regular	1 oz	15.0	138	98%
ranch	1 oz	20.0	180	100%
Thousand Island	1 oz	14.0	140	90%
■ **SOUP**				
bean & pasta	1 serving	7.2	174	37%
minestrone	1 serving	1.3	90	13%
GODFATHER'S PIZZA				
■ **GOLDEN CRUST PIZZA**				
cheese				
small	⅙ pizza	8.0	213	34%
medium	⅛ pizza	9.0	229	35%
large	1/10 pizza	11.0	261	38%
combo				
small	⅙ pizza	12.0	273	40%
medium	⅛ pizza	13.0	283	41%
large	1/10 pizza	15.0	322	42%
■ **ORIGINAL PIZZA**				
cheese				
mini	¼ pizza	4.0	138	26%
small	⅙ pizza	7.0	239	26%
medium	⅛ pizza	8.0	242	30%
large	1/10 pizza	8.0	271	27%
combo				
mini	¼ pizza	5.0	164	27%
small	⅙ pizza	11.0	299	33%
medium	⅛ pizza	12.0	318	34%
large	1/10 pizza	12.0	332	33%
STUFFED PIZZA				
cheese				
small	⅙ pizza	11.0	310	32%
medium	⅛ pizza	13.0	350	33%
large	1/10 pizza	16.0	380	38%
combo				
small	⅙ pizza	20.0	430	42%
medium	⅛ pizza	23.0	480	43%
large	1/10 pizza	26.0	520	45%

Food and Description	Amount	Fat Grams	Total Calories	% Fat Calories
HARDEE'S				
■ **BEVERAGES**				
chocolate shake	1 shake	5.0	370	12%
peach shake	1 shake	4.0	390	9%
strawberry shake	1 shake	4.0	420	9%
vanilla shake	1 shake	5.0	350	13%
■ **BREAKFAST**				
Big Country Breakfast				
w/bacon	1 serving	43.0	740	52%
w/sausage	1 serving	61.0	930	59%
biscuits				
apple cinnamon 'n' raisin	1 serving	8.0	200	36%
bacon, egg, & cheese	1 serving	31.0	530	53%
bacon & egg	1 serving	27.0	490	50%
biscuit 'n' gravy	1 serving	28.0	510	49%
country ham	1 serving	22.0	430	46%
ham	1 serving	20.0	400	45%
ham, egg, & cheese	1 serving	27.0	500	49%
rise 'n' shine	1 serving	21.0	390	48%
sausage	1 serving	31.0	510	55%
sausage & egg	1 serving	35.0	560	56%
ultimate omelet	1 serving	30.0	530	51%
Frisco breakfast sandwich/ham	1 serving	22.0	480	41%
hash rounds	1 serving	14.0	230	55%
margarine/butter blend	1 serving	4.0	35	100%
orange juice	11 fl oz	–	140	–
pancakes	3 pancakes	2.0	280	6%
w/1 sausage patty	1 serving	16.0	430	34%
w/2 bacon strips	1 serving	9.0	350	23%
syrup	1 serving	–	120	–
■ **BURGERS & BEEF**				
cheeseburger				
bacon cheeseburger	1 burger	36.0	600	54%
quarter pound	1 burger	25.0	490	46%
regular	1 burger	13.0	300	39%
hamburger				
big deluxe	1 burger	30.0	530	51%
big Hardee burger w/cheese	1 burger	43.0	680	57%
Frisco	1 burger	50.0	760	59%
mushroom 'n' Swiss	1 burger	27.0	520	47%
regular	1 burger	9.0	250	32%
roast beef sandwich/regular	1 sandwich	11.0	270	37%
■ **CHICKEN, FISH, & HAM**				
chicken fillet sandwich	1 sandwich	15.0	420	32%
fisherman's fillet sandwich	1 sandwich	22.0	500	40%
fried chicken				
breast	1 serving	15.0	370	36%
leg	1 serving	7.0	170	37%

Food and Description	Amount	Fat Grams	Total Calories	% Fat Calories
thigh	1 serving	15.0	330	41%
wing	1 serving	8.0	200	36%
grilled marinated chicken breast sandwich	1 sandwich	9.0	290	28%
hot ham 'n' cheese sandwich	1 sandwich	13.0	350	33%
■ CONDIMENTS (*See also* Salads & Dressing in this section)				
gravy	1.5 oz	–	20	–
■ DESSERT				
big cookie	1 cookie	12.0	280	39%
cool twist cone				
chocolate	1 cone	2.0	180	10%
vanilla	1 cone	2.0	170	11%
vanilla/chocolate	1 cone	2.0	180	10%
cool twist sundae				
hot fudge	1 sundae	6.0	290	19%
strawberry	1 sundae	2.0	210	9%
■ SALADS & DRESSING				
salad dressing				
French	1 pkt	–	70	–
ranch	1 pkt	29.0	290	90%
Thousand Island	1 pkt	23.0	250	83%
garden salad	1 serving	13.0	210	56%
grilled chicken salad	1 serving	3.0	150	18%
side salad	1 serving	–	25	–
■ SIDE ORDERS (*See also* Salads & Dressing in this section)				
coleslaw	4 oz	20.0	240	75%
French fries	small	10.0	240	38%
	medium	15.0	350	39%
	large	18.0	430	38%
mashed potatoes	4 oz	–	70	–
JACK-IN-THE-BOX				
■ BEVERAGES				
chocolate milk shake	1 small	6.0	390	14%
Coca-Cola				
classic	1 small	–	190	–
Diet Coke	1 small	–	1	–
coffee	1 small	–	5	–
Dr. Pepper	1 small	–	190	–
iced tea	1 small	–	–	–
milk/2% reduced fat	8.5 fl oz	5.0	120	38%
orange juice	6.5 fl oz	–	80	–
Ramblin' Root Beer	1 small	–	240	–
Sprite	1 small	–	190	–
strawberry milk shake	1 small	7.0	330	19%
vanilla milk shake	1 small	7.0	350	18%
■ BREAKFAST				
Breakfast Jack	1 serving	12.0	300	36%
Country Crock spread	1 serving	3.0	25	100%

Food and Description	Amount	Fat Grams	Total Calories	% Fat Calories
grape jelly	1 pkt	–	40	–
hash browns	1 serving	11.0	160	62%
pancake platter	1 serving	12.0	400	27%
syrup	1 pkt	–	120	–
sausage croissant	1 croissant	48.0	670	64%
scrambled egg pocket	1 pocket	21.0	430	44%
sourdough breakfast sandwich	1 sandwich	20.0	380	47%
supreme croissant	1 croissant	36.0	570	57%
■ BURGERS & BEEF				
cheeseburger				
bacon bacon	1 burger	45.0	710	57%
regular	1 burger	15.0	320	42%
double	1 burger	24.0	450	48%
ultimate	1 burger	79.0	1030	69%
hamburger				
Colossus	1 burger	84.0	1100	69%
grilled sourdough	1 burger	43.0	670	58%
Outlaw	1 burger	40.0	720	50%
quarter pound	1 burger	27.0	510	48%
regular	1 burger	11.0	280	35%
Jumbo Jack				
plain	1 burger	32.0	560	51%
w/cheese	1 burger	40.0	650	55%
Monterey roast beef sandwich	1 sandwich	30.0	540	50%
■ CHICKEN & FISH				
chicken sandwich				
Caesar	1 sandwich	26.0	520	45%
chicken fajita pita	1 sandwich	8.0	290	25%
grilled fillet	1 sandwich	19.0	430	40%
regular	1 sandwich	18.0	400	41%
spicy crispy	1 sandwich	27.0	560	43%
supreme	1 sandwich	36.0	620	52%
The Really Big Chicken Sandwich	1 sandwich	56.0	900	56%
chicken strips/breaded	4 pieces	13.0	290	40%
	6 pieces	20.0	450	40%
chicken teriyaki bowl	1 bowl	1.5	580	2%
fish supreme sandwich	1 sandwich	34.0	590	52%
■ CONDIMENTS (See also Salads & Related Items in this section)				
catsup	1 pkt	–	10	–
cheese				
American	1 slice	3.5	45	70%
Swiss-style	1 slice	3.0	40	68%
dipping sauce				
BBQ	1 pkt	–	45	–
buttermilk house	1 pkt	13.0	130	90%
sweet & sour	1 pkt	–	40	–
tartar	1 pkt	15.0	150	90%
guacamole	1 pkt	4.0	50	55%

Food and Description	Amount	Fat Grams	Total Calories	% Fat Calories
hot sauce	1 pkt	–	5	–
mayonnaise	1 pkt	17.0	155	99%
mustard				
Chinese hot	1 pkt	–	5	–
regular	1 pkt	–	5	–
salsa	1 pkt	–	10	–
sour cream	1 pkt	6.0	60	90%
soy sauce	1 pkt	–	5	–
■ DESSERT				
cheesecake				
chocolate chip cookie dough	1 slice	18.0	360	45%
plain	1 slice	18.0	310	52%
hot apple turnover	1 turnover	19.0	350	40%
■ SALADS & RELATED ITEMS				
croutons	1 serving	2.0	50	36%
garden chicken salad	1 serving	9.0	200	41%
salad dressing				
blue cheese	1 pkt	18.0	210	77%
buttermilk house	1 pkt	30.0	290	93%
Italian/low-calorie	1 pkt	1.5	25	54%
Thousand Island	1 pkt	24.0	250	86%
side salad	1 serving	4.0	70	51%
■ SIDE ORDERS (*See also* Salads & Related Items in this section)				
bacon & cheddar potato wedges	1 serving	58.0	800	65%
egg roll	3 pieces	24.0	440	49%
	5 pieces	41.0	750	65%
French fries	small	11.0	220	45%
	regular	17.0	350	44%
	jumbo	19.0	400	43%
	super scoop	29.0	590	44%
jalapeños/stuffed	7 pieces	27.0	420	58%
	10 pieces	39.0	600	59%
onion rings	1 serving	23.0	380	54%
seasoned curly fries	1 serving	20.0	360	50%
■ TACOS				
super	1 taco	17.0	281	54%
regular	1 taco	11.0	187	53%
KENNY ROGERS ROASTERS				
■ CHICKEN & TURKEY				
chicken pot pie	1 pot pie	33.0	708	42%
¼ chicken				
dark meat				
w/skin	4.35 oz	16.7	271	55%
skinless	3.29 oz	7.3	169	39%
white meat				
w/skin	4.7 oz	10.7	244	40%
skinless	3.74 oz	2.3	144	14%

Food and Description	Amount	Fat Grams	Total Calories	% Fat Calories
½ chicken				
w/skin	9.06 oz	27.5	515	48%
skinless	7.03 oz	9.5	313	27%
sliced turkey breast	4.5 oz	2.2	158	13%
■ SALADS & DRESSING				
chicken Caesar salad	1 serving	8.7	285	27%
roasted chicken salad	1 serving	10.3	292	32%
salad dressing				
blue cheese	2.5 oz	39.0	370	95%
buttermilk ranch	2.5 oz	48.0	430	100%
Caesar	2.5 oz	36.0	340	95%
honey French	2.5 oz	29.0	350	75%
honey mustard	2.5 oz	28.0	320	79%
Italian/fat-free	2.5 oz	–	35	–
Thousand Island	2.5 oz	33.0	330	90%
■ SANDWICHES				
BBQ chicken pita	1 sandwich	7.2	400	16%
chicken Caesar pita	1 sandwich	34.8	606	52%
roasted chicken pita	1 sandwich	35.3	685	46%
turkey sandwich	1 sandwich	12.0	385	28%
■ SIDE ORDERS (*See also* Salads & Dressing in this section)				
baked sweet potato	1 serving	0.3	263	1%
cinnamon apples	1 serving	5.0	200	23%
coleslaw	1 serving	15.5	225	62%
corn muffin	1 muffin	8.0	175	41%
corn niblets	1 serving	0.7	112	6%
corn on the cob	1 piece	0.8	68	11%
cornbread stuffing	1 serving	18.6	326	51%
creamy Parmesan spinach	1 serving	5.5	119	42%
honey baked beans	1 serving	1.0	150	6%
Italian green beans	1 serving	8.2	116	64%
macaroni & cheese	1 serving	5.8	197	26%
pasta salad				
regular	1 serving	11.6	236	44%
sour cream & dill	1 serving	16.3	233	63%
potato salad	1 serving	27.3	390	63%
potatoes				
garlic parsley	1 serving	12.0	259	42%
real mashed	1 serving	14.4	295	44%
rice pilaf	1 serving	4.7	173	24%
side salad	1 serving	0.3	23	12%
steamed vegetables	1 serving	0.3	48	6%
tomato-cucumber salad	1 serving	2.2	123	16%
zucchini & squash Santa Fe	1 serving	4.5	70	58%
■ SOUP				
chicken noodle	1 cup	1.1	55	18%
	1 bowl	1.8	91	18%

Food and Description	Amount	Fat Grams	Total Calories	% Fat Calories
KENTUCKY FRIED CHICKEN				
extra tasty crispy				
breast	1 piece	28.0	470	54%
drumstick	1 piece	11.0	190	52%
thigh	1 piece	25.0	370	61%
wing	1 piece	13.0	200	59%
hot & spicy				
breast	1 piece	35.0	530	59%
drumstick	1 piece	11.0	190	52%
thigh	1 piece	27.0	370	66%
wing	1 piece	15.0	210	64%
nuggets & sauce				
nuggets only	3.4 oz	18.0	284	57%
sauce				
barbeque	1 oz	<1.0	35	13%
honey	1 oz	–	49	–
mustard	1 oz	<1.0	36	23%
sweet & sour	1 oz	<1.0	58	9%
original recipe				
breast	1 piece	24.0	400	54%
drumstick	1 piece	9.0	140	58%
thigh	1 piece	18.0	250	65%
wing	1 piece	10.0	140	64%
tender roast				
breast				
w/skin	1 piece	10.8	251	39%
skinless	1 piece	4.3	169	23%
drumstick				
w/skin	1 piece	4.3	97	40%
skinless	1 piece	2.4	67	32%
thigh				
w/skin	1 piece	12.0	207	52%
skinless	1 piece	5.5	105	47%
wing w/skin	1 piece	7.7	121	57%
other				
chicken pot pie	1 pot pie	42.0	770	49%
crispy strips	3 pieces	15.8	261	54%
hot wings	6 pieces	33.0	471	63%
■ SANDWICHES				
Colonel's chicken sandwich	1 sandwich	22.0	497	40%
BBQ flavored chicken sandwich	1 sandwich	8.0	256	28%
■ SIDE ORDERS				
BBQ baked beans	1 serving	3.0	190	14%
buttermilk biscuit	1 biscuit	10.0	180	50%
coleslaw	1 serving	9.0	180	45%
corn on the cob	1 piece	3.0	180	15%
garden rice	1 serving	1.5	120	11%
green beans	1 serving	1.5	45	30%

Food and Description	Amount	Fat Grams	Total Calories	% Fat Calories
macaroni & cheese	1 serving	8.0	180	40%
mashed potatoes & gravy	1 serving	6.0	120	45%
mean greens	1 serving	3.0	70	39%
potato salad	1 serving	14.0	230	55%
potato wedges	1 serving	13.0	280	42%
red beans & rice	1 serving	3.0	130	21%

KRYSTAL

■ BEVERAGE

chocolate shake	16 fl oz	10.0	275	33%

■ BREAKFAST

biscuits				
bacon	1 biscuit	17.0	306	50%
bacon, egg, & cheese	1 biscuit	26.0	423	55%
country ham	1 biscuit	17.0	334	46%
egg	1 biscuit	19.0	327	52%
gravy	1 biscuit	26.0	419	56%
plain	1 biscuit	12.0	244	44%
sausage	1 biscuit	30.0	437	62%
donuts				
iced				
chocolate	1 donut	11.0	212	47%
vanilla	1 donut	9.0	196	41%
plain	1 donut	9.0	150	54%
pancakes	3 pancakes	12.0	212	51%
Sunriser	1 serving	17.0	259	59%

■ BURGERS & HOT DOGS

Burger Plus				
plain	1 burger	26.0	415	56%
w/cheese	1 burger	31.0	473	59%
cheeseburger				
bacon	1 burger	34.0	521	59%
cheese Krystal	1 burger	10.0	167	54%
double cheese Krystal	1 burger	18.0	337	48%
hamburger				
Big K	1 burger	35.0	540	58%
double Krystal	1 burger	14.0	277	45%
Krystal	1 burger	7.0	158	40%
Pups				
chili	1 hot dog	10.0	162	55%
chili cheese	1 hot dog	13.0	211	55%
corn	1 hot dog	14.0	214	59%
plain	1 hot dog	9.0	160	51%

■ DESSERT

apple pie	1 slice	10.0	300	30%
lemon meringue pie	1 slice	9.0	340	24%
pecan pie	1 slice	23.0	450	46%

Food and Description	Amount	Fat Grams	Total Calories	% Fat Calories
■ **SANDWICH**				
crispy crunchy chicken	1 sandwich	24.0	467	46%
■ **SIDE ORDERS**				
chili	8 oz	8.0	218	33%
	12 oz	12.0	327	33%
fries				
Krys Kross				
plain	1 serving	29.0	486	54%
chili cheese	1 serving	39.0	625	56%
w/cheese	1 serving	31.0	516	54%
regular	small	13.0	262	45%
	regular	18.0	353	46%
	large	23.0	463	45%
LION'S CHOICE				
■ **DESSERT**				
vanilla yogurt	4 oz	–	80	–
■ **SANDWICHES**				
roast beef	5 oz	12.0	332	33%
turkey	5 oz	9.0	276	29%
■ **SIDE ORDER**				
French fries	3.5 oz	5.8	163	32%
LITTLE CAESAR'S PIZZA				
■ **PIZZA**				
Pan!Pan!				
baby	1 pizza	24.0	615	35%
medium				
cheese	1 slice	6.0	180	30%
pepperoni	1 slice	7.7	200	35%
Pizza!Pizza!/round				
cheese	1 slice	7.0	201	31%
pepperoni	1 slice	8.7	220	36%
■ **SALADS & DRESSING**				
antipasto salad	1 serving	11.8	176	60%
Caesar salad	1 serving	5.4	140	35%
Greek salad	1 serving	9.6	168	51%
salad dressing				
blue cheese	1.5 oz	14.0	160	79%
Caesar	1.5 oz	17.0	183	84%
French	1.5 oz	15.7	166	85%
Greek	1.5 oz	30.0	270	100%
Italian				
fat-free	1.5 oz	–	15	–
regular	1.5 oz	21.0	200	95%
ranch	1.5 oz	22.0	221	90%
Thousand Island	1.5 oz	17.0	183	84%
tossed salad	1 serving	3.0	116	23%

Food and Description	Amount	Fat Grams	Total Calories	% Fat Calories
■ SANDWICHES				
cold/deli-style				
ham & cheese	1 sandwich	35.0	735	43%
Italian	1 sandwich	37.0	740	45%
veggie	1 sandwich	29.0	647	40%
hot/oven-baked				
Cheeser	1 sandwich	39.5	825	43%
Meatsa	1 sandwich	55.5	1036	48%
pepperoni	1 sandwich	47.0	900	47%
supreme	1 sandwich	46.0	895	46%
veggie	1 sandwich	24.0	670	32%
■ SIDE DISHES (*See also* Salads & Dressing in this section)				
crazy bread	1 piece	3.4	106	29%
crazy sauce	1 serving	0.4	74	5%
LONG JOHN SILVER'S				
■ BEVERAGE				
Diet Coke	8 fl oz	–	1	–
■ CONDIMENTS				
honey mustard sauce	0.42 oz	–	20	–
catsup	0.32 oz	–	10	–
lettuce	1 serving	–	8	–
malt vinegar	0.18 oz	–	–	–
margarine	1 tsp	4.0	35	100%
salad dressing				
French/fat-free	1.5 oz	–	50	–
Italian	1 oz	14.0	130	97%
ranch				
fat-free	1.5 oz	–	50	–
regular	1 oz	18.0	170	95%
Thousand Island	1 oz	10.0	110	82%
shrimp sauce	0.42 oz	–	15	–
sour cream	1 serving	6.0	60	90%
sweet & sour sauce	0.42 oz	–	20	–
tartar sauce	0.42 oz	1.5	35	39%
■ ENTRÉES				
chicken				
batter-dipped	1 piece	6.0	120	45%
flavorbaked				
à la carte	1 piece	3.0	110	25%
over rice w/baked potato & green beans	1 meal	7.5	448	15%
over rice w/side salad	1 meal	7.0	275	23%
popcorn	1 serving	14.0	250	50%
clams/batter-dipped	3 oz	17.0	300	51%
fish				
batter-dipped	1 piece	11.0	170	58%

Food and Description	Amount	Fat Grams	Total Calories	% Fat Calories
flavorbaked				
à la carte	1 piece	2.5	90	25%
over rice w/baked potato & green beans	1 meal	9.5	518	17%
over rice w/side salad	1 meal	9.0	345	23%
popcorn	1 serving	14.0	290	43%
fish & chicken combo/flavorbaked/over rice w/baked potato & green beans	1 meal	10.0	538	17%
shrimp				
batter-dipped	1 piece	2.5	35	64%
popcorn	1 serving	15.0	280	48%
■ SANDWICHES				
chicken/flavorbaked	1 sandwich	10.0	290	31%
fish				
batter-dipped/w/o sauce	1 sandwich	13.0	320	37%
flavorbaked	1 sandwich	14.0	320	39%
ultimate	1 sandwich	21.0	430	44%
■ SIDE ORDERS				
baked potato	1 potato	–	210	–
cheese sticks	1 serving	9.0	160	51%
coleslaw	1 serving	6.0	140	39%
corn cobbette				
w/butter	1 piece	8.0	140	51%
w/o butter	1 piece	0.5	80	6%
fries	1 serving	15.0	250	54%
green beans	1 serving	0.5	30	13%
hushpuppy	1 piece	2.5	60	38%
rice pilaf	1 serving	3.0	140	19%
side salad	1 serving	–	25	–

MACHEEZMO MOUSE
■ BURRITOS

Food and Description	Amount	Fat Grams	Total Calories	% Fat Calories
chicken	1 burrito	11.0	580	17%
chili	1 burrito	11.0	605	16%
combo	1 burrito	12.0	630	17%
veggie	1 burrito	8.0	655	11%
■ CONDIMENTS & ACCOMPANIMENTS				
beans	1 oz	–	35	–
Boss Sauce	1 oz	–	30	–
broccoli	1 oz	–	4	–
cheese	1 oz	5.0	81	56%
chicken	1 oz	1.0	35	26%
chili	1 oz	1.0	43	21%
chips	1 serving	6.0	140	39%
cilantro	1 oz	–	8	–
el bento	1 serving	1.0	77	12%
enchilada sauce	1 oz	–	6	–
Famouse #5	1 serving	5.0	585	8%

Food and Description	Amount	Fat Grams	Total Calories	% Fat Calories
fresh greens	1 oz	–	2	–
guacamole	1 oz	3.0	100	27%
marinated veggies	1 oz	<1.0	10	45%
Mexican cheese	1 oz	8.0	100	72%
mustard dressing	1 oz	<1.0	25	18%
nacho grande	1 serving	44.0	855	46%
rice	1 oz	<1.0	45	10%
salsa	1 oz	–	4	–
sour cream	1 oz	3.0	35	77%
tortilla				
corn	2 pieces	–	90	–
flour	2.5 oz	3.0	200	14%
wheat	2.5 oz	3.0	200	14%
■ DESSERT				
nonfat yogurt	1 oz	<1.0	20	23%
■ EL BENTO				
deluxe	1 serving	7.0	740	9%
Kid	1 serving	1.0	235	4%
■ ENCHILADAS				
chicken	1 enchilada	16.0	545	26%
chili	1 enchilada	16.0	560	26%
veggie	1 enchilada	14.0	635	20%
■ QUESADILLAS				
Kid				
cheese	1 serving	13.0	360	33%
chicken	1 serving	15.0	430	31%
snack				
cheese	1 serving	13.0	377	31%
chicken	1 serving	15.0	450	30%
■ RICE & BEANS				
rice, beans, salad	1 meal	<1.0	344	1%
rice, beans, broccoli	1 meal	<1.0	328	1%
■ SALADS				
chicken	1 serving	11.0	445	22%
chicken power	1 serving	1.0	275	3%
veggie power	1 serving	<1.0	200	2%
veggie taco	1 serving	14.0	655	19%
■ TACOS				
snack				
chicken	1 serving	8.0	290	25%
chili	1 serving	8.0	310	23%
veggie	1 serving	6.0	290	19%
Kid				
cheese	1 serving	5.0	285	16%
chicken	1 serving	7.0	355	18%
veggie deluxe	1 serving	6.0	665	8%

Food and Description	Amount	Fat Grams	Total Calories	% Fat Calories
MAZZIO'S PIZZA				
■ **APPETIZERS**				
garlic bread w/cheese	2 slices	35.0	700	45%
meat nachos	1 serving	21.0	500	38%
■ **PASTA**				
chicken Parmesan	1 serving	19.0	590	29%
fettuccine Alfredo	small	28.0	440	57%
meat lasagna	small	25.0	460	49%
spaghetti	small	10.0	290	31%
■ **PIZZA**				
deep pan/medium				
cheese	1 slice	13.0	350	33%
combo	1 slice	18.0	410	40%
pepperoni	1 slice	17.0	380	40%
Pan sausage	1 slice	22.0	430	46%
original crust/medium				
cheese	1 slice	8.0	260	28%
combo	1 slice	13.0	320	37%
pepperoni	1 slice	11.0	280	35%
sausage	1 slice	16.0	350	41%
thin crust/medium				
cheese	1 slice	9.0	220	37%
■ **SANDWICHES**				
BBQ beef & cheddar	1 sandwich	24.0	580	37%
chicken & cheddar	1 sandwich	24.0	570	38%
ham & cheese	1 sandwich	39.0	790	44%
submarine/deluxe	1 sandwich	43.0	810	48%
McDONALD'S				
■ **BEVERAGES**				
apple juice	6 fl oz	–	80	–
chocolate shake/low-fat	1 small	5.0	340	13%
Coca-Cola				
classic	12 fl oz	–	110	–
	16 fl oz	–	150	–
	21 fl oz	–	210	–
	32 fl oz	–	310	–
Diet Coke	12 fl oz	–	1	–
	16 fl oz	–	1	–
	21 fl oz	–	2	–
	32 fl oz	–	3	–
milk/1% low-fat	8 fl oz	2.5	110	23%
orange drink/Hi-C	12 fl oz	–	120	–
	16 fl oz	–	160	–
	21 fl oz	–	240	–
	32 fl oz	–	350	–
orange juice	6 fl oz	–	80	–

Food and Description	Amount	Fat Grams	Total Calories	% Fat Calories
Sprite	12 fl oz	–	110	–
	16 fl oz	–	150	–
	21 fl oz	–	210	–
	32 fl oz	–	310	–
strawberry shake/low-fat	1 small	5.0	340	13%
vanilla shake/low-fat	1 small	5.0	340	13%
■ BREAKFAST				
apple bran muffin/fat free	1 muffin	–	170	–
biscuit				
bacon, egg, & cheese	1 biscuit	26.0	440	53%
plain	1 biscuit	13.0	260	45%
sausage	1 biscuit	29.0	430	61%
sausage & egg	1 biscuit	35.0	520	61%
breakfast burrito	1 burrito	20.0	320	56%
Cheerios	1 pkg	1.0	70	13%
cinnamon roll	1 roll	20.0	400	45%
Danish				
apple	1 Danish	16.0	360	40%
cheese	1 Danish	22.0	410	48%
cinnamon raisin	1 Danish	22.0	430	46%
raspberry	1 Danish	16.0	400	36%
Egg McMuffin	1 McMuffin	13.0	290	40%
English muffin w/spread	1 muffin	2.0	140	13%
hash brown potatoes	1 serving	8.0	130	55%
hot cakes				
plain	1 serving	7.0	310	20%
w/margarine & syrup	1 serving	16.0	580	25%
pork sausage	1 serving	16.0	170	85%
Sausage McMuffin				
regular	1 McMuffin	23.0	360	58%
w/egg	1 McMuffin	29.0	440	59%
scrambled eggs	1 serving	12.0	170	64%
Wheaties	1 pkg	0.5	80	6%
■ BURGERS				
Arch Deluxe				
w/bacon	1 burger	34.0	610	50%
w/o bacon	1 burger	31.0	570	49%
Big Mac	1 burger	28.0	530	48%
cheeseburger	1 burger	14.0	320	39%
hamburger	1 burger	10.0	270	33%
Quarter Pounder				
regular	1 burger	21.0	510	53%
w/cheese	1 burger	30.0	530	51%
■ CHICKEN & FISH				
Chicken McNuggets & sauce				
McNuggets	4 pieces	11.0	190	52%
	6 pieces	17.0	290	53%
	9 pieces	26.0	430	54%

Food and Description	Amount	Fat Grams	Total Calories	% Fat Calories
sauce				
barbecue	1 pkt	–	45	–
honey	1 pkt	–	45	–
honey mustard	1 pkt	4.5	50	81%
hot mustard	1 pkt	3.5	60	46%
sweet & sour	1 pkt	–	50	–
Fillet-O-Fish sandwich	1 sandwich	16.0	350	40%
McChicken sandwich	1 sandwich	30.0	510	53%
McGrilled Chicken Classic sandwich	1 sandwich	4.0	260	14%
■ DESSERT				
apple pie	1 pie	13.0	260	45%
ice cream				
hot caramel sundae	1 serving	3.0	310	9%
hot fudge lowfat sundae	1 serving	5.0	290	15%
strawberry lowfat sundae	1 serving	1.0	240	4%
vanilla low-fat cone	1 cone	0.5	120	4%
McDonaldland cookies	1 pkg	9.0	260	31%
nuts for sundaes	1 serving	3.5	40	79%
■ SALADS & RELATED ITEMS				
bacon bits	1 pkg	1.0	15	60%
chef salad	1 serving	11.0	210	47%
croutons	1 pkg	1.5	50	27%
fajita chicken salad	1 serving	6.0	160	34%
garden salad	1 serving	4.0	80	45%
salad dressing				
blue cheese	1 pkg	17.0	190	80%
vinaigrette/lite	1 pkg	2.0	50	36%
ranch	1 pkg	21.0	230	82%
red French/low-calorie	1 pkg	8.0	160	45%
Thousand Island	1 pkg	13.0	190	67%
side salad	1 serving	2.0	45	40%
■ SIDE ORDERS (*See also* Salads & Related Items in this section)				
French fries	small	10.0	210	43%
	large	22.0	450	44%
	super size	26.0	540	43%
MRS. WINNER'S				
■ BREAKFAST				
biscuit	1 biscuit	12.6	243	47%
breakfast steak	1 serving	19.6	252	70%
chicken fillet/breaded	1 serving	6.2	154	36%
country ham	1 serving	3.6	61	53%
egg	1 serving	3.4	53	58%
orange juice/Minute Maid	6 fl oz	–	80	–
sausage patty	1 serving	16.0	172	84%
■ CHICKEN				
rotisserie/skinless				
dark meat quarter	4.3 oz	10.0	215	42%

Food and Description	Amount	Fat Grams	Total Calories	% Fat Calories
white meat quarter	5.2 oz	9.0	240	34%
■ SIDE ORDERS				
biscuit	1 biscuit	12.6	243	47%
broccoli pasta salad	3 oz	11.0	175	57%
coleslaw	3.5 oz	7.0	135	47%
green beans	3.5 oz	<1.0	30	15%
honey yeast roll	1 roll	3.5	200	16%

1 POTATO 2 POTATO
■ POTATOES

Cajun shrimp	1 potato	1.0	258	3%
chicken & creamy mushroom	1 potato	10.0	353	25%
chicken stir-fry	1 potato	3.0	328	8%
crab & broccoli	1 potato	6.0	335	16%
four cheeses & vegetables	1 potato	13.0	400	29%
Santa Fe black bean	1 potato	9.0	350	23%
Southwestern grilled chicken	1 potato	4.0	286	13%
spinach soufflé	1 potato	9.0	310	26%
veggie & herb	1 potato	2.0	243	7%

PERKINS
■ BREAKFAST

hash brown potatoes	3 oz serving	2.5	100	23%
muffins				
apple	1 muffin	24.0	543	40%
banana nut	1 muffin	29.0	586	45%
blueberry	1 muffin	23.0	506	41%
bran	1 muffin	17.0	478	32%
carrot	1 muffin	23.0	560	37%
chocolate chocolate chip	1 muffin	26.0	548	43%
corn	1 muffin	17.0	683	22%
cranberry nut	1 muffin	28.0	558	45%
98% fat-free	1 muffin	1.0	495	2%
oat bran	1 muffin	16.0	513	28%
plain	1 muffin	26.0	586	40%
omelettes				
country club				
omelette only	1 serving	79.0	935	76%
w/hash browns	1 serving	82.0	1033	71%
deli ham & cheese				
omelette only	1 serving	79.0	962	74%
w/hash browns	1 serving	82.0	1063	69%
Denver w/fruit cup	1 serving	6.5	235	25%
everything				
omelette only	1 serving	53.5	700	69%
w/hash browns	1 serving	56.0	800	63%
Granny's country				
omelette only	1 serving	81.5	940	78%

Food and Description	Amount	Fat Grams	Total Calories	% Fat Calories
w/hash browns	1 serving	89.0	1245	64%
ham & cheese				
omelette only	1 serving	51.5	745	62%
w/hash browns	1 serving	54.0	745	65%
mushroom & cheese				
omelette only	1 serving	60.0	690	78%
w/hash browns	1 serving	62.5	788	71%
seafood w/fruit cup	1 serving	5.7	270	19%
pancakes				
buttermilk	3 pancakes	12.0	445	24%
harvest grain w/low-calorie syrup	5 pancakes	3.5	475	7%
short stack	3 pancakes	2.0	270	7%
toast w/margarine & grape jelly	1 piece	12.0	220	49%
■ DESSERT				
apple pie				
regular	1 slice	26.0	520	45%
sweetened w/Equal	1 slice	24.0	420	51%
cherry pie				
regular	1 slice	26.0	570	41%
sweetened w/Equal	1 slice	24.0	425	51%
coconut cream pie	1 slice	33.0	435	68%
French silk pie	1 slice	37.0	550	61%
lemon meringue pie	1 slice	16.0	395	36%
peanut butter brownie pie	1 slice	35.0	455	69%
pecan pie	1 slice	26.0	669	35%
■ SALADS				
chef	1 mini	11.0	215	46%
dinner/lite	1 serving	2.0	105	17%
■ SANDWICH				
vegetable pita stir-fry				
sandwich only	1 serving	9.0	305	27%
w/coleslaw	1 serving	18.0	440	37%
w/coleslaw & pasta salad	1 serving	32.5	625	47%
w/pasta salad	1 serving	24.0	495	44%

PETER PIPER PIZZA
■ PIZZA

Food and Description	Amount	Fat Grams	Total Calories	% Fat Calories
bacon				
Express Lunch Pizza	⅛ pizza	6.5	182	32%
extra large pie	½₂ pizza	10.7	311	31%
large pie	⅛ pizza	11.4	331	31%
medium pie	⅛ pizza	8.6	249	31%
small pie	⅛ pizza	7.6	217	32%
beef				
Express Lunch Pizza	⅛ pizza	5.0	165	27%
extra large pie	½₂ pizza	7.8	280	25%
large pie	⅛ pizza	8.0	296	24%
medium pie	⅛ pizza	6.0	222	24%

Food and Description	Amount	Fat Grams	Total Calories	% Fat Calories
small pie	⅛ pizza	5.4	194	25%
black olive				
Express Lunch Pizza	⅛ pizza	4.4	157	25%
extra large pie	1⁄12 pizza	6.8	265	23%
large pie	⅛ pizza	7.0	279	23%
medium pie	⅛ pizza	5.0	209	22%
small pie	⅛ pizza	4.6	182	23%
cheese				
Express Lunch Pizza	⅛ pizza	4.0	152	24%
	1 pizza	15.7	608	23%
extra large pie	1⁄12 pizza	6.0	257	21%
	1 pizza	73.0	3078	21%
large pie	⅛ pizza	6.0	270	20%
	1 pizza	49.5	2160	21%
medium pie	⅛ pizza	4.6	203	20%
	1 pizza	37.0	1620	21%
small pie	⅛ pizza	4.0	177	20%
	1 pizza	24.5	1059	21%
extra cheddar				
Express Lunch Pizza	⅛ pizza	6	180	30%
extra large pie	1⁄12 pizza	9.0	290	28%
large pie	⅛ pizza	9	306	26%
medium pie	⅛ pizza	6.4	224	26%
small pie	⅛ pizza	5.7	196	26%
extra mozzarella				
Express Lunch Pizza	⅛ pizza	5.5	174	28%
extra large pie	1⁄12 pizza	9.0	300	27%
large pie	⅛ pizza	10.0	320	28%
medium pie	⅛ pizza	7.0	236	27%
small pie	⅛ pizza	5.7	198	26%
green pepper				
Express Lunch Pizza	⅛ pizza	4.0	153	24%
extra large pie	1⁄12 pizza	6.0	259	21%
large pie	⅛ pizza	6.0	272	20%
medium pie	⅛ pizza	4.6	204	20%
small pie	⅛ pizza	4.0	178	20%
ham				
Express Lunch Pizza	⅛ pizza	4.0	156	23%
extra large pie	1⁄12 pizza	6.0	261	21%
large pie	⅛ pizza	6.4	276	21%
medium pie	⅛ pizza	4.8	207	21%
small pie	⅛ pizza	4.0	180	20%
jalapeño				
Express Lunch Pizza	⅛ pizza	4.0	153	24%
extra large pie	1⁄12 pizza	6.0	259	21%
large pie	⅛ pizza	6.0	266	20%
medium pie	⅛ pizza	4.6	205	20%
small pie	⅛ pizza	4.0	178	20%

Food and Description	Amount	Fat Grams	Total Calories	% Fat Calories
mushroom				
Express Lunch Pizza	⅛ pizza	4.0	153	24%
extra large pie	½2 pizza	6.0	259	21%
large pie	⅛ pizza	4.0	181	20%
medium pie	⅛ pizza	4.7	204	21%
small pie	⅛ pizza	4.0	178	20%
onion				
Express Lunch Pizza	⅛ pizza	4.0	153	23%
extra large pie	½2 pizza	6.0	258	21%
large pie	⅛ pizza	6.0	271	20%
medium pie	⅛ pizza	4.6	204	20%
small pie	⅛ pizza	4.0	177	20%
pepperoni				
Express Lunch Pizza	⅛ pizza	5.5	168	29%
extra large pie	½2 pizza	8.8	284	28%
large pie	⅛ pizza	9.0	308	26%
medium pie	⅛ pizza	7.0	229	28%
small pie	⅛ pizza	6.0	198	27%
pineapple				
Express Lunch Pizza	⅛ pizza	4.0	154	23%
extra large pie	½2 pizza	6.0	260	21%
large pie	⅛ pizza	6.0	274	20%
medium pie	⅛ pizza	4.7	206	21%
small pie	⅛ pizza	4.0	179	20%
salami				
Express Lunch Pizza	⅛ pizza	5.0	164	27%
extra large pie	½2 pizza	7.5	273	25%
large pie	⅛ pizza	7.8	288	24%
medium pie	⅛ pizza	6.0	216	25%
small pie	⅛ pizza	5.0	189	24%
sausage				
Express Lunch Pizza	⅛ pizza	5.8	178	29%
extra large pie	½2 pizza	8.0	284	25%
large pie	⅛ pizza	8.4	300	25%
medium pie	⅛ pizza	6.0	224	24%
small pie	⅛ pizza	5.6	197	26%
tomato				
Express Lunch Pizza	⅛ pizza	4.0	153	24%
extra large pie	½2 pizza	6.0	257	21%
large pie	⅛ pizza	6.0	275	20%
medium pie	⅛ pizza	4.7	204	21%
small pie	⅛ pizza	4.0	177	20%
PIZZA HUT				
■ PIZZA				
Big Foot				
cheese	1 slice	6.0	186	29%
pepperoni	1 slice	7.0	205	31%

Food and Description	Amount	Fat Grams	Total Calories	% Fat Calories
pepperoni, mushroom, & Italian sausage	1 slice	8.0	214	34%
hand-tossed/medium				
beef	1 slice	9.0	260	31%
cheese	1 slice	7.0	235	27%
ham	1 slice	5.0	213	21%
Italian sausage	1 slice	11.0	267	37%
meat lover's	1 slice	11.0	314	32%
pepperoni	1 slice	8.0	238	30%
pepperoni lover's	1 slice	14.0	306	41%
pork topping	1 slice	10.0	268	34%
supreme	1 slice	12.0	284	38%
super supreme	1 slice	13.0	296	40%
veggie lover's	1 slice	6.0	216	25%
pan				
medium				
beef	1 slice	13.0	286	45%
cheese	1 slice	11.0	261	38%
ham	1 slice	9.0	239	34%
Italian sausage	1 slice	15.0	293	46%
meat lover's	1 slice	18.0	340	48%
pepperoni	1 slice	12.0	265	41%
pepperoni lover's	1 slice	17.0	332	46%
pork topping	1 slice	14.0	294	43%
super supreme	1 slice	17.0	323	47%
supreme	1 slice	15.0	311	43%
veggie lover's	1 slice	10.0	243	37%
personal				
pepperoni	1 pizza	28.0	637	40%
supreme	1 pizza	34.0	722	42%
stuffed crust/ham/medium	⅛ pizza	13.0	396	30%
thin 'n crispy/medium				
beef	1 slice	11.0	229	43%
cheese	1 slice	8.0	205	35%
ham	1 slice	7.0	184	34%
Italian sausage	1 slice	12.0	236	46%
meat lover's	1 slice	13.0	288	41%
pepperoni	1 slice	10.0	215	42%
pepperoni lover's	1 slice	16.0	289	50%
pork topping	1 slice	12.0	237	46%
super supreme	1 slice	14.0	270	47%
supreme	1 slice	13.0	257	46%
veggie lover's	1 slice	16.0	289	50%
triple decker/ham/medium	⅛ pizza	17.0	402	38%

PONDEROSA

■ **BEVERAGES**

Food and Description	Amount	Fat Grams	Total Calories	% Fat Calories
coffee/black	6 fl oz	–	2	–

Food and Description	Amount	Fat Grams	Total Calories	% Fat Calories
milk				
chocolate	8 fl oz	8.5	208	37%
whole	8 fl oz	8.6	159	49%
tea/unsweetened	6 fl oz	–	2	–
■ **CONDIMENTS**				
BBQ sauce	1 Tbs	–	25	–
cheese sauce	4 Tbs	2.0	52	35%
cheese spread	1 oz	6.7	98	62%
cocktail sauce	2 Tbs	1.0	34	26%
gravy				
brown	4 Tbs	1.0	25	36%
turkey	4 Tbs	<1.0	25	7%
herb-garlic cheese spread	1 Tbs	10.0	100	90%
lemon	1 wedge	–	3	–
margarine				
liquid	1 Tbs	11.0	100	100%
whipped	1 Tbs	1.2	34	32%
salad oil	1 Tbs	14.0	120	100%
sour cream	1 Tbs	2.5	26	87%
spaghetti sauce	4 oz	4.0	110	33%
sweet & sour sauce	1 oz	<1.0	37	12%
tartar sauce	1 oz	10.5	95	100%
■ **DESSERT**				
banana pudding	1 oz	2.4	52	42%
ice milk				
chocolate	3.5 oz	2.9	152	17%
vanilla	3.5 oz	2.6	150	16%
mousse				
chocolate	1 oz	4.4	78	51%
strawberry	1 oz	4.6	74	56%
strawberry glaze	1 oz	–	37	–
topping				
caramel	1 oz	<1.0	100	6%
chocolate	1 oz	<1.0	89	3%
strawberry	1 oz	<1.0	71	3%
whipped	1 oz	6.4	80	72%
vanilla wafer	2 cookies	1.0	35	26%
■ **ENTRÉES**				
chicken				
breast	1 serving	2.1	98	19%
wings	2 pieces	9.0	213	38%
fish				
baked/Bake'n Broil	1 serving	13.0	230	51%
fried	1 serving	9.0	190	43%
fish nuggets	1 piece	1.7	31.0	49%
halibut/broiled	1 serving	2.4	170	13%
hot dog	1 hot dog	13.0	144	81%
roughy/broiled	1 serving	4.8	138	31%

Food and Description	Amount	Fat Grams	Total Calories	% Fat Calories
salmon/broiled	1 serving	2.7	192	13%
scrod/baked	1 serving	1.0	120	8%
sirloin tips/precooked	5 oz	8.2	473	16%
steak				
chopped/precooked	4 oz	16.2	225	65%
	5.3 oz	21.5	296	65%
Kansas city strip/precooked	5 oz	5.7	138	37%
New York strip/precooked	8 oz	10.5	314	30%
	10 oz	14.5	384	34%
porterhouse/precooked	16 oz	30.9	640	43%
rib-eye/precooked	5 oz	12.8	219	53%
	6 oz	14.2	282	45%
sirloin/precooked	7 oz	10.8	241	40%
T-bone/precooked	8 oz	8.5	178	43%
teriyaki/precooked	5 oz	3.1	174	16%
	10 oz	18.4	444	37%
steak kabobs/precooked/meat only	3 oz	4.8	153	28%
steak sandwich	1 sandwich	11.1	408	24%
shrimp				
fried	7 pieces	0.5	231	2%
mini	6 pieces	1.7	47	33%
swordfish/broiled	1 serving	9.4	271	31%
trout/broiled	1 serving	3.9	228	15%
■ SALAD BAR ITEMS				
apple				
fresh	1 medium	1.0	80	11%
canned	4 oz	–	90	–
apple ring/spiced	4 oz	–	100	–
applesauce	4 oz	–	80	–
banana	1 medium	<1.0	87	2%
banana chips	2 oz	1.3	25	47%
beets/diced	4 oz	<1.0	55	7%
breadstick				
Italian	1 piece	1.0	100	9%
sesame	2 pieces	–	35	–
broccoli	1 oz	<1.0	9	90%
cabbage				
green	1 oz	–	9	–
red	1 oz	–	1	–
cantaloupe	1 wedge	–	13	–
celery	1 oz	–	4	–
cheese/imitation/shredded	1 oz	7.0	90	70%
cherry peppers	2 pieces	<1.0	7	26%
chicken salad	3.5 oz	15.4	213	65%
chow mein noodles	0.2 oz	1.2	25	43%
coconut/shredded	0.2 oz	1.9	25	68%
cottage cheese	4 oz	5.0	120	38%
crackers/melba snacks	2 pieces	–	18	–

Food and Description	Amount	Fat Grams	Total Calories	% Fat Calories
croutons	1 oz	3.7	115	29%
cucumber	1 oz	–	4	–
eggs/hard-cooked/diced	2 oz	6.6	94	63%
fruit cocktail	4 oz	<1.0	97	2%
garbanzo beans	1 oz	–	102	–
gelatin/plain	4 oz	–	71	–
granola	0.2 oz	1.0	24	38%
grapes	10 pieces	<1.0	34	5%
ham/diced	2 oz	10.0	120	75%
honeydew melon	1 wedge	<1.0	25	7%
lettuce	1 oz	–	5	–
macaroni salad	3.5 oz	11.7	335	31%
mushrooms	1 oz	–	8	–
olives				
black	1 olive	<1.0	4	90%
green	1 olive	<1.0	3	90%
onion/red or yellow	1 oz	–	11	–
orange	1 piece	–	45	–
pasta salad/premade	3.5 oz	11.7	269	39%
peaches/canned	4 oz	–	70	–
peanuts/granulated	0.2 oz	2.3	30	69%
pears/canned	4 oz	<1.0	98	5%
pepper/green	1 oz	–	6	–
pickles				
dill spears	0.14 oz	–	<1	–
sweet chips	0.14 oz	–	4	–
pineapple				
canned/tidbits	4 oz	<1.0	95	2%
fresh/wedges	1 wedge	–	11	–
potato salad	3.5 oz	5.9	126	42%
radish	1 oz	–	4	–
scallion	1 piece	–	7	–
spinach	1 oz	–	7	–
sprouts				
alfalfa	1 oz	–	10	–
bean	1 oz	–	10	–
strawberries	2 oz	<1.0	14	13%
sunflower seeds	0.2 oz	2.8	32	79%
tomato	1 oz	–	6	–
turkey/julienne	1 oz	<1.0	29	19%
turkey-ham salad	3.5 oz	12.8	186	62%
watermelon	1 wedge	<1.0	111	7%
yogurt				
fruit	4 oz	1.0	115	8%
vanilla	4 oz	2.0	110	16%
■ SIDE DISHES (*See also* Salad Bar Items in this section)				
baked beans	4 oz	6.0	170	32%
baked potato	1 serving	<1.0	145	3%

Food and Description	Amount	Fat Grams	Total Calories	% Fat Calories
carrots	3.5 oz	–	31	–
cauliflower/breaded	4 oz	1.0	115	8%
corn	3.5 oz	<1.0	90	5%
green beans	3.5 oz	–	20	–
macaroni & cheese	1 oz	<1.0	17	26%
mashed potatoes	1 serving	<1.0	62	3%
okra/breaded	4 oz	1.0	124	7%
onion rings/breaded	4 oz	8.8	213	37%
pasta shells	2 oz	<1.0	78	3%
peas	3.5 oz	<1.0	67	4%
potato wedges	1 serving	6.0	130	42%
rice pilaf	1 serving	4.0	160	34%
roll				
dinner	1 roll	3.4	184	17%
sourdough	1 roll	1.0	110	8%
spaghetti	2 oz	<1.0	78	3%
stuffing	4 oz	11.0	230	43%
tortilla chips	1 oz	8.0	150	48%
winter mix	3.5 oz	–	25	–
zucchini/breaded	4 oz	<1.0	102	6%

POPEYE'S CHICKEN & BISCUITS
■ CHICKEN & SHRIMP

Food and Description	Amount	Fat Grams	Total Calories	% Fat Calories
chicken				
mild				
breast	1 piece	15.9	270	53%
leg	1 piece	7.3	120	55%
thigh	1 piece	22.7	300	68%
wing	1 piece	10.7	160	60%
nuggets	1 serving	32.0	410	70%
spicy				
breast	1 piece	15.9	270	53%
leg	1 piece	7.3	120	55%
thigh	1 piece	22.7	300	68%
wing	1 piece	10.7	160	60%
shrimp	1 serving	16.4	250	59%

■ DESSERT

Food and Description	Amount	Fat Grams	Total Calories	% Fat Calories
apple pie	1 slice	15.8	290	49%

■ SIDE ORDERS

Food and Description	Amount	Fat Grams	Total Calories	% Fat Calories
biscuit	1 biscuit	15.0	250	54%
Cajun rice	1 serving	5.4	150	32%
coleslaw	1 serving	11.2	149	68%
corn on the cob	1 piece	3.0	127	21%
French fries	1 serving	12.2	240	46%
onion rings	1 serving	19.3	310	56%
potatoes & gravy	1 serving	6.0	100	54%
red beans & rice	1 serving	17.0	270	57%

Food and Description	Amount	Fat Grams	Total Calories	% Fat Calories
QUINCY'S				
■ **BREAKFAST**				
bacon	1 serving	3.0	35	77%
corned beef hash	1 serving	15.0	210	64%
country ham	1 serving	6.0	90	60%
escalloped apples	1 serving	2.0	120	15%
oatmeal	1 serving	2.0	175	10%
pancakes	1 serving	3.0	95	28%
sausage gravy	1 serving	6.0	70	77%
sausage links	1 serving	22.0	225	88%
scrambled eggs	1 serving	7.0	95	66%
steak fingers	1 serving	25.0	360	63%
syrup	1 oz	–	75	–
■ **CONDIMENTS**				
margarine	2 Tbs	22.0	200	100%
salad dressing				
blue cheese	1 oz	16.0	155	93%
French				
light	1 oz	4.0	85	42%
regular	1 oz	12.0	125	86%
honey mustard	1 oz	6.0	100	54%
Italian				
creamy/light	1 oz	4.0	65	55%
light	1 oz	2.0	20	90%
regular	1 oz	14.0	135	93%
Parmesan peppercorn	1 oz	14.0	150	84%
ranch	1 oz	11.0	110	90%
Thousand Island/light	1 oz	4.0	65	55%
■ **DESSERT**				
banana pudding	1 serving	12.0	240	45%
brownie pudding cake	1 serving	5.0	310	15%
cobbler				
apple	1 serving	8.0	255	28%
cherry	1 serving	8.0	410	18%
peach	1 serving	8.0	305	24%
cookie				
chocolate chip	1 cookie	5.0	60	75%
sugar	1 cookie	3.0	60	45%
topping				
hot caramel	1 oz	1.0	105	9%
hot fudge	1 oz	4.0	105	34%
pineapple	1 oz	–	70	–
yogurt/frozen	1 serving	2.0	135	13%
■ **ENTRÉES**				
beef stir-fry	16 oz	77.0	950	73%
chicken				
grilled	regular	2.0	125	14%
	large	3.0	250	11%

Food and Description	Amount	Fat Grams	Total Calories	% Fat Calories
homestyle/fillet	6 oz	24.0	410	53%
stir-fry	15.75 oz	66.0	780	76%
chopped beef steak	5.75 oz	34.0	470	65%
fillet of beef	5.5 oz	12.0	330	33%
hamburger/quarter pound	1 burger	20.0	410	44%
prime rib	8 oz	46.0	570	73%
	16 oz	93.0	1145	73%
sirloin tips	4 oz	9.0	240	34%
steak				
country style	5 oz	29.0	380	69%
rib-eye	7.25 oz	60.0	670	81%
	9.5 oz	78.0	870	81%
sirloin	petite	37.0	450	74%
	regular	54.0	650	75%
	large	70.0	850	74%
sizzlin strip	9.5 oz	37.0	595	56%
T-bone	14 oz	170.0	1610	95%
trout/grilled	6 oz	12.0	300	36%
■ SANDWICHES				
country style steak sandwich	1 sandwich	29.0	520	50%
grilled chicken sandwich	1 sandwich	5.0	305	15%
■ SIDE ORDERS				
baked potato/w/o butter	1 serving	–	370	–
black-eyed peas	4 oz	1.0	75	12%
broccoli				
plain	10 oz	1.0	110	8%
w/cheese sauce	12 oz	13.0	250	47%
broccoli & rice casserole	4 oz	5.0	100	45%
cabbage/steamed	4 oz	4.0	85	42%
carrots/steamed	4 oz	4.0	85	42%
corn				
on the cob	1 piece	1.0	140	6%
whole kernel	4 oz	6.0	110	49%
cornbread	1 piece	5.0	140	32%
green beans	1 serving	1.0	25	36%
hashrounds	1 serving	14.0	230	54%
macaroni & cheese	4 oz	9.0	165	49%
mashed potatoes	4 oz	<1.0	70	6%
mushrooms	1 serving	12.0	115	94%
new potatoes	4 oz	11.0	190	52%
pinto beans	4 oz	–	70	–
refried beans	4 oz	7.0	140	45%
rice pilaf	3.5 oz	2.0	105	17%
squash	4 oz	10.0	110	82%
turnip greens	4 oz	6.0	75	72%
vegetable medley	4 oz	<1.0	35	13%
yams/candied	4 oz	10.0	250	36%

Food and Description	Amount	Fat Grams	Total Calories	% Fat Calories
■ SOUP				
chili w/beans	1 serving	11.0	235	42%
clam chowder	1 serving	9.0	180	45%
cream of broccoli	1 serving	10.0	170	53%
vegetable beef	1 serving	2.0	90	20%
RALLY'S				
■ BEVERAGES				
chocolate shake	1 shake	12.0	411	26%
Coca-Cola				
Diet Coke	16 fl oz	–	1	–
	32 fl oz	–	2	–
regular	16 fl oz	–	120	–
	32 fl oz	–	216	–
Dr. Pepper	16 fl oz	–	120	–
	32 fl oz	–	216	–
Fanta				
orange	16 fl oz	–	147	–
	32 fl oz	–	264	–
root beer	16 fl oz	–	130	–
	32 fl oz	–	234	–
iced tea	16 fl oz	–	3	–
	32 fl oz	–	6	–
Ramblin' Root Beer	16 fl oz	–	147	–
	32 fl oz	–	264	–
Sprite	16 fl oz	–	119	–
strawberry/banana shake	1 shake	11.0	399	25%
vanilla shake	1 shake	11.0	320	31%
■ BURGERS & SAUSAGE				
cheeseburger				
bacon	2 burgers	40.3	622	58%
double	1 burger	49.0	733	60%
Rallyburger				
regular	1 burger	25.0	435	52%
w/cheese	1 burger	29.4	485	55%
smokin' sausage				
plain	1 sausage	39.6	724	49%
w/chili	1 sausage	62.0	830	67%
■ CHICKEN				
chicken sandwich	1 sandwich	30.8	530	52%
■ COMBINATION MEALS				
large combo meal				
regular	1 meal	40.5	970	38%
w/cheese	1 meal	45.0	1018	40%
regular combo meal				
regular	1 meal	32.7	715	41%
w/cheese	1 meal	37.2	765	44%

Food and Description	Amount	Fat Grams	Total Calories	% Fat Calories
■ **MEXICAN FOOD**				
chili	8 oz	19.0	340	50%
taco/soft	1 taco	10.0	223	40%
■ **SIDE ORDERS**				
fries	regular	7.8	158	44%
	large	15.6	317	44%
RAX				
■ **BEVERAGES**				
chocolate yogurt shake	1 shake	11.0	420	24%
strawberry yogurt shake	1 shake	11.0	410	24%
vanilla yogurt shake	1 shake	11.0	330	30%
■ **SALADS & DRESSING**				
Caesar side salad	1 serving	2.0	40	45%
gourmet garden salad	1 serving	9.0	220	37%
grilled chicken Caesar salad	1 serving	5.0	160	28%
salad dressing				
blue cheese	1 serving	16.0	145	99%
buttermilk ranch	1 serving	20.0	175	100%
Catalina/fat-free	1 serving	–	50	–
creamy Caesar	1 serving	15.0	140	96%
honey French	1 serving	5.0	140	32%
Italian/fat-free	1 serving	–	15	–
ranch/fat-free	1 serving	–	60	–
Thousand Island	1 serving	13.0	130	90%
vinaigrette	1 serving	4.0	70	51%
side salad	1 serving	4.0	40	90%
■ **SANDWICHES**				
barbecue beef				
hold the mayo & oil	1 sandwich	10.0	315	29%
regular	1 sandwich	19.5	400	44%
BBC (beef, bacon, & cheddar)	1 sandwich	51.0	720	64%
cheddar melt				
hold the mayo & oil	1 sandwich	15.6	283	50%
regular	1 sandwich	22.6	346	59%
deluxe				
hold the mayo & oil	1 sandwich	13.0	325	36%
regular	1 sandwich	34.6	521	60%
grilled chicken				
hold the mayo & oil	1 sandwich	7.0	285	22%
regular	1 sandwich	33.5	526	57%
Jr. deluxe				
hold the mayo & oil	1 sandwich	8.0	215	33%
regular	1 sandwich	25.0	370	61%
mushroom melt	1 sandwich	37.5	600	56%
Philly melt	1 sandwich	32.0	540	53%
regular Rax				
hold the mayo & oil	1 sandwich	13.0	305	38%

Food and Description	Amount	Fat Grams	Total Calories	% Fat Calories
regular	1 sandwich	22.0	390	51%
turkey				
hold the mayo & oil	1 sandwich	4.0	230	16%
regular	1 sandwich	32.0	485	59%
turkey-bacon club	1 sandwich	46.5	680	62%
■ SIDE ORDERS				
baked potato				
cheese	1 potato	–	270	–
cheese & bacon	1 potato	18.5	336	50%
cheese & broccoli	1 potato	–	281	–
plain	1 potato	–	207	–
w/butter	1 potato	11.3	306	33%
w/sour topping	1 potato	4.0	257	14%
■ SOUP				
chicken noodle	1 serving	1.0	115	8%
chili	1 serving	9.5	160	53%
cream of broccoli	1 serving	4.0	95	38%
RED LOBSTER				
■ APPETIZERS				
Lighthouse selections				
shrimp cocktail				
regular	3 oz	0.5	80	6%
colossal	5.9 oz	1.5	140	10%
regular				
calamari	1 serving	22.0	350	57%
chicken fingers	1 serving	18.0	390	42%
crab add-on	1 serving	1.0	60	15%
crab & shrimp cakes	1 serving	24.0	480	45%
lobster quesadilla	1 serving	47.0	760	56%
mozarella cheesticks	1 serving	46.0	730	57%
mushrooms				
fresh/fried	1 serving	51.0	790	58%
lobster-stuffed	1 serving	26.0	400	59%
stuffed	1 serving	27.0	420	58%
Parmesan zucchini	1 serving	40.0	620	58%
shrimp				
chilled/in the shell	6 oz	1.5	110	12%
cocktail/shelled	6 pieces	0.5	50	9%
■ ENTRÉES				
Lighthouse selections				
chicken breast				
garlic herb-seared	13.2 oz	10.0	500	18%
honey BBQ	13.4 oz	11.0	510	19%
spicy grilled	13.2 oz	10.0	500	18%
chicken salad/grilled/ w/fat-free ranch dressing	20.3 oz	7.0	270	23%
cod/baked cod	14.2 oz	10.0	450	20%

Food and Description	Amount	Fat Grams	Total Calories	% Fat Calories
haddock/baked	14.2 oz	11.0	460	22%
king crab legs	9 oz	3.5	200	16%
mahi mahi/lemon-pepper grilled	14.2 oz	10.0	460	20%
Maine lobster/live	9.2 oz	1.5	190	7%
rock lobster tail/broiled	8 oz	6.0	200	27%
shrimp & scallops/seared	18.6 oz	13.0	610	19%
snow or Dungeness crab legs	7 oz	2.0	140	13%
regular				
Admiral's Feast	1 serving	52.0	1060	44%
Atlantic cod/haddock/baked	1 serving	6.0	220	25%
broiled fisherman's platter	1 serving	23.0	600	35%
broiled seafarer's platter	1 serving	19.0	450	38%
catfish Santa Fe	1 serving	9.0	340	24%
chicken				
breast				
grilled	1 serving	7.0	230	26%
teriyaki grilled	1 serving	7.0	240	26%
fresco	1 serving	73.0	1320	50%
smothered	1 serving	31.0	530	53%
chicken salad/grilled/w/fat-free ranch dressing/lunch entrée	20.3 oz	7.0	270	23%
clam strips	1 serving	39.0	720	49%
crab Alfredo	1 serving	66.0	1170	51%
fish & shrimp combo	1 serving	35.0	730	43%
flounder fillet/baked/lunch entrée	11.6 oz	6.0	350	15%
lobster, shrimp, & scallop scampi	1 serving	33.0	870	34%
mahi mahi/lemon-pepper grilled	1 serving	7.0	240	26%
Maine lobster/live				
steamed	1 serving	1.0	160	6%
stuffed	1 serving	10.0	430	21%
Neptune's Feast	1 serving	62.0	1210	46%
New York strip steak	1 order	34.0	560	55%
New York strip steak & fried shrimp	1 order	46.0	780	53%
New York strip steak & rock lobster tail	1 order	31.0	570	49%
rock lobster tail/broiled	1 tail	6.0	190	28%
shrimp				
carbonara	1 serving	76.0	1290	53%
large/fried	1 serving	27.0	500	49%
Milano	1 serving	65.0	1190	49%
popcorn	1 serving	37.0	580	57%
shrimp & chicken	1 serving	15.0	340	40%
shrimp combo	1 serving	23.0	380	54%
shrimp feast	1 serving	24.0	470	46%
snow crab legs	1 serving	2.0	110	16%
■ SOUP				
bayou style seafood gumbo	6 oz	4.0	120	30%
broccoli cheese soup	1 serving	9.0	160	51%
clam chowder	6 oz	5.0	130	35%

Food and Description	Amount	Fat Grams	Total Calories	% Fat Calories
ROY ROGERS				
■ **BREAKFAST**				
bagel				
cinnamon raisin	1 bagel	1.0	300	3%
plain	1 bagel	2.0	300	6%
big country breakfast platter				
w/bacon	1 serving	43.0	740	52%
w/ham	1 serving	39.0	710	49%
w/sausage	1 serving	60.0	920	59%
biscuit				
bacon	1 biscuit	23.0	420	49%
bacon & egg	1 biscuit	26.0	470	50%
cinnamon 'n raisin	1 biscuit	18.0	370	44%
ham & cheese	1 biscuit	24.0	450	48%
ham & egg	1 biscuit	23.0	460	45%
ham, egg, & cheese	1 biscuit	27.0	500	49%
hashrounds	1 serving	14.0	230	55%
orange juice	11 fl oz	–	140	–
pancakes				
pancakes only	3 pancakes	2.0	280	6%
w/bacon	1 serving	9.0	350	23%
w/sausage	1 serving	16.0	430	33%
sourdough ham, egg, & cheese				
plain	1 serving	21.0	390	48%
regular	1 serving	24.0	480	45%
sausage	1 serving	31.0	510	55%
sausage & egg	1 serving	35.0	560	56%
■ **BURGERS & BEEF**				
cheeseburger				
bacon	1 burger	28.0	490	51%
¼ pound	1 burger	22.0	470	42%
regular	1 burger	13.0	300	39%
sourdough bacon	1 burger	18.0	730	22%
hamburger				
¼ pound	1 burger	18.0	430	38%
regular	1 burger	9.0	260	31%
roast beef sandwich	1 sandwich	4.0	260	14%
■ **CHICKEN & FISH**				
chicken fillet sandwich	1 sandwich	24.0	500	43%
chicken nuggets	6 pieces	18.0	290	56%
	9 pieces	29.0	460	57%
fisherman's fillet	1 sandwich	21.0	490	39%
fried chicken				
breast	1 piece	15.0	370	36%
thigh	1 piece	15.0	330	41%
wing	1 piece	8.0	200	36%
grilled chicken sandwich	1 sandwich	11.0	340	29%

Food and Description	Amount	Fat Grams	Total Calories	% Fat Calories
Roy's Roaster/¼ chicken				
dark meat				
skinless	1 serving	10.0	190	47%
w/skin	1 serving	34.0	490	62%
white meat				
skinless	1 serving	6.0	190	28%
w/skin	1 serving	29.0	500	52%
sourdough grilled chicken sandwich	1 sandwich	21.0	500	38%
■ CONDIMENTS				
gravy	1.5 oz	–	20	–
■ DESSERT				
hot fudge sundae	1 sundae	10.0	320	28%
strawberry shortcake	1 piece	21.0	480	39%
strawberry sundae	1 sundae	6.0	260	21%
vanilla frozen yogurt	1 cone	4.0	180	20%
■ SALADS				
garden	1 serving	9.0	190	43%
grilled chicken	1 serving	4.0	120	30%
side	1 serving	–	20	–
■ SIDE DISHES (*See also* Salads in this section)				
baked beans	5 oz	2.0	160	11%
baked potato				
plain	1 potato	1.0	130	9%
w/margarine	1 serving	13.0	240	11%
w/margarine & sour cream	1 serving	19.0	300	57%
coleslaw	5 oz	25.0	295	76%
cornbread	1 piece	17.0	310	49%
French fries	regular	15.0	350	39%
	large	18.0	430	38%
mashed potatoes	5 oz	–	92	–
SHONEY'S				
■ BREAKFAST				
bacon	3 strips	9.4	109	78%
biscuit	1 biscuit	8.0	170	42%
blueberry muffin	1 serving	7.0	214	29%
country gravy	3 oz	9.8	114	77%
croissant	1 biscuit	16.0	260	55%
egg/fried	1 serving	14.7	159	83%
grits	1 serving	3.2	57	51%
ham/breakfast	2 slices	2.0	59	31%
hash browns	1 serving	3.0	90	30%
home fries	1 serving	3.7	115	29%
honey bun	1 bun	14.0	265	48%
pancake/6" dia	1 serving	<1.0	91	2%
sausage	1 patty	9.6	103	84%
sirloin/charbroiled	6 oz	24.5	357	62%
syrup/low-calorie	2.2 oz	–	98	–

Food and Description	Amount	Fat Grams	Total Calories	% Fat Calories
toast w/butter	2 slices	5.2	163	29%
■ BURGERS				
All-American	1 burger	32.6	501	59%
bacon	1 burger	40.0	591	61%
mushroom-Swiss	1 burger	41.7	616	61%
old-fashioned	1 burger	28.2	470	54%
Shoney burger	1 burger	35.7	498	65%
■ CONDIMENTS (See also Salads & Dressing in this section)				
BBQ sauce	1 serving	1.0	41	22%
cocktail sauce	1 serving	–	36	–
sweet & sour sauce	1 serving	–∙	58	–
tartar sauce	1 serving	7.7	84	83%
■ DESSERT				
apple pie à la mode	1 serving	23.0	492	42%
carrot cake	1 serving	26.0	500	47%
hot fudge cake	1 serving	19.7	522	34%
hot fudge sundae	1 serving	22.0	451	44%
strawberry pie	1 serving	16.7	332	45%
strawberry sundae	1 serving	19.0	380	45%
walnut brownie à la mode	1 serving	33.7	576	53%
■ ENTRÉES				
beef patty/light	1 serving	22.9	289	71%
chicken				
charbroiled	1 serving	7.4	239	28%
Hawaiian	1 serving	7.4	262	25%
chicken tenders	1 serving	20.4	388	47%
country fried steak	1 serving	27.2	449	55%
fish				
baked	1 serving	1.4	170	7%
light fried	1 serving	14.4	297	44%
fish & chips w/fries	1 serving	34.8	639	49%
fish & shrimp	1 serving	25.5	487	47%
Italian feast	1 serving	19.6	500	35%
lasagna	1 serving	9.8	297	30%
liver & onions	1 serving	22.9	411	50%
seafood platter	1 serving	28.0	566	45%
shrimp				
bite-size	1 serving	24.7	387	57%
boiled	1 serving	1.0	93	10%
charbroiled	1 serving	3.0	138	20%
shrimp sampler	1 serving	22.7	412	50%
shrimper's feast	regular	22.2	383	52%
	large	33.3	575	52%
spaghetti	1 serving	16.3	496	30%
steak				
half o'pound	1 serving	34.4	435	71%
rib-eye	8 oz	50.5	605	75%
sirloin	6 oz	24.5	357	62%

Food and Description	Amount	Fat Grams	Total Calories	% Fat Calories
steak 'n shrimp				
w/charbroiled shrimp	1 serving	22.6	361	56%
w/fried shrimp	1 serving	32.7	507	58%
■ SALADS & DRESSING				
ambrosia salad	¼ cup	3.3	75	40%
apple grape surprise salad	¼ cup	–	19	–
beet onion salad	¼ cup	1.3	25	47%
broccoli/cauliflower salad	¼ cup	8.5	98	78%
broccoli/cauliflower/carrot salad	¼ cup	4.4	53	75%
broccoli/cauliflower/ranch salad	¼ cup	6.4	65	89%
carrot apple salad	¼ cup	9.0	99	82%
coleslaw	¼ cup	5.0	69	65%
cucumber salad/lite	¼ cup	–	12	–
Don's pasta salad	¼ cup	4.6	82	50%
fruit delight salad	¼ cup	1.6	54	27%
Italian vegetable salad	¼ cup	–	11	–
kidney bean salad	¼ cup	2.0	55	33%
macaroni salad	¼ cup	13.9	207	60%
mixed fruit salad	¼ cup	–	37	–
mixed squash salad	¼ cup	4.0	49	73%
oriental salad	¼ cup	2.7	79	31%
pea salad	¼ cup	5.5	73	68%
rotelli pasta salad	¼ cup	4.0	78	46%
salad dressing				
Biscayne/low-calorie	2 Tbs	1.0	62	15%
blue cheese	2 Tbs	13.0	117	100%
French				
regular	2 Tbs	12.0	124	87%
rue	2 Tbs	10.0	122	74%
honey mustard	2 Tbs	17.0	165	93%
Italian				
creamy	2 Tbs	15.0	135	100%
golden	2 Tbs	15.0	141	96%
Weight Watchers	2 Tbs	–	10	–
ranch	2 Tbs	10.0	95	95%
Thousand Island	2 Tbs	13.0	130	90%
Seigan salad	¼ cup	3.6	72	45%
snow salad	¼ cup	4.0	72	50%
spaghetti salad	¼ cup	4.6	81	51%
spring salad	¼ cup	2.9	38	69%
summer salad	¼ cup	11.6	114	92%
three bean salad	¼ cup	5.0	96	47%
Waldorf salad	¼ cup	5.2	81	58%
■ SANDWICHES				
baked ham	1 sandwich	10.3	290	32%
charbroiled chicken	1 sandwich	17.0	451	34%
chicken fillet	1 sandwich	21.2	464	41%
country fried	1 sandwich	25.8	588	39%

Food and Description	Amount	Fat Grams	Total Calories	% Fat Calories
fish	1 sandwich	12.7	323	35%
grilled bacon & cheese	1 sandwich	28.2	440	58%
grilled cheese	1 sandwich	16.9	302	50%
ham club on whole wheat	1 sandwich	35.5	642	50%
patty melt	1 sandwich	41.7	640	59%
Philly steak	1 sandwich	44.0	673	59%
Reuben	1 sandwich	34.7	596	52%
Slim Jim	1 sandwich	23.9	484	44%
turkey club on whole wheat	1 sandwich	32.7	635	46%

■ SIDE DISHES (*See also* Salads & Dressing in this section)

baked potato	1 serving	<1.0	264	1%
French fries	3 oz	7.5	189	36%
	4 oz	9.9	252	35%
Grecian bread	1 serving	2.2	80	25%
mushrooms/sautéed	3 oz	6.5	75	78%
onion rings	1 piece	3.0	52	52%
onions/sautéed	2.5 oz	2.0	37	49%
rice	3.5 oz	3.7	137	24%

■ SOUP

bean	6 oz	1.0	63	14%
beef cabbage	6 oz	3.0	86	31%
broccoli/cauliflower	6 oz	9.2	124	67%
cheddar chowder	6 oz	2.3	91	23%
cheese Florentine ham	6 oz	7.8	110	64%
chicken gumbo	6 oz	2.0	60	30%
chicken noodle	6 oz	1.4	62	20%
chicken rice	6 oz	<1.0	72	6%
clam chowder	6 oz	5.4	94	52%
corn chowder	6 oz	4.7	148	29%
cream of broccoli	6 oz	4.6	75	55%
cream of chicken	6 oz	8.9	136	59%
cream of chicken vegetable	6 oz	1.3	79	15%
onion	6 oz	2.0	29	62%
potato	6 oz	3.4	102	30%
tomato Florentine	6 oz	1.0	63	14%
tomato vegetable	6 oz	<1.0	46	6%
vegetable beef	6 oz	1.5	82	16%

SIZZLER

■ CONDIMENTS

buttery dipping sauce	1½ oz	37.0	330	100%
cocktail sauce	1½ oz	–	40	–
guacamole	1 oz	4.0	42	86%
hibachi sauce	1½ oz	–	57	–
Malibu sauce	1½ oz	31.0	283	99%
margarine/whipped	1½ Tbs	12.0	105	100%
marinara sauce	1 oz	–	13	–
nacho cheese sauce	1 oz	10.0	120	75%

Food and Description	Amount	Fat Grams	Total Calories	% Fat Calories
salsa	1 oz	–	7	–
sour dressing	2 Tbs	6.0	60	90%
	1½ oz	9.0	89	91%
tartar sauce	1½ oz	17.0	170	90%
■ **DESSERT BAR ITEMS**				
chocolate & vanilla soft-serve frozen dessert	4 oz	4.0	136	26%
chocolate syrup	1 oz	–	90	–
strawberry topping	1 oz	–	70	–
whipped topping	1 Tbs	1.0	12	–
■ **ENTRÉES**				
chicken				
breast				
hibachi w/pineapple	5 oz	3.0	193	14%
lemon-herb	5 oz	3.0	140	19%
Santa Fe	5 oz	3.0	150	18%
patty/Malibu	1 patty	19.0	310	55%
hamburger/meat, bun, lettuce, & tomato	1 burger	33.0	626	47%
salmon	8 oz	12.0	247	44%
shrimp				
broiled	5 oz	6.0	150	36%
fried	4 shrimp	2.0	223	81%
mini	4 oz	1.0	152	6%
scampi	5 oz	3.0	143	19%
steak	6 oz	20.0	316	57%
	8 oz	27.0	421	58%
	9.5 oz	32.0	500	58%
swordfish	8 oz	14.0	315	40%
■ **SALADS & SALAD BAR ITEMS**				
alfalfa sprouts	¼ cup	–	2	–
avocados	½ avocado	15.0	153	88%
bacon bits	1 Tbs	2.0	27	67%
bean sprouts	¼ cup	–	–	–
beets	¼ cup	–	13	–
bell peppers	2 oz	–	8	–
broccoli	½ cup	–	12	–
cantaloupe	½ cup	–	28	–
carrot & raisin salad	2 oz	10.0	130	69%
carrots	¼ cup	–	12	–
cherry tomatoes	¼ cup	–	12	–
Chinese chicken salad	2 oz	2.0	54	33%
cottage cheese	2 oz	1.0	51	18%
cucumber	2 oz	–	7	–
egg/hard-cooked	1 oz	3.0	44	61%
garbanzo beans	¼ cup	1.0	63	14%
grapes	½ cup	–	29	–
honeydew melon	½ cup	–	30	–
jicama	2 oz	–	13	–

Food and Description	Amount	Fat Grams	Total Calories	% Fat Calories
kidney beans	¼ cup	–	52	–
kiwifruit	2 oz	–	35	–
lettuce,				
iceberg	1 cup	–	7	–
romaine	1 cup	–	9	–
Mediterranean minted fruit salad	2 oz	–	29	–
Mexican fiesta salad	2 oz	–	54	–
olives	1 oz	6.0	62	87%
onion/red	2 Tbs	–	8	–
peaches	¼ cup	–	34	–
peas	¼ cup	–	31	–
pineapple	½ cup	–	38	–
potato salad				
old fashioned	2 oz	5.0	84	54%
red herb	2 oz	9.0	121	67%
mushrooms	¼ cup	–	4	–
red cabbage	¼ cup	–	6	–
salad dressing				
blue cheese	1 oz	12.0	111	97%
honey mustard	1 oz	16.0	160	90%
Italian				
lite	1 oz	–	14	–
Parmesan	1 oz	10.0	100	90%
Japanese rice vinegar	1 oz	–	10	–
ranch				
reduced calorie	1 oz	8.0	90	80%
regular	1 oz	12.0	120	90%
Thousand Island	1 oz	15.0	143	94%
seafood Louis pasta salad	2 oz	2.0	64	28%
seafood salad	2 oz	3.0	56	48%
spicy jicama salad	2 oz	–	16	–
spinach	½ cup	–	6	–
strawberries	½ cup	–	22	–
teriyaki beef salad	2 oz	2.0	49	37%
tuna pasta salad	2 oz	10.0	133	68%
turkey ham	1 oz	5.0	62	73%
watermelon	½ cup	–	28	–
zucchini	¼ cup	–	5	–
■ SIDE ORDERS & APPETIZERS (See also Salads & Salad Bar Items in this section)				
baked potato/flesh only	4 oz	–	105	–
cheese toast	1 piece	21.0	273	69%
chicken wings	1 oz	4.0	73	49%
fettuccine	2 oz	1.0	80	11%
focaccia bread	2 pieces	7.0	108	58%
French fries	4 oz	12.0	358	30%
meatballs	4 meatballs	11.0	157	63%
potato skin	2 oz	8.0	160	45%
refried beans	¼ cup	1.0	62	15%

Food and Description	Amount	Fat Grams	Total Calories	% Fat Calories
rice pilaf	6 oz	5.0	256	18%
saltine crackers	2 crackers	1.0	25	36%
spaghetti	2 oz	–	80	–
taco filling	2 oz	9.0	103	79%
taco shell	1 shell	2.0	50	36%
■ SOUP				
broccoli cheese	4 oz	9.0	139	58%
chicken noodle	4 oz	1.0	31	29%
clam chowder	4 oz	6.0	118	46%
minestrone	4 oz	–	36	–
vegetable sirloin	4 oz	2.0	60	30%

SONIC
■ BURGERS & HOT DOGS

Food and Description	Amount	Fat Grams	Total Calories	% Fat Calories
cheese coney				
extra long				
plain	1 coney	39.0	635	55%
w/onions	1 coney	39.2	640	55%
regular				
plain	1 coney	23.3	358	59%
w/onions	1 coney	23.3	361	58%
cheeseburger				
bacon	1 burger	38.6	548	63%
mini	1 burger	14.4	281	46%
chili pie	1 piece	22.6	327	62%
corn dog	1 corn dog	15.0	280	48%
hamburger				
hickory	1 burger	15.7	314	45%
mini	1 burger	11.0	246	24%
#1				
plain	1 burger	26.6	409	59%
w/cheese	1 burger	32.4	479	61%
#2				
plain	1 burger	15.7	323	43%
w/cheese	1 burger	21.5	393	49%
hot dog/regular	1 hot dog	15.3	258	53%
jalapeño burger/double meat & cheese	1 burger	40.6	638	57%
Super Sonic burger/double meat & cheese				
w/mayo	1 burger	51.5	730	63%
w/mustard	1 burger	40.7	644	57%
■ SANDWICHES				
BLT	1 sandwich	19.3	322	54%
chicken				
breaded	1 sandwich	24.7	455	49%
grilled	1 sandwich	4.3	215	18%
fish	1 sandwich	7.0	277	23%
grilled cheese	1 sandwich	17.0	288	53%
steak	1 sandwich	41.6	631	59%

Food and Description	Amount	Fat Grams	Total Calories	% Fat Calories
■ **SIDE ORDERS**				
French fries				
plain	regular	8.3	233	32%
	large	11.2	315	32%
w/cheese	large	20.7	420	44%
onion rings	regular	26.5	404	59%
	large	37.8	577	59%
Tater Tots				
plain	1 serving	7.0	150	42%
w/cheese	1 serving	13.0	220	53%
STEAK & SHAKE				
■ **BEVERAGES**				
chocolate shake	1 shake	37.8	608	56%
coffee	6 fl oz	–	2	–
Dr. Pepper	10.5 fl oz	–	137	–
hot chocolate	6 fl oz	18.6	686	24%
tea				
hot	7 fl oz	–	4	–
iced	7.5 fl oz	–	6	–
lemon drink	1 small	–	86	–
milk/whole	8 fl oz	7.9	146	49%
orange drink	1 small	–	83	–
orange juice	7 fl oz	<1.0	105	3%
root beer	10 fl oz	–	115	–
strawberry shake	1 shake	40.0	648	56%
vanilla shake	1 shake	38.4	619	56%
■ **BURGERS & CHILI**				
chili & oyster crackers	1 serving	14.0	337	37%
chili mac & 4 saltines	1 serving	12.4	311	36%
chili 3 ways & 4 saltines	1 serving	16.0	402	36%
steakburger				
regular				
plain	1 burger	7.1	277	23%
w/cheese	1 burger	13.3	353	34%
super				
plain	1 burger	12.0	375	29%
w/cheese	1 burger	18.3	451	37%
triple				
regular	1 burger	17.0	474	32%
w/cheese	1 burger	29.5	626	42%
■ **DESSERT**				
apple Danish	1 Danish	23.8	391	55%
apple pie				
à la mode	1 piece	25.5	549	42%
plain	1 piece	17.65	407	39%
brownie	1 piece	11.5	258	40%
brownie fudge sundae	1 sundae	35.2	645	49%

Food and Description	Amount	Fat Grams	Total Calories	% Fat Calories
cheesecake				
plain	1 piece	11.0	368	27%
w/strawberries	1 piece	11.4	386	26%
cherry pie				
à la mode	1 piece	21.6	476	41%
plain	1 piece	13.8	334	37%
Coca-Cola float	1 serving	17.2	514	30%
hot fudge nut sundae	1 sundae	34.4	530	58%
lemon float	1 serving	18.6	555	30%
lemon freeze	1 serving	24.9	548	41%
orange float	1 serving	16.8	502	30%
orange freeze	1 serving	23.8	516	42%
root beer float	1 serving	16.7	529	28%
strawberry sundae	1 sundae	21.7	330	59%
vanilla ice cream	1½ scoops	11.7	213	49%
■ SALADS				
chef salad	1 serving	17.6	313	51%
lettuce & tomato salad w/1 oz Thousand Island dressing	1 serving	15.3	168	82%
low-calorie platter	1 serving	13.7	293	42%
■ SANDWICHES				
baked ham	1 sandwich	22.0	451	44%
egg	1 sandwich	9.9	275	32%
ham & egg	1 sandwich	17.2	434	36%
toasted cheese	1 sandwich	13.3	250	48%t
■ SIDE ORDERS				
baked beans	1 serving	3.7	173	19%
cottage cheese	½ cup	3.6	94	35%
French fries	1 serving	10.2	211	44%
lettuce & tomato	1 serving	–	4	–
SUBWAY				
■ CONDIMENTS				
bacon	2 slices	4.0	45	80%
cheese	2 triangles	3.0	41	66%
mayonnaise dressing				
light	1 tsp	2.0	18	100%
regular	1 tsp	4.0	37	100%
mustard	2 tsp	–	8	–
olive oil blend	1 tsp	5.0	45	100%
vinegar	1 tsp	–	1	–
■ DESSERT				
cookies				
chocolate chip	1 cookie	8.0	161	45%
chocolate chip M&M	1 cookie	8.0	162	44%
chocolate chip walnut	1 cookie	9.0	165	49%
chocolate chunk	1 cookie	7.0	160	39%
double chocolate Brazil nut	1 cookie	11.0	200	50%

Food and Description	Amount	Fat Grams	Total Calories	% Fat Calories
oatmeal raisin	1 cookie	6.0	147	37%
peanut butter	1 cookie	9.0	169	48%
sugar	1 cookie	9.0	178	46%
toffee crunch	1 cookie	8.0	153	47%
white chocolate chip	1 cookie	8.0	166	43%
white chocolate macadamia nut	1 cookie	10.0	174	52%
■ SALADS & RELATED ITEMS				
bread bowl for salad	1 serving	4.0	290	12%
roasted chicken breast fillet salad	1 serving	3.0	143	19%
salad dressing/2-oz pkts				
French				
fat-free	1 pkt	–	15	–
regular	1 pkt	5.0	65	83%
Italian				
creamy	1 pkt	6.0	65	83%
fat-free	1 pkt	–	5	–
ranch				
fat-free	1 pkt	–	12	–
regular	1 pkt	9.0	87	93%
Thousand Island	1 pkt	6.0	65	83%
Subway club salad	1 serving	3.0	123	22%
Subway seafood & crab salad				
made w/light mayonnaise dressing	1 serving	8.0	155	46%
regular	1 serving	17.0	238	64%
tuna salad				
made w/light mayonnaise dressing	1 serving	13.0	194	60%
regular	1 serving	31.0	345	81%
turkey breast salad	1 serving	2.0	99	18%
veggie delite salad	1 serving	1.0	45	20%
■ SANDWICHES				
6" sub				
cold				
classic Italian BMT	1 sandwich	21.0	434	44%
cold cut trio	1 sandwich	12.0	347	31%
ham	1 sandwich	4.0	273	13%
roast beef	1 sandwich	6.0	299	18%
Subway club	1 sandwich	6.0	300	18%
Subway seafood & crab				
made w/light mayo/no cheese	1 sandwich	10.0	333	27%
regular	1 sandwich	19.0	415	41%
tuna				
made w/light mayo/no cheese	1 sandwich	15.0	372	36%
regular	1 sandwich	33.0	522	57%
turkey breast	1 sandwich	4.0	276	13%
turkey breast & ham	1 sandwich	4.0	275	13%
veggie delite	1 sandwich	3.0	223	12%
hot				
meatball	1 sandwich	15.0	411	33%

Food and Description	Amount	Fat Grams	Total Calories	% Fat Calories
roasted chicken breast fillet	1 sandwich	5.0	321	14%
steak & cheese	1 sandwich	10.0	363	25%
Subway melt	1 sandwich	12.0	361	30%
deli-style sandwich				
jumbo				
bologna	1 sandwich	27.0	446	54%
ham	1 sandwich	5.0	259	17%
roast beef	1 sandwich	9.0	335	24%
Subway seafood & crab				
made w/light mayo/no cheese	1 sandwich	13.0	348	34%
regular	1 sandwich	27.0	472	51%
tuna				
made w/light mayo/no cheese	1 sandwich	22.0	406	49%
regular	1 sandwich	47.0	632	67%
turkey breast	1 sandwich	6.0	290	19%
junior				
bologna	1 sandwich	11.0	270	37%
ham	1 sandwich	4.0	208	17%
roast beef	1 sandwich	5.0	232	19%
Subway seafood & crab				
made w/light mayo/no cheese	1 sandwich	6.0	238	23%
regular	1 sandwich	11.0	279	35%
tuna				
made w/light mayo/no cheese	1 sandwich	9.0	257	32%
regular	1 sandwich	18.0	332	49%
turkey breast	1 sandwich	4.0	218	17%

TACO BELL
■ BURRITOS

Food and Description	Amount	Fat Grams	Total Calories	% Fat Calories
bean				
light	1 burrito	6.0	330	16%
regular	1 burrito	12.0	391	28%
beef	1 burrito	19.0	432	40%
big beef supreme	1 burrito	25.0	525	43%
chicken				
light	1 burrito	6.0	290	19%
regular	1 burrito	13.0	345	34%
chicken supreme				
light	1 burrito	10.0	410	22%
regular	1 burrito	23.0	520	40%
chili cheese	1 burrito	18.0	391	41%
combination	1 burrito	17.0	412	37%
7-layer				
light	1 burrito	9.0	440	18%
regular	1 burrito	21.0	485	39%
steak supreme	1 burrito	23.0	500	41%
supreme/light	1 burrito	8.0	350	21%

Food and Description	Amount	Fat Grams	Total Calories	% Fat Calories
■ **CONDIMENTS**				
guacamole	1 pkt	3.0	36	75%
jalapeño peppers	1 serving	–	20	–
nacho cheese sauce	1 serving	4.0	51	71%
pico de gallo	1 serving	–	6	–
ranch dressing	1 pkt	14.0	136	93%
salsa	1 pkt	–	27	–
sauce				
green	1 serving	–	4	–
picante	1 pkt	–	3	–
red	1 serving	–	10	–
sour cream	1 pkt	4.0	44	82%
taco sauce				
hot	1 pkt	–	2	–
medium	1 pkt	–	–	–
■ **NACHOS & MISCELLANEOUS**				
Mexican pizza	1 serving	38.0	574	60%
Meximelt/beef	1 serving	14.0	262	48%
nachos				
BellGrande	1 serving	34.0	633	48%
regular	1 serving	18.0	345	47%
supreme	1 serving	18.0	364	45%
■ **SALADS**				
taco salad				
light				
w/chips	1 serving	19.0	550	31%
w/o chips	1 serving	9.0	330	25%
regular	1 serving	55.0	838	59%
■ **SIDE ORDERS**				
cinnamon twist	1 serving	6.0	139	26%
pintos & cheese	1 serving	9.0	190	43%
rice/seasoned	1 serving	3.0	110	25%
■ **TACOS & TOSTADAS**				
taco				
chicken/soft				
light	1 taco	5.0	180	25%
regular	1 taco	10.0	223	40%
plain				
original				
light	1 taco	5.0	140	32%
regular	1 taco	11.0	180	55%
soft				
light	1 taco	5.0	180	25%
regular	1 taco	11.0	223	44%
steak/soft	1 taco	9.0	217	37%
supreme				
original				
light	1 taco	5.0	160	28%

Food and Description	Amount	Fat Grams	Total Calories	% Fat Calories
regular	1 taco	15.0	225	60%
soft	1 taco	15.0	268	50%
tostada	1 tostada	11.0	242	41%

TACO TIME
■ BURRITOS
bean				
crisp	1 burrito	17.0	391	39%
soft				
regular	1 burrito	21.0	547	35%
w/o cheese	1 burrito	14.0	462	27%
casita				
regular	1 burrito	32.0	602	48%
w/o sour cream	1 burrito	26.0	537	44%
w/o sour cream or cheese	1 burrito	17.0	427	36%
combo				
soft				
regular	1 burrito	24.0	550	39%
w/o cheese	1 burrito	17.0	465	33%
meat				
crisp	1 burrito	20.0	393	46%
soft				
regular	1 burrito	26.0	552	42%
w/o cheese	1 burrito	19.0	467	37%
veggie				
regular	1 burrito	20.0	535	34%
w/o sour cream	1 burrito	17.0	502	30%
w/o sour cream or cheese	1 burrito	12.5	477	24%

■ CONDIMENTS & INDIVIDUAL INGREDIENTS
beef	2.5 oz	9.7	115	76%
casa sauce	1 oz	–	40	–
cheese	¾ oz	7.0	85	74%
chicken	3 oz	3.0	135	20%
chips	2 oz	12.0	239	45%
E-sauce	1 oz	–	14	–
guacamole	1 oz	5.0	50	90%
hot sauce	1 oz	–	10	–
lettuce	½ oz	–	2	–
Mexican dressing	2 oz	–	20	–
ranchero salsa	2 oz	<1.0	18	40%
sour cream	1 oz	6.0	65	83%
sour cream dressing	1.5 oz	12.0	135	80%
taco shell				
11" dia	1 shell	2.5	175	13%
6" dia	1 shell	2.0	78	12%
Thousand Island dressing	1 oz	10.0	107	84%
tomato	½ oz	–	3	–

Food and Description	Amount	Fat Grams	Total Calories	% Fat Calories
tortilla				
flour				
regular				
8" dia	1 tortilla	2.5	107	21%
10" dia	1 tortilla	4.6	199	21%
fried				
8" dia	1 tortilla	9.5	170	50%
10" dia	1 tortilla	14.6	209	63%
wheat/6" dia	1 tortilla	2.0	50	36%
■ SALADS				
chicken taco				
w/sour cream dressing	1 serving	31.0	571	49%
w/o sour cream dressing	1 serving	19.0	436	39%
w/o sour cream dressing & cheese	1 serving	14.5	381	34%
side salad				
w/o dressing	1 serving	7.0	106	59%
w/o dressing & cheese	1 serving	2.5	51	44%
taco				
w/sour cream dressing	1 serving	21.0	447	42%
w/o sour cream dressing	1 serving	16.0	347	41%
w/o sour cream dressing & cheese	1 serving	9.0	262	31%
veggie				
w/o dressing	1 serving	17.0	357	43%
w/o dressing & cheese	1 serving	12.5	302	37%
■ SIDE ORDERS				
crustos	1 serving	15.0	373	36%
empañada/cherry	1 empañada	9.0	250	32%
Mexican brown rice	1 serving	2.0	160	11%
Mexi-fries	regular	17.0	266	58%
	large	34.0	532	58%
refritos				
regular	1 serving	18.0	378	43%
w/o cheese	1 serving	11.0	293	34%
■ TACOS				
cheeseburger				
regular	1 taco	30.0	589	46%
w/o Thousand Island dressing	1 taco	20.0	482	37%
w/o Thousand Island dressing & cheese	1 taco	13.0	397	29%
chicken/soft				
regular	1 taco	12.0	390	28%
w/o cheese	1 taco	7.5	335	20%
plain	1 taco	13.0	218	54%
soft flour				
regular	1 taco	19.0	416	41%
w/o cheese	1 taco	12.0	331	33%
■ TOSTADAS				
tostada delight				
w/meat	1 tostada	30.0	560	48%

Food and Description	Amount	Fat Grams	Total Calories	% Fat Calories
w/o sour cream	1 tostada	24.0	495	44%
w/o sour cream & cheese	1 tostada	17.0	410	37%
tostada w/meat				
regular	1 tostada	22.0	409	48%
w/o cheese	1 tostada	15.0	324	42%

WENDY'S
■ BEVERAGES

Food and Description	Amount	Fat Grams	Total Calories	% Fat Calories
coffee	6 fl oz	–	–	–
cola	1 small	–	90	–
diet cola	1 small	–	–	–
hot chocolate	6 fl oz	3.0	80	34%
lemonade	1 small	–	90	–
lemon-lime	1 small	–	90	–
milk/2% reduced fat	8 fl oz	4.0	110	33%
tea/hot or iced	6 fl oz	–	–	–

■ BUNS

Food and Description	Amount	Fat Grams	Total Calories	% Fat Calories
kaiser	1 bun	3.0	190	14%
sandwich	1 bun	2.5	160	14%

■ BURGERS

Food and Description	Amount	Fat Grams	Total Calories	% Fat Calories
big bacon classic on kaiser bun	1 burger	33.0	610	49%
cheeseburger				
bacon/junior	1 burger	21.0	410	46%
regular				
deluxe junior	1 burger	16.0	360	40%
junior	1 burger	13.0	320	37%
kid's meal/2 oz	1 burger	13.0	320	37%
hamburger				
junior	1 burger	10.0	270	33%
kid's meal	1 burger	10.0	270	33%
single				
plain	1 burger	16.0	350	40%
w/everything	1 burger	20.0	420	43%
hamburger patty				
junior	1 patty	7.0	100	63%
¼ lb	1 patty	13.0	200	59%

■ CHICKEN

Food and Description	Amount	Fat Grams	Total Calories	% Fat Calories
breaded chicken sandwich	1 sandwich	18.0	440	37%
chicken club sandwich	1 sandwich	23.0	500	41%
chicken fillet				
breaded	1 piece	12.0	230	47%
grilled	1 piece	2.5	70	32%
crispy chicken nuggets & sauce				
nuggets only	6 pieces	20.0	280	64%
sauce				
barbecue	1 pkg	–	50	–
honey	1 pkg	–	45	–
sweet & sour	1 pkg	–	45	–

Food and Description	Amount	Fat Grams	Total Calories	% Fat Calories
sweet mustard	1 pkg	1.0	50	18%
grilled chicken sandwich	1 sandwich	7.0	290	22%
■ CHILI, CHEESE, & CRACKERS				
cheddar cheese/shredded	2 Tbs	6.0	70	77%
chili	8 oz	7.0	210	30%
	12 oz	10.0	310	29%
crackers	2 pieces	0.5	25	18%
■ CONDIMENTS (*See also* Salads & Salad Bar Items; Super Bar Items in this section)				
American cheese				
regular	1 slice	5.0	70	64%
junior	1 slice	4.0	45	80%
bacon	1 piece	2.5	30	75%
honey mustard/low-calorie	1 tsp	1.5	25	54%
catsup	1 serving	–	10	–
mayonnaise	1 serving	3.0	30	90%
mustard	1 serving	–	–	–
onion	1 serving	–	–	–
pickles	1 serving	–	–	–
sour cream	1 pkt	6.0	60	90%
■ DESSERT				
chocolate chip cookie	1 cookie	11.0	270	37%
chocolate pudding	¼ cup	3.0	70	34%
frosty-dairy	12 oz	10.0	340	26%
	16 oz	13.0	460	25%
	20 oz	17.0	570	27%
vanilla pudding	¼ cup	3.0	70	34%
■ SALADS & SALAD BAR ITEMS				
alfalfa sprouts	½ cup	–	4	–
applesauce/chunky	2 Tbs	–	30	–
bacon bits	2 Tbs	2.5	45	50%
breadstick	1 piece	3.0	130	21%
broccoli	¼ cup	–	–	–
cantaloupe	1 piece	–	15	–
carrots	¼ cup	–	5	–
cauliflower	¼ cup	–	–	–
cheese/shredded	2 Tbs	4.0	50	72%
chicken salad	2 Tbs	5.0	70	64%
chow mein noodles	¼ cup	2.0	35	51%
coleslaw	2 Tbs	3.0	45	60%
cottage cheese	2 Tbs	1.5	30	45%
croutons	2 Tbs	1.0	30	30%
cucumber	2 slices	–	–	–
deluxe garden salad	1 serving	6.0	110	49%
egg/hard-cooked	2 Tbs	3.0	40	68%
green peas	2 Tbs	–	15	–
green peppers	2 pieces	–	–	–
grilled chicken salad	1 serving	8.0	200	36%
honeydew melon	1 piece	–	20	–

Food and Description	Amount	Fat Grams	Total Calories	% Fat Calories
lettuce				
iceberg	1 cup	–	10	–
romaine	1 cup	–	10	–
mushrooms	¼ cup	–		
orange	2 slices	–	15	–
Parmesan blend	2 Tbs	4.0	70	51%
pasta salad	2 Tbs	–	25	–
peaches	1 piece	–	15	–
pepperoni/sliced	6 pieces	3.0	30	90%
pineapple chunks	4 pieces	–	20	–
potato salad	2 Tbs	7.0	80	79%
red onion	3 rings	–	–	–
salad dressing				
blue cheese	2 Tbs	19.0	170	100%
French				
fat-free	2 Tbs	–	30	–
regular	2 Tbs	10.0	120	75%
sweet red	2 Tbs	10.0	130	69%
ranch/Hidden Valley				
reduced fat	2 Tbs	5.0	60	75%
regular	2 Tbs	10.0	90	90%
Italian/reduced fat	2 Tbs	3.0	40	68%
Italian Caesar	2 Tbs	16.0	150	96%
salad oil	2 Tbs	14.0	130	97%
Thousand Island	2 Tbs	13.0	130	90%
wine vinegar	1 Tbs	–	–	–
seafood salad	¼ cup	4.0	70	51%
side salad				
Caesar	1 serving	5.0	110	41%
regular	1 serving	3.0	60	45%
strawberries	1 berry	–	10	–
strawberry-banana dessert	⅓ cup	–	110	–
sunflower seeds & raisins	2 Tbs	5.0	80	56%
taco salad	1 serving	30.0	590	46%
tomato wedges	1 piece	–	5	–
turkey ham	2 Tbs	4.0	50	72%
watermelon	1 piece	–	20	–
■ SIDE ORDERS				
baked potato				
bacon & cheese	1 serving	18.0	540	30%
broccoli & cheese	1 serving	14.0	470	27%
cheese	1 serving	23.0	570	36%
chili & cheese	1 serving	24.0	620	35%
plain	1 serving	–	310	–
sour cream & chives	1 serving	6.0	380	14%
French fries	small	13.0	260	45%
	medium	19.0	380	45%
	biggie	23.0	460	45%

Food and Description	Amount	Fat Grams	Total Calories	% Fat Calories
■ SUPER BAR ITEMS				
Alfredo sauce	¼ cup	1.5	30	45%
cheese sauce	¼ cup	1.0	25	36%
macaroni & cheese	½ cup	6.0	130	42%
picante sauce	2 Tbs	–	10	–
refried beans	¼ cup	3.0	80	34%
rice/Spanish	¼ cup	1.0	60	15%
rotini	½ cup	2.0	90	20%
sour topping/imitation	2 Tbs	5.0	60	75%
spaghetti sauce				
meat sauce	¼ cup	1.5	45	30%
regular	¼ cup	–	30	–
taco chips	8 pieces	7.0	120	53%
taco meat	2 Tbs	4.0	80	45%
taco sauce	2 Tbs	–	10	–
taco shell	1 shell	4.0	60	60%
tortilla/flour	1 tortilla	2.5	110	20%
WHATABURGER				
■ BEVERAGES				
chocolate shake	12 fl oz	9.0	365	22%
Coca-Cola				
Cherry Coke	16 fl oz	–	150	–
classic	16 fl oz	–	140	–
Diet Coke	16 fl oz	–	1	–
coffee				
black	1 small	–	5	–
w/1 pkt cream	1 small	1.0	15	60%
w/1 pkt sugar	1 small	–	20	–
Dr. Pepper	16 fl oz	–	140	–
iced tea	16 fl oz	–	3	–
milk/2% reduced fat	1 serving	4.5	115	35%
orange juice	6 fl oz	–	80	–
root beer	16 fl oz	–	160	–
Sprite	16 fl oz	–	140	–
strawberry shake	12 fl oz	9.0	350	23%
vanilla shake	12 fl oz	9.5	325	26%
■ BREAKFAST				
biscuit				
bacon	1 biscuit	20.0	360	50%
egg & cheese	1 biscuit	26.5	435	55%
egg, cheese, & bacon	1 biscuit	33.0	515	58%
egg, cheese, & sausage	1 biscuit	42.0	600	63%
gravy	1 biscuit	27.5	480	52%
plain	1 biscuit	13.5	280	43%
sausage	1 biscuit	29.0	450	58%
blueberry muffin	1 muffin	8.0	240	30%

Food and Description	Amount	Fat Grams	Total Calories	% Fat Calories
breakfast platter				
w/bacon	1 serving	44.0	695	57%
w/sausage	1 serving	53.0	785	61%
breakfast on a bun				
plain	1 serving	28.0	455	55%
w/bacon	1 serving	19.5	365	48%
egg omelette sandwich	1 sandwich	13.0	290	40%
hash browns	1 serving	9.0	150	54%
pancakes				
pancakes only	3 pancakes	6.0	260	21%
w/sausage	1 serving	21.0	425	44%
scrambled eggs	2 eggs	15.0	189	71%
■ BURGERS				
Justaburger	1 burger	11.5	275	38%
Whataburger				
junior	1 burger	12.0	300	36%
regular	1 burger	26.0	298	39%
small bun, w/o oil	1 burger	19.0	410	42%
■ CHICKEN & FISH				
chicken strips	2 pieces	5.5	120	41%
grilled chicken sandwich				
regular	1 sandwich	14.0	445	28%
small bun/w/mustard/no oil or dressing	1 sandwich	3.0	300	9%
w/o oil or salad dressing	1 sandwich	5.5	358	14%
w/o salad dressing	1 sandwich	8.5	385	20%
Whatacatch sandwich	1 sandwich	25.0	467	48%
Whatachick'n sandwich	1 sandwich	23.0	500	41%
■ CONDIMENTS				
bacon	1 slice	3.5	40	79%
butter	1 serving	4.0	36	100%
cheese slice	1 small	4.0	50	72%
	1 large	7.5	90	75%
chicken gravy	3 oz	4.5	75	54%
grape jelly	1 serving	–	45	–
honey	1 serving	–	25	–
jalapeño pepper	1 pepper	–	3	–
margarine	1 serving	3.0	25	100%
picante sauce	1 serving	–	5	–
sour cream	2 oz	12.0	125	86%
strawberry jam	1 serving	–	40	–
syrup	1 serving	–	180	–
■ DESSERT				
apple turnover	1 turnover	11.0	215	46%
cookies				
chocolate chunk	1 cookie	16.0	250	58%
macadamia nut	1 cookie	16.0	270	53%
oatmeal raisin	1 cookie	7.0	222	28%
peanut butter	1 cookie	13.5	260	47%

Food and Description	Amount	Fat Grams	Total Calories	% Fat Calories
■ **MEXICAN FOOD**				
fajita				
beef	1 fajita	12.0	326	33%
chicken	1 fajita	7.0	275	23%
taquito				
potato	1 taquito	22.0	450	44%
sausage	1 taquito	26.0	445	53%
w/bacon	1 taquito	16.0	335	43%
■ **SALADS & RELATED ITEMS**				
club crackers	1 pkg	1.0	30	30%
croutons	1 pkg	1.0	30	30%
garden salad	1 serving	0.5	55	8%
grilled chicken salad	1 serving	1.5	150	9%
salad dressing				
French	1 pkt	21.0	260	73%
ranch	1 pkt	33.0	320	93%
Thousand Island	1 pkt	12.0	160	68%
vinaigrette/lite	1 pkt	2.0	40	45%
Texas toast	1 slice	4.5	150	27%
■ **SIDE ORDERS**				
baked potato				
plain	1 serving	0.5	310	1%
w/broccoli & cheese	1 serving	10.0	453	20%
w/cheese	1 serving	16.5	510	29%
French fries	junior	12.0	221	49%
	regular	18.0	332	49%
	large	124.5	445	50%
onion rings	regular	19.0	330	52%
	large	29.0	495	53%
WHITE CASTLE				
■ **BREAKFAST**				
sausage & egg sandwich	1 sandwich	22.0	322	62%
sausage sandwich	1 sandwich	12.0	196	55%
■ **BUN**				
white bun	1 bun	<1.0	74	6%
■ **BURGERS**				
cheeseburger	1 burger	11.0	200	50%
hamburger	1 burger	8.0	161	45%
■ **CHICKEN & FISH**				
chicken sandwich	1 sandwich	7.5	186	36%
fish sandwich/w/o tartar sauce	1 sandwich	5.0	155	29%
■ **CONDIMENTS**				
onion chips	3.3 oz	17.0	329	47%
tartar sauce	1 Tbs	8.0	72	100%
■ **SIDE ORDERS**				
French fries	regular	15.0	301	45%
onion rings	regular	13.0	245	48%

PERSONAL FOOD DIARY

Date	Food	Amount	Fat Grams	Total Calories	% Fat Calories